KINDLING 5

ADVANCES IN BEHAVIORAL BIOLOGY

Recent Volumes in This Series

Volume 36 NOVEL APPROACHES TO THE TREATMENT OF ALZHEIMER'S DISEASE
Edited by Edwin M. Meyer, James W. Simpkins, and Jyunji Yamamoto

Volume 37 KINDLING 4
Edited by Juhn A. Wada

Volume 38A BASIC, CLINICAL AND THERAPEUTIC ASPECTS OF ALZHEIMER'S AND PARKINSON'S DISEASES
Volume 1
Edited by Toshiharu Nagatsu, Abraham Fisher, and Mitsuo Yoshida

Volume 38B BASIC, CLINICAL AND THERAPEUTIC ASPECTS OF ALZHEIMER'S AND PARKINSON'S DISEASES
Volume 2
Edited by Toshiharu Nagatsu, Abraham Fisher, and Mitsuo Yoshida

Volume 39 THE BASAL GANGLIA III
Edited by Giorgio Bernardi, Malcolm B. Carpenter, Gaetano Di Chiara, Micaela Morelli, and Paolo Stanzione

Volume 40 TREATMENT OF DEMENTIAS: A New Generation of Progress
Edited by Edwin M. Meyer, James W. Simpkins, Jyunji Yamamoto, and Fulton T. Crews

Volume 41 THE BASAL GANGLIA IV: New Ideas and Data on Structure and Function
Edited by Gérard Percheron, John S. McKenzie, and Jean Féger

Volume 42 CALLOSAL AGENESIS: A Natural Split Brain?
Edited by Maryse Lassonde and Malcolm A. Jeeves

Volume 43 NEUROTRANSMITTERS IN THE HUMAN BRAIN
Edited by David J. Tracey, George Paxinos, and Jonathan Stone

Volume 44 ALZHEIMER'S AND PARKINSON'S DISEASES: Recent Developments
Edited by Israel Hanin, Mitsuo Yoshida, and Abraham Fisher

Volume 45 EPILEPSY AND THE CORPUS CALLOSUM 2
Edited by Alexander G. Reeves and David W. Roberts

Volume 46 BIOLOGY AND PHYSIOLOGY OF THE BLOOD–BRAIN BARRIER: Transport, Cellular Interactions, and Brain Pathologies
Edited by Pierre-Olivier Couraud and Daniel Scherman

Volume 47 THE BASAL GANGLIA V
Edited by Chihiro Ohye, Minoru Kimura, and John S. McKenzie

Volume 48 KINDLING 5
Edited by Michael E. Corcoran and Solomon L. Moshé

A Continuation Order Plan is available for this series. A continuation order will bring delivery of each new volume immediately upon publication. Volumes are billed only upon actual shipment. For further information please contact the publisher.

KINDLING 5

Edited by

Michael E. Corcoran

University of Saskatchewan
Saskatoon, Saskatchewan, Canada

and

Solomon L. Moshé

Albert Einstein College of Medicine
Bronx, New York

Deb —
Happy reading
MEC

PLENUM PRESS • NEW YORK AND LONDON

Library of Congress Cataloging-in-Publication Data

On file

Proceedings of the Fifth International Conference on Kindling, held June 27–30, 1996, in Victoria, British Columbia, Canada

ISBN 0-306-45805-5

A Division of Plenum Publishing Corporation
233 Spring Street, New York, N.Y. 10013

10 9 8 7 6 5 4 3 2 1

Printed in the United States of America

To Juhn A. Wada, the Thunderbird of Kindling

PREFACE

The last Kindling Conference was organized by Dr. Juhn Wada and held at the University of British Columbia, Vancouver, B.C., in 1989. In the intervening years, research on kindling has proceeded at an explosive pace and significant advances have been made in our understanding of the molecular biological, anatomical, and physiological substrates of kindling, as well as in our appreciation of the age-dependent effects and complex behavioral consequences of kindling, its sensitivity to drugs, and its relevance to the clinical epilepsies. In order to review these developments and to provide researchers with an opportunity to interact face to face and discuss the issues that preoccupy us all, we organized the Fifth International Conference on Kindling, in Victoria, B.C., in the summer of 1996. Most of the stalwarts in kindling research were invited, as were a number of investigators whose research on kindling has become prominent in the past few years. We continue to miss the late Graham Goddard, the discoverer of kindling, and were saddened by the recent death of Eric Lothman, a prolific researcher and clinician who would have been a prominent participant. We were deeply disturbed to learn of the death of Frank Morrell, one of the earliest kindlers and an eminent neurologist, who died several months after our conference. We also regret that several of our colleagues were unable to attend the conference: Robert Ackermann, Tallie Baram, Robert De Lorenzo, Lewis Haberly, Gregory Holmes, Gildas Le Gal La Salle, Frank Morrell and Leyla de Toledo Morrell, Robert Post, Mitsumoto Sato, and Thomas Sutula.

The organization of Kindling 5 was slightly different from the past kindling conferences, in that the talks were loosely organized into themes, with each session being followed by a general discussion. In keeping with past conferences, however, we have attempted to capture the gist of the discussions that followed the presentations. The discussions are often more revealing than the formal presentations, and if nothing else they convey some of the informality of the dialogue among a group of researchers who know each other well.

Kindling 5 was dedicated to the keynote speaker, Dr. Juhn Wada, who is Professor Emeritus of Psychiatry and Neurological Sciences at the University of British Columbia. Everybody knows Dr. Wada. He is one of the preeminent epileptologists in the world, having contributed insightful and important research and clinical practice for over 40 years. He is the originator of the carotid amytal test for cerebral dominance, and he performed research with various "animal models" that anticipated aspects of kindling. In 1972 he turned his attention to kindling and became one of its most ardent boosters and one of the most prolific researchers in the field. He also was the driving force behind the first four International Conferences on Kindling, and it is fair to say that the prominence of kindling is in no small measure attributable to his influence.

Dr. Wada has been the recipient of many honours and awards. He was one of the organizers of and President of the Canadian League Against Epilepsy. He was President of the American Epilepsy Society, and he used his office to promote the recruiting of basic scientists as members of AES. In recognition of his many contributions to humanity, in 1992 he was made an Officer of the Order of Canada, entitling him to append the initials "O.C." after his name. In 1995 the Japanese Government awarded him the Order of the Sacred Treasure, Gold and Silver Star, in recognition of his exemplary efforts to promote and expand relations between Canada and Japan in the medical field.

We want to thank the following sponsors for very generously providing the financial support that has made Kindling 5 possible:

- Parke Davis (Warener-Lambert Co.)
- CIBA-GENEVA
- Hoechst Marion Roussel, Inc.
- Bloorview Epilepsy Research Program (University of Toronto)
- Abbott Laboratories
- Wyeth-Ayerst Laboratories
- McNeil Pharmaceutical Corp.
- Wallace Laboratories

We also thank a number of people whose outstanding efforts enabled the conference to run smoothly. Several graduate students from the Department of Psychology, University of Victoria, assisted in the technical aspects of the conference: Lisa Armitage had the responsibility of transcribing discussions unexpectedly thrust on her at the last possible instant before the conference began, and she responded heroically by keeping an online record of the gist of the discussions. She also did much of the transcribing to hard copy after the conference. Darren Hannesson was responsible for the taping of the discussions and kept notes on who said what and when. This responsibility too came at the last minute. Paul Mohapel did a first rate job as the projector guy, handling the task without any major glitches, and even found time to ask a few pertinent questions. The organization of the molecular details of the conference was handled by several people from Conference Management, Division of Continuing Studies, University of Victoria: Mary O'Rourke quarterbacked the whole operation from the outset. We could not have done it without her, and she has our eternal gratitude. Nieves Forcada-Ausio helped with many of the organizational details, as did Sarah D'Aeth, who also was present for the entire conference and cracked the whip regarding adjourning for meals, submitting manuscripts, and regulating the air conditioning. Charlene Quinn and Victoria Emery provided critical background support. They all made the conference a reality. Finally, we thank all the kindlers, without whom there would not have been a Fifth International Conference on Kindling.

Michael E. Corcoran and Solomon Moshé

CONTENTS

BEHAVIORAL EFFECTS OF KINDLING

DRUGS AND KINDLING

1

GENETIC PREDISPOSITION AND KINDLING SUSCEPTIBILITY IN PRIMATES

Juhn A. Wada

Divisions of Neurosciences and Neurology
The University of British Columbia
Vancouver, British Columbia, Canada V6T 2A1

1. INTRODUCTION

Among patients with temporal lobe epilepsy with a focus in identical anatomical locations, some patients have non-convulsive seizures exclusively, even when medication is withdrawn, while others begin with generalized convulsive seizures which readily recur when medication is reduced. Between these two extremes, there are those patients who display partial motor seizure without ever developing secondary generalization. The reason for such differences is not known. A less favorable prognosis has been suggested for those partial epilepsy patients with generalized seizures than for those without[14,26,27]. Furthermore, convulsive evolution in partial seizure is reported to be the major factor for a serious morbidity in status epilepticus[6]. An understanding of the mechanisms underlying convulsive evolution and its bilateralization/generalization is important since once they are defined, it may be possible to modify them for therapeutic or prophylactic purposes. However, due to the complexity and diversity of both etiologic and genetic factors in human epilepsy little progress has been made in our understanding, which is largely dependent on studies in animal models, of the underlying mechanisms. One of these models, kindling, has proved to be an ideal one for partial onset secondarily generalized seizure[28]. In this model, we have become accustomed to assessing the degree of kindling susceptibility by the speed with which convulsive development and its bilateralization/generalization occur. In general, once a day amygdaloid (AM) stimulation results in secondarily generalized convulsion in about two weeks in rodents, four weeks in cats, and 6–10 months in rhesus monkeys. Some strain difference has been noted within the same species as to the kindling rate[24,46]. In our laboratory we also noted, for example, that black hooded rats tend to kindle faster than Wister rats. Indeed, the potential contribution of genetic susceptibility has been studied by subjecting strains of mice[17], gerbils[2] and audiogenic rats to kindling[4] assessing resultant evidence of interaction between kindling and intrinsic seizure predisposition.

Kindling 5, edited by Corcoran and Moshé.
Plenum Press, New York, 1998.

2. LANDMARKS OF KINDLING SUSCEPTIBILITY

In our feline kindling study we have encountered some animals that require four months to kindle. Most frequently, it is due to a delay of the convulsive evolution of AM onset limbic seizure, but at times it is the result of delayed bilateralization/generalization. When neither an age factor nor a systemic disease is involved, and histological examination excludes technical error, participation of intrinsic or genetic factors needs to be considered. In our primate kindling study we also noted significant species variation in kindling and kindled seizure. Naturally, the interpretation of group differences must be guarded since the population involved is small and no precise information is available as to their origin and family background. Nonetheless, some startling differences in the kindling profile emerged from among the five primate species we have studied. These are: the speed of convulsive development and generalization, the ultimate quality of kindled seizure, and the extent of both positive and negative transhemispheric transfer effects.

Figure 1 illustrates the general chronological features in primates and Table 1 summarizes the differential features of amygdaloid (AM) kindling in five primate species. The primate species studied are: photosensitive Papio papio (PP) and Papio cynocephalus (PC), non-sensitive Papio hamadryas (PH), Macaca fuscata (MF), and Macaca mulatta (MM). Two differences are immediately apparent, i.e., speed of kindling and quality of kindled seizure.

For both Stage 3 convulsive evolution and Stage 4 convulsive bilateralization, the mean number of daily AM stimulations required is 33 and 47, respectively, for baboons and 120 and 186, respectively, for monkeys. Both after discharge (ADT) and generalized seizure triggering thresholds (GST) are much higher in baboons (means of 371 and 151 μA, respectively) than in monkeys (means of 196 and 88 μA, respectively), indicating that this remarkable discrepancy must represent a difference in excitability of structures outside of the AM participating in kindling. In addition, bisymmetrical and bisynchronous Stage 5 seizures, implying equal temporal and spatial ictal involvement of both frontocentral cortical areas, develop only in photosensitive baboons PP and PC[5,36]. This is in striking contrast to a

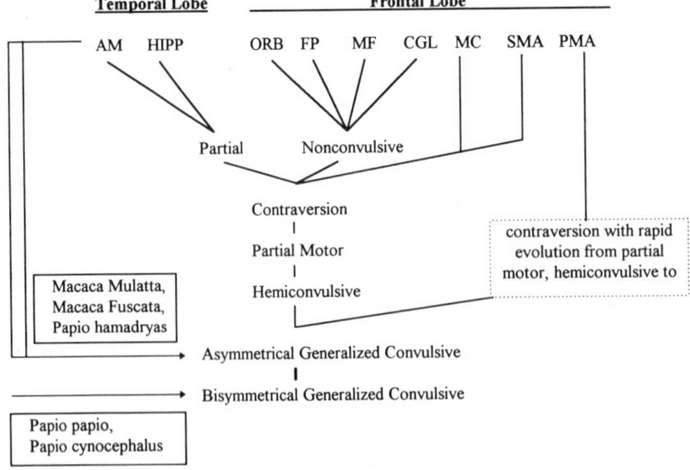

Figure 1. General chronological profile of primate kindling. Abbreviations: AM: amygdala, Hipp: hippocampus, ORB: orbital, FP: frontal polar, MF: mesial frontal, CGL: cingulate, MC: motor cortical, SMA: supplementary motor area, PMA: premotor area.

Table 1. Profile of amygdaloid kindling in primates

	Primate species				
	PP	PC	PH	MF	MM
ϕ Generalized onset convulsive response to s.c. Bemegride (mg/kg)	4.0		11		16.5
Number of stimulations required for:					
Stage 3: Partial motor seizure	11	24	65	106	154
		(33)		(120)	
Stage 4: Secondary generalization	22	32	87	177	196
		(47)		(186)	
Stage 5: Bisymmetrical convulsion	72	71	–	–	–
% of animal with seizure stage instability	0	0	40	100	100
Sustained kindling suppression at secondary site	+		–	–	–

Abbreviations: PP: *Papio papio*, PC: *Papio cynocephalus*, PH: *Papio hamadryas*, MF: *Macaca fuscata*, MM: *Macaca mulatta*, ( ) = Mean Score, ϕ = Following electrode implantation but before kindling.

markedly asymmetrical final Stage 4 seizure in the non-photosensitive baboon PH and in monkeys suggesting a major functional difference in the mechanism of convulsive bilateralization/generalization between photosensitive and non-sensitive primates.

Another striking difference is the persistent seizure stage stability in the photosensitive baboons in contrast to the remarkable seizure stage instability in the nophotosensitive PH and monkeys. This difference becomes manifest with Stages 3 and 4 development. Therefore, the presence or absence of this instability suggests a difference in the strength of limbic motor linkage underlying convulsive evolution and its generalization between species.

At the secondary site, the chronological profile of accelerated kindling (positive transfer effect) is also significantly different among the species (Table 2). Thus, kindled

Table 2. Transhemispheric positive and negative transfer effects

			Secondary site kindling				
				Positive transfer			
			Negative transfer (sustained kindling suppression)	Abrupt onset kindled seizure			Sequential accelerated kindling
Brain site	Species	AD		Isolated	Sustained		
Amygdala	PP	+	+	+			
	PH	+			+	or	+
	MF	+	+		+	or	+
	MM	+					+
Frontal pole		+	+				
	PP	+	+				
Mesial frontal	PC	+	+				
	MM	+	+				
Cingulate	PP	+	+				
Premotor	PP	+			+		
Supplementary motor	MM	+			+		
	PP	+			+		

Abbreviations: PP: *Papio papio*, PC: *Papio cynocephalus*, PH: *Papio hamadryas*, MF: *Macaca fuscata*, MM: *Macaca mulatta*, AD = After discharge generation.

seizure in its final form may evolve abruptly from Stage 0 skipping the intermediate stages within one week in PP and some PH, while an orderly sequential development through Stages 1 to 4, requiring many more days, is the rule in monkeys and some PH. Furthermore, the pattern of seizure kindled at the secondary site has been described to be a perfect mirror image of the primary site kindled one both in cats and primates except for PH and MF. In some PH, the convulsive pattern of both Stages 3 and 4 is identical to that of the primary site kindled one. In all MFs, Stage 3 seizure is a mirror image but as it evolves to Stage 4 it reverts back to a pattern identical to that of the primary site kindled one. All the above findings suggest a significant species difference in the impact of the primary site kindling on the secondary site convulsive evolution and its bilateralization /generalization. An additional difference is the sustained suppression of seizure development in kindling at the secondary site in PP and some MF[13,34]. The powerful nature of this suppression is indicated in one primary site kindled PP (W229) which failed to show seizure development for eight months at the secondary site (Wada, unpublished data). Subsequently, however, this animal abruptly developed Stage 4 on the 249th day and then Stage 5 the next day. Since 6, 23, and 84 days were required for Stages 3, 4, and 5 development, respectively, at the primary site in this animal and since positive transfer effect persists for three years in this species[28], it appears that the positive transfer effect was masked by a more powerful but slowly decaying suppressive effect in this animal.

A combination of both positive and suppressive effects has been observed in PP and some MF but some PP showed either positive or suppressive effects alone. On the other hand, PH showed either a very abrupt or a sequential pattern while MM showed only a sequential pattern. Therefore, the pattern of secondary site kindling appears to be determined by a balance between the intensity of positive and suppressive effects. Again, the target of both positive (facilitation) and negative (suppression) effects appears to be the site(s) of the anatomical substratum underlying convulsive evolution and its generalization. Finally, the quality of the final stage kindled generalized seizure is different: only PP and PC showed bisymmetrical onset seizure, while the rest was clearly asymmetrical onset with a slow sequential march and secondary generalization, indicating a significant difference in the spatial and temporal process of bilateralization/generalization.

All the above findings indicate: a) a spectrum of kindling susceptibility ranging from maximal (PP and PC) to minimal (MM) with PH and MF in between; and b) the anatomical mechanism underlying both convulsive evolution and its bilateralization/generalization are the underpinning of this susceptibility spectrum. Therefore, some of our recent observations on the potential anatomical substrata underlying these processes are briefly reviewed below.

2.1. Convulsive Evolution

Insight into the possible anatomy of convulsive evolution came from our study of photosensitivity in PP[43,44]. Since bilateral occipital corticectomy including the primary visual receiving area eliminates photosensitivity, it became clear that the geniculo-occipital system is critical for a photoconvulsive response to occur. Because the visual afferents must access the motor mechanism for a photosensitive response to occur and since the fronto-rolandic cortex is the site of genetically dictated neurophysiological abnormality in this species[22], it was hypothesized that the occipito-frontal association pathway is involved for behavioural expression of photosensitivity. Deep bilateral coronal transection of the hemispheres above the sylvian fissure at the parietal junction in PP reduced but did not eliminate photosensitivity[44]. This finding suggested the possible involvement of an unknown subcortical structure which has connections with both the occipital and the frontal cortices for photically induced seizure to occur. Among a number of potential candidate sites, the claustrum appeared attractive since it has reciprocal connections with both the visual and the frontal cortices in this species[24]. Therefore, the claustrum appears strategically located between the visual afferent and the motor efferent for organized action.

We found that unilateral claustral lesioning in D,L-allylglycine treated cats transformed photically induced bisymmetrical onset generalized convulsive seizure into a partial onset secondarily generalized one, beginning in the non-lesioned hemisphere[15]. This finding is now replicated in the photosensitive PP[39]. Since both photically-induced and AM kindling-induced convulsion begins with initial facial involvement, we tested the hypothesis that the claustrum is also involved in convulsive evolution in AM kindling. It was found that unilateral claustral lesioning ipsilateral to AM stimulation in feline kindling or kindled seizure did not prevent or eliminate convulsive seizure development. However, the convulsive seizure was now a complete mirror image of the expected or the established one, beginning in the non-lesioned hemisphere and becoming secondarily generalized[16]. Thus, transhemispheric migration of AM onset limbic seizure to the non-lesioned hemisphere was necessary for convulsive evolution to take place. For cross-species validation we examined the effect of claustral lesioning ipsilateral to the kindled amygdala or the cingulate cortex in PP[39]. In this primate series, unilateral claustral lesioning effectively eliminated the convulsive component of partial onset secondarily generalized seizure, leaving the non-convulsive component intact (Figure 2). Unlike the findings in cats, only an isolated transhemispheric migration of discharge occurred in one cingulate-kindled animal with a mirror image convulsive seizure, suggesting a significant species difference between the feline and primate species in this regard (Figure 2, top).

The above findings confirmed that the claustrum is the critical anatomical substratum for convulsive evolution of partial seizure originating in the amygdala or the cingulate cortex in both cats and primates. Since claustral lesioning contralateral to stimulation has no effect on generalization of convulsive seizure originating in the non-lesioned hemisphere, it is clear that the claustrum is not involved in the mechanism of secondary generalization.

Finally, the specific frontocentral area to which the claustrum projects for convulsive evolution is not known. Although the convulsive seizure induced by photic stimulation and AM and CG kindling commences in the face, the cortical face area is an unlikely specific claustral target since kindling of the rolandic face area is extremely difficult with no electroclinical recruitment despite over 300 daily generations of AD (Wada and Sakai, unpublished data). A line of evidence suggests that the premotor cortical area may be the primary target for the following reasons: (a) convulsive development in AM kindling is associated with contraversion; (b) selective resection of the premotor cortical area ipsilateral to AM kindling does not prevent but markedly delays the onset of convulsive evolution[36], and (c) hemi- and then generalized convulsive evolution is extremely rapid in premotor cortical kindling even in the non-predisposed MM[1].

2.2. Convulsive Bilateralization and Generalization

Bisection of the forebrain commissures and more specifically the anterior two thirds of the corpus callosum not only prevents convulsive bilateralization in kindling but also transforms generalized kindled convulsion to hemiconvulsion in rats[18–20,38], cats[39,43], monkeys[41] and baboons[27,3]. Although convulsive generalization does occur in baboons with complete forebrain bisection if persistently kindled,[34] it is obvious that the corpus callosum is the major, if not exclusive, anatomical substratum for convulsive bilateralization and generalization.

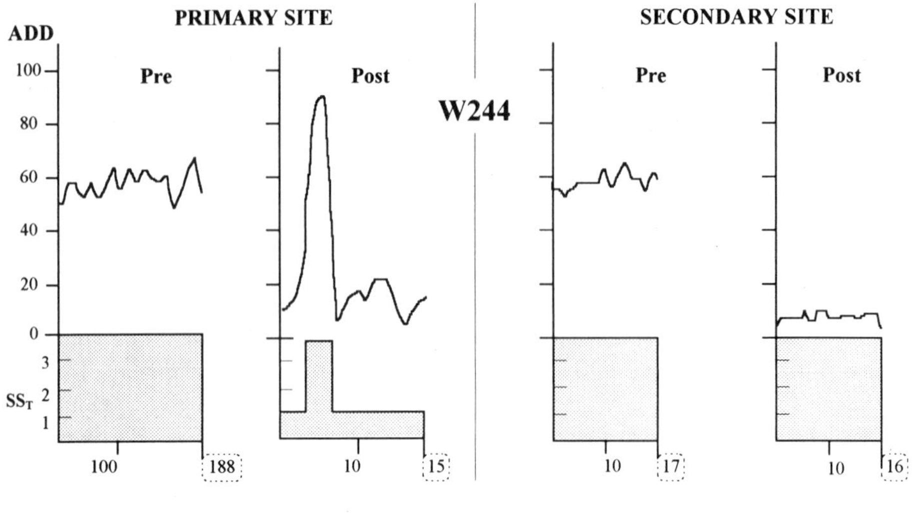

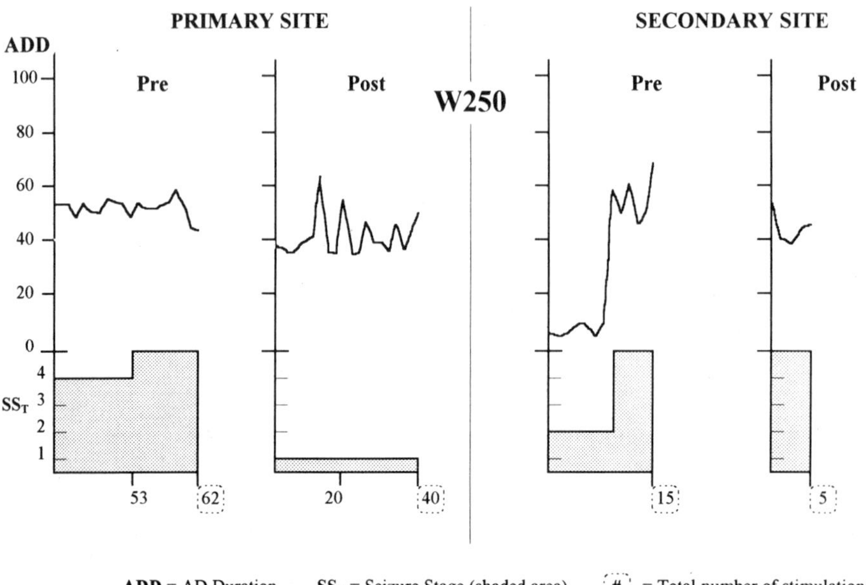

ADD = AD Duration SS_T = Seizure Stage (shaded area)   # = Total number of stimulations

Figure 2. Effect of claustral lesion on cingulate (top) and amygdaloid (bottom) kindled seizure in *Papio papio*.

Throughout our primate studies, we were impressed with the qualitative difference in seizure development and developed seizure between bisected PP and MM (Table 3). Thus, the speed of Stage 3 convulsive onset becomes three times faster in MM, while it becomes slower in predisposed PP when compared with intact animals. In these bisected animals, the speed of the convulsive march for completion of the hemiconvulsive seizure was entirely opposite between PP and MM: 4.5 times slower in the former and twice as fast in MM, respectively, when compared with intact animals. These findings suggest a differential functioning of the corpus callosum in the two species, being largely inhibitory in MM and dysfunctional in PP, thus allowing mutual facilitation (disinhibition) between

Table 3. Differential effect of callosal bisection on amygdaloid kindling and kindled seizure in *Papio papio* and *Macaca mulatta*

	Papio papio		*Macaca mulatta*	
Convulsive seizure	Intact	Bisected	Intact	Bisected
Development	Rapid	Slow	Slow	Rapid
Ictal march	Rapid	Slow	Slow	Rapid
Intensity	+++	+	+	++

the two frontocentral regions leading to rapid bisymmetrical, bisynchronous Stage 5 seizure development in the latter species.

2.3. Transhemispheric Positive Transfer Effect

Kindling at one brain site accelerates subsequent kindling at a distant but synaptically related structure.[9] The anatomical substratum for this transhemispheric positive transfer effect remains enigmatic. The pioneering study of McIntyre showed forebrain bisection including the massa intermedia had no effect on positive transfer effect in rats. The finding, therefore, suggested the probable participation of the brain stem.[20] In rodents, however, extensive bisection of the midbrain to the pons failed to eliminate positive transfer effect,[3] while lesioning of the massa intermedia by localized ibotenic acid injection into the massa intermedia eliminated the positive transfer effect (Ehara and Wada, in preparation). In cats, electrolytic lesioning of the thalamic reticular nucleus, medialis dorsalis[30] and the centrum medianum[10] ipsilateral to AM kindling eliminates it. On the other hand, bisection of the massa intermedia has no effect,[13] but, its lesioning by either electrolytic means[10] or localized injection of ibotenic acid[7] eliminates positive transfer effect. The ineffectiveness of complete midsaggital bisection of the massa intermedia in PP has also been confirmed (Sakai/Wada, unpublished data).

Most recently, we found that midsagittal bisection of the midbrain to the pons in cats completely abolishes positive transfer effect (Hamada and Wada, in preparation). This finding is now replicated in the Japanese monkey Macaca fuscata undergoing amygdaloid kindling (Hiyoshi, Wada, Kudo et al., in preparation) (Table 4). The findings suggest the importance of the brain stem for this effect and is consistent with our previous observation that lesioning of the midbrain reticular formation prevents development of positive transfer effect.[30] Taking into consideration the fact that forebrain commissure bisection reduces positive transfer effect in cats,[8,43] PP[34] and MM,[41] the anatomical mechanisms underlying this effect appear to be the vertically oriented neuronal system extending from the brain stem to the cerebral cortex with the non-specific thalamic system playing an important role. It remains to be seen whether the same mechanism applies to kindling of brain structures other than the AM. For example, the mechanisms underlying positive transfer effect between rodent AM and hippocampal kindling are not the same.[21] Similarly, we now have some evidence indicating that the mechanisms underlying AM and temporal neocortical kindling in the Japanese monkey Macaca fuscata may not be the same (Hiyoshi, Wada, Kudo et al, in preparation).

2.4. Transhemispheric Negative Transfer (Sustained Seizure Suppression) Effect

Although secondary site kindling will result in the early emergence of kindled seizures, the quality of the secondary site kindling and kindled seizure is significantly differ-

Table 4. Effect of various procedures on transhemispheric positive transfer effect in amygdaloid kindling

Procedure	Structure	Rat	Cat	MM	MF	PP
Bisection	Corpus callosum	+	–	–		–
	Massa intermedia	+	+			+
	Midbrain—pons	+	–		–	
Ibotenic acid lesioning	Massa intermedia	–	–			
Electrolytic lesioning	Massa intermedia		–			
	Medialis dorsalis		–			
	Centrum medianum		–			
	Reticular nucleus		–			
	Midbrain reticular formation	+	–			

Primates: MM = *Macaca mulatta*; MF = *Macaca fuscata*; PP = *Papio papio*

ent from that of the primary site kindled one. Thus, after discharge is largely lateralized to the secondary site hemisphere and the latency for onset of both convulsive evolution and secondary generalization are significantly longer, suggesting a much slower process in the secondary site hemisphere when compared with that of the primary site. This negative transfer effect is transient and said to decay in about two weeks in rodents[22]. In cats, however, it lasts for one year[11]. It should be noted that the presence of the negative transfer effect does not prevent seizure development and that even when the positive transfer effect is absent kindling takes place at the secondary site with a speed similar to that expected at the primary site[10,11]. Therefore, the failure of seizure development for 3–8 months as observed in PP represents an active and persistent suppression of convulsive evolution[31,37]. A similar persistent antiepileptogenic effect observed at the secondary site AM only in PP has also been identified to occur in kindling of the frontal polar, the mesial frontal, and the cingulate cortices in the same species[29,40,43]. However, it was found that this persistent antiepileptogenic effect which lasted for over three months at the mesial frontal cortical kindling was also shared not only by predisposed PC but also by MM with no predisposition[43] (Table 2).

Until recently, the above mentioned profound suppression of seizure development has never been observed in species other than the primates and therefore, it was considered to be a primate specific effect. Recently, however, we found that a powerful and enduring antiepileptogenic effect can be had by cingulate cortical kindling in cats (Wada and Hirayasu, in preparation). Among a number of brain sites so far subjected to kindling in cats, the cingulate cortex is the only area to show this effect. Therefore, it is possible that this suppression is unique to kindling of the mesial hemispheric cortical areas in both cats and primates regardless of seizure predisposition. Results of our preliminary study of the effects of picrotoxin, phentolamine, and theophyline on this suppressed state suggest the possible involvement of GABAergic and α-adrenergic receptors (Sakai and Wada, unpublished data).

Many questions remain unanswered. However, our findings confirm that repeated seizures lead to a modification of brain function which manifests itself not only in enduringly enhanced seizure susceptibility but also in persistent and powerful antiepileptogenicity. Since kindling occurs in all the species of animals so far examined it must represent a neurobiological principle of mammalian brain function, and thus kindling-induced persistent failure of kindling is most likely attained at the expense of physiological cerebral function. It is obvious that kindling-induced reorganization of brain function can be expressed not only in overtly apparent ictal manifestation but also in very subtle and sustained interictal disturbances. As a long term potentiation-like process participates in kindling, it would not be surprising if a long term depression-like process is also activated by kindling. This view has some indirect support from our observation that kindling of predisposed baboons rarely leads to fatal status epilepticus. Further characterization and identification of the mechanisms underlying this kindling-induced persistent suppression of kindling are obviously warranted.

3. SUMMARY

Review of the amygdaloid kindling profile in five different primate species identified the speed of both convulsive onset and its bilateralization and the quality of kindled seizure as the critical ictal features which define position of each species in the spectrum of kindling susceptibility. Our studies to this date suggest that the claustrum and the corpus callosum are responsible for convulsive evolution and bilateralization, respectively. Thus, genetically dictated susceptibility of one or both of these structures appears to be the determinant of the kindling profile unique to each primate species. In this spectrum, Macaca mulatta is at the minimal end while Papio papio and Papio cynocephalus are at the maximal end, with Papio hamadryas and Macaca fuscata in between and sharing traits from both the minimal and maximal ends. From this perspective, permissiveness of the claustrum and callosal dysfunction are considered to be responsible for the extraordinary speed of kindling and the bisymmetrical onset of kindled seizure in predisposed baboons, Papio papio and Papio cynocephalus.

Transhemispheric positive transfer effect has often been regarded as evidence for secondary epileptogenesis. However, there has not been any evidence that it is due to enhanced excitability of the non-kindled hemisphere. Rather, this effect appears to be entirely dependent on the vertically-oriented neuronal system extending from the brain stem to the cerebral cortex of the kindled hemisphere in which the non-specific thalamus appears to play an important role.

In amygdaloid kindling, persistent suppression of seizure development at the secondary site occurs only in Papio papio. The same suppressive effect had been observed in frontal polar kindling in the same species. More recently, kindling of mesial frontal and cingulate cortices was also found to induce the same effect not only in predisposed Papio papio and Papio cynocephalus but also in non-predisposed Macaca mulatta and in cats. Mechanisms underlying this kindling-induced profound and long-lasting antiepileptogenic effect remain to be elucidated.

ACKNOWLEDGMENTS

This work was supported by grants from the Medical Research Council of Canada and Vancouver Society for Epilepsy Research. The author thanks Kim Eyrl for her technical assistance.

REFERENCES

1. Baba, H., Sakai, S. and Wada, J.A., Premotor (area 6) cortical kindling in primates: Senegalese baboon (*Papio papio*) and rhesus monkey, In Wada, J.A. (Ed) *Kindling 3*, Raven Press, New York, 1986 447–469.
2. Cain, P. and Corcoran, M.E., Kindling in the seizure-prone and seizure resistant Mongolian gerbil, *Electroenceph. Clin. Neurophysiol.*, 49 (1980) 360–365.

3. Chiba, S. and Wada, J.A., Amygdala kindling in rats with brain stem bisection, *Brain Res.*, 682 (1995) 50–54.
4. Coffey, L.L., Reith, M.E.A., Chen, N.H., Mishra, P.K. and Jobe, P.C., Amygdala kindling of forebrain seizures and the occurrence of brain stem seizures in genetically epilepsy-prone rats, *Epilepsia*, 37 (1996) 188–197.
5. Corcoran, M.E., Cain, D.P. and Wada, J.A., Amygdaloid kindling in Papio cynocephalus and subsequent recurrent spontaneous seizures, *Folia Psychiatrica et Neurologica Japonica*, 38 (1984) 151–159.
6. DeLorenzo, R.J., Pellock, J.M. Towne, A.R. and Buggs, J.G., Epidemiology of status epilepticus, *J. Clin. Neurophysiol.*, 12 (1995) 316–325.
7. Ehara, T. and Wada, J.A., Midline thalamus and amygdaloid kindling, In Wada, J.A. (Ed) *Kindling 4*, Raven Press, New York, (1990) 409–422.
8. Fukuda, H., Wada, J.A., Riche, D. and Naquet, R., Role of the corpus callosum and hippocampal commissure on transfer phenomenon in amygadaloid kindled cats, *Exp. Neurol.*, 98 (1987) 189–197.
9. Goddard, G.V., McIntyre, D.C. and Leech, C.K., A permanent change in brain function resulting from daily stimulation, *Exp. Neurol.*, 25 (1969), 295–330.
10. Hiyoshi, T. and Wada, J.A., Midline thalamic lesion and feline amygdaloid kindling. I. Effect of lesion placement prior to kindling, *Electroenceph. Clin. Neurophysiol.*, 70 (1988) 325–338.
11. Hiyoshi, T. and Wada, J.A., Lasting nature of both transfer and interference in amygdaloid kindling in cats: observation upon stimulation with 11 month rest following primary site kindling, *Epilepsia*, 33 (1992) 222–227.
12. Hiyoshi, T., Wada, J.A., Kudo, T., Amano, K., Yagi, K. and Seino, M., Amygdaloid kindling in the Japanese monkey Macaca fuscata. I: Electroclinical seizure development and developed seizure, *Epilepsia*, In press.
13. Ishibashi, M. and Wada, J.A., Division of massa intermedia has no effect in feline amygdaloid kindling, *Epilepsia*, 31 (1990) 632.
14. Juul-Jensen, P. and Foldspang, A., Natural history of epileptic seizures, *Epilepsia*, 24 (1983) 297–312.
15. Kudo, T. and Wada, J.A., Effect of unilateral claustral lesion on intermittent light stimulation-induced convulsive response in D,D-allylglycine treated cats, *Electroenceph. Clin. Neurophysiol.*, 95 (1995) 63–68.
16. Kudo, T. and Wada, J.A., Claustrum and amygdaloid kindling, In Wada, J.A. (Ed) *Kindling 4*, Plenum Press, New York, 1990 397–408.
17. Leech, C.K. and McIntyre, D.C., Kindling rates in inbred mice: an analog to learning ? *Behaviour Biol.*, 16 (1976) 439–452.
18. McCaughran J.A. Jr., Corcoran, M.E. and Wada, J.A., Development of kindling amygdaloid seizures after section of the forebrain commissures in rats, *Folia Psychiatrica et Neurologica Japonica*, 30 (1976) 65–71.
19. McCaughran, J.A., Corcoran, M.E. and Wada, J.A., Role of the forebrain commissures in amygdaloid kindling in rats, *Epilepsia*, 19 (1978), 19–33.
20. McIntyre, D.C., Split brain rat: transfer and interference of kindled amygdala convulsions, In Wada, J.A. (Ed) *Kindling*, Raven Press, New York, (1996) 85–102.
21. McIntyre, D.C., Forebrain commissure and limbic kindling, In Reeves, A.J. (Ed) *Epilepsy and the corpus callosum 2*, Plenum Press, New York, 1995 79–89.
22. McIntyre, D.C. and Goddard, G.V., Transfer, interference and spontaneous recovery of convulsions kindled from the rat amygdala, *Electroenceph. Clin. Neurophysiol.*, 35 (1973) 533–543.
23. Naquet, R., Silva-Comte, C. and Menini, C., Implication of the frontal cortex in paroxysmal manifestations (EEG and EMG) induced by light stimulation in the Papio papio, In: Speckmann, E.J. and Elger, C.E. (Eds.) *Epilepsy and motor system*, Urban and Schwarzenberg, Munich, 1983 220–237.
24. Racine, R.J., Burhnam, W.M. and Gartner J.G., Rates of motor seizure development in rats subjected to electrical brain stimulation: strain and interstimulus interval, *Electroenceph. Clin. Neurophysiol.*, 35 (1973) 553–556.
25. Riche, D. and Lanoir, J., Some claustro-cortical connections in the cat and baboon as studied by retrograde horseradish peroxidase transport, *J. Comp. Neurol.*, 177 (1978) 435–444.
26. Rodin, E.A., *The prognosis of patients with epilepsy*, Charles C, Thomas, Springfield, Ill., 1968.
27. Schmidt, D., Jing-Jane, T. and Jang, D., Generalized tonic-clonic seizures in patients with complex partial seizures: Natural history and prognostic relevance, *Epilepsia*, 24 (1983), 43–48.
28. Wada, J.A. Preface. Wada, J.A. *Kindling*, Raven Press, New York. 1976.
29. Wada, J.A., Amygdaloid and frontal cortical kindling in subhuman primates. In Girgis, M. and Kiloh, L.G. (Eds.) *Limbic epilepsy and the dyscontrol syndrome*, Elsevier, Amsterdam, (1980) 133–147.
30. Wada, J.A., Secondary cerebral functional alterations examined in the kindling model of epilepsy. In Mayerdorf, A. and Schmidt, R.P. (Eds.) *Secondary epileptogenesis*, Raven Press, New York (1982) 45–114.
31. Wada, J.A., Erosion of kindled epileptogenesis and kindling induced long-term seizure suppressive effect in primates, In J.A. Wada (Ed) *Kindling 4*, Raven Press, New York, 1990, 383–396.

32. Wada, J.A., Forebrain convulsive mechanisms examined in the primate model of generalized epilepsy: emphasis on the claustrum. In Malafosse, A., Genton, P., Hirsch, E. et al (Eds.) *Idiopathic generalized epilepsies: clinical, experimental and genetic aspects*, John Libby, London, (1994) 349–374.
33. Wada, J.A. and Komai, T., Effect of anterior two thirds callosal bisection upon bisymmetrical and bisynchronous generalized convulsions kindled from amygdala in epileptic baboon, Papio papio, In Reeves, A.G. (Ed) *Epilepsy and the corpus callosum*, Plenum Press, New York, 1985 75–98.
34. Wada, J.A. and Mizoguchi, T., Limbic kindling in the forebrain bisected photosensitive baboon Papio papio. *Epilepsia*, 25 (1984) 278–287.
35. Wada, J.A and Naquet, R., Examination of neural mechanisms involved in photogenic seizure susceptibility in epileptic Senegalese baboon, Papio papio, *Epilepsia*, 13 (1972) 344.
36. Wada, J.A. and Okamoto, M., The differential role of the mesial and lateral frontal cortices in amygdaloid kindling and kindled seizure in Senegalese baboons, Papio papio, Wada, J.A. (Ed.) *Kindling 3*, Raven Press, New York (1986) 409–426.
37. Wada, J.A. and Osawa, T., Spontaneous recurrent seizure state induced by daily electric amygdaloid stimulation in Senegalese baboons Papio papio, *Neurology*, 26 (1976) 273–28.
38. Wada, J.A. and Sato, M., The generalized convulsive seizure state induced by daily electrical stimulation of the amygdala in split brain cats, *Epilepsia*, 16 (1975) 417–430.
39. Wada, J.A. and Tsuchimochi, H., Claustral activation of hemispheric motor mechanism in partial seizure, *Epilepsia*, 33 (1992) 37.
40. Wada, J.A. and Tsuchimochi, H., Cingulate kindling in Senegalese baboons, Papio papio, *Epilepsia*, 36 (1995) 1142–1151.
41. Wada, J.A., Mizoguchi, T. and Komai, S., Cortical motor activation in amygdaloid kindling: observations in nonepileptic monkeys with anterior two thirds callosal section, In Wada, J.A. (Ed) *Kindling 2*, (1981) 235–248.
42. Wada, J.A., Mizoguchi, T. and Komai, S., Kindling epileptogenesis in orbital and mesial frontal cortical areas of subhuman primates, *Epilepsia*, 26 (1985) 472–479.
43. Wada, J.A., Nakashima, T. and Kaneko, Y, Forebrain bisection and feline amygdaloid kindling, *Epilepsia*, 23 (1982) 521–530.
44. Wada, J.A., Terao, A. and Booker, H.E., Longitudinal correlative analysis of photosensitive baboons, Papio papio, *Neurology*, 22(1972) 1272–12885.
45. Wada, J.A., Naquet, R., Cartier, J., Chaharmasson, G. and Menini, C., Further examination of neural mechanisms involved in photogenic seizure susceptibility in the epileptic Senegalese baboon, Papio papio, *Electroenceph. Clin. Neurophysiol.*, 35 (1973) 786.
46. Wauquier, A. Ashton, D. and Mellis, W., Behavioural analysis of amygdaloid kindling in beagle dogs and the effects of clonazepam, diazepam, phenobarbital, diphenylhydantoin and flunarizine on seizure manifestation, *Exp. Neurol.*, 64 (1979) 579–586.

GENERAL DISCUSSION 1

K. Gale: Juhn, the data you showed on the claustrum are really exciting and very interesting in terms of that being an area that may be able to translate some of the sensory input into motor output procedures. Did you do any experiments where you lesioned the claustrum bilaterally to see whether that could completely prevent both the ipsilateral as well as the contralateral manifestations?

J. Wada: No we have not done that. I thought if we did probably we would kill the animals. When you make bilateral lesions, often the animals' condition very badly deteriorates, and I didn't want to have that for a chronic experiment.

K. Gale: One thing that occurred to me was that you could do the lesion on one side and then allow the kindling to progress to the other side. And so it would seem that perhaps at that point it would be interesting to lesion the contralateral.

J. Wada: Yes, this in progress.

J. Pinel: Juhn, in the work that you have done with the development of spontaneous motor convulsions, have you noticed any predictors of this? For example, do the animals that reach class 5 elicited convulsions more quickly also reach the spontaneous state more quickly, or were there things in the interictal behaviour of the animals that would predict the emergence of these spontaneous seizures?

J. Wada: "Spontaneous" implies it is totally unpredicatble. I have not found any way of predicting which animal might develop seizures spontaneously. There is a tremendous spectrum among primates, which can produce rapid interictal spike discharge versus little or no discharge. For example, the papio cynocephalus studied by Michael Corcoran had literally no or minimal interictal discharge and yet emitted spontaneous generalized convulsions. So this is no indicator. We looked at many other aspects, but found no preditor.

J. Pinel: We've reached the same conclusions, studying the development of spontaneous seizures in rats.

J. Wada: And that's where the vague notion of genetic predisposition comes in. Of course this is a very dangerous thing for me to say because, knowing nothing about genetics and knowing that our population is so small that our findings could be due to sampling error, this could possibly explain our results. How can I explain, for example, cats usually kindled within about twenty to twenty-five days, the normal kindling, yet we have cats which required more than three months to kindle and others requiring only 12 days, and yet there was no technical error in terms of electrode placement. I also wondered if the animals themselves have strange diseases of some kind, and so we subjected to them very serious survey of their health condition but found nothing. So that I must conclude that there is a tremendous spectrum, and this spectrum must represent the distribution of a genetic predisposition.

F. Lopez da Silva: Enjoyed very much your talk. I was just wondering about these spontaneous seizures—whether on behavioural and electrographic dimensions, the spontaneous seizures are similar to or different from those that you trigger by your kindling stimulation.

J. Wada: Oh yes, they are identical.

F. Lopez da Silva: You never found any different pattern?

J. Wada: The only difference is in Papio papio. In some Papio papio, when it's kindled to stage 5, stimulation immediately triggers a beautiful bisymmetrical bisynchronous seizure. There's no way you can tell, looking at the record of behaviour, that it is not triggered. But some animals show a lag, in terms of showing a partial seizure for a few seconds, then onto this the bisymmetrical, bisynchronous pattern develops. But when you examine some of these animals' spontaneous seizures, they are often identical to the kindled pattern, or they may be just bisymmetrical and bisynchronous onset, indicating possibly that these seizures reflect the predisposed nature of the species that is boosted up by the kindling process. But excluding Papio papio, the majority of the spontaneous seizures we have documented are identical to the kindled ones.

A. Fernandez-Guardiola: You remember the work of Bert, in Africa, who was one of the first to discover photosensitivity. But there is something more than species- specific or genetic factors at work, because he found that the baboons in the west were less sensitive than the baboons in the east, and maybe there is an ecological factor involved in this. Also, do Papio papio show photosensitivity during sleep?

J. Wada: Second question first. We haven't really studied photosensitivity during sleep, but I can tell you when animals are at a drowsy state, or at repose, eyes closed and awake (judging from the EEG), cortical stimulation does not elicit a convulsive response, and the same with photic stimulation, unless you arouse them, in which case they immediately go into photoconvulsive seizure. So I would suspect that an animal would be protected from photosensitivity. And I would agree that photosensitivity depends on where an animal lives. I don't know how to interpret it, even in Senegal, where our Papio papio came from. The animals we have been using are from Casamatch region, and these animals are known to have a very high sensitivity. This is an area which is sandwiched by two rivers, and if you go beyond this river, photosensitivity just drops like this, and we haven't studied these groups.

2

IDIOSYNCRASIES OF LIMBIC KINDLING IN DEVELOPING RATS

Kurt Z. Haas,[1] Ellen F. Sperber,[2] Barbara Benenati,[2] Patric K. Stanton,[1,2] and Solomon L. Moshé[1,2,3]

[1]Department of Neuroscience
[2]Department of Neurology
[3]Department of Pediatrics
Albert Einstein College of Medicine
1410 Pelham Parkway South
Bronx, New York 10461-1602

While expression of the basic kindling phenomena appears to be the same regardless of age, kindling in developing rats differs significantly from adult kindling in a number of characteristics which may shed light on age-dependent differences in human epilepsy[4,26], (Baram this volume). At all ages (older than postnatal day [PN] 7), repeated electrical stimuli delivered to limbic structures lead to the progression from focal to generalized seizures, increase in afterdischarge (AD) duration, and a permanent alteration in seizure susceptibility. However, there are age-dependent differences in the rates of kindling development and kindling potential of specific limbic sites, motor seizure expression, interactions between kindled foci, and effects of kindling on dentate synaptic transmission and morphologic hippocampal alterations. These differences correlate well with the heightened seizure susceptibility of the young, their predisposition to multifocal seizures, and the resistance of the immature hippocampus to seizure-induced hippocampal injury.

1. DEVELOPMENTAL KINDLING IN THE AMYGDALA, HIPPOCAMPUS, PIRIFORM CORTEX, AND DEEP ENDOPIRIFORM NUCLEUS

The rate of kindling development is more rapid in immature rats, compared to adults[4,26,29]. This trend is often evident as a faster progression from focal to generalized seizures. At the same time, kindling rates in different brain regions vary in adult rats, and this difference has been attributed to the relative epileptogenicity of these sites[13]. We have characterized kindling rates in a number of brain regions in immature rats, to determine if

Kindling 5, edited by Corcoran and Moshé.
Plenum Press, New York, 1998.

Table 1. Adult rats: number of stimulations (x±SE) required for the development of stage 5 seizures[33] as a function of limbic site

Amygdala	Dorsal hippocampus	DEN	Piriform cortex
12.9 ± 1.5 n=18	21.4 ± 3.4* n=7	12.6 ± 1.3 n=7	13.3 ± 1.8 n=4

Data obtained from Zhao and Moshé[38] and Haas et al.[16]
*Significantly different from the other 3 groups.

the heightened seizure susceptibility seen early in development is specific for a particular kindled site, or represents a more general characteristic of the immature rat brain. We stimulated a number of regions in the 16 day old rat including the amygdala, hippocampus, piriform cortex, deep endopiriform nucleus (DEN) and dorsal to the DEN (dDEN).

In the adult rat, the piriform cortex is very prone to developing seizures and has been shown to be rapidly involved in kindled seizures initiated elsewhere[19,21,22,34]. The DEN is a region of the anterior, or pre-, piriform cortex, termed the 'area tempestas' by Gale and colleagues[11,32], which they showed to be a site where seizures can be readily initiated with very low concentrations of chemical convulsants[32]. Furthermore, kindled seizures initiated in other limbic sites can be suppressed by DEN injections of glutamate receptor antagonists[9] or the GABA transaminase inhibitor gamma-vinyl-GABA (GVG).[36] Kindling rates of both the piriform cortex and DEN are among fastest of any brain regions studied[13,17,38], although the kindling rates in the piriform cortex vary depending on both the layer and anterior/posterior site stimulated[19]. Table 1 shows that, in the adult rat, kindling rates are similar in the amygdala, DEN and superficial piriform cortex (located ventral to the DEN)[38], whereas the hippocampus kindles more slowly[13,16].

To study kindling in these regions in the developing rat, we implanted electrodes in various sites on PN 14, and stimulations were given over two days (PN 16 and 17). Since rats at this age do not demonstrate kindling refractoriness[29], stimulations were delivered every 15 minutes. Comparison of rates of kindling development between the piriform cortex, DEN, dDEN, amygdala, and hippocampus demonstrated that the amygdala, hippocampus, piriform cortex and dDEN kindled at the same rate, while kindling in the DEN was significantly faster. Figure 1 shows the mean kindling stages at each stimulation trial for all 5 regions, indicating the remarkable similarity between all sites except for the DEN. AD durations were also similar between the amygdala, hippocampus, piriform cortex and above the DEN, while the ADs from DEN stimulation were significantly longer.

The data indicate that, in 2 week old rats, most of the limbic regions kindle at the same rate except for the DEN, which kindles faster than any other region tested. The

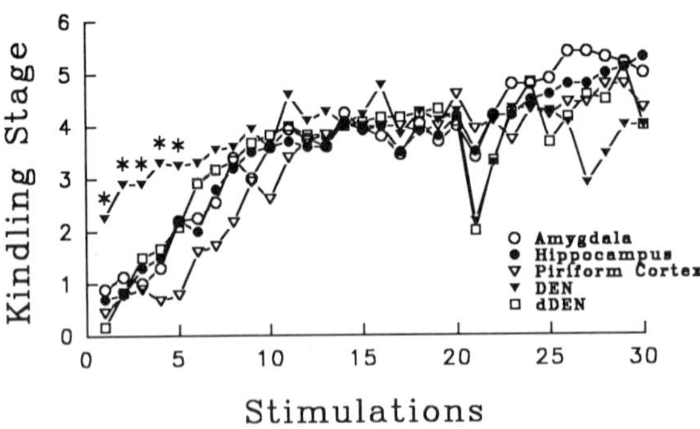

Figure 1. Comparison of the rate of kindling development in various limbic sites in two-week old rats. In contrast to kindling in adults, the hippocampus kindled at the same rate as the amygdala, piriform cortex and dDEN. The DEN kindled at a faster rate than the other 4 groups.

increased susceptibility of the 2 week old DEN should be contrasted to the findings in adults, in which the DEN exhibited a similar kindling rate to other adjacent regions, as well as the amygdala. The second important finding is that, in 2 week old rats, the dorsal hippocampus kindled as easily as most other limbic regions. This was not the case in adults, in which the hippocampus kindled much slower than other regions. The similarity of kindling rates of several limbic sites in 2 week old rats may be due to the more rapid generalization of seizures throughout the immature brain, and may contribute to the earlier appearance of bilateral seizures compared to adults[15,16,26].

2. DEVELOPMENTALLY-SPECIFIC KINDLING STAGES, INCLUDING EXPRESSION OF SEVERE KINDLED SEIZURES AND SPONTANEOUS SEIZURES

Kindling in the piriform cortex, DEN, amygdala, and hippocampus elicited the same types of motor seizure behaviors in immature rats, some of which are seldom, or never seen in adults. For example, in adults, the kindling stage 3 of the Racine scale, unilateral forelimb clonus, is typically followed by stage 4, synchronous bilateral forelimb clonus[33]. However, in immature rats, unilateral forelimb clonus progresses to bilateral asynchronous forelimb clonus. This age-specific expression of bilateral, but asynchronous motor seizures, which we have called stage 3.5, may be due to the incomplete development or myelination of the corpus callosum[14,18].

More dramatic seizure behaviors elicited with relatively few stimuli (less than 30) in immature rats are severe kindled seizures, which involve wild running and jumping with vocalizations. We have called this behavior stage 6, since it typically follows stage 4 or 5 seizures[15]. A recording of the AD associated with a stage 6 seizure in an immature rat is presented in Figure 2, along with an AD from an adult given the same number of stimula-

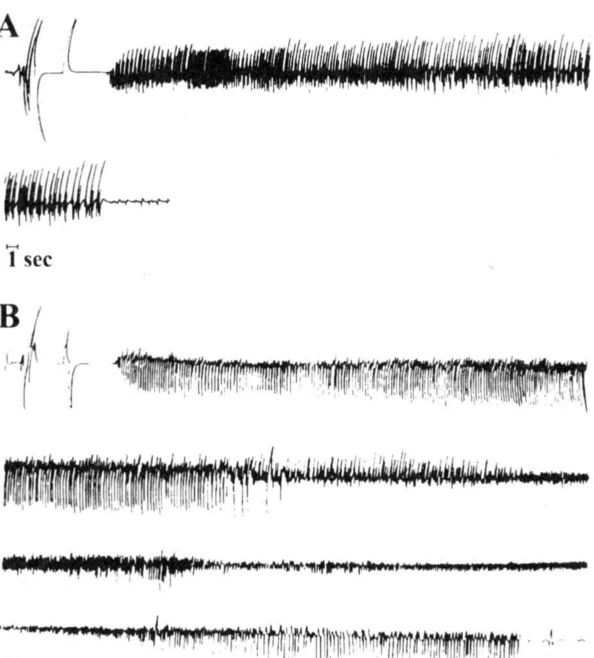

Figure 2. A. Afterdischarge (AD) recorded in the hippocampus associated with a stage 5 seizure in an adult rat given 24 kindling stimuli. B. Representative AD from the hippocampus of a 16-day-old rat pup, accompanying a stage 6 seizure, elicited by kindling stimulation number 24.

tions, demonstrating the longer duration of ADs associated with these severe seizures in young rats. After the appearance of stage 6 seizures, kindled seizures can continue to increase in severity and in some rats, stage 6 is followed by continuous tonus, which we term stage 7. In immature rats, these severe seizures were elicited with less than 30 stimuli from all brain regions tested.

The expression of severe kindled seizures in immature rats after relatively few stimuli differs markedly from kindling in adults, which do not normally express severe kindled seizures at all. Instead, kindled motor behavior typically plateaus at stage 5. Kindled seizures similar to stage 6 and 7 have been reported in adult rats, but only after delivering more than 100 stimulations[31]. In addition to more readily expressing severe kindled seizures, in a few immature rats, kindling with less than 30 stimuli resulted in the appearance of spontaneous seizures (see also Baram, this volume). As with severe seizures, kindling-induced spontaneous seizures in adults have only been reported after far larger numbers of stimuli[24]. The more rapid appearance of stage 6 and stage 7 seizures early in development suggests a heightened tendency of seizures to spread in the immature brain. It has been proposed that brainstem structures may be the substrate of stage 6 and 7 seizures[5]. In collaboration with Bob Ackermann, we used the 2-deoxyglucose (2-DG) technique[1] to map the structures metabolically active during the expression of stage 6 and 7 seizures in 2 week old rats. Preliminary results of these studies suggest that the increases in 2-DG uptake are confined to rhinencephalic structures, arguing against the involvement of brain stem structures in severe seizures in 2 week old rats.

Alternatively, the rapid appearance of stage 6 and 7 seizures could be due to the delayed development of brain circuits that normally limit the spread of seizures in adults. The GABAergic substantia nigra-cortex circuit[30] and ascending noradrenergic pathways[2,3,6,23,35] (Burchfiel, Applegate this volume) are two such circuits.

3. INTERACTION BETWEEN KINDLING AT TWO FOCI

An intriguing aspect of the kindling model is that multiple kindling foci in the same brain can interact. A phenomenon called positive transfer occurs when the presence of an initial kindling focus enhances the rate of kindling at a second kindling focus[13]. In contrast, when two foci are kindled at the same time by alternating stimuli between sites at subsequent trials, a seizure-suppression mechanism, called kindling antagonism, occurs[7,15]. Instead of the concurrent development of kindling at both foci, kindling at one focus progresses from focal to generalized seizure stages, while kindling at the second focus is suppressed, resulting in only focal seizures. The study of kindling antagonism has been restricted to adult animals, and it has been attributed to contributing to the low incidence of multifocal seizures in adults. Multifocal seizures, however, are more common early in life, and therefore, it is an intriguing hypothesis that kindling antagonism may be reduced in young animals.

In order to examine the interaction between two kindling foci in the immature rat, electrodes were implanted in both the amygdala, and either contralateral or ipsilateral hippocampus, in the same animals. Stimulations were delivered to one of the two foci on alternating trials. Figure 3 illustrates our findings from this concurrent kindling of the amygdala and hippocampus in PN 16–17 day rats. In contrast to the retardation of kindling development seen in adults, alternating stimuli between two foci in immature rats produced a positive transfer between sites, resulting in faster kindling rates at both sites compared to kindling at each individual focus[15,16]. Kindling at each focus using the alter-

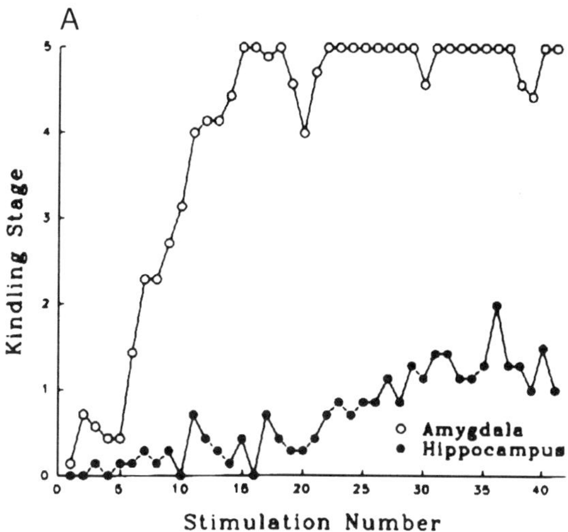

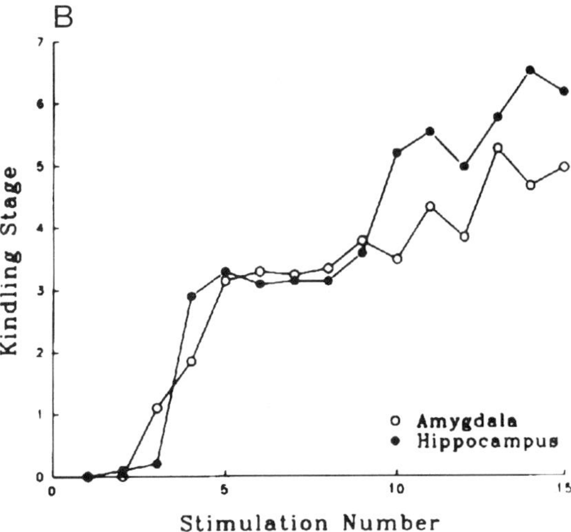

Figure 3. A. In adult rats, alternating kindling stimulations between the amygdala and hippocampus results in kindling antagonism. Mean seizure stages demonstrate the retardation of kindling development in the hippocampus. B. Mean seizure stages of 16–17-day-old rat pups in response to alternating kindling stimulations between the amygdala and hippocampus. In contrast to the kindling antagonism produced by alternate kindling in adults, positive transfer occurs between concurrently kindled foci in immature rats. [Figure modified with permission from *Brain Research* (1992) 68: 140–3.]

nating paradigm was approximately twice as fast as kindling at each site alone. The lack of kindling antagonism in immature rats suggests that the mechanisms underlying the seizure-suppression associated with kindling antagonism in adult rats may be nonfunctional during development. This is consistent with the hypothesis that the lack of kindling antagonism may be responsible for the preponderance of multifocal seizures in the young[15,16].

It has been suggested that noradrenergic projections to the forebrain may play a role in kindling antagonism in adult rats, since depletion of brain norepinephrine (NE) levels with 6-hydroxydopamine reduces kindling antagonism[2]. NE has also been implicated in another form of kindling-induced seizure-suppression, known as kindling refractoriness[23]. Kindling refractoriness is the slowing of the rate of kindling produced by decreasing the interval between each kindling stimulation trial. In adult rats, intervals between kindling stimuli shorter than a few hours reduce the rate of kindling. It has been shown that hourly stimulations produce kindling at a slower rate than daily stimuli, and an interval of 15 minutes severely retards or completely prevents kindling[13,29].

In contrast to the strong seizure refractoriness found in adult rats, we have shown that 2-week-old rats fail to demonstrate any kindling refractoriness when stimuli are delivered at short intervals. Kindling rates in immature rats are not altered by use of stimulus intervals of 1 hour or 15 minutes[29]. It is possible that the mechanism underlying kindling postictal refractoriness and kindling antagonism are related, since both appear to require the neurotransmitter norepinephrine[2,23]. It is a reasonable hypothesis that the immaturity of noradrenergic transmission in the first few postnatal weeks in the rat[26] underlies the lack of both kindling antagonism and kindling refractoriness.

4. DEVELOPMENTAL KINDLING DOES NOT PRODUCE LONG-TERM ALTERATIONS OF DENTATE SYNAPTIC TRANSMISSION

It was first demonstrated by Maru and Goddard that kindled seizures in adult rats induce an increase of synaptic inhibition on dentate granule cells[20]. This enhancement of inhibition is rapid, beginning within 24 h after a single kindling-induced AD, and can last for a number of weeks[10,12,25]. The role of enhanced dentate inhibition in the process of kindling is not clear. It may contribute to the kindling phenomenon, or be a compensatory response to kindled seizures. To further address this question, we examined dentate synaptic transmission after kindling in immature rats using the *in vitro* hippocampal slice preparation and paired-pulse stimulation of the perforant path synapses on dentate granule cells. Two weeks following completion of kindling in PN 16–17 rats, hippocampal slices were prepared from both kindled rats and age-matched controls. While perforant path-evoked paired-pulse inhibition of granule cells two weeks after kindling in adult rats was markedly enhanced, kindling in PN 16–17 rats produced no such alterations in inhibition.

Figure 4A illustrates the normal triphasic paired-pulse profile in both control adult and immature rat hippocampal slices, which is composed of early and late paired-pulse inhibition, separated by paired-pulse facilitation. Figure 4B demonstrates the increase of paired-pulse inhibition and loss of paired-pulse facilitation following kindling in adults. In contrast to adults, kindling in the immature rat produced no alterations of the paired-pulse profile (Fig. 4B). These results indicate that the developing brain is resistant to kindling-induced long-term alterations in granule cell inhibition. Furthermore, this shows that enhanced inhibition is not an obligatory component of the process of kindling, but is more likely an age-dependent compensatory response to seizures. In further support of this notion, we have also observed a resistance of immature dentate inhibition to seizure-induced changes due to two other convulsants, kainic acid and flurothyl.

5. SEIZURE-INDUCED SYNAPTIC REORGANIZATION

Sutula et al.[37] first demonstrated that, in adult rats, kindling can induce aberrant synaptic reorganization of the mossy fibers in the inner molecular layer of the dentate gyrus. It is, as yet, unclear whether this synaptic reorganization labeled by Timm stain is due to cell loss of mossy fiber target cells as suggested by Cavazos[8]. Recent studies (Racine, this volume and the discussion) suggest that this synaptic reorganization can occur in the absence of any discernible cell loss. It has, however, been speculated that the synaptic reorganization of mossy fibers may be partially responsible for the permanence of kindling.

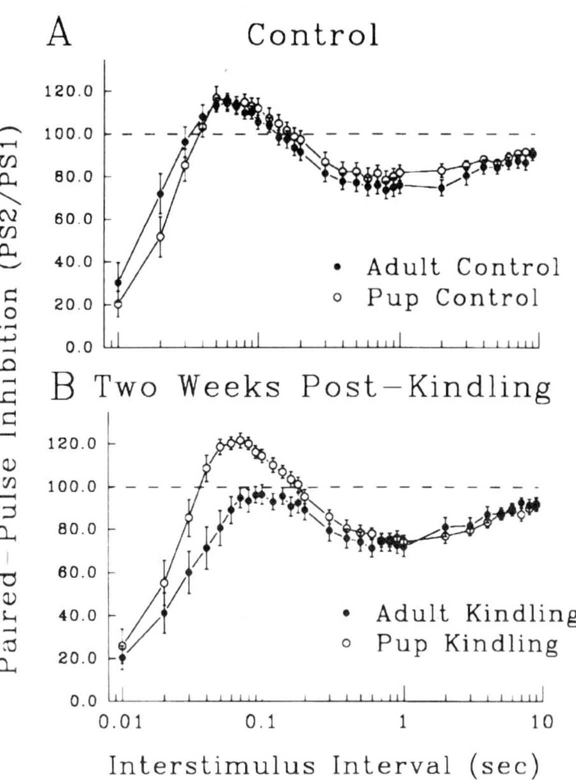

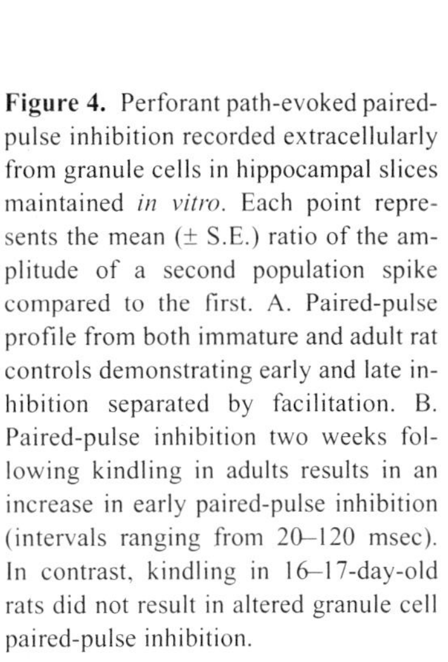

Figure 4. Perforant path-evoked paired-pulse inhibition recorded extracellularly from granule cells in hippocampal slices maintained *in vitro*. Each point represents the mean (± S.E.) ratio of the amplitude of a second population spike compared to the first. A. Paired-pulse profile from both immature and adult rat controls demonstrating early and late inhibition separated by facilitation. B. Paired-pulse inhibition two weeks following kindling in adults results in an increase in early paired-pulse inhibition (intervals ranging from 20–120 msec). In contrast, kindling in 16–17-day-old rats did not result in altered granule cell paired-pulse inhibition.

Once induced in two-week old rats, kindling is permanent. Adult rats previously kindled as rat pups at PN 16, rekindle faster than naive controls either at the same (initial) kindling site or a contralateral site[27,28]. To determine whether the permanence of kindling in developing rats is associated with synaptic reorganization of mossy fibers, we kindled two-week old rats from the amygdala or dorsal hippocampus until the rats exhibited several stage 6 seizures. The rats were sacrificed 2 weeks after the completion of kindling, a time point of intense synaptic reorganization of the mossy fibers in kindled adult rats. The extent of synaptic reorganization was assessed using the Timm method as described by Sutula[37]. In contrast, to the adult findings, we found no synaptic reorganization of mossy fibers following kindling in PN 16 rats. These results suggest that synaptic reorganization of the mossy fibers may not be the substrate for the permanence of kindling, because, in developing rats, kindling is permanent even when synaptic reorganization in the dentate has not occurred (Figure 5).

6. CONCLUSIONS

The data outlined here describe a number of age-dependent properties of kindling which may underlie the heightened seizure susceptibility and propensity to multifocal seizures of the immature brain. The similarity of kindling rates of different brain regions, rapid expression of severe as well as spontaneous seizures, and the positive transfer between alternately kindled foci all indicate that seizures more easily propagate through these structures in the immature brain compared to adults. Our results also indicate that the DEN in the immature rat, unlike the adult, is a site with a heightened sensitivity to kin-

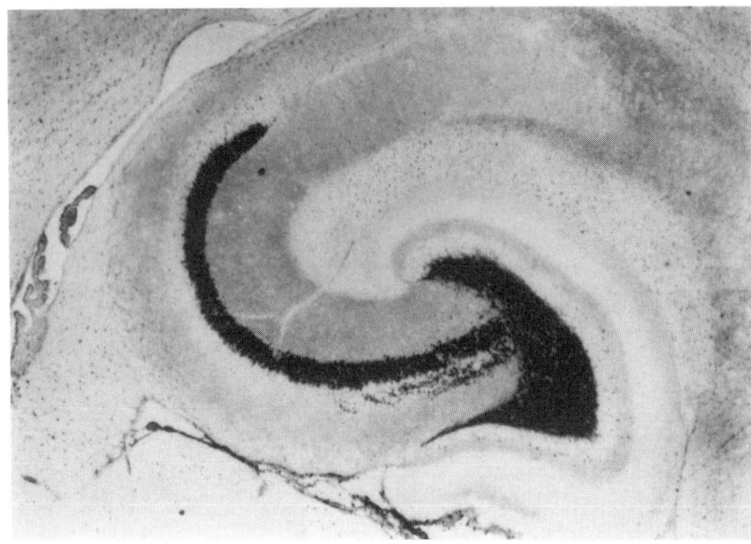

Figure 5. Timm silver-sulfide stain of the hippocampus two weeks following amygdala kindling in a 16–17 day old rat pup. Dark granular positive Timm staining is restricted to the normal mossy fiber termination zones, including the hilus and CA3 pyramidal cell proximal dendrites. No abnormal supragranular staining was observed in the dentate gyrus, indicating that kindling in immature rats is not associated with mossy fiber synaptic reorganization to this region as it is in adults.

dling, and may therefore play a role in epileptogenesis at this age. The absence of kindling antagonism with multifocal kindling in developing rats also demonstrates a lack of seizure-suppression mechanisms which normally suppress multiple focal seizures in adults. In addition, we have also found that kindling in the immature rat does not result in the kind of long-term alterations in dentate synaptic transmission seen after kindling in adults. Furthermore, kindling in developing rats does not produce any changes in synaptic connectivity of the dentate gyrus although it produces a persistent increase in seizure susceptibility into adulthood. The observations may shed light on the mechanisms involved in epileptogenesis and consequences of kindling. The age-related differences must be taken into account in the design of appropriate treatment of age-specific seizure disorders.

ACKNOWLEDGMENTS

This work was supported in part by the NIH training grant T32DK07513 (KZH), the Klingenstein Foundation, the Office of Naval Research (PKS), NINDS research grant NS-20253 (SLM), and NINDS research grant NS-30387 (EFS).

REFERENCES

1. Ackermann, R. F., Moshé, S. L. and Albala, B. J. (1989) Restriction of enhanced [2–14C]deoxyglucose utilization to rhinencephalic structures in immature amygdala-kindled rats. *Experimental Neurology*, 104: 73–81.
2. Applegate, C. D., Burchfiel, J. L. and Konkol, R. J. (1986) Kindling antagonism: effects of norepinephrine depletion on kindled seizure suppression after concurrent, alternate stimulation in rats. *Experimental Neurology*, 94: 379–90.

3. Applegate, C. D., Konkol, R. J. and Burchfiel, J. L. (1987) Kindling antagonism: a role for hindbrain norepinephrine in the development of site suppression following concurrent, alternate stimulation. *Brain Research*, 407: 212–22.
4. Baram, T. Z., Hirsch, E. and Schultz, L. (1993) Short-interval amygdala kindling in neonatal rats. *Brain Research. Developmental Brain Research*, 73: 79–83.
5. Browning, R. A. (1986) Neuroanatomical localization of structures responsible for seizures in the GEPR: lesion studies. *Life Sciences*, 39: 857–67.
6. Burchfiel, J. L., Applegate, C.D. and Konkol, R.J. Kindling antagonism: a role for norepinephrine in seizure suppression. In: "Kindling 3", edited by J.A. Wada. New York. Raven Press,1986, pp. 213–229.
7. Burchfiel, J. L., Serpa, K. A. and Duffy, F. H. (1982) Kindling antagonism: interactions of dorsal and ventral entorhinal cortex with the septum during concurrent kindling. *Brain Research*, 238: 3–12.
8. Cavazos, J. E. and Sutula, T. P. (1990) Progressive neuronal loss induced by kindling: a possible mechanism for mossy fiber synaptic reorganization and hippocampal sclerosis [published erratum appears in Brain Res 1991 Feb 8;541(1):179]. *Brain Research*, 527: 1–6.
9. Croucher, M. J., Bradford, H. F., Sunter, D. C. and Watkins, J. C. (1988) Inhibition of the development of electrical kindling of the prepyriform cortex by daily focal injections of excitatory amino acid antagonists. *European Journal of Pharmacology*, 152: 29–38.
10. de Jonge, M. and Racine, R. J. (1987) The development and decay of kindling-induced increases in paired-pulse depression in the dentate gyrus. *Brain Res*, 412: 318–328.
11. Gale, K. (1988) Progression and generalization of seizure discharge: anatomical and neurochemical substrates. *Epilepsia*, 29: S15–34.
12. Gilbert, M. E. (1991) Potentiation of inhibition with perforant path kindling: an NMDA-receptor dependent process. *Brain Research*, 564: 109–16.
13. Goddard, G. V., McIntyre, D. C. and Leech, C. K. (1969) A permanent change in brain function resulting from daily electrical stimulation. *Experimental Neurology*, 25: 295–330.
14. Gravel, C. and Hawkes, R. (1990) Maturation of the corpus callosum of the rat: I. Influence of thyroid hormones on the topography of callosal projections. *Journal of Comparative Neurology*, 291: 128–46.
15. Haas, K. Z., Sperber, E. F. and Moshe, S. L. (1990) Kindling in developing animals: expression of severe seizures and enhanced development of bilateral foci. *Brain Research. Developmental Brain Research*, 56: 275–80.
16. Haas, K. Z., Sperber, E. F. and Moshe, S. L. (1992) Kindling in developing animals: interactions between ipsilateral foci. *Brain Research. Developmental Brain Research*, 68: 140–3.
17. Honack, D., Wahnschaffe, U. and Loscher, W. (1991) Kindling from stimulation of a highly sensitive locus in the posterior part of the piriform cortex. Comparison with amygdala kindling and effects of antiepileptic drugs. *Brain Research*, 538: 196–202.
18. Kristensson, K., Zeller, N. K., Dubois-Dalcq, M. E. and Lazzarini, R. A. (1986) Expression of myelin basic protein gene in the developing rat brain as revealed by in situ hybridization. *Journal of Histochemistry & Cytochemistry*, 34: 467–73.
19. Loscher, W., Ebert, U., Wahnschaffe, U. and Rundfeldt, C. (1995) Susceptibility of different cell layers of the anterior and posterior part of the piriform cortex to electrical stimulation and kindling: comparison with the basolateral amygdala and "area tempestas". *Neuroscience*, 66: 265–76.
20. Maru, E. and Goddard, G. V. (1987) Alteration in dentate neuronal activities associated with perforant path kindling III. Enhancement of synaptic inhibition. *Exp Neurol*, 96: 46–60.
21. McIntyre, D. C., Kelly, M. E. and Armstrong, J. N. (1993) Kindling in the perirhinal cortex. *Brain Research*, 615: 1–6.
22. McIntyre, D. C. and Plant, J. R. (1993) Long-lasting changes in the origin of spontaneous discharges from amygdala-kindled rats: piriform vs. perirhinal cortex in vitro. *Brain Research*, 624: 268–76.
23. McIntyre, D. C., Rajala, J. and Edson, N. (1987) Suppression of amygdala kindling with short interstimulus intervals: effect of norepinephrine depletion. *Experimental Neurology*, 95: 391–402.
24. Milgram, N. W., Michael, M., Cammisuli, S., Head, E., Ferbinteanu, J., Reid, C., Murphy, M. P. and Racine, R. (1995) Development of spontaneous seizures over extended electrical kindling. II. Persistence of dentate inhibitory suppression. *Brain Research*, 670: 112–20.
25. Milgram, N. W., Yearwood, T., Khurgel, M., Ivy, G. O. and Racine, R. (1991) Changes in inhibitory processes in the hippocampus following recurrent seizures induced by systemic administration of kainic acid. *Brain Research*, 551: 236–46.
26. Moshé, S. L. (1981) The effects of age on the kindling phenomenon. *Developmental Psychobiology*, 14: 75–81.
27. Moshé, S. L. and Albala, B. J. (1982) Kindling in developing rats: persistence of seizures into adulthood. *Brain Research*, 256: 67–71.

28. Moshé, S. L. and Albala, B. J. (1983) Maturational changes in postictal refractoriness and seizure susceptibility in developing rats. *Annals of Neurology*, 13: 552–7.
29. Moshé, S. L., Albala, B. J., Ackermann, R. F. and Engel, J., Jr. (1983) Increased seizure susceptibility of the immature brain. *Brain Research*, 283: 81–5.
30. Moshé, S. L., Brown, L. L., Kubova, H., Veliskova, J., Zukin, R. S. and Sperber, E. F. (1994) Maturation and segregation of brain networks that modify seizures. *Brain Research*, 665: 141–6.
31. Pinel, J. P. and Rovner, L. I. (1978) Electrode placement and kindling-induced experimental epilepsy. *Experimental Neurology*, 58: 335–46.
32. Piredda, S. and Gale, K. (1985) A crucial epileptogenic site in the deep prepiriform cortex. *Nature*, 317: 623–5.
33. Racine, R. J. (1972) Modification of seizure activity by electrical stimulation. II. Motor seizure. *Electroencephalography & Clinical Neurophysiology*, 32: 281–94.
34. Racine, R. J., Mosher, M. and Kairiss, E. W. (1988) The role of the pyriform cortex in the generation of interictal spikes in the kindled preparation. *Brain Research*, 454: 251–63.
35. Stanton, P. K. (1992) Noradrenergic modulation of epileptiform bursting and synaptic plasticity in the dentate gyrus. *Epilepsy Research—Supplement*, 7: 135–50.
36. Stevens, J. R., Phillips, I. and de Beaurepaire, R. (1988) gamma-Vinyl GABA in endopiriform area suppresses kindled amygdala seizures. *Epilepsia*, 29: 404–11.
37. Sutula, T., He, X. X., Cavazos, J. and Scott, G. (1988) Synaptic reorganization in the hippocampus induced by abnormal functional activity. *Science*, 239: 1147–50.
38. Zhao, D. Y. and Moshé, S. L. (1987) Deep prepiriform cortex kindling and amygdala interactions. *Epilepsy Research*, 1: 94–101.

DISCUSSION OF SOLOMON MOSHÉ'S PAPER

R. Adamec: This is a methodological question. Could there be any anesthetic confound?

S. Moshé: We have kindled adults and pup days postoperatively, at a time when all rats were awake and alert.

R. Adamec: Some anesthetics have metabolites.

S. Moshé: We used ketamine.

R. Adamec: You mentioned that sometimes there are vocalizations during seizures. Have you tried measuring tones?

S. Moshé: No.

J. McNamara: You looked at sprouting in 15 day old rats. How much time elapsed before the animals were killed?

S. Moshé: We have killed the pups at different time points, from 2 weeks to months. There was no mossy fiber sprouting.

J. McNamara: Did you look at rekindling?

S. Moshé: Rats kindled as pups rekindle faster in adulthood than naive rats.

J. McNamara: The rate of kindling in P15 rats is equivalent in the dorsal hippocampus and the amygdala. This is different from in the mature rat. Why do you think that is?

S. Moshé: There are many differences, including the precocious development of excitatory synapses, pruning, changes in local and distant connectivity.

W. M. Burnham: Do other parts of the limbic system kindle at the same rate in 15-day-old rats?

S. Moshé: The amygdala and hippocampus, but not the area tempestas.

W. M. Burnham: Do the jumping seizures look a bit subcortical? We study the rats in a suspended harness, so that we can see both tonus and clonus.

S. Moshé: I agree. However, our 2DG studies have failed to show any brainstem uptake during jumping seizures.

K. Gale: You showed the uptake of 2-deoxyglucose in the supra-kindled animals. Did the substantia nigra light up?

S. Moshé: No, 2DG uptake was confined to the rhinencephalic structures.

K. Gale: When alternating stimulation between the amygdala and hippocampus, is it correct that you found no kindling antagonism?

S. Moshé: Not only was there no antagonism, we found an actual facilitation. This may be due to a decrease of noradrenaline in the immature brain.

J. Engel: Kindling is a progressive phenomenon. Did the kindling you observed in rat pups start out with clinical signs?

S. Moshé: It began with prolonged AD, and manifestations appeared in 2 to 3 stimulations. Because it is difficult to look at mouth clonus, we have missed some early signs. In area tempestas we observed faster kindling to stage 3. After that point it was similar to other regions.

F. Lopes da Silva: Did you perform a neuronal count of the dentate gyrus comparing young and old rats?

S. Moshé: Not yet.

F. Lopes da Silva: From your data, would you conclude that sprouting is counteracting the effects of kindling—that is, is it protective and in younger rats you don't see that?

S. Moshé: We have not looked at it like that. The point I am trying to make is that the permanence of kindling is not necessarily correlated with the changes in the dentate gyrus, such as sprouting.

3

LONG-TERM EFFECTS OF KINDLING ON LEARNING AND MEMORY IN THE DEVELOPING BRAIN

Matthew Sarkisian, Pushpa Tandon, and Gregory L. Holmes

Department of Neurology
Harvard Medical School
Children's Hospital
Boston, Massachusetts

1. INTRODUCTION

One of the pressing questions in pediatric epilepsy is whether seizures cause brain damage. Determining the relative contribution of variables such as seizure type, frequency, duration, age of onset, etiology, and drug effects makes it difficult to assess the role of seizures *per se* in neurological sequelae. Because of the inherent difficulties in determining the effects of seizures using clinical data, animal models can provide insights into the mechanism of seizure-induced damage.

Prior research in our laboratory, using a variety of animal models, has demonstrated that the long-term effects of seizures may be age-dependent. Kainic acid-induced status epilepticus resulted in long-term deficits in learning, memory, behavior and seizure susceptibility in mature rats but had no discernible effect in rats ≤ 20 days of age[32]. Continuous hippocampal stimulation, a model of limbic status epilepticus, causes long-term adverse effects on cognition in pubescent and mature rats but not prepubescent animals[34]. Likewise, pilocarpine-induced seizures result in greater cognitive impairment in immature rats than mature animals[16].

While these studies demonstrated the long-term adverse effects of prolonged seizures in the mature brain, it is not known whether there are age-related differences in the cognitive effects of recurrent seizures. Since many children and adults have recurrent seizures despite treatment with antiepileptic drugs, this is an area of significant clinical interest. To determine whether there are age-related differences in outcome following repetitive seizures we evaluated the effects of repetitive kainic acid (KA) seizures on immature and mature rats. Our goals in the study were twofold: firstly we wished to determine whether recurrent administration of KA leads to a progressive decrease in latency and increase in severity, i.e. a kindling effect; secondly we wanted to determine the long term effects of repetitive seizures on subsequent learning in immature and mature animals.

Kindling 5, edited by Corcoran and Moshé.
Plenum Press, New York, 1998.

2. METHODS

2.1. Water Maze

Prior to administration of KA animals were pre-trained in the water maze Group A consisted of P15 rats (n = 16) who were assigned to KA-treatment and controls (n = 8). Group B consisted of P55 rats who were assigned to KA-treatment (n = 12) and controls (n = 7).

A circular swimming pool made from a galvanized stock water tank (117 cm diameter × 50 cm high) was filled to a depth of 25 cm. with water at a temperature of 26 ± 1°C. The pool was illuminated by overhead fluorescent lights and kept in a permanent location throughout the study. Four points on the rim of the pool were designated as north, south, east and west. On day one, the rats were placed in the pool for 60 seconds of habituation to the apparatus with no platform present ("free swim"). Starting on day 2 and continuing through day 5, rats were trained for 24 trials (6 trials per day) to locate and escape onto a plexiglass platform (8 cm × 8 cm) placed 1.5 cm under the water. The bath was made opalescent by the addition of powdered milk. At the start of each trial, the rat was held facing the perimeter and dropped into the pool to ensure immersion. Entry from the N, S, E or W points was varied in a quasi-random order. Latencies to escape onto the platform were recorded[20,21]. The design of the study tests the ability of an animal to learn and remember the spatial location of the escape platform using only visual cues and measures hippocampal integrity[3,20,22,33].

Following completion of the water maze the rats received serial injections of KA, an analogue of glutamic acid, which when given either systemically or intracerebrally to animals results in a condition similar to human temporal lobe epilepsy[25]. Group A received injections of KA (10 mg/kg) on P20, P22, P24, and P26 while controls received equal volume injections of saline. Immediately following all of the injections, rats were placed into individual plastic cages and their behavior coded every 10 minutes for two hours. Time to forelimb clonus was recorded. Animals that did not have forelimb clonus by 120 minutes were arbitrarily given a time of 120 minutes. Group B received KA (14 mg/kg/day) on P60, P62, P64, and P66 while controls received equal volume injections of saline. As with the younger animals, behavior was coded every 10 minutes for two hours.

Following the last injection of KA the animals in both age groups were returned to cages until water maze testing was repeated in Group A at P60 and Group B at P100.

2.2. EEG

To monitor EEG changes following KA, a subset of rats at P16 and P56 had electrodes placed into the dorsal hippocampus. Following a four day recovery period the animals received serial injections of KA using the same dosages and schedule as described above.

3. RESULTS

3.1. Behavioral Changes Following KA

The response of serial injections of KA was significantly different in the two age groups. In the rats receiving injections starting at P20 there was a decrease in seizure severity and increase in latency with serial injections. Forelimb clonus occurred in 13 of 19 rats (68.4%) with the first KA injection, 4 of 19 rats (21%) with the second injection, 5 of 19 rat (26%) with the third injection, and in none of the 19 rats with the fourth injection. In addition, there was an increasing latency to forelimb clonus with the four injections ($F = 12.49$, $p \leq 0.001$) (Fig. 1a). None of the P20 rats died with serial injections of KA. In the rats receiving KA beginning at P60 there was an increasing severity of seizures and mortality with serial injections. Forelimb clonus occurred in 8 of 12 rats (66.7%) with the first KA injection, 5 of 8 rats (62.5%) with the second injection, 7 of 7 rats (100%) with the third injection, and in 1 of 6 rats (16.7%) with the fourth injection. There was a mortality rate of 33% (4 of 12 rats) following the first injection, 12.5% (1 of 8 rats) following the second injection, 14% (1 of 7 rats), and 0% following the fourth injection. Except for the fourth injection, there was a mild decrease in latency to forelimb clonus with the four injections ($F = 12.49$, $p \leq 0.001$) (Fig. 1b).

3.2. EEG Changes Following KA

Ictal discharges, defined as rhythmic epileptiform discharges, occurred on all four days of KA injection in both Group A and B. However, in the immature rats the ictal discharges on days 3–4 were sporadic and poorly sustained when compared to the older rats in which ictal discharges were virtually continuous on each day of injection (Figure 2).

3.3. Changes in Water Maze Performance Following KA

There were no differences in learning the position of the platform in the water maze in rats assigned to the KA or control groups in either the P15 or P55 rats. However, following KA, there were significant differences in the age group in performance in the water maze. There were no differences in learning the position of the water maze platform between animals receiving serial injections of KA beginning at P20 and the controls

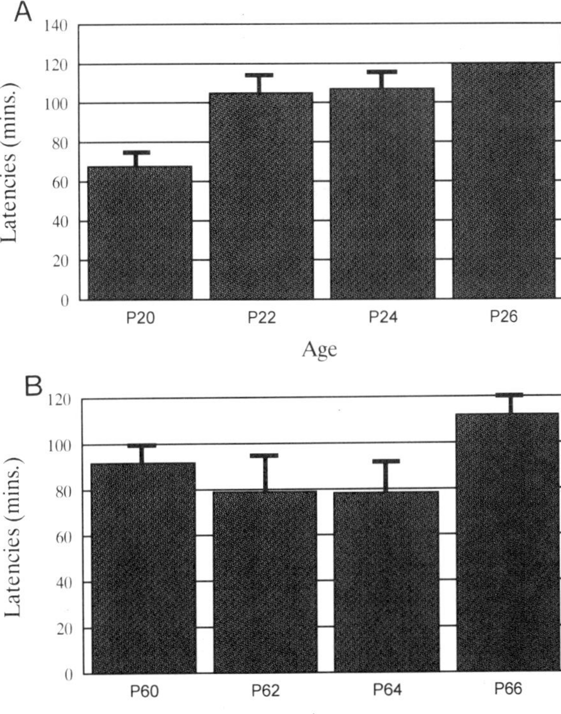

Figure 1. a. Latency to forelimb clonus following serial injections of KA beginning at P20; b. Latency to forelimb clonus following serial injections of KA beginning at P60.

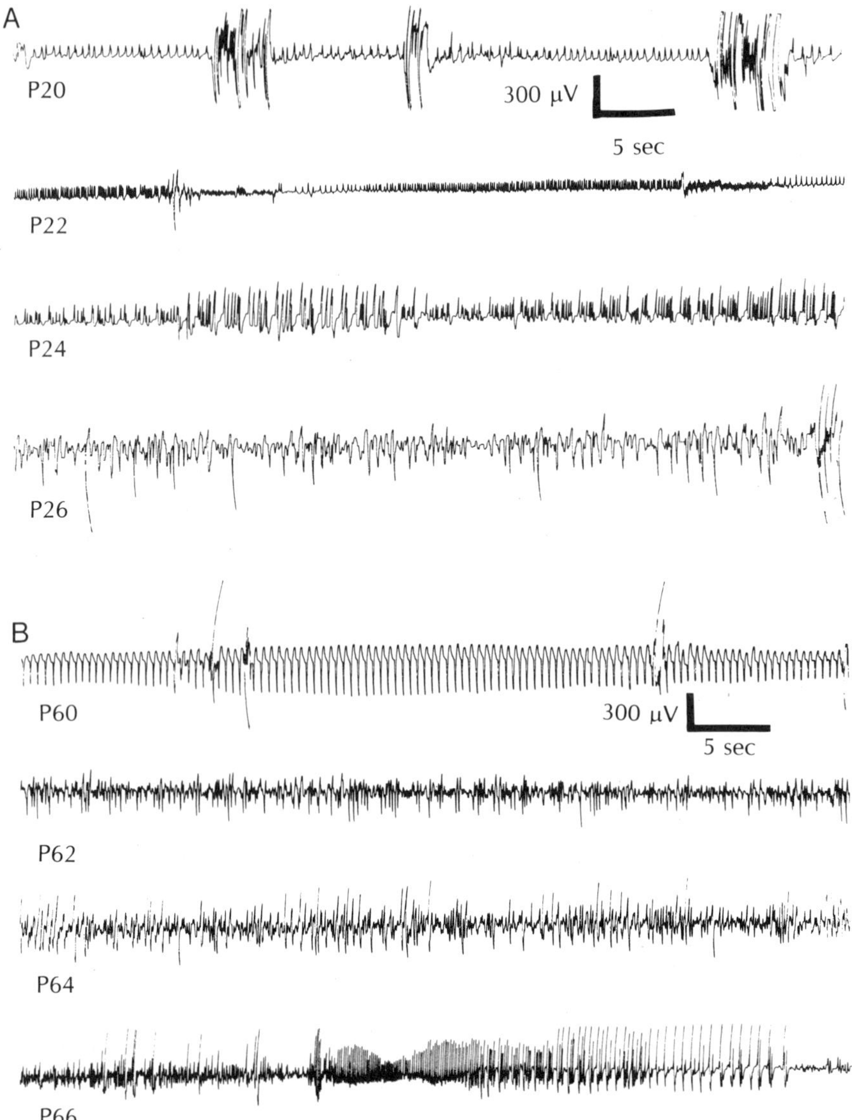

Figure 2. a. EEG changes in the immature rats with serial injections of KA; b. EEG changes in the mature rats with serial injections of KA. The ictal discharges in the immature rats were more continuous than those in the immature rats.

(F = 0.011; p = 0.917) (Fig. 3a). However, in rats receiving KA beginning at P60 there was a significant impairment in latency to platform (F = 20.256; p<0.001) (Fig. 3b).

4. DISCUSSION

This study demonstrates that the effect of serial administration of KA is highly age-dependent. KA caused severe and prolonged seizures in both the immature and mature animals with the first injection. However, there was a modest kindling effect in the mature

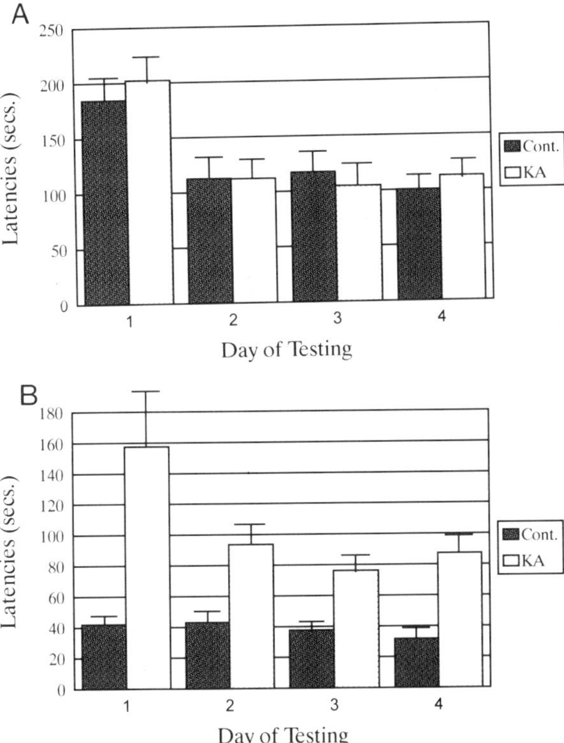

Figure 3. A. Time to platform in rats following serial administration of KA at P20; B. Time to platform in rats following serial administration of KA at P60.

animals as evidenced by a decrease in latency and increase in severity of the seizures with serial injections whereas in the immature animals, the situation was the opposite where serial injections of KA resulted in decreased severity of the seizures. This lack of progression of the seizures in the young rats occurred despite the presence of ictal discharges following all four injections of KA. These results are in concordance with prior work from our laboratory where we found that daily injections of low dose KA to P25 rats resulted in tolerance, with a progressive decrease in duration of EEG ictal discharges and severity of the seizures[29].

Whether repetitive seizures leads to subsequent cognitive effects is dependent on a number of factors. Our study suggests that one important variable is age of the animal. However, other variables are important in determining whether kindling affects subsequent cognition. These factors include the method used for kindling, timing of the kindling in relationship to the learning task, and type of learning task.

Whether the agent used to kindle leads to histological damage appears to play a role in whether cognitive impairment occurs. Animals with histological changes following kindling are more likely to have impairment in learning and memory than animals without such lesions. In this study, despite prolonged and intense seizures, KA in the immature rats produced no discernible hippocampal lesions or any deficits in water maze performance. However KA in mature rats leads to widespread lesions, particularly in the hippocampus, amygdala, piriform, and entorhinal cortex[2,13,30] and severe deficits in learning the position of the water maze. Supporting this concept is the study of Letty et al.[13] who found that electrical amygdala kindling resulted in no histological lesions or effects on subsequent learning, while a single injection of intraamygdala KA, which resulted in widespread histological damage, caused significant deficits in memory in a radial-arm maze.

However, cognitive impairment can occur following repetitive seizures, despite the lack of apparent histological damage. Neill and colleagues[26] administered a convulsant dosage of flurothyl three times daily to P15 rats three times a day for five consecutive days. When the rats were fully mature, they underwent behavioral testing using the water maze and auditory quality or location discrimination. With serial flurothyl administration seizure duration increased and latency to seizure decreased progressively with each exposure. Compared to controls, flurothyl-treated rats had impaired performance in the water maze and on a task of auditory location, but not on quality discrimination. These deficits occurred despite the lack of any histological damage. However it should be noted that the authors did not quantify cell number in the animals. Similarly, Holmes et al.[10] subjected genetically epilepsy prone rats (GEPRs) to 66 audiogenic seizures between 45–75 days of age, administered at a rate of 2–3 stimulations a day. Compared to controls, GEPRs reached criteria less frequently in the T-maze, required longer times to find the platform in the Morris water maze, were less active in the open field, less aggressive in the home cage intruder test, and more irritable and aggressive in the handling test. While no major histological lesions were seen, no detailed histological analysis was performed.

Another factor that may be important in determining whether repetitive seizures alter memory and learning is the timing of the seizures during task acquisition. There are a number of reports which have demonstrated impairment of working or reference memory in spatial tests after hippocampal, amygdala, septal, or perforant path kindling[11,14,15,17]. Following pre-training in the 8-arm maze, Leung and colleagues[14,15] kindled rats in the hippocampus and then measured relearning. Compared to non-stimulated controls[14] and rats subjected to low-frequency stimulations[15] kindled rats had significant deficits in memory. Lopes da Silva et al.[17] also performed hippocampal kindling following training in the 8-arm maze. The authors found that both working (short-term) and reference (long-term) memory were impaired by the kindling.

However, a number of studies have demonstrated that kindling does not appear to impair memory when kindling either precedes or follows the learning task[5,7,18,19,28]. For example, Holmes and colleagues[9] evaluated the long-term effects of kindling in P20, P40, and P60 day-old rats using hippocampal electrical stimulations. Rats were kindled to stage 5 seizures and then received an additional 15 seizures using the same kindling stimulation. At age 80 days, animals were tested in the Morris water maze and open field test, a measure of activity level. No differences were noted in time to platform in the water maze or activity level in the open field test between the kindled rats and controls in any of the three age groups. Likewise, Letty and colleagues[13] also found that mature rats undergoing amygdala kindling had no deficits in the radial-arm maze, a test of spatial memory.

The type of task used to study deficits in memory and learning is also important. Following pentylenetetrazol (PTZ) or amygdala-kindling, impairment of learning was task specific[1]. Rats undergoing PTZ-kindling were significantly impaired in two-way active avoidance learning while amygdala-kindled rats did not differ from controls. However, in brightness discrimination, the situation was reversed with the PTZ-treated animals performing well and amygdala-treated animals having deficits. We have found that following a single episode of pilocarpine-induced status epilepticus animals can have a normal performance in the water maze yet have significant impairment in auditory discrimination learning[27].

The relationship between age and seizure-induced sequelae is of considerable interest since, contrary to some clinical impressions, the immature brain appears to be less vulnerable to seizure-induced brain damage than the mature brain following prolonged seizures.[4,8,12,31,34]. In this study, we demonstrated that immature rats had no measurable problems in learning and memory following four injections of KA while mature rats had significant deficits. While the immature brain may be less vulnerable to both prolonged and recurrent seizures, it is important to note that the immature brain is not immune to seizure-induced damage. Both prolonged[6] and recurrent seizures[26] can lead to deficits during development. Furthermore, kindling in immature animals results in a lasting increase in seizure susceptibility[23,24].

ACKNOWLEDGMENTS

Supported by a grant from the NINDS (NS27984) to GLH.

REFERENCES

1. Becker A, Grecksch G, Rüthrich H-L, Pohle W, Marx B, Matthies H: Kindling and its consequences on learning in rats. *Behav Neural Biol* 1992;57:37–43
2. Ben-Ari Y, Tremblay E, Ottersen OP: Injections of kainic acid into the amygdaloid complex of the rat: An electrographic, clinical and histological study in relation to the pathology of epilepsy. *Neuroscience* 1980;5:515–528
3. Bures J, Buresova O: Spatial Memory in Animals. in John RJ (ed): *Machinery of the Mind.* Boston, Birkäuser, 1990, pp 291–310
4. Cavalheiro EA, Silva DF, Turski WA, Calderazzo-Filho LS, Bortolotto ZA, Turski L: The susceptibility of rats to pilocarpine-induced seizures is age-dependent. *Dev Brain Res* 1987;37:43–58
5. Feasy-Truger KJ, Kargl L, ten Bruggencate G: Differential effects of dentate kindling on working and reference spatial memory in the rat. *Neurosci Lett* 1993;151:25–28
6. Franck JE, Schwartzkroin PA: Immature rabbit hippocampus is damaged by systemic but not intraventricular kainic acid. *Dev Brain Res* 1984;13:219–227
7. Greenough WT, West RW, De Vogd TJ: Subsynaptic plate perforations: changes with age and experience in the rat. *Science* 1978;202:1096–1098
8. Hirsch E, Baram TZ, Snead OC, III: Ontogenic study of lithium-pilocarpine-induced status epilepticus in rats. *Brain Res* 1992;583:120–126
9. Holmes GL, Chronopoulos A, Stafstrom CE, Mikati MA, Thurber SJ, Hyde PA, Thompson JL: Effects of kindling on subsequent learning, memory, behavior, and seizure susceptibility. *Dev Brain Res* 1993;73:71–77
10. Holmes GL, Thompson JL, Marchi TA, Gabriel PS, Hogan MA, Carl FG, Feldman DS: Effects of seizures on learning, memory, and behavior in the genetically epilepsy-prone rat. *Ann Neurol* 1990;27:24–32
11. Knowlton BJ, Shapiro ML, Olton DS: Hippocampal seizures disrupt working memory performance but not reference memory acquisition. *Behav Neurosci* 1989;103:1144–1147
12. Lee CL, Hrachovy RA, Smith KL, Frost JD, Jr., Swann JW: Tetanus toxin-induced seizures in infant rats and their effects on hippocampal excitability in adulthood. *Brain Res* 1995;677:97–109
13. Letty S, Lerner-Natoli M, Rondouin G: Differential impairments of spatial memory and social behavior in two models of limbic epilepsy. *Epilepsia* 1995;36:973–982
14. Leung LS, Boon KA, Kaibara T, Innis NK: Radial maze performance following hippocampal kindling. *Behav Brain Res* 1990;40:119–129
15. Leung LS, Shen B: Hippocampal CA1 evoked response and radial 8-arm maze performance after hippocampal kindling. *Brain Res* 1991;555:353–357
16. Liu Z, Gatt A, Mikati M, Holmes GL: Long-term behavioral deficits following pilocarpine seizures in immature rats. *Epilepsy Res* 1995;19:191–204
17. Lopes da Silva FH, Gorter JA, Wadman WJ: Kindling of the hippocampus induces spatial memory deficits in the rat. *Neurosci Lett* 1986;63:115–120
18. McNamara RK, Kirkby RD, dePace GE, Corcoran ME: Limbic seizures, but not kindling, reversibly impair place learning in the Morris water maze. *Behav Brain Res* 1992;50:167–175
19. Morrell H, De Toledo-Morrell L: Kindling as a model of neuronal plasticity. in Wada JA (ed): *Kindling 3.* New York, Raven Press, 1986, pp 17–36
20. Morris R: Development of a water maze procedure for studying spatial learning in the rat. *J Neurosci Meth* 1984;11:47–60

21. Morris RGM: Synaptic plasticity and learning: selective impairment of learning in rats and blockade of long-term potentiation *in vivo* by the N-methyl-D-aspartate receptor antagonist AP5. *J.Neurosci.* 1989;9:3040–3057
22. Morris RGM, Garrud P, Rawlins JNP, O'Keefe J: Place navigation impaired in rats with hippocampal lesions. *Nature* 1982;297:681–683
23. Moshé SL, Albala BJ: Kindling in developing rats: persistence of seizures into adulthood. *Dev Brain Res* 1982;4:67–71
24. Moshé SL, Albala BJ: Maturational changes in postictal refractoriness and seizure susceptibility in developing rats. *Ann Neurol* 1983;13:552–527
25. Nadler JV: Kainic acid as a tool for the study of temporal lobe epilepsy. *Life Sci* 1981;29:2031–2042
26. Neill J, Liu Z, Sarkisian M, Tandon P, Yang Y, Stafstrom C, Holmes GL: Recurrent seizures in immature rats: effect on auditory and visual discrimination. *Dev Brain Res* 1996;(in press)
27. Neill JC, Liu Z, Gatt A, Mikati M, Holmes GL: Pilocarpine-induced seizures impair acquisition rate of auditory discriminations using location cues. *Soc Neurosc Abst* 1993;19:394(abstract)
28. Nieminen AS, Sirviö J, Teittinen K, Pitkänen A, Airaksinen MM, Riekkinen P: Amygdala kindling increased fear-response, but did not impair spatial memory in rats. *Physiol Behav* 1992;51:845–849
29. Roberts RC, Ribak CE: IV. Anatomical changes of the GABAergic system in the inferior colliculus of the genetically epilepsy-prone rat. *Life Sci* 1986;39:789–798
30. Schwob JE, Fuller T, Price JL, Olney JW: Widespread patterns of neuronal damage following systemic or intracerebral injections of kainic acid: A histological study. *Neuroscience* 1980;5:991–1014
31. Sperber EF, Haas KZ, Stanton PK, Moshé SL: Resistance of the immature hippocampus to seizure-induced synaptic reorganization. *Dev Brain Res* 1991;60:88–93
32. Stafstrom CE, Holmes GL, Chronopoulos A, Thurber S, Thompson JL: Age-dependent cognitive and behavioral deficits following kainic acid-induced seizures. *Epilepsia* 1993;34:420–432
33. Sutherland RJ, Whishaw IQ, Kolb B: A behavioural analysis of spatial localization following electrolytic, kainate or colchicine-induced damage to the hippocampus. *Behav Brain Res* 1983;7:133–153
34. Thurber S, Chronopoulos A, Stafstrom CE, Holmes GL: Behavioral effects of continuous hippocampal stimulation in the developing rat. *Dev Brain Res* 1992;68:35–40

SHORT INTERVAL ELECTRICAL AMYGDALA KINDLING IN INFANT RATS

The Paradigm and Its Application to the Study of Age-Specific Convulsants

Tallie Z. Baram,[1] Edouard Hirsch,[2] and Linda Schultz[1]

[1]Departments of Pediatrics, Anatomy, and Neurobiology and Neurology
University of California, Irvine
Irvine, California, USA
[2]INSERM U 398
Strasbourg, France

1. ABSTRACT

Kindling is a powerful paradigm for investigating seizure generation, propagation and generalization. Kindling has been extensively utilized as a model of limbic seizures in the adult rat, and its reproducibility and precision are also particularly useful for the study of epilepsy in the developing brain. In the juvenile rat (>15 days), the refractory period between stimuli is much shorter than in the adult, potentially reflecting the increased excitability of the immature brain during this developmental period. "Rapid" or short-interval amygdala kindling of juvenile rats has been characterized and studied extensively.

The neuropeptide, corticotropin releasing hormone (CRH), produces limbic seizures in adult rodents, with a latency of 7–9 hours. The temporal and behavioral similarities between CRH-induced seizures and electrical amygdala kindling have suggested a common mechanism. In the infant rat (7–14 days), intracerebroventricular (icv) administration of picomolar doses of CRH produces amygdala-origin prolonged seizures with a very short latency (two minutes). The goals of studies described in this report were: a) to determine whether the rapid amygdala kindling paradigm could be applied to infant rats. b) to characterize the behavioral and electrical parameters of the kindling paradigm at this age. c) to study the interaction of CRH-induced seizures and amygdala kindling during infancy in the rat.

Using the short-interval-kindling method, Stage 5 behavioral seizures were achieved even in 7-day-old pups. However, the progression of behavioral kindling was different from that of older rats, and the correlation between electrographic after-discharges and behavioral stages was inversely related to age. Reliable, progressive amygdala afterdis-

Kindling 5, edited by Corcoran and Moshé.
Plenum Press, New York, 1998.

charges were difficult to ascertain in many animals prior to postnatal day 9. Spontaneous seizures occurred relatively frequently in younger age groups. Administration of a specific blocker of CRH receptors either icv or into the amygdala did not alter the rate of kindling development. Once stage 5 seizures were achieved, blocking CRH-receptors did not affect the expression of these seizures.

In conclusion, electrical amygdala kindling using short inter-stimulus intervals is a reliable and reproducible paradigm in rats during the second postnatal week, suggesting significant functional maturity of the amygdala-limbic circuitry at this age. The data provide no evidence for a mechanistic interaction between amygdala kindling and amygdala-origin CRH-induced seizures in the developing rat.

2. INTRODUCTION

Kindling has been proposed as a measure of excitability of the involved neuronal circuits[1–3]. Since the seminal manuscript by Goddard[1], the kindling paradigm has proven immensely useful as a model of epilepsy and of neuronal plasticity in adult rats[2,3]. Kindling-evoked afterdischarges may reflect the susceptibility of an interconnected group of neurons to generate synchronized, potentially epileptic activity[3]. The rate of progression of behavioral kindling stages from focal, through unilateral, to generalized phenomena provides a measure of both inhibitory and excitatory mechanisms in seizure propagation[2–4].

The amygdala kindling paradigm has been extensively utilized in immature rats, older than 15 days[4–8]. In this age group, the "refractory period" is much shorter than that in adult rats[4,6,9]. Therefore, immature rats are capable of developing afterdischarges and generalized seizures following several hours of stimulation at intervals of 15 minutes. This forms the basis for the short interval or "rapid" amygdala kindling paradigm. In a series of studies[5,6,8], Moshe et al. characterized the electrical amygdala kindling model in the immature rat. They determined that the minimal current required for generation of afterdischarges (afterdischarge threshold) in 15-day-old rats was higher than in older animals.[5] In their hands, only 75% of rats at that age could be kindled. Other authors[10] concluded that 10- and 14-day old rats could not be kindled consistently.

A number of experimental approaches suggest that during infancy (the second week of life) the rat brain is highly susceptible to induction of seizures.[11–13] The precise mechanisms underlying this observation are not fully understood. The rapid kindling model, using stimulus intervals of 15 minutes, results in a fully kindled brain within several hours. This should permit assessment of susceptibility to seizure-induction on a specific postnatal day, which is critical during a period of rapid brain growth and maturation.[14] Aside from providing a powerful tool for the study of seizure-susceptibility in the developing brain in general, kindling may be particularly useful in understanding specific issues of developmental epilepsy[5,14]. For example, it may provide insight into the mechanisms of the age-specific potency and rapidity of the "natural" convulsant peptide, corticotropin releasing hormone (CRH)[15,16].

CRH has been shown to excite neurons both in vivo and in vitro[17–23]. The peptide produces neuronal depolarization in CA1 and CA3 hippocampal pyramidal cells in the slice preparation[17–19]. CRH administered into the cerebral ventricles (icv) of mature rats causes epileptiform discharges in the amygdala[20,21], which spread to the hippocampus. The latency to the onset of these discharges is one to three hours, and over 3–7 hours, behavioral and electrographic seizures develop. The doses needed for seizure generation in adult rats are 1.5 to 15 nanomole[20,21]. We have reported that CRH is a far more rapid-acting and potent convulsant in the neonatal (first postnatal week) and infant rat (second postnatal week)[24–27]. The latency to seizures onset is less than two minutes, and convulsant doses are as low as 0.075 nanomole.

The long latency of CRH induced seizures in adult rodents, and their behavioral resemblance to kindling, suggested a potential participation of endogenous CRH, present in high concentration in several amygdala nuclei, in the kindling process[20,21,28]. The interaction of synthetic CRH administration with the development and expression of kindled seizures in the immature rat have not been studied. This report focuses on the response of infant rats to repeated amygdala stimulation at short (15 minute) intervals[29]. We demonstrate the progressive behavioral and electrical kindling stages, and the achievement of stage 5 seizures in infant rats. Rate of kindling and the onset and incidence of spontaneous seizures are discussed, as well as the application of the model to evaluate the mechanisms of CRH-induced seizures.

3. MATERIALS AND METHODS

3.1. Animals

Pregnancy-timed, Sprague-Dawley derived rats were obtained from Zivic-Miller, (Zelionple, PA). They were housed under a 12-hour light/dark cycle, and fed ad libitum. Delivery times were monitored and were accurate to within 12 hours, and the day of birth was considered day zero. The pups were kept with the mothers, and litters were culled to 12 pups. Infant rats were subjected to surgery 24–48 hours prior to kindling (24 hours for the younger rats, 48 hours for 9 days and older)[24,25,29]. Kindling was carried out starting between 9:00 and 9:30 am, to avoid potential diurnal variation in the rate of kindling development[28]. All experiments were carried out in normothermic shielded chambers[24,25,30] and were approved by the institutional Animal Care Committee.

3.2. Surgical Procedures

Electrodes were implanted under halothane anaesthesia[31], using an infant-rat stereotaxic apparatus, as previously described[24,25,29]. Bipolar twisted wire electrodes, (Plastics One, Roanoke, VA) with a wire diameter of 0.1–0.15 mm and vertical inter-tip distance of 0.5–1.0 mm) were inserted through a burr-hole and aimed at the basolateral nucleus of the amygdala. Electrodes were anchored to the skull with an acrylic cement "cap" attached also to one or two screws. The coordinates for the basolateral amygdala nucleus are age dependent, and have been published elsewhere.[29] Subsequent to each experiment, an electrolytic lesion (5–15 mAmp, 5–10 seconds) was generated, and electrode placement was verified. Animals were decapitated; brains were removed onto dry ice and blocked. Sequential 20 micron coronal sections were stained with cresyl violet.

For infusion of CRH or of the CRH antagonist, a stainless steel cannula was inserted into the cerebral lateral ventricle (icv) at the time of electrode placement[24,25]. For infusions and recording from the central nucleus of the amygdala, an electrode/cannula (315G; MS 303/2, Plastics One, VA) directed to the ACE replaced both electrode and icv cannula.

3.3. Administration of CRH and a CRH Antagonist

Alpha-helical CRH-(9–41), (4–6 μg) and CRH itself (0.3 nanomole) were administered icv via the chronic cannula in 1–2 microliters using a micro-infusion pump. Control animals were given saline/dye vehicle. Cannula placement and presence of dye in third ventricle were verified for each animal.

3.4. Short Interval Kindling Technique

The kindling paradigm was modified from Haas[8] as described[29]. Briefly, the kindling stimulus consisted of a one-second train of 60 Hz monophasic current, or a 3-second train of 400 μA peak-to-peak current, generated by an A-M isolated pulse stimulator (model 2100) and visualized using a Tektronix 5111a oscilloscope. Baseline EEGs were recorded for five minutes, as well as two-minute or longer samples immediately after each stimulation. Pups were stimulated at 15-minute intervals. Since infant rats (7–12 days) displayed a unique sequence of kindling-induced behaviors, a kindling scale was generated for them, based on the one defined by Moshe's group[4,8] for older pups (Table 1). The rate of kindling development was assessed by measuring afterdischarges duration after each stimulation, and the number of stimulations needed for the achievement of each kindling stage.

The presence of "spontaneous" seizures was determined as well. The latter were defined as stage 4 or 5 behaviors occurring, de novo, more than 4 minutes after the most recent stimulation. Rats with spontaneous seizures were usually stimulated once subsequent to the initial seizure, in an attempt to assess the length of the refractory period between the seizure and subsequent stimulation. These rats were then observed for several hours without further stimulation. All pups with "spontaneous" seizures continued to manifest them intermittently until the end of the experiment.

3.5. Analysis of the Rapid Kindling Experiments

Of 51 infant rats, correct placement of electrodes was achieved in 41 (nine 7-day, nine 8-day, ten 9-day, five 10- and eight 12-day-old). Only animals with correct placement were included in the analysis. Animals were combined into three age groups: 7–8 days (n = 18), 9–10 days (n = 15) and 12 days old (n = 8). Pooled data are presented as mean values ± standard error of the mean (SEM). Significance of difference among groups was analyzed using Mann-Whitney's rank sum test.

3.6. Interactions of CRH and Rapid Kindling: Experimental Design and Analysis

3.6.1. Does Acute Pretreatment with CRH Antagonist into the Cerebral Ventricles Alter the Rate of Kindling Development? Rats aged 10–13 days (n=17) were infused with CRH antagonist 15 minutes prior to initiation of kindling. The time of administration and the dose were appropriate for blocking CRH receptors as determined by prevention of CRH induced seizures[24].

Table 1. Stages of kindling-induced behaviors in infant rats

Stage	Days 7–9	Days 11–12
0	Behavior arrest	Behavior arrest
1	Head bob/facial movement	Head bob/facial movement
2	"Chewing"/neck flexion	Neck flexion "chewing"
3	Vigorous lick/limb rotation	Unilateral clonus/body flexion
3.5	Unilateral clonus*	Alternating clonus
4	Rearing (rare)	Forepaw rotation/bilateral clonus/rearing
5	Tonic extension	Loss of balance/extension

*Alternating clonus was seen rarely in 7-day-old rats.
(Adapted from ref. 29, with permission.)

3.6.2. Does Acute Pretreatment with CRH Antagonist into the Amygdala Alter the Rate of Kindling Development? 11-day-old pups (n=6) were infused with alpha-helical CRH-(9–41) via a double lumen electrode/cannula 15 minutes prior to kindling.

3.6.3. Does Chronic Pretreatment with a CRH Receptor Blocker Alter Kindling Development? Pups (n=4) were implanted with osmotic pumps on postnatal days 9–10, and kindled on postnatal day 12.

3.6.4. Does CRH Antagonist Alter the Expression of Kindled Seizures? CRH receptor blocker (4 μg) was administered to rat pups (n=6) once afterdischarge duration was 60 seconds.

3.6.5. Does "Chronic" Pretreatment with CRH Facilitate Kindling? Rat pups were given CRH (0.3 nanomole) icv four times on postnatal days 9–12, and were kindled on postnatal day 12. They were compared to sham-infused controls.

3.6.6. Does Acute Pre-Administration of CRH Facilitate Kindling? Rat pups were infused with CRH immediately prior to the first kindling stimulus. Since the behavioral seizures induced by CRH resemble those of kindling (Table 2), the CRH infused group was compared to controls only for EEG parameters (duration of afterdischarges).

For all these experiments, control and experimental groups with verified electrode and cannula placement were compared for the number of stimulations needed to achieve afterdischarges longer than 60 seconds, for the progression of behavioral kindling stages and for the number of stimulation needed to achieve stage 5 seizures.

4. RESULTS

The spectrum of progressive, stimulation-induced behaviors was age-dependent. In 7–9-day-old rats, as in those aged 10–12 days, behavior arrest and head/face movements were observed initially. Subsequent stages in the youngest group (7–9 days) consisted of tonic neck-flexion or forelimb rotation, followed by forelimb clonus (Table 1). Further, alternating clonus, prominent in 10–12-day-old pups (as well as in older rats[8]) was infrequent. The behavioral seizures observed after CRH closely resembled the sequence of kindling stages (Table 2), suggesting common propagation pathways.

Inter-animal variability was greater in 7–9-day-old rats than in older pups (Table 3); the number of stimulations required for each behavioral stage differed substantially. Overall, 7–8-day-old animals progressed faster to stage 3 (4.94 ± 0.5 stimulations; n =18) than

Table 2. Comparison of CRH- and kindling-induced behavioral stages in infant rats

	Behavior	
Stage	Kindling	CRH Seizures
0	Behavior arrest	—
1	Head bob, facial movement	Jaw myoclonus
2	"Chewing"/neck flexion	Licking, chewing
3	Unilateral clonus	Forepaw clonus
3.5	Alternating clonus	"Swimming"
4	Limb rotation, bilateral clonus	—
5	Loss of balance, extension	Loss of balance

Table 3. Rate of kindling in infant rats per number of stimulations for each stage of kindling

Age (days)	n	Behavioral stage 1	2	3	4[#]	5
7–8	18	1.3 ± 0.1	2.9 ± 0.4	4.9 ± 0.5	8.2 ± 0.7	11.7 ± 0.6
9–10	15	1.3 ± 0.1	2.3 ± 0.3	5.8 ± 0.6	11.3 ± 1.0*	17.2 ± 0.7*
12	8	1.1 ± 0.1	3.1 ± 0.5	5.6 ± 0.8	11.5 ± 1.1*	20.4 ± 0.5*

Values are mean ± s.e.m. *Significantly different than 7–8 days ($p < 0.005$). [#]Stage 3.5 or stage 4 in the 7–8-day-old group.

10–12-day-old pups (5.7 ± 0.6 stimulations: n = 23). Kindling rate of the younger group to behavioral stage 4 was rapid; a mean of 8.2 stimulations at 7–8 days versus 11.5 stimulations in 12-day-old pups ($p < 0.005$, and Table 3).

The current of 400 μA was above threshold for the 9–12-day-old rats, and resulted in after-discharges. In younger rats, using a longer train duration (suggested by E. W. Lothman, personal communication) yielded discernible afterdischarges in most pups, though with a more variable contour (Figure 1). 9-day-old rats tended to have longer after discharge duration after each stimulation than 12-day-old ones (Figure 1).

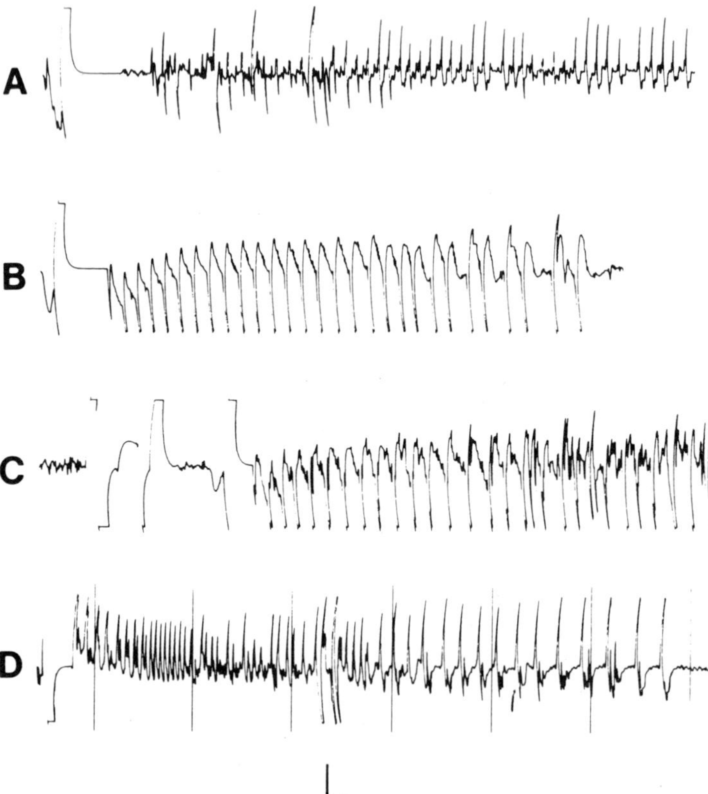

Figure 1. Afterdischarges in 7–12-day-old infant rats subjected to short-interval stimulation. A. 7-day-old rat, subsequent to the fifth stimulation. B. 9-day-old rat, fifth stimulation. C. 10-day-old rat, 19th stimulation. D. 12-day-old rat, 17th stimulation. Horizontal bar = 1 sec. Vertical bar = 10 uV in A, 20 uV in B, C, 40 uV in D. (From ref 29, with permission.).

Table 4. "Spontaneous" seizures during kindling in infant rats

Age (days)	Number of rats with seizures (%)	Median stimulation number at onset (range)
7–8	9/18 (50)	11 (5–12)
9–10	7/14 (50)	17 (15–19)
12	2/8 (25)	19,19

From ref. 29, with permission.

Spontaneous seizures were observed with an earlier onset and a higher incidence in the youngest animals (Table 4). The incidence of such seizures was 50% in 7–8-day-old animals. They occurred subsequent to kindling stage 3.5–5, and persisted until the termination of the experiment (2–3 hours).

None of the manipulations of CRH-induced neurotransmission, either chronically or acutely, altered the rate of kindling development. For example, pre-treatment with CRH immediately prior to kindling did not decrease the number of stimulations needed for achievement of afterdischarge duration of 60 seconds (7 stimulations in both control and experimental groups). Further, pre-treatment with CRH antagonist did not suppress the expression of kindled seizures: i.e., when given after afterdischarge duration reached 60 seconds, the antagonist did not prevent further increases in afterdischarge duration, or the achievement of stage 5 seizures. The number of experimental animals per group was too small to entirely exclude the possibility of a small (10–25%) effect of CRH or the antagonist on the parameters measured. The significance of such potential, relatively low-magnitude effects in view of substantial inter-animal variability in the rate of kindling in the developing rat, is questionable.

5. DISCUSSION

These studies demonstrate that the rapid kindling paradigm can be used in the infant rat, during the second postnatal week. The model is a powerful tool with several advan-

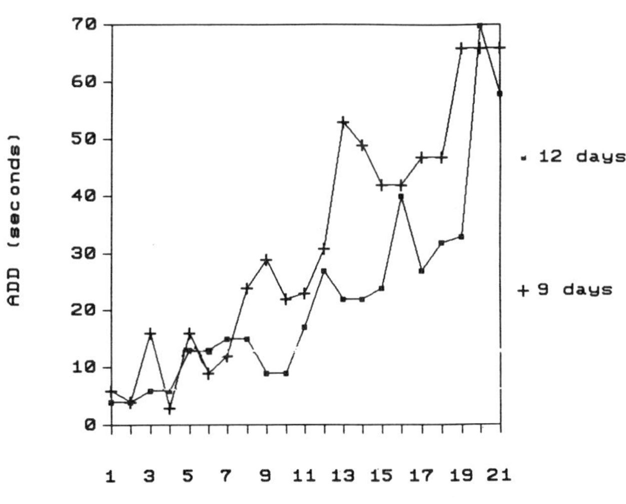

Figure 2. Correlation of afterdischarge duration and stimulation number in 9- and 12-day-old infant rats. See text for details of kindling paradigm (from ref. 29, with permission).

tages: 1) It is a measure of susceptibility to seizure generation at a specific, single age-point, which is of paramount importance in studying rapidly developing infant rats. 2) It provides a well characterized, reproducible model, with several quantitative parameters, permitting comparison of control and experimental groups. 3) Amygdala kindling relies on limbic mechanisms of seizure propagation—which is useful for studies of limbic or "temporal lobe epilepsy" models during development. 4) The paradigm is also age-specific, and is thus attractive for study of age-specific convulsants with overlapping neuroanatomic substrates, such as CRH-induced seizures.

Both amygdala[5,6,8,32,33] and hippocampal[7,34] rapid kindling paradigms have been well characterized in "suckling" or "weanling" rats (older than 15 days). Haas et al. devised a behavioral scale to account for the different progression of stimulation induced seizures in the immature brain[8]. Amygdala kindling has been used to assess the effect of anatomical, metabolic and hormonal[35] inputs on seizure susceptibility in the immature rat[4,32,33]. We demonstrate that this experimental model can be extended to rats during the second post-natal week (infant rats). Gilbert and Cain[10] were unable to induce amygdala kindling in 10-day-old rats, and only "weak stage 3" response in 14-day-old rats. The authors used kindling parameters similar to ours, but applied stimuli at 2 hour intervals, which may account for their results. Further, the afterdischarge threshold is higher in younger rats[5]. Eliciting afterdischarges at this age depends on a composite of the magnitude and the duration of the stimulating current (unpublished observations, and E.W. Lothman, personal communication). We utilized a current of 400 μA, which is suprathreshold for the 15-day-old rat. The ability to obtain afterdischarges in 7–8-day-old was enhanced by increasing train duration to 3–4 seconds. These pups progressed to stage 5 seizures.

Fully kindled rats (subsequent to three or more stage 5 seizures) may develop spontaneous seizures[9]. The likelihood of such events increases with the number of stimulations[36]. Spontaneous seizures occurred with high frequency in the kindled infant rats, and required relatively few stimulations. Furthermore, even within the limited spectrum of ages studied, the frequency of spontaneous seizures correlated inversely to age. This is consistent with an increased excitability and susceptibility to seizures of the immature brain[4,6,11–13,33].

The infant rapid amygdala kindling process, as opposed to amygdala kindling in the adult, was not influenced by alteration of CRH-mediated neurotransmission. Ehlers[20] described the long latency to the onset of seizures induced by CRH in mature rodents. A single administration of CRH produced a sequence of behaviors similar to the behavioral stages of kindling. It was hypothesized that CRH could be a kindling stimulus for the development of limbic seizures[20,21,28]. Weiss et al., using mature male Sprague-Dawley rats, studied the effect of CRH on the development of kindling[21]. Large doses of CRH were given daily for five days, followed by daily electrical kindling. On the first two days, CRH resulted in behavioral seizures and in afterdischarge-like activity on amygdala EEG. CRH effect diminished after the third and fourth injections, and no seizures occurred after the fifth. Pre-administration of CRH, however, significantly accelerated the development of stage 3 seizures (after 8.2 stimulations versus 16.1 in vehicle-treated rats). Afterdischarge duration throughout the kindling process was significantly longer in CRH pre-treated rats. The data were interpreted to suggest a role for endogenous CRH in limbic excitability, and a mechanistic interaction with the kindling process.

In the infant, administration of a single, low dose (e.g., 0.15 nanomole) of CRH results in limbic seizures with behavioral progression similar to the stages of kindling[24,25] (Table 2). It was therefore not possible to study the alteration of behavioral stages of rapid kindling by pre-administration of CRH. However, no effect of CRH on afterdischarge duration was evident. Blocking of CRH receptors with doses of alpha-helical CRH which are sufficient to prevent CRH-induced seizures, altered neither the behavioral nor the EEG (afterdischarge duration) aspects of kindling development. Although lack of effect does not exclude a synergistic interaction between rapid kindling and CRH in the infant rat, our data do not indicate the presence of such interaction.

The large doses of CRH administered in adult rat studies can be expected to act peripherally, on CRH receptors in the pituitary[15,16], elevating the levels of plasma ACTH and glucocorticoids. Glucocorticoids clearly augment kindling development: Indeed, the Lewis rat strain which is deficient in CRH production kindles more slowly, an effect largely reversible by corticosterone[28]. Therefore, the apparent interaction of CRH and kindling in the adult may be due to elevated plasma glucocorticoids[21,28]. The low doses of CRH producing seizures in the infant rat do not increase plasma cortcosterone[24]. Seizures, including those produced by CRH, are stressful, and elevate plasma corticosterone transiently. Glucocorticoid receptors are present in the amygdala and hippocampus of the infant rat[37], yet, as discussed above, neither CRH nor a CRH receptor blocker altered the rate of kindling development.

In summary, rapid electrical amygdala kindling over several hours is possible during the second postnatal week in the rat. The short refractory period and the high frequency of "spontaneous" seizures are consistent with enhanced excitability of limbic circuitry during this developmental stage. Brain development in the 7–12-day-old rat roughly corresponds to that of the newborn and infant human. This experimental paradigm should thus permit further study of mechanisms of epilepsy development during this critical and highly vulnerable age.

ACKNOWLEDGMENTS

This manuscript is dedicated to the memory of E.W. Lothman, for his guidance and support. Studies were supported in part by NIH NS 01307 and NS28912, and by an Epilepsy foundation of America research award (T.Z.B).

REFERENCES

1. Goddard, G.V., McIntyre, D. and Leech, C.K., A permanent change in brain function resulting from daily electrical stimulation. Exp. Neurol., 25 (1969) 295–330.
2. Lothman, E.W., Bertram, E.H., III and Stringer, J. L., Kindling, a model of epilepsy, in: Functional anatomy of hippocampal seizures, Prog. Neurobiol., 37 (1991) 1–82.
3. McNamara, J.O., Byrne, M.C., Dashieff, R.M. and Fitz, J.G., The kindling model of epilepsy: a review. Prog. Neurobiol., 15 (1980) 139–159.
4. Moshe, S.L., The ontogeny of seizures and substantia nigra modulation, In P. Kellaway and J.L. Noebels (Eds.), Problems and concepts in developmental neurophysiology, Baltimore, The Johns Hopkins Press, 1989, pp. 247–261.
5. Moshe, S.L., Sharpless, N.S. and Kaplan, J., Kindling in developing rats: variability of afterdischarge thresholds with age, Brain Res., 211 (1981) 190–195.
6. Moshe, S.L., Albala, B.J., Ackerman, R.F. and Engel, J., Jr., Increased seizure susceptibility of the immature brain, Dev. Brain Res., 7 (1983) 81–85.
7. Holmes, G.L., and Thompson, J.L., Rapid kindling in the prepubescent rat, Brain Res., 433 (1987) 381–384.
8. Haas, K.Z., Sperber, E.F. and Moshe, S.L., Kindling in developing animals: expression of severe seizures and enhanced development of bilateral foci. Dev. Brain Res., 56 (1990) 275–280.
9. Racine, R.J., Burnham, W. M. and Gartner, J. G., First trial motor seizures triggered by amygdaloid stimulation in the rat. Electroencephal. Clin. Neurophysiol. 35 (1973) 487–494.

10. Gilbert, M.E. and Cain, D.P., A developmental study of kindling in the rat. Dev. Brain Res., 2 (1982) 321–328.
11. Swann, J.W., Smith, K.L., Gomez, C.M. and Brady, R.J., The ontogeny of hippocampal local circuits and focal epileptogenesis. Epilepsy Res., supp. 9 (1992) 115–125.
12. Shinnar, S. and Moshe, S.L. Age specificity of seizure expression in genetic epilepsies. In: Anderson, E.E., Hauser, W.A., Leppik, I.E., Noebels, J.L., Rich, S.S., eds. Genetic Strategies in Epilepsy Research. Elsevier 1991;69–85
13. Sperber, E.F., Stanton, P.K., Haas, K., Ackerman, R.F. and Moshe, S.L. Developmental differences in the neurobiology of epileptic brain damage in: Mol. Neurobiol. Epilepsy, Elsevier, pp 67–81;1992
14. Woodbury, D.M. Significance of animal models of epilepsy for evaluation of anti-epileptic drug therapy in children. In: Antiepileptic Drug Therapy in Pediatrics. P.L. Morselli, C.E. Pippinger, J.K. Penry, Eds. Raven Press, New York, 349–362, 1983
15. Vale, W., Spiess, J., Rivier, C. et al., Characterization of a 41-residue ovine hypothalamic peptide that stimulates secretion of corticotropin and Beta-endorphin. Science, 213 (1981) 1394–1397.
16. Sawchenko, P.E., Imaki, T., Potter, E., Kovacs, K., Imaki, J. and Vale, W. The functional neuroanatomy of corticotropin releasing factor. CIBA Foundation Symp. 172:5–21;1993.
17. Aldenhoff, J.B., Gruol, D.L., Rivier, J. et al., Corticotropin-releasing factor decreases postburst hyperpolarization and excites hippocampal neurons. Science 221 (1983) 875–877.
18. Smith, B.N. and Dudek, F.E. Age-related epileptogenic effects of corticotropin releasing hormone in the isolated CA1 region of rat hippocampal slices. J. Neurophysiol. 72 (1994) 2328–2333.
19. Hollrigel, G., Baram, T.Z. and Soltesz, I. Corticotropin Releasing Hormone decreases inhibitory synaptic transmission in the hippocampus of infant rats Soc. Neurosci. Abst. (submitted)
20. Ehlers, C.L., CRF effects on EEG activity: Implications for the modulation of normal and abnormal brain states. In E.B. De Souza and C.B. Nemeroff (Eds.), Corticotropin-releasing factor: Basic and Clinical Studies of a Neuropeptide, CRC, Boca Raton, 1990, pp. 233–248.
21. Weiss, S.R.B., Post, R.M., Gold, P.W., Chrousos, G., et al CRF-induced seizures and behavior: interaction with amygdala kindling Brain Res. 372 (1986) 345–351.
22. Fox, E.A. and Gruol, D.L. CRF suppresses the afterhyperpolarization in cerebellar Purkinje neurons Neurosci. Lett., 149 (1993) 103–107.
23. Valentino, R,J,, Page, M.E. and Curtis, A.L. Activation of noradrenergic locus ceruleus neurons by hemodynamic stress is due to local release of CRF. Brain Res., 555(1991) 25–34
24. Baram, T.Z. and Schultz, L., CRH is a rapid and potent convulsant in the infant rat, Dev. Brain Res., 61 (1991) 97–101.
25. Baram, T.Z., Hirsch, E., Snead, O.C. III and Schultz, L., CRH induced seizures in the infant brain originate in the amygdala. Ann. Neurol., 31 (1992) 488–494.
26. Baram, T.Z. and Ribak, C.E., Peptide-induced infant status epilepticus causes neuronal death and synaptic reorganization. NeuroReport 6 (1995) 277–280
27. Ribak, C.E. and Baram, T.Z. Selective death of hippocampal CA3 pyramidal cells with mossy fiber afferents after CRH- induced status epilepticus in infant rats. Dev. Brain Res. 91 (1996) 245–251.
28. Weiss, G.K., Castillo, N. and Fernandez, M. Amygdala kindling is altered in rats with a deficit in the responsiveness of the HPA axis Neurosci. Lett., 157 (1993) 91–94
29. Baram, T.Z., Hirsch, E. and Schultz, L. Short-interval amygdala kindling in neonatal rats. Dev. Brain Res. 73 (1993) 79–83
30. Baram, T.Z. and Hirsch, E. EEG recording in neonatal rats: Some pitfalls and solutions. Dendron, 1 (1992) 39–46
31. Cain, D.P., Raithby, A. and Corcoran, M.E., Urethane anesthesia blocks the development and expression of kindled seizures. Life Sci., 44 (1989) 1201–1206.
32. Holmes, G.L. and Weber, D.A., Effects of ACTH on seizure susceptibility in the developing brain Ann. Neurol., 20 (1986) 82–88.
33. Lee, S.S., Murat, R. and Matsuura S., Effects of Hypoglycemia on kindling seizures in suckling rats, Exp. Neurol., 99 (1988) 142–153.
34. Michelson, H.B. and Lothman, E.W., An ontogenic study of kindling using rapidly recurring hippocampal seizures, Dev. Brain Res., 61 (1991) 79–85.
35. Cain, D.P., Plant, J., Rouleau S., Corcoran, M.E., Failure to kindle seizures after repeated intracerebral administration of arginine vasopressin. Life Sci., 38 (1986) 985–989.
36. Pinel, J.P. and Rovnar, L.I., Electrode placement and kindling-induced experimental epilepsy, Exp. Neurol. 58 (1978) 335–346.
37. Yi, S.J., Masters, J.N. and Baram, T.Z. Glucocorticoid receptor-mRNA ontogeny in the fetal and postnatal rat brain Mol. Cell. Neurosci. 5 (1994) 385–393.

5

ONTOGENY OF TEMPORAL LOBE EPILEPSY IN AMYGDALA-KINDLED KITTENS

Phenomenology, Treatment Alternatives, and Basic Mechanisms of Sleep-Waking State Seizure Activity

Margaret N. Shouse,[1,2,3*] James Langer,[1] Paul Farber,[1] Michael Bier,[1,2,3] Orly Alcalde,[1] and Ronald Szymusiak[1,2,3]

[1]Sleep Disturbance Research (151A3)
VA Medical Center, Sepulveda California 91413
[2]Department of Neurobiology, School of Medicine
[3]Department of Medicine, School of Medicine
UCLA, Los Angeles, California 90063

1. INTRODUCTION

This chapter addresses three topics. First, we depict the features of a unique developmental model of spontaneous temporal lobe epilepsy (TLE) in amygdala-kindled kittens. Second, we report recent advances in potential treatment alternatives via focal and extra-focal microinfusion of anti-epileptic agents as well as mechanisms which could explain them. Third, we suggest mechanisms that could account for the spontaneous increase in seizure discharge propagation during non-rapid-eye-movement (NREM) sleep, including the transition into rapid-eye-movement (REM).

1.1. Developmental TLE

Many epilepsies are considered developmental since they typically begin between infancy and adolescence[5,7], but the timing of interictal seizure activity is similar regardless of the type of seizure disorder or age at onset[7,23]. Interictal seizure discharge is most likely to spread during NREM and is least likely to do so during REM when compared to waking in human and infra-human species[4,23]. Localization-related epilepsies are distinguished from primary generalized seizure disorders in that ictal seizure discharge, particularly when accompanied by secondary generalized tonic-clonic convulsions (GTCs), most often

* Correspondence: M.N. Shouse, Ph.D., 2242 South Bentley Avenue, Los Angeles, CA 90064-1940.

Kindling 5, edited by Corcoran and Moshé.
Plenum Press, New York, 1998.

occur in NREM sleep and the REM sleep transition[23]. Secondary generalized TLE is the "prototypic pure sleep epilepsy," as nearly 60% of these patients have GTCS in NREM or the REM transition[7].

We have developed a model of spontaneous sleep epilepsy, using the amygdala kindling technique in kittens[19,21,22]. Kindled kittens resemble human counterparts since GTCs most often occur in NREM and the REM transition and least often occur during stable REM. In contrast, partial and complex-partial seizures can happen at any time. Figure 1 illustrates a focal onset spontaneous GTC originating from amygdala in the transition from slow-wave-sleep (SWS) into REM. These spontaneous seizures and their distribution in the sleep-wake cycle persist to adulthood. The model thus affords a unique opportunity to study novel treatment alternatives as well as basic mechanisms of seizure-prone and seizure-resistant sleep and waking states.

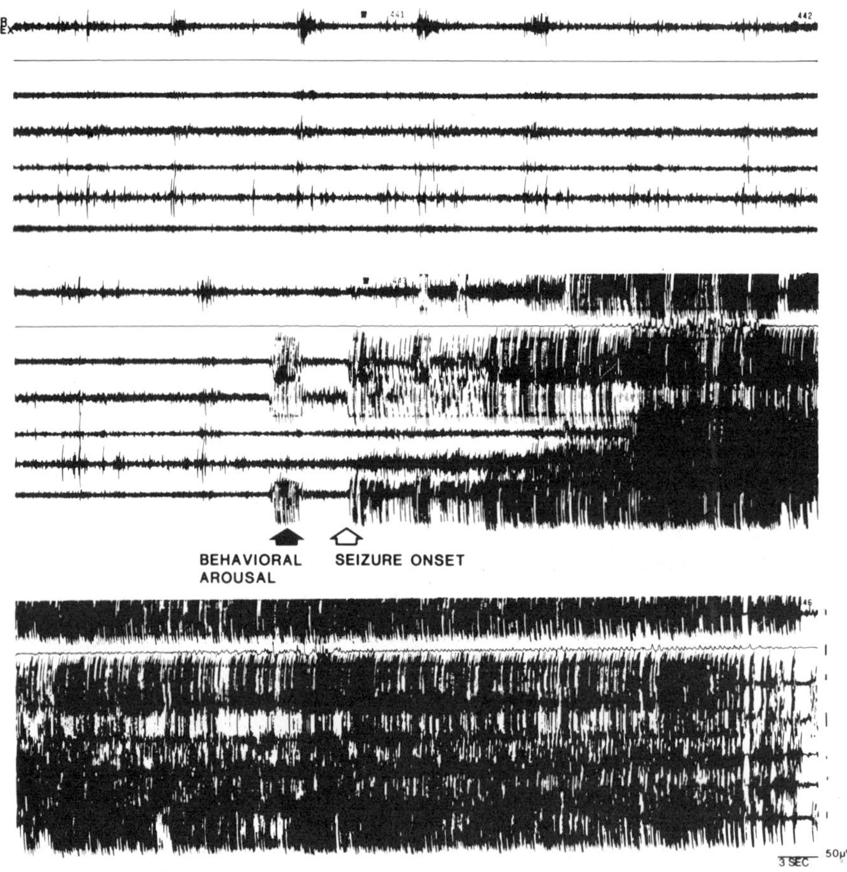

Figure 1. A continuous 3-min recording showing a spontaneous convulsion during the transition from slow-wave-sleep (SWS) into rapid-eye-movement (REM) sleep in an amygdala-kindled kitten. The top tracing illustrates SWS indexed by high-density sleep spindles over motor cortex. The middle tracing indicates the transition from SWS to REM indexed by reduced EEG spindles with continued ponto-geniculo-occipital (PGO) discharge. Focal onset occurred in the amygdala bilaterally (unfilled arrow) and appeared to be preceded by what may have been a paroxysmal amygdaloid discharge with motor accompaniment (behavior arousal, filled arrow, note increase in EMG activity). The bottom tracing shows the remainder of the convulsion. Abbreviations: EOG=electroculogram; AMY=amygdala; LGN=lateral geniculate nucleus; EMG=electromyogram. Paper speed=10mm/sec. (Reprinted from 25).

1.2. Microinfusion Studies

We chose to study agents modifying norepinephrine (NE) release NE because changes in NE cell discharge and release are among the best documented factors in regulation of seizures[3,15,17] and are also implicated in sleep-waking state changes[8,28]. Locus ceruleus (LC) cells discharge at progressively reduced rates during NREM and the transition into REM. Declining NE release at these times could provide a natural mechanism for seizure generalization in sleep. LC projects also to forebrain diffusely[9] and could encourage spread of ictal discharge from any site. However, the LC also innervates the amygdala directly in cats[12] and could affect focal and secondary seizure propagation monosynaptically.

Figure 2 shows initial results from studies of effects of microinfusion of noradrenergic agents into either amygdala[20,27] or pons[24,27]. Preliminary microinfusion findings suggested that the NE agonist clonidine (CLON) not only blocked waking seizures but also normalized sleep (not shown) in epileptic kittens, whereas the NE agonist idazoxan (IDA) had the opposite effects at both microinfusion sites (n=6 kittens per site). The illustration depicts microinfusion effects of CLON and IDA on amygdala-kindled afterdischarge (AD) and GTC seizure thresholds. Values are expressed as mean percent change from sham control thresholds obtained before and after microinfusions (1μL) of vehicle (saline) at the beginning and end of the experiment as well as after low, medium and high doses of CLON or IDA (n=1 infusion per dose). CLON dosages were 1.4, 7.3 and 14.66 μg/uL or 5.5, 27.5 and 55.0 nmol. IDA dosages were 0.33, 0.66 and 1.32 μg/uL or 1.38, 2.75 and 5.5 nmol. Order of drugs administered, as well as dosages of CLON and IDA infusions, and site of microinfusions were partially counterbalanced. CLON increased AD and GTC seizure threshold, whereas IDA reduced AD and GTC seizure thresholds at both infusion sites. Effects were also dose-dependent in both cases, but more potent after pontine than amygdala infusion[24]. Thus, α-2 agents had the same effects on sleep (not shown) and seizures after microinfusion, as reported rlsewhere after microinfusion of IDA[1,17,18] and CLON[17,18,30]. Figures 3 and 4 are EEG illustrations showing effects of pontine microinfusion of IDA on evoked amygdala GTC seizure threshold (Fig. 3) and of CLON on a kitten suffering status epilepticus (Fig. 4).

The microinfusion effects are nevertheless puzzling, as NE agonists and antagonists have been shown to affect autoreceptors in a way that can have opposing effects on NE release (e.g., ref. 31). Accordingly, one might have expected CLON to reduce NE release, thus decreasing amygdala kindled seizure thresholds, whereas IDA could have had the opposite effects. This did not happen here, nor did it occur in several other microinfusion studies, some using equivalent or higher dosages of the same α-2 agonists and/or antagonists in pons[1,11] or amygdala[18], where pre-synaptic autoreceptors also exist. It is difficult to reconcile these in vivo findings with in vitro receptor physiology findings. We cannot meaningfully comment on this apparent paradox until concurrent receptor binding studies are performed. We also cannot eliminate non-adrenergic imidazoline receptor binding as a factor in our findings[2].

We can discuss other factors which could have contributed to our observations. Three options are addressed below.

a. One possibility is ventricular invasion of microinfused agents. The histology[24] appears to refute this hypothesis because the electrode and infusion needle placements are sufficiently distant from the ventricular system at both sites in all six kittens. Also, the latency between infusion and threshold testing was brief (10/min). The general rule is 1 cubic mm diffusion per μl infused. Pearson product moment correlations (*r*) compared millimeter distance from nearest ventricle

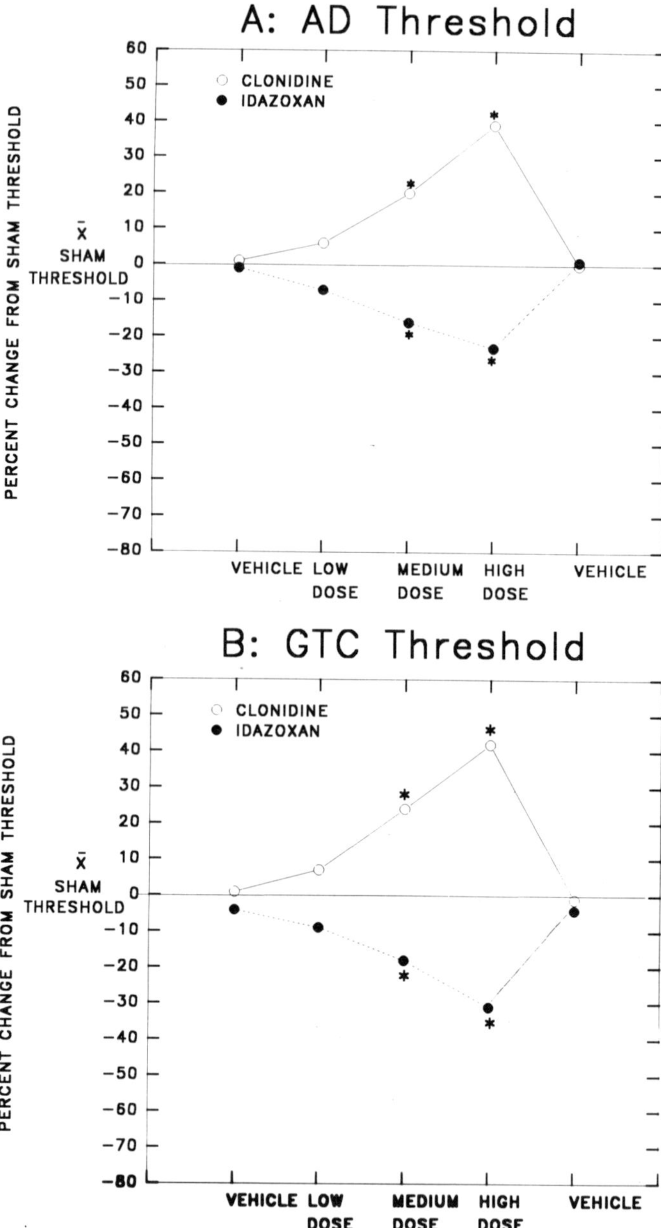

Figure 2. Effects of amygdala (left) and pontine (right) microinfusion of the a-2 adrenoreceptor agonist clonidine (CLON) and the a-2 adrenoreceptor antagonist idazoxan (IDA) on amygdala-kindled seizure thresholds to afterdischarge (A; top) and generalized tonic-clonic convulsions (B; bottom). Values are expressed as mean percent change from sham control thresholds (needle insertion only) obtained before and after microinfusions (1μL) of vehicle (saline) at the beginning and end of the experiment as well as after low, medium and high doses of CLON or IDA (n = 1 infusion per dose). Dosages were: CLON (5.5, 27.5, and 55.0 nmol) or IDA (1.38, 2.75, and 5.5 nmol). Order of administered drugs and dosages was partially counterbalanced. Three of 6 kittens had the CLON series first, and 3 had the IDA series first at each microinfusion site. Order of dosages was medium, high and low in 2 kittens per drug. Two kittens had a low, medium and high dosage sequence, whereas 2 had a high,

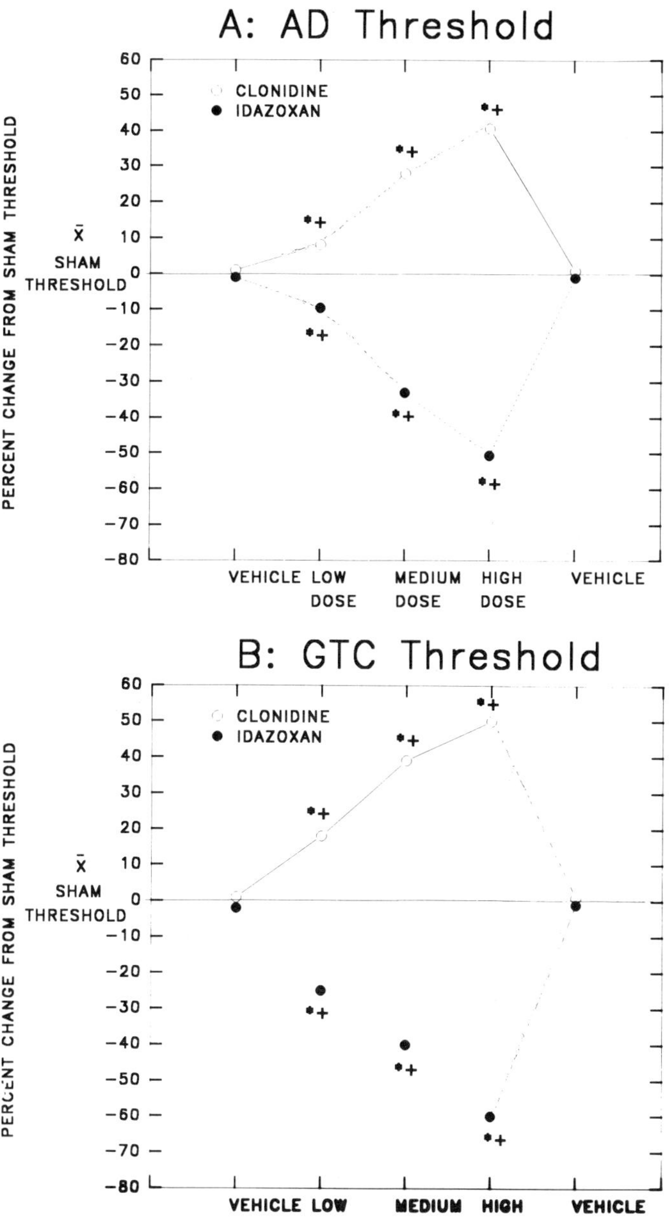

medium and low dosage sequence. Two-way analyses of variance (ANOVAs) with repeated measures on one variable were applied to percentile data for CLON vs. IDA. This is an A(B×S) design in which A is the non-repeated measure (infusion sites) and B is the repeated measure (intra-subject response over time). Post-hoc comparisons were independent or dependent t-tests. Statistical results were highly significant in all cases. CLON increased AD and GTC seizure thresholds, whereas IDA reduced AD and GTC seizure thresholds after microinfusion at both sites. Results were dose-dependent. Effects were more pronounced after pontine than amygdala microinfusion. For amygdala infusion, * = $p < .05$ from vehicle; for pontine microinfusion, * = $p < .01$ from vehicle; + = $p < .01$ between doses. (Reprinted from 24).

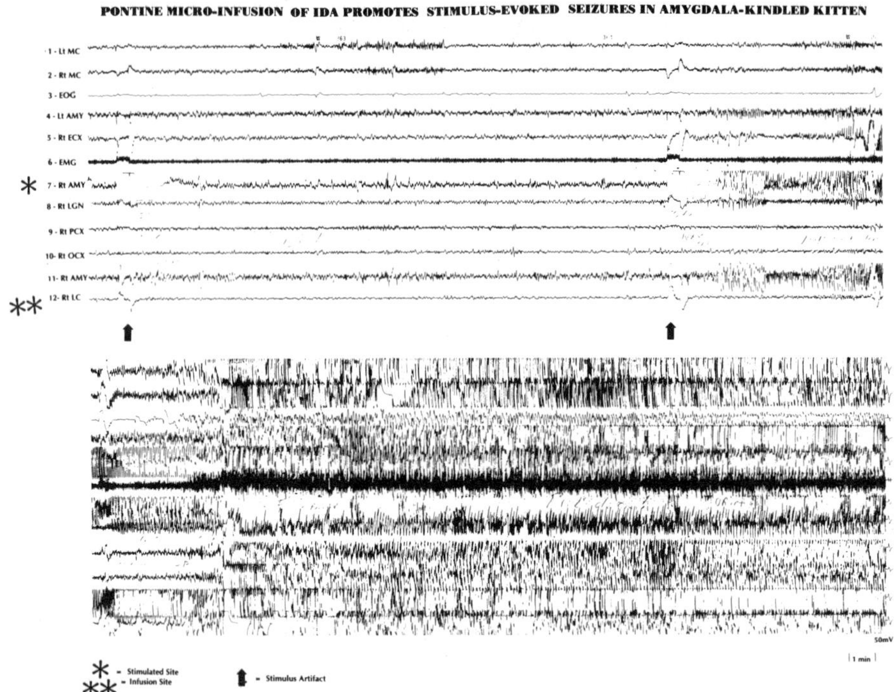

Figure 3. Continuous recording showing effects of pontine microinfusion of IDA (1.32 μg/ml; ** = infusion site) on stimulus-evoked AD in the ipsilateral amygdala (* = stimulated amygdala). Stimulus artifact is indicated by the arrows. Post-infusion threshold was 41% below that for focal AD obtained after mean sham control thresholds conducted the day before and the day after this microinfusion. Thus, IDA not only lowered focal AD threshold, but also augmented seizure discharge propagation. Recording speed = 10 mm/sec. Abbreviations: Lt = left; Rt = right; MC = motor cortex; EOG = electrooculogram; AMY = amygdala; ECX = entorhinal cortex; EMG = electromyogram; LGN = lateral geniculate nucleus; PCX = posterolateral cortex; OCX = occipital cortex; LC = locus ceruleus. Paper speed = 10 mm/s.

to percentile threshold data. Values never exceeded 0.002, df=4, p=ns. While we can not conclusively rule out ventricular invasion in the present results, our findings suggest a neuronal rather than a ventricular mechanism.

b. A second possibility is that the pontine microinfusion effects may have been mediated by post-synaptic action of NE-containing terminals in amygdala. This "neuronal hypothesis" would be consistent with LC stimulation effects on amygdala kindled seizures[32] and with reports that partial LC lesions cause a 71% reduction in amygdaloid NE concentrations[10]. Also, there is a higher concentration of NE-containing neurons in LC complex than NE-containing terminals in the amygdala, a factor which may explain larger pontine vs. amygdala microinfusion effects.

c. A third, and perhaps most likely alternative that might explain greater pontine than amygdala microinfusion effects is that other pontine cell populations affected the outcome. For example, increases or decreases in pontine NE secretion can have contrasting effects upon discharge of adjacent pontine cholinergic neurons[28]. However, pontine NE and Ach discharge rates sometimes coincide, including wakefulness[9]. Increased release of both transmitters can have antiepileptic properties, whereas reduced release can be proconvulsant[3,26]. Therefore, a combination of *in-*

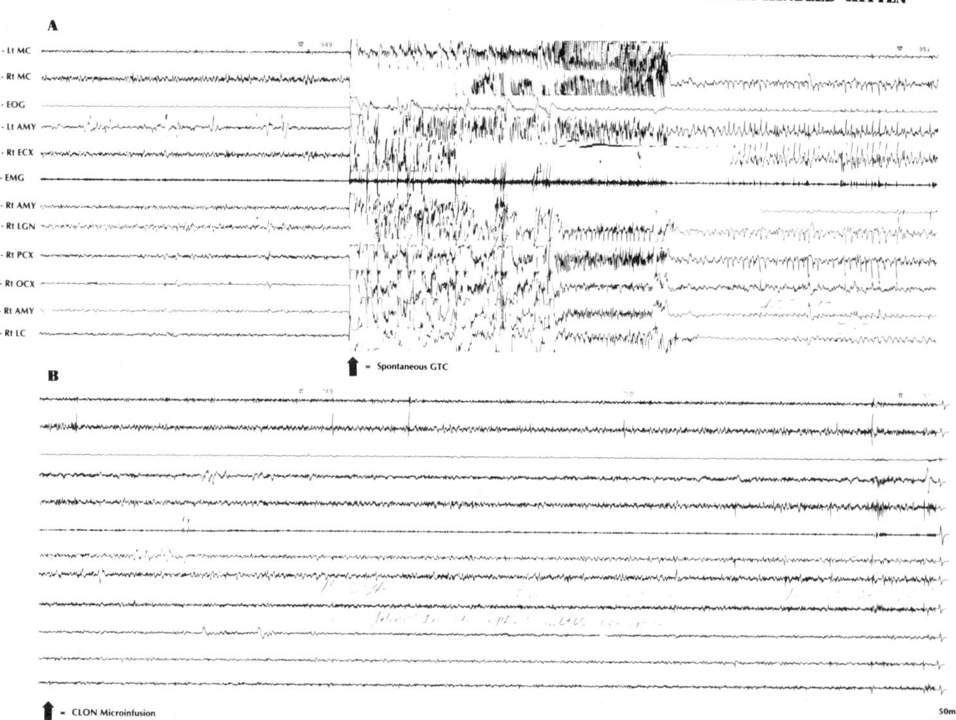

Figure 4. Effect of pontine microinfusion of CLON (14.66 μg/ml) on spontaneous convulsive status epilepticus 24-h after a stimulus-evoked seizure. At (a), continuous recording of spontaneous GTC, onset of which is indicated by the arrow. At (b), continuous 3-min recording after pontine microinfusion, indicated by the arrow, performed during a post-ictal phase 24-h after onset of spontaneous GTCs. While it is conceivable that the convulsion stopped spontaneously, we have observed numerous cases of convulsive status in amygdala-kindled kittens. None survived or stopped seizing without medical intervention. Paper speed = 10 mm/sec.

creased NE and Ach or of *reduced* NE and Ach release could act synergistically, thus accounting for larger, contrasting CLON vs. IDA pontine microinfusion effects on amygdala kindled seizure susceptibility during wakefulness.

Figures 5 and 6 illustrate that cholinergic cells can influence seizure discharge propagation in adult cats kindled as kittens. Figure 5 shows that a PGO spike in lateral geniculate nucleus (LGN), thought to be driven by choninergic cells of the pontine tegmentum[13,29], can also trigger a convulsions in the REM transition[25]. Figure 6 shows that photic stimulation can evoke epileptiform PGO-like activity in LGN and amygdala that not only outlasts the stimulus but also culminated in a GTC[25].

1.3. Mechanisms of Seizure-Prone and Seizure Resistant Sleep Wake-States

The timing of GTCs in the REM transition points to brainstem mediation, as the "ultradian" basic-rest-activity-cycle, defined by cyclic REM onset in sleep, persists only in the brainstem after midcollicular transection. Subsequent studies revealed that the generators of REM sleep and its transition exist within the pontine tegmentum, and substantial evidence implicated this region in sleep-related seizure activity (e.g., ref. 28).

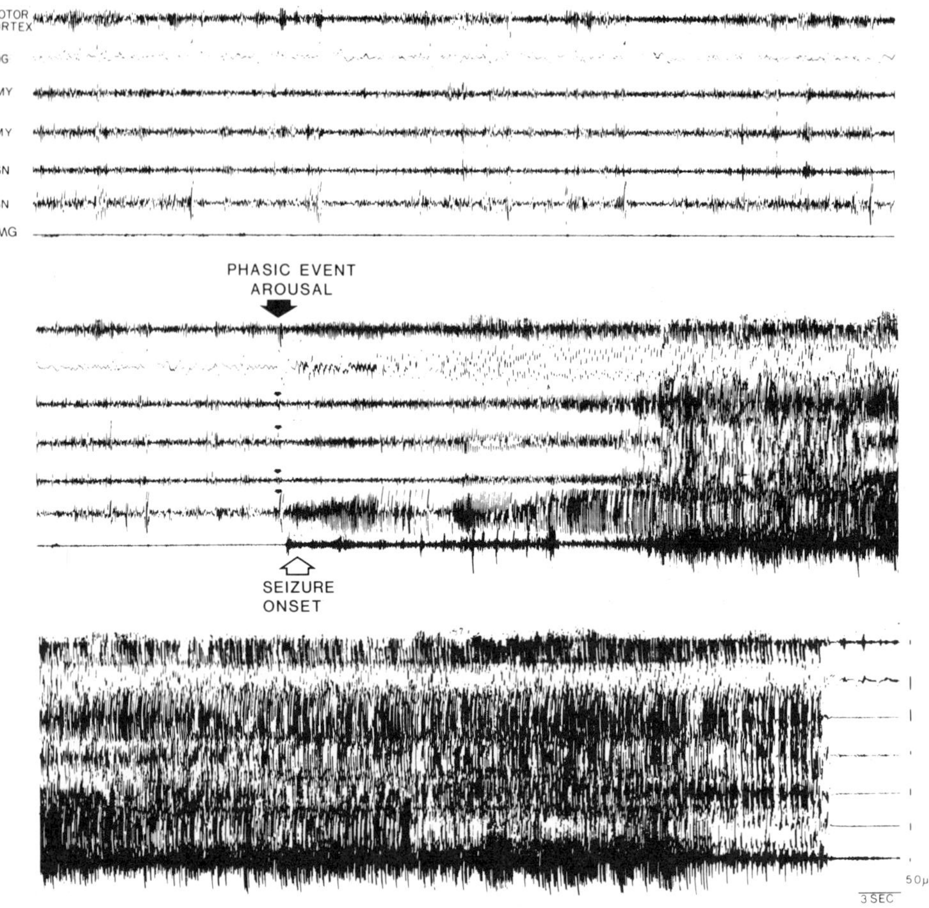

Figure 5. A continuous, 3-min tracing showing a spontaneous generalized tonic-clonic convulsion during the REM sleep transition. The REM transition begins in the middle tracing with EEG desynchronization and increased density of eye movements with ponto-geniculo-occipital (PGO) activity ipsilateral to the kindling electrode [second lateral geniculate nucleus (LGN) channel]. The convulsion was initiated or preceded by epileptiform discharges in various EEG channels associated with phasic ocular movement [electrooculogram (EOG) channel] and high-voltage,epileptiform PGO discharge in the second LGN channel. Paper speed was 10 mm/s. (Reprinted from 25).

An executive mechanism for REM onset and maintenance is still unspecified. However, at least three cell populations in the pons interact to generate various components of sleep and arousal, including the tonic and phasic events of transitional and stable REM sleep[6,8,28]. The neural groups are: 1) noradrenergic cells in the vicinity of locus ceruleus (LC), 2) serotonergic cells in the dorsal raphe nucleus (DRN) and 3) cholinergic cells in the pedunculopontine and laterodorsal tegmentum (PPT & LDT).

These pontine cells exhibit characteristic electrical activity and transmitter release properties during seizure-prone sleep states when compared to wakefulness. For example, LC, DRN and PPT/LDT neurons discharge at progressively reduced rates at NREM onset and sustain reduced discharge patterns throughout stable NREM[6]. Reduced release of NE, 5-hydroxytryptamine (5-HT) and acetylcholine (Ach) may encourage synchronous EEG discharge patterns and secondary generalized TLE at this time, since experimental suppression of these transmitters promotes NREM sleep[6] as well as kindled seizures (see ref. 23 for a review).

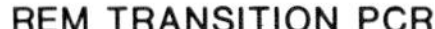

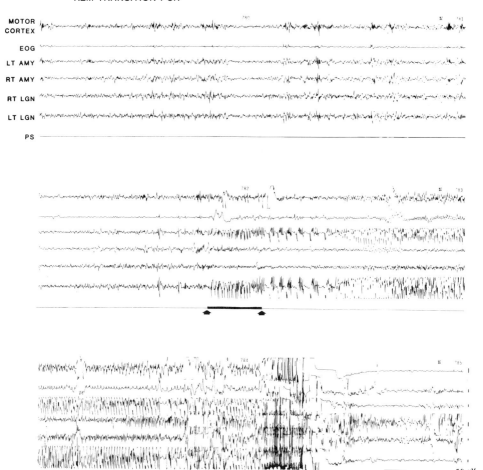

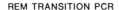

Figure 6. A continuous 3 min tracing showing a photoconvulsive response during a transition from slow-wave-sleep (SWS) to rapid-eye-movement (REM) sleep in an amygdala-kindled kitten. The top tracing shows SWS, indexed by high density sleep spindles in cortical and subcortical sites. The middle tracing indicates the beginning of the transition into REM, as indexed by reduced EEG amplitude, increased eye movement (EOG or electrooculogram) and onset of ponto-geniculo-occipital (PGO) waves in left amygdala (AMY) and lateral geniculate nucleus (LGN). The arrows indicate photic stimulation (PS) delivered at a rate of 15/sec. During PS, epileptiform PGOs were evident in left AMY and LGN. Following PS, epileptiform complexes persisted and assumed the appearance of abnormal k-complexes in the kindled left amygdala and the ipsilateral LGN. These events culminated in a generalized tonic-clonic (GTC) convulsion. The bottom tracing shows conclusion of the GTC. Paper speed = 10mm/sec. (Reprinted from 25).

Noradrenergic and serotonergic cell discharge rates further decline during the transition from NREM to REM sleep, whereas cholinergic cells in PPT and LDT discharge at progressively higher rates and exhibit a bursting pattern during the transition into REM (e.g., ref. 28). Bursting of cholinergic cells might further favor seizure generalization in the transition, since pontine cholinergic projections appear to generate proconvulsant phasic events of the REM transition, notably PGO waves[13,28,29].

On the other hand, the cell discharge and chemical trends seen during the REM transition, including reduced noradrenergic cell activity, reach their peak during stable REM sleep[28] which is antiepileptic for all generalized seizure events. This apparent inconsistency may be related to the role of reduced NE release in generating seizure resistant components of REM. Electrical silence of noradrenergic cells at this time promotes activity of adjacent neurons, notably cholinergic, to induce the intense EEG desynchronization and lower motor neuron inhibition of REM. We have linked seizure-resistant actions of REM to these tonic EEG and motor components[26]. These tonic events distinguish stable REM from NREM and the REM transition and might explain contrasting effects on seizure discharge propagation at these times as follows:

a. During NREM many cells in the brain discharge synchronously[23]. Lasting oscillations of rhythmic burst-pause firing patterns result in convergent synaptic actions. Via temporal and spatial summation, synchronous synaptic effects, whether excitatory or inhibitory, are likely to augment the magnitude of post-synaptic responses, including epileptic ones. This is particularly relevant to secondary generalized convulsions originating from focal epileptic neurons. Unlike cells generating the spike-wave complexes associated with absence seizures[4], focal epileptic neurons are both hyperexcitable and lack adequate inhibitory mechanisms[4,16], rendering them more susceptible to seizure discharge propagation during NREM. The surge of afferent excitatory input associated with phasic events like PGO spikes in the REM transition may simply exacerbate the inherent hyper-responsiveness of focal epileptic neurons, further increasing the probability of seizure discharge propagation (Figs. 5 and 6). Culmination in secondary generalized GTCs may be attributable to the presence of antigravity muscle tone in NREM and the REM transition, which permits seizure related movement[26].
b. During REM, many cells in the brain discharge asynchronously[28]. The divergent synaptic signals of asynchronous discharge patterns, due to reduced temporal and spatial summation, are less likely to augment seizure discharge magnitude or propagation. Highly localized seizure discharge persists in REM, often in conjunction with phasic events, but profound lower motor inhibition of REM creates virtual paralysis and blocks seizure-related movement. Evidence supporting this conceptualization derives from several sources, including experimental dissociation of REM sleep components[23,26]. Figure 7 shows REM sleep before and after dissociation techniques. Figure 8 shows effects of these techniques on penicillin epilepsy. The anti-cholinergic agent atropine induces a SWS-like EEG synchronization in REM and selectively abolishes REM sleep protection against EEG seizure discharge propagation, whereas lesions of pons, particularly peri-LC alpha, selectively abolish lower motor neuron inhibition and protection against clinical motor accompaniment in REM sleep. Paradoxically, then, the differential interaction of these pontine cell populations may contribute not only to seizure-prone components of NREM and the REM transition but also to the antiepileptic properties of REM.

2. CONCLUSIONS

2.1. Developmental Epilepsy Model

We discovered a model of spontaneous TLE in amygdala-kindled kittens. The kittens display spontaneous "sleep epilepsy," which persists to adulthood.

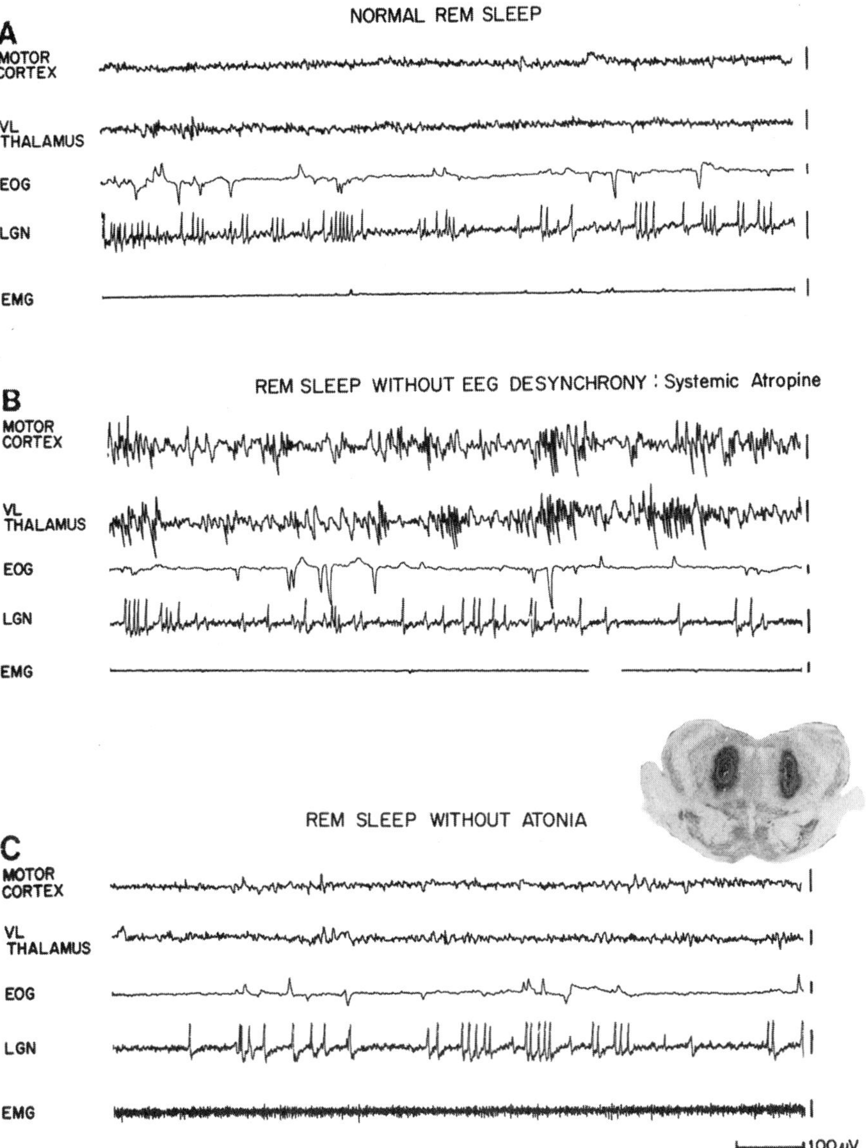

Figure 7. The top tracing (a) shows normal REM sleep, evidenced by EEG desynchronization and atonia with periodic bursts of phasic events, including rapid eye movements and ponto-geniculo-occipital (PGO) spikes. The middle tracing (b) shows that systemic atropine selectively abolishes EEG desynchronization. Instead, there is SWS sleep-like EEG with synchronized background and sleep spindles. However, atonia is intact as are eye movements and PGO spikes. Clustering of PGOs is diminished as customarily reported. The bottom tracing (c) shows that a pontine lesion selectively eliminates atonia. Note presence of tonic EMG activity in the bottom channel of this tracing. Paper speed = 10 mm/s. (Reprinted from 26).

2.2. Microinfusion Effects and Mechanisms

Microinfusion of the noradrenergic agonist CLON suppressed spontaneous and evoked seizures, whereas the noradrenergic antagonist IDA increased evoked seizure sus-

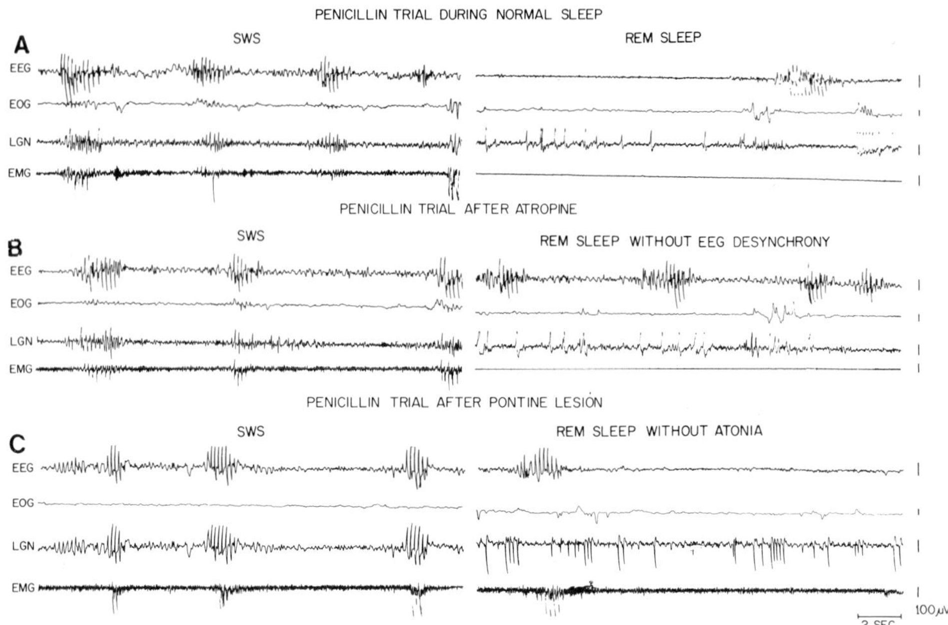

Figure 8. Systemic penicillin epilepsy during SWS (left), the equivalent of NREM in humans, and REM sleep (right) before and after dissociation of REM sleep components. The top tracing (a) shows frequent spike-wave activity in SWS with clinical accompaniment (see discharge in the EMG channel). Rare spike-wave paroxysms occur in REM without clinical accompaniment. The middle tracing (b) shows that the anti-cholinergic agent atropine abolishes differences between SWS and REM in EEG synchrony and spike-wave discharge, but there is still no clinical accompaniment in REM, presumably because atonia is intact. The bottom tracing (c) shows that pontine lesions which abolish atonia selectively block clinical motor accompaniment. Paper speed = 10 mm/s. (Reprinted from 26).

ceptibility. Magnitude of effects was significantly greater after pontine than amygdala infusion, possibly because suppression of noradrenergic cell discharge in LC affected local post-synaptic NE release at the focus and/or at extra-focal sites. Alternatively, infusion of NE-modulating agents may have activated autoreceptors in the pontine tegmentum, which influence adjacent cholinergic and serotonergic cells. These cells are implicated both in amygdala kindled seizure susceptibility and also in onset of seizure-prone and seizure-resistant sleep states.

2.3. Seizure-Prone vs. Seizure-Resistant Sleep-State Mechanisms

We propose that synchronous cellular discharge patterns during NREM, thought to result from reduced NE, Ach and serotonin (5-HT) release, increase the magnitude and spread of post-synaptic responses, including epileptic discharge. The further decline in noradrenegic and possibly serotonergic cell activity in the REM transition increases bursting of cholinergic cells, which generate proconvulsant phasic events such as PGO spikes, at this time. Presence of skeletal muscle tone permits clinical accompaniment. During stable REM, asynchronous cell discharge, thought to result from tonic reduction of NE and possibly 5-HT with increased Ach release, discourages synchronous post-synaptic responses, thus preventing spread of epileptic seizure discharge. Skeletal motor paralysis during REM prevents clinical motor accompaniment.

2.4. Clinical Relevance

Regardless of mechanism, the microinfusion technique could ultimately provide a treatment alternative for the prevalent but medically refractory TLE seizure disorder without attendant complications of systemic medication or surgical resection.

ACKNOWLEDGMENTS

Supported by the Department of Veterans Affairs.

REFERENCES

1. Bier, M.J. and McCarley, R.W., REM-enhancing effects of the adrenergic antagonist idazoxan infused into the medial pontine reticular formation of the freely moving cat, Brain Res., 634 (1994) 333–338.
2. Brown, C.M., MacKinnon, A.C., McGrath, J.C., Spedding, M. and Kilpatrick, A.T., 2 adrenoreceptor subtypes and imidazoline-like binding sites in the rat brain, Br. J. Pharmacol., 99 (1990) 803–809.
3. Corcoran, M.E. and Mason, S.T., Role of forebrain catecholamines in amygdaloid kindling, Brain Res., 190 (1980) 473–484.
4. Gloor P., Generalized epilepsy with spike-wave discharge: A reinterpretation of its electroencephalographic and clinical manifestations, Epilepsia, 20 (1979) 571–588.
5. Hauser, W.A. and Kurland, L.T., The epidemiology of epilepsy in Rochester, Minnesota, 1935 through 1967, Epilepsia, 16 (1975) 1–66.
6. Jacobs, B.L., Overviewiew of the activity of monoaminergic neurons across the sleep-wake cycle. In: Wauquier, A. Monti, J.M., Gaillard, J.M. and Radusovacki, M., (Eds.) Sleep; Neurotransmitters and Neuromodulators. N.Y., Raven Press, 1985; pp. 1–14.
7. Janz D., The grand mal epilepsies and the sleeping-waking cycle, Epilepsia, 3 (1962) 69–109.
8. Jones, B. E., Basic mechanisms of sleep-wake states. In: Meir H. Kryger, Thomas Roth and William C. Dement (Eds.). Principles and Practice of Sleep disorders Medicine, 2nd.(Ed). W. B. Saunders Co., Philadelphia, (1994), pp. 145–162.
9. Jones, B.E. and Moore, R.W., Ascending projections of the locus coeruleus in the rat II. Autoradiographic Study, Brain Res., 127 (1977) 23–53.
10. Kubaik, P. and Zagrodzka, J., DSP-4 lesion of locus coeruleus does not affect spontaneous predatory behavior in cats, Acta. Neurobiologiae Exp., 53 (1993) 525–534.
11. Leppavuori, A., Putkonen, P.T.S. and Stenberg, D., Sedation and suppression of paradoxical sleep in the cat after clonidine, Acta. Physiol. Scand. Suppl., 440 (1976) 60.
12. McBride, R.I., Sutin, J., Projections of the Locus Coeruleus and Adjacent Pontine Tegmentum in the Cat, J. Comp. Neurol, 165 (1976) 265–284.
13. McCarley, R.W., Nelson, J.P. and Hobson, J.A., Ponto-geniculo-occipital (PGO) burst neurons: Correlational evidence for neuronal generators of PGO waves, Science, 20 (1978) 269–272.
14. McIntyre, D.C. and Guigna, L., Effect of clonidine on amygdala kindling in normal and 6-hydroxydopamine-pretreated rats, Exp. Neurol., 99 (1988) 96–106.
15. McIntyre D.C., Saari, M. and Pappas, B.A., Potentiation of amygdala in adult or infant rats by injection of 6-hydroxydopamine, Exp. Neurol., 63 (1979) 527–544.
16. McNamara J.O., Cellular and molecular basis of epilepsy, J. Neurosci., 14 (1994) 3413–3425.
17. Pelletier, M. and Corcoran, M.E., Intra-amydgaloid infusions of clonidine retard kindling, Brain Res., 598 (1992) 51–58.
18. Pelletier, M. and Corcoran, M.E., Infusions of α-2 noradrenergic agonists and antagonists into the amygdala: Effects on kindling, Brain Res., 632 (1993) 29–35.
19. Shouse, M.N., Langer, J.V., and Dittes, P.R., Spontaneous sleep epilepsy in amygdala kindled kittens: A preliminary report, Brain Res., 535 (1990)163–168.
20. Shouse, M.N., Bier, M., Langer, J., Alcalde, O., Richkind, M. and Szymusiak, R., The alpha-2 agonist clonidine suppresses seizures, whereas the alpha-2 antagonist idazoxan promotes seizures: A microinfusion study in amygdala kindled kittens, Brain Res., 648 (1994) 352–356.
21. Shouse, M.N., Langer, J.V., and Dittes, P.R., The ontogeny of feline temporal lobe epilepsy: II. Stability of spontaneous sleep epilepsy in amygdala-kindled kittens, Epilepsia, 33 (1992) 789–798.

22. Shouse, M.N., King, A., Langer, J., Vreeken, T. King. K. and Richkind, M., The ontogeny of feline temporal lobe epilepsy: kindling a spontaneous seizure disorder in kittens, Brain Res., 525 (1990) 215–224.
23. Shouse, M.N., Martins da Silva, A. and Sammaritano, M., Circadian rhythm, sleep, and epilepsy, J. Clin. Neuro. Physiol., 13 (1996) 1–19.
24. Shouse, M.N., Langer J., Bier M., Farber, P.R., Alcalde O., Moghimi, R., Richkind M. and Szymusiak, R., The alpha-2 adrenoreceptor agongonist clonidine suppresses seizures, whereas the alpha-2 adrenoreceptor antagonist idazoxan promotes seizures in amygdala-kindled kittens: A comparison of amygdala and pontine microinfusion effects, Epilepsia, 1996, in press.
25. Shouse, M.N., Langer, J. Alcalde, O, Szymusiak, R. and Bier, M. Paroxysmal arousals in amygdala-kindled kittens: Could they be subclinical seizures? Epilepsia, 36 (1995) 290–300.
26. Shouse, M.N., Siegel, J.M., Wu, M.F., Szymusiak, R.S. and Morrison, A.R. Mechanisms of seizure suppression during REM sleep in cats, Brain Res., 505 (1989) 271–282.
27. Shouse, M.N., Langer J., Bier M., Farber, P.R., Alcalde O., Moghimi, R., Richkind M. and Szymusiak, R., The alpha-2 adrenoreceptor agonist clonidine suppresses seizures, whereas the alpha-2 adrenoreceptor antagonist idazoxan promotes seizures: Pontine microinfusion studies of amygdala-kindled kittens, Brain Res., 1996, in press.
28. Siegel, J. S., Brainstem mechanisms generating REM sleep. In: Meir H. Kryger, Thomas Roth and William C. Dement (Eds.) Principles and Practice of sleep disorders medicine, 2nd. Ed. Philadelphia, W. B. Saunders Co., 1994, pp. 125–144.
29. Steriade, M., Pare, D., Datta, M., Oakson, G., Curro-Dossi, R., Different cellular types in mesopontine cholinergic nuclei related to ponto-geniculo-occipital waves, J. Neurosci., 10 (1990) 2560–2579.
30. Tononi, G., Pompeiano, M. and Cirelli C., Suppression of desynchronized sleep through microinjection of the alpha 2-adrenergic agonist clonidine in the dorsal pontine tegmentum of the cat, Pflugers Archiv. Euro. J. of Physiol., 418 (1991) 512–8.
31. Trevor, D., L'Heureux, R., Carter, C. and Scatton, B., Presynaptic alpha-2 adrenoceptors play a major role in the effects of idazoxan on cortical noradrenaline release (as measured by in vivo dialysis) in the rat, J. Pharmacol. Exp. Therap., 241 (1987) 642–649.
32. Weiss, G.K., Lewis, J., Jimenez-Rivera Vigil, A. and Corcoran, M.E., Antikindling effects of locus ceruleus stimulation: Mediation by ascending noradrenergic projections, Exp. Neurol., 108 (1990) 136–140.

DISCUSSION OF MARGARET SHOUSE'S PAPER

J. McNamara: Were those cats receiving the microinfusions previously kindled?

M. Shouse: Yes, we were measuring effects of infusions on seizure thresholds. It's very difficult to look at spontaneous seizures, to predict their onset. We are starting to do some slower infusions now, and we have had one case where we were able to stop status epilepticus with a clonidine microinfusion. If we can get this microinfusion thing working, both on evoked and spontaneous seizures, we have ourselves a very nice treatment alternative for medically managing temporal-lobe epilepsy that is notoriously medically refractory. This could end up providing a handy alternative to complications attendant to systemic medication and to surgical resection.

J. McNamara: Just a comment on that. There's work been done by a lot of people with norepinephrine, Michael Corcoran, Olle Lindvall, and so on, who have shown effects mainly on the development of the process of kindling, not on the expression.

M. Shouse: We just didn't find that. It's a difference that we have reported and commented on; I can't explain it.

J. McNamara: What percentage of cats, when kindled as kittens, exhibit spontaneous seizures?

M. Shouse: All of them!

J. McNamara: What about cats that undergo electrode implantation but no stimulation as kittens, what percentage of them are having spontaneous seizures?

M. Shouse: They don't have seizures of any kind. Maybe Dr. Wada can comment on this, but you kindle an adult cat and you are lucky to see a spontaneous seizure even if you over-kindle them as John Pinel does with his rodents.

J. McNamara: The genetic factor of the kindled cats...

M. Shouse: That's an interesting thing that we have been looking at. We were getting all of our cats from UC Davis, that was our first batch, and I think we had about sixty percent develop convulsive status—they all developed some kind of spontaneous seizure as we subsequently learned. But when they developed some kind of a virus in their colony, we had to go to other sources, and the proportions just changed. I presume that is related to some sort of a genetic factor. We haven't really sorted it out yet but I'm ready to confess that I think that that is a factor.

B. Adamec: I'm interested in your barking cat. Is that the only one you've seen it in?

M. Shouse: The only one I've seen it in so far.

B. Adamec: No sound?

M. Shouse: No sound.

B. Adamec: That looks very familiar to me, only I see it at the onset of a partial hippocampal seizure and it is associated with a cry that is called a lonesome cry. You can hear cats do that in the colony at night.

M. Shouse: The vocalization you just described is actually a component of most kindled seizures, while you're doing the stimulation it's part of the evoked seizure. We can see that too. But this cat never made a peep.

B. Adamec: But some cats are very silent. Is this cat vocal normally?

M. Shouse: Yes.

GENERAL DISCUSSION 2

C. Applegate: I just have one comment about Dr. Moshé's 2-DG data. I guess in other brainstem seizure models, 2-DG does show changes in brainstem labelling. In our hands the pattern of c-fos labelling in the brainstem strictly depends on the kind of seizure that an adult animal has. If they have a clonic seizure with no tonic manifestations, the brainstem is clean of c-fos labelling, but as soon as they show running-bouncing seizures then the brainstem lights up. So that's an interesting difference.

S. Moshé: That's why I mentioned the flurothyl data. In the flurothyl model you can maintain status epilepticus and severe seizures for 45 minutes. We injected the deoxyglucose in these animals after they developed status epilepticus. In this model there was increased uptake of the deoxyglucose in brainstem structures, with the exclusion of the substantia nigra. These data are different from the data with kindling, in which we never saw any deoxyglucose uptake in brainstem structures. The difference between the two methods is in the creation of the seizure. In kindling, the animals experienced 3 or 4 brief seizures, not a prolonged period of status epilepticus.

C. Applegate: Just to continue the question. You got no labelling in the substantia nigra regardless of the hemisphere stimulated?

S. Moshé: We did not see any increased uptake in the substantia nigra.

J. Stripling: I just wanted to ask some more about your rapid kindling in the piriform cortex. You had placements just dorsal to the endopiriform. I assume you are in the claustrum?

S. Moshé: Yes, it is.

J. Stripling: The endopiriform has a marked rostrocaudal extent. Did you notice any patterns or differences in the electrode placements?

S. Moshé: When we initially analysed the data, I thought there may be an anterior-posterior difference in the kindling rate. When we redid the experiments, the data did not support an anterior-posterior difference. That is why we bunched the data together.

J. Stripling: So you got rapid kindling anywhere along the anterior-posterior axis?

S. Moshé: There may have been an animal that was faster. I really drove the student nuts, because I wanted to know if there was an anterior-posterior difference. It did not turn out to be the case.

M. Gilbert: I have a question about your late paired-pulse depression and your failure to find that in your kindled animals. Were those animals kindled as pups and then tested as adults? Was it *in vivo* or *in vitro?*

S. Moshé: The experiments were performed in vitro. The rat pups were kindled at PN16, then were allowed to grow for another two weeks. At that point, they were sacrificed. Half of the brain was used for histological analysis, while the other half was used for in vitro experiments.

M. Gilbert: I'd like to make a comment about your failure to see late paired-pulse depression in your adult kindled animals. There's a very strong stimulus dependancy in late paired-pulse depression; so if you stimulated at or near maximal stimulus intensities you may not see late paired-pulse depression and that could account for the discrepancy between your findings and those of others.

S Moshé: The point that I tried to make was that by using the same paradigm in kainic acid-induced status epilepticus and in kindling we found differences in paired-pulse inhibition. Animals exposed to kainic-acid status epilepticus had increased early and late inhibition while animals exposed to kindling showed mostly increases in early inhibition. This may be due to the fact that the changes in late inhibition that are observed with kindling are not sustained; so it is possible that when we tested the animals at two weeks the late inhibition changes had disappeared.

S. Leung: I presume you don't find any behavioural differences in your kindled rat pups, as you say there's no mossy fiber sprouting, no paired-pulse depression in vitro, and I suppose they don't show any behavioral deficits.

S. Moshé: Animals kindled early in life and rekindled in adulthood are more susceptible to kindled seizures either from the same amygdala or contralateral amygdala. The way we did this experiment is as follows: We kindled animals at PN15 and 16, and then we removed the electrodes. We sutured the scalp and allowed the rats to grow to about 60 days, when the were reimplanted with new electrodes either ipsilateral or contralateral to the initial kindling site. All animals kindled faster than controls within 2 or 3 stimulations. We did not do any behavioral testing at the time that the animals were growing. Greg Holmes has performed such studies and he has exposed rats to various behavioral tasks. His data indicate that animals exposed to seizures early in life do not show any behavioral deficits, while animals exposed to seizures at a later stage have such deficits. It should be pointed out that in the kainic acid model there seems to be a relationship between the occurrence of spontaneous seizures and the appearance of morphological or neurophysiological changes in the dentate. It appears that spontaneous seizures will appear after the age of 20 to 25 days, the first age at which consistent pathological changes can be observed in the hippocampus.

C. Applegate: I just wanted to follow up on Jim McNamara's question to Dr. Shouse, which is that if you apply noradrenergic agonists to a fully-kindled animal you don't influence the seizure expression at all. In your model you're able to affect the seizure expression rather profoundly, and I was wondering if you could just speculate whether that means that these spontaneous seizures have a very different mechanism from kindled seizures?

M. Shouse: I'm not really sure. There are a couple of things I didn't mention. One of them is that we can get seizures that literally start off in the amygdala, in the focus, during sleep and the REM transition, and just look exactly as though we had stimulated them. What we also get, which I think is probably similar to what Nico Moshé was talking about, is multifocal epilepsy. We were first seeing seizures in the geniculate, but nobody really believes they started there, everyone believes they started in the pons because that's really what runs the geniculate. So the answer is, I think the kindling process is different in immature animals because, for whatever reason, they are just more vulnerable. Perhaps they lack the development of the inhibitory systems that are required. We haven't looked into, but there's a reason for it and ultimately we'll come up with it.

6

LASTING PROLONGATION OF NMDA CHANNEL OPENINGS AFTER KINDLING

Istvan Mody* and David N. Lieberman

Departments of Neurology and Physiology
Reed Neurological Research Center
UCLA School of Medicine
710 Westwood Plaza
Los Angeles, California 90095-1769

1. INTRODUCTION

Central synapses undergo specific lasting structural or functional alterations. This property, also referred to as plasticity, is an essential property of synaptic transmission. Proper central nervous system development, function, and, unfortunately, malfunction leading to specific brain disorders would be unthinkable without plastic alterations at the level of synapses. An essential consequence of plasticity at the synaptic level is the altered gain of synaptic transmission, resulting in an increase or a decrease in synaptic strength. An excessively increased excitatory synaptic drive may induce aberrant discharges in neurons easily convertible into epilepsy at the network level. Probing the basic mechanisms of epileptogenesis has furnished evidence consistent with highly conserved means of plastic neuronal alterations regardless of the experimental models or species involved. Several cellular and molecular neuronal changes appear to be common to human temporal lobe epilepsy (TLE) and to various experimental chronic epilepsy models.[43] The more conserved an alteration in neuronal function, across boundaries of species and experimental models, the more likely the resultant change in neuronal excitability should have a fundamental role in the pathogenesis of TLE.

Of the many experimental animal models of TLE, kindling-induced epilepsy, stands out as a model in which several modifications have been resolved in detail at wide range of levels: neuronal networks, single neurons, synapses, and even single channels.[28,32] Here we will focus on the possible mechanisms underlying the plasticity of glutamate receptors of the NMDA type during kindling-induced epileptogenesis. The cellular and molecular bases of the changes in NMDA channel function may be shared with human TLE. In the

* e-mail: mody@ucla.edu

Kindling 5, edited by Corcoran and Moshé.
Plenum Press, New York, 1998.

near future, identification of specific alterations in neuronal excitability common to human TLE and to experimental TLE models is expected to result in major breakthroughs in our understanding of the basis for the altered cellular and synaptic properties in epilepsies.

2. THE NMDA RECEPTOR

Fast excitatory neurotransmission in the mammalian CNS primarily results from the activation of ionotropic or ligand-gated glutamate receptors.[8,11,42] Initially these receptors were classified depending on the preferred synthetic agonist into AMPA, KA and NMDA type receptors. The NMDA receptor is a remarkable member of the glutamate receptor family bearing peculiar characteristics clearly distinguishing it from the rest of the glutamate-gated channels.[5,25] Its block by Mg^{2+} at membrane potentials close to the resting potential of neurons and the relief provided by depolarization has long implicated the NMDA receptor in the generation of epileptiform activity.[6,30] A notable sensitivity to glycine fueled speculations about it being a receptor for two distinct amino acids: glutamate and glycine. Most importantly for its profound involvement in neuronal plasticity, it is among the few glutamate receptors allowing Ca^{2+} to enter nerve cells and to produce lasting alterations in their excitability. On the basis of these properties, the NMDA channels are ideally suited to fulfill the role of a neuronal coincidence detector,[44] an important function for paving the road toward the consistent activation of entire neuronal networks.

Through cloning various glutamate receptor subunits, molecular biological studies have recently uncovered specific subunit assemblies with various degrees of homology (Fig. 1) corresponding to each type of the previously pharmacologically identified glutamate receptors.[11,42] For example, the NMDA type of receptor (NMDAR) has five different subunits, NMDAR1, and NMDA2A-D, which can assemble to form functional NMDA channels. The exact nature and stoichiometry of assembly of these subunits at individual synapses is poorly understood, but studies using expression systems have shown that the various subunit combinations result in channels with very distinct properties.[7,35,46] To further complicate the picture, the gene encoding the NMDAR1 exhibits three potential regions of alternative splicing: one 21 amino acid segment at the N-terminus (N1), and two exons encoding 37 (C1) and 38 (C2) amino acids respectively at the C-terminus.[56] Depending which exon is spliced in or out, eight different NMDAR1 variants may result (denoted in a binary notation as $NMDAR1_{000}$ to $NMDAR1_{111}$). These splice variants differ significantly in their sensitivity to agonists, glycine, Zn^{2+} and polyamines.[56]

The epileptogenic potential of NMDA receptor activation was recognized early on following the discovery of specific glutamate receptor subtypes. NMDA receptor antagonists are potent antiepileptics; unblocking NMDA receptors by lowering the extracellular

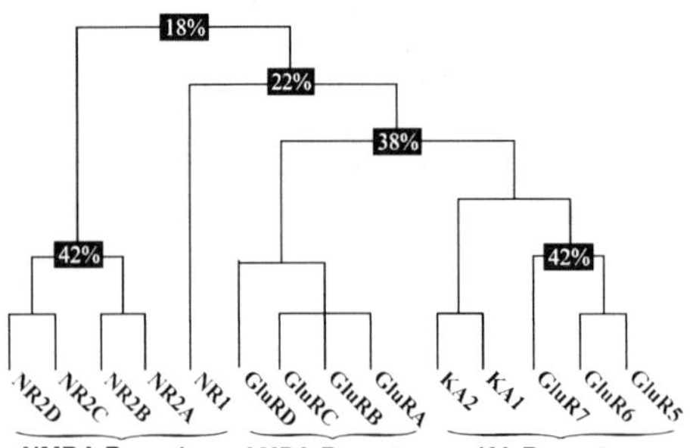

Figure 1. Homology tree of the ionotropic glutamate receptors. These receptors can be divided into three functional and pharmacological categories: kainate receptors, AMPA receptors and NMDA receptors. The numbers in the boxes indicate the percent homology in the amino acid sequence of the various glutamate receptor subunits. The splice variants have been omitted for clarity.

Mg^{2+} concentration causes epileptiform activity; and regardless of the experimental paradigm used, there is generally a strong correlation between the activation of NMDA receptors and epileptiform events.[6,27,30] The abundance of NMDA receptors in the normal brain and their undisputed involvement in normal brain development and plasticity presented a paradox. If this was true, how could the normal brain be free of epilepsy? Something had to happen in the epileptic brain ultimately resulting in the enhanced activation of NMDA receptors. In other words, the NMDA receptors coincidence detectors and hence key players in neuronal plasticity, had to experience some plastic alterations themselves (lately termed metaplasticity[1]) sufficiently increasing their function to cause epileptogenesis.

The kindling-induced enhanced recruitment into synaptic transmission of previously "dormant" NMDA receptors on dentate gyrus (DG) granule cells (GC)[31,33] was the first clue for the presence of such plasticity in TLE. These findings were substantiated in follow-up electrophysiological and biochemical studies.[28,29,32] We have also shown at the single channel level this enhanced NMDA function to be manifested by prolonged openings, bursts, clusters and superclusters of NMDA channel activity,[17] and by an increased agonist potency.[18] Our findings are also consistent with a change in the Mg^{2+} block, *i.e.*, a reduced affinity of the channel pore to Mg^{2+} at depolarized potentials, and have demonstrated an enhanced phosphorylation state of the channels after kindling.[17]

One of the remarkable characteristics of kindling-induced changes in the pharmacology of NMDA receptors is the persistence of the alterations for longer than one month of a seizure-free period.[19,26,55] The question was whether these pharmacological changes had functional counterparts. We have recently completed a study examining the persistence in the increased duration of NMDA channel openings. The NMDA channel openings were still prolonged when recorded 28 days and 60 days after the last kindling stimulus (Fig. 2). There were no differences between the prolonged openings 2–3 days, 28 days, or even 60 days after the last seizure. These prolonged openings also resemble the behavior of

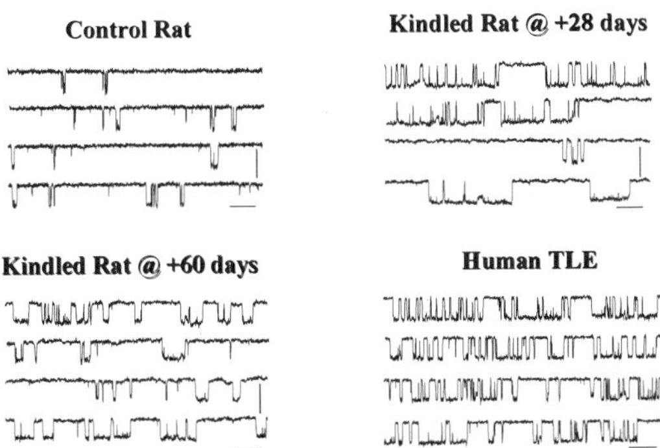

Figure 2. Prolongation of NMDA channel openings in kindled granule cells 28 and 60 days following the last kindled seizure, and in a human TLE patient. Each panel illustrates four successive traces of 250 ms each showing the openings of NMDA channels (downward deflections) in the absence of extracellular Mg^{2+} with 5 mM glycine and L-aspartic acid (500 nM) in the cell-attached pipette (holding was –60 mV on the intracellular side). Note the dramatic prolongation of the openings in the kindled granule cells, and the long bursting periods in the human TLE neuron. Recordings were obtained in granule cells acutely dissociated from electrode-implanted controls and kindled animals with at least 20 stage 5 motor seizures. The averages of the opening characteristics of NMDA channels were all significantly different ($p<0.01$ paired two-tailed t-test) from controls both at 28 and 60 days after the last kindled seizure. No differences were noted in single channel conductance. Note the characteristic increase in the "burstiness" of the kindled channels, particularly evident in the human TLE granule cell. Calibration bars: 5 pA and 25 ms.

NMDA channels observed in granule cells dissociated from TLE patients who have undergone therapeutic surgical resection of the hippocampus (Fig. 2). The longevity of the altered NMDA channel function in the absence of further kindled seizures is consistent with the prolonged NMDA channel openings being part of the "kindled state" rather than being a short-lived consequence of temporal lobe seizure activity. The results also indicate that, unless the turnover rate of NMDA channels is dramatically slowed down in kindling, the mechanism(s) responsible for the dramatic prolongation of NMDA channel openings must affect all receptors newly inserted into the membrane. As discussed below, some likely possibilities include the synthesis of novel ("epileptic") NMDA receptor subunits,[19] or lasting alterations in the regulatory mechanisms governing NMDA channel function such as protein kinases or phosphatases,[21,47,51,53] or other regulatory proteins such as PSD-95[16] or calmodulin.[9]

The lasting changes in NMDA channel function after kindling are present in spite of no apparent persistent changes in mRNA levels for any of the five known NMDAR subunits (R1 and R2A-D),[15,19] (and Soltesz, Monyer, and Mody, unpublished observations), although some short term changes in message can be observed.[37] A significant kindling-induced difference related to NMDA receptors is found, however, in the hippocampal CA3 region. The binding of two competitive NMDA receptor antagonists, 3-[(±)-2-(carboxypiperazine-4-yl)] [1,2–^{3}H-]propyl-1-phosphonic acid (^{3}H-CPP) and *cis*-4-(phosphonomethyl)-2–^{3}H-piperidinecarboxylate (^{3}H-CGS-19755) is remarkably distinct: an increase in ^{3}H-CPP binding 28 days after the last kindled seizure is not paralleled by an increase in ^{3}H-CGS-19755 binding.[19] These findings, together with the good correspondence between the binding profiles of various NMDA ligands and the specific subunit distribution of NMDA receptors,[4] raise the possibility that a novel, hitherto uncharacterized type of NMDA receptor may have emerged after kindling. To date little is known about how these changes affecting NMDA receptor function occur and how they can persist for a long time.

One possibility, albeit inconsistent with the presently available experimental evidence, is a seizure-induced alteration in the stoichiometry of assembly of different NMDAR subunits. Considering the rapid turnover rate of NMDARs[45,50] it is unlikely for changes in receptor assembly to outlive the last kindled seizure by more than two months. Another possibility, independent of subunit stoichiometry but related to alterations in NMDAR subunits, is the insertion of novel alternatively spliced NMDARs into the hetero-pentameric receptors following kindling. To date no published data are available concerning the levels of various alternatively spliced NMDAR1 subunits following kindling, but preliminary observations are consistent with such alterations.[49] If NMDAR1 splicing were altered in epilepsy, one of the most exciting consequences would be the change in the effects of certain NMDAR modulators and ligands, including antagonists, depending on the splice variant. Previously negative modulators of NMDARs may become potentiators and *vice versa*, while some compounds may lose their effectiveness altogether. Consistent with this hypothesis, it has been difficult to reconcile how several competitive and non-competitive NMDA receptor antagonist become much less effective against kindled seizures.[13,23,30,45,54] For example, the NMDA channel blocker memantine (1-amino-3,5-dimethyladamantane), originally an anticonvulsant, is converted into a proconvulsant after kindling.[22] If these puzzling findings reflect some changes in the molecular structure of NMDARs, then understanding the nature of the molecular alterations and the precise sensitivity to modulators will aid us in developing antiepileptic drugs with specific actions on modified and unique "epileptic" receptors.

The different effect of Zn^{2+} on NMDAR1 splice variants raises another important question relevant to human TLE and TLE models with significant Zn^{2+}-containing mossy fiber sprouting. Zinc can block native NMDA channels in cultured neurons,[25] but mutation of a single amino acid residue can drastically decrease Zn^{2+}-sensitivity.[41] Worse still, certain splice variants of NMDAR1 are potentiated instead of being inhibited by Zn^{2+}.[10,56] The known potentiation of AMPA receptors by Zn^{2+},[36,39] the Zn^{2+}-induced block of kindled $GABA_A$ receptors[3] (see below), and the possibility of kindled NMDARs becoming insensitive or even enhanced by Zn^{2+}, would put this cation into an extremely critical position for controlling neuronal excitability in the epileptic dentate gyrus. Since the sprouted mossy fibers elevate the total extrapolated Zn^{2+} content of the dentate gyrus to about 150% of control,[34] the enhanced Zn^{2+} release into the molecular and granule cell layers may block $GABA_A$ receptors and potentiate NMDA and non-NMDA receptor activity all at the same time. This combined effect could have an extremely epileptogenic potential particularly during repetitive activity in the mossy fibers known to efficiently release the cation.[2,12]

As an alternative hypothesis to the modification in the *structure* of NMDA receptors, it is possible that the plasticity does not occur at the level of the receptor subunits but rather at the level of the numerous regulatory mechanisms controlling the *function* of NMDA channels. Lasting covalent modifications through phosphorylation or dephosphorylation of ligand-gated channels are known to be effective means of regulating their function.[40] Our recent findings have unveiled the control of NMDA channel openings through the activation of a calmodulin-dependent phosphatase (calcineurin or PP2B).[20] These results have since been corroborated in tissue culture, and have been extended to the regulation of synaptically mediated NMDA responses.[38,47] We wanted to know if inhibition of the intracellular phosphatase responsible for the control of NMDA channel function will still affect the prolonged openings seen in kindled neurons. Surprisingly, perfusion of okadaic acid (10 mM) had no effect on the openings of kindled NMDA channels (Fig.3), but prolonged the channel openings recorded in the electrode-implanted and age matched

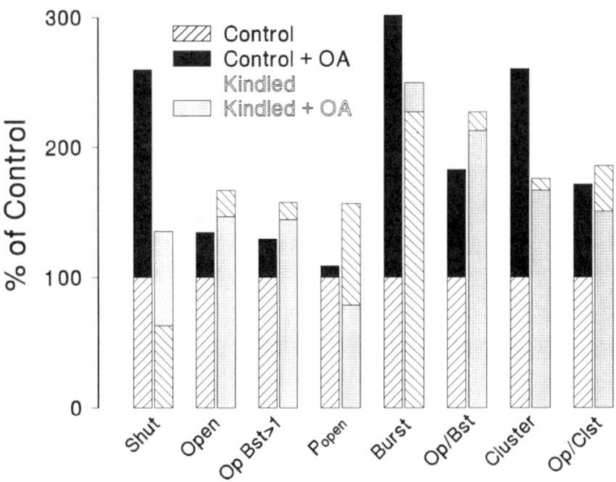

Figure 3. The phosphatase inhibitor okadaic acid (OA; 10 μM) can no longer prolong NMDA channel openings in kindled neurons. Control NMDA channel parameters (from left to right: mean shut time, mean open time, mean open time in bursts with more than one opening, open probability, mean burst length, mean number of openings per burst, mean cluster duration, and mean number of openings per cluster) are taken as 100% (///// shaded bars). The effect of OA on these parameters is illustrated by the black bars. For example OA increased the mean burst duration of NMDA channel openings to 300% of control. The effect of kindling is depicted by the \\\\\ shaded bars and should be compared to controls (/////). OA had no significant effect on the already prolonged kindled NMDA channel openings (gray shaded bars), and in some cases, such as the mean cluster length, it actually *decreased* their duration. Similar data were obtained with the specific calcineurin inhibitor FK-506 (not shown). These findings are consistent with a possible impairment of the calcineurin-dependent negative feedback exerted on NMDA channel openings.

controls[21] much like previously described.[20] This experimental evidence supports the hypothesis that the regulation of NMDA receptors by the calcium/calmodulin dependent phosphatase calcineurin (PP2B)[20,47] is altered after kindling. It is possible that comparable functional rather than structural alterations of NMDA receptors will be found in granule cells recorded in the human TLE dentate gyrus, where NMDA receptor mediated synaptic excitability is enhanced.[14,24,48]

3. CONCLUSIONS

In summary, the kindling model of TLE shows a significant amount of metaplasticity, characterized by plastic changes in receptors such as NMDA which themselves are actively involved in shaping neuronal plasticity. The evidence to date indicates that the plasticity of the NMDA receptors on kindled granule cells does not involve any structural modifications, but rather a lasting reduction in the negative feedback exerted by calcium ions via the CaM-dependent phosphatase calcineurin. It remains to be determined whether the loss of calcineurin-dependent regulation of NMDA channels after kindling is a consequence of reduced levels of calcineurin or a loss of calcineurin function. Since other enzymes such as calmodulin and superoxide dismutase (Wang et al., 1996) are potent regulators of calcineurin activity, the loss of calcineurin per se need not be postulated in the "kindled state". Nevertheless, the altered regulatory mechanisms of NMDA channel function in TLE should constitute important future targets for pharmacological approaches aimed at preventing epileptogenesis.

ACKNOWLEDGMENTS

The technical assistance of B. Oyama is very much appreciated. The research presented here was supported by grants from the NIH/NINDS. DNL was supported by a Howard Hughes MD PhD Predoctoral Fellowship.

REFERENCES

1. Abraham, W.C. and Bear, M.F., Metaplasticity: the plasticity of synaptic plasticity, *TINS*, 19 (1996) 126–130.
2. Assaf, S.Y. and Chung, S.H., Release of endogenous Zn^{2+} from brain tissue during activity, *Nature*, 308 (1984) 734–736.
3. Buhl, E.H., Otis, T.S., and Mody, I., Zinc-induced collapse of augmented inhibition by GABA in a temporal lobe epilepsy model, *Science*, 271 (1996) 369–373.
4. Buller, A.L., Larson, H.C., Schneider, B.E., Beaton, J.A., Morrisett, R.A., and Monaghan, D.T., The molecular basis of NMDA receptor subtypes: native receptor diversity is predicted by subunit composition, *J. Neurosci.* 14 (1994) 5471–5484.
5. Collingridge, G.L. and Watkins, J.C., The NMDA Receptor, Oxford: Oxford University Press, (1994).
6. Dingledine, R., McBain, C.J. and McNamara, J.O., Excitatory amino acid receptors in epilepsy, *Trends in Pharmacol. Sci.*, 11 (1990) 334–338.
7. Ebralidze, A.K., Rossi, D.J., Tonegawa, S. and Slater, N.T., Modification of NMDA receptor channels and synaptic transmission by targeted disruption of the NR2C gene, *J. Neurosci.*, 16 (1996) 5014–5025.
8. Edmonds, B., Gibb, A.J. and Colquhoun, D., Mechanisms of activation of glutamate receptors and the time course of excitatory synaptic currents, *Ann. Rev. Physiol.*, 57 (1995) 495–519.
9. Ehlers, M.D., Zhang, S., Bernhardt, J.P. and Huganir, R.L., Inactivation of NMDA receptors by direct interaction of calmodulin with the NR1 subunit, *Cell*, 84 (1996) 745–755.

10. Hollmann, M., Boulter, J., Maron, C., Beasley, L., Sullivan, J., Pecht, G. and Heinemann, S., Zinc potentiates agonist-induced currents at certain splice variants of the NMDA receptor, *Neuron*, 10 (1993) 943–954.
11. Hollmann, M. and Heinemann, S., Cloned glutamate receptors, *Annu. Rev. Neurosci.*, 17 (1994) 31–108.
12. Hönack, D. and Löscher, W., Kindling increases the sensitivity of rats to adverse effects of certain antiepileptic drugs, *Epilepsia*, 36 (1995) 763–771.
13. Isokawa, M. and Levesque, M.F., Increased NMDA responses and dendritic degeneration in human epileptic hippocampal neurons in slices, *Neurosci. Lett.*, 132 (1991) 212–216.
14. Kamphuis, W., Hendriksen, H., Diegenbach, P.C. and Lopes da Silva, F.H., *N*-methyl-D-aspartate and kainate receptor gene expression in hippocampal pyramidal and granular neurons in the kindling model of epileptogenesis, *Neuroscience*, 67 (1995) 551–559.
15. Köhr, G., De Koninck, Y. and Mody, I., Properties of NMDA receptor channels in neurons acutely isolated from epileptic (kindled) rats, *J. Neurosci.*, 13 (1993) 3612–3627.
16. Köhr, G. and Mody, I., Kindling increases *N*-methyl-D-aspartate potency at single *N*-methyl-D-aspartate channels in dentate gyrus granule cells, *Neuroscience*, 62 (1994) 975–981.
17. Kornau, H.C., Schenker, L.T., Kennedy, M.B. and Seeburg, P.H., Domain interaction between NMDA receptor subunits and the postsynaptic density protein PSD-95, *Science*, 269 (1995) 1737–1740.
18. Kraus, J.E., Yeh, G.C., Bonhaus, D.W., Nadler, J.V. and McNamara, J.O., Kindling induces long-lasting expression of a novel population of NMDA receptors in hippocampal region CA3, *J. Neurosci.*, 14 (1994) 4196–4205.
19. Lieberman, D.N. and Mody, I., Regulation of NMDA channel function by endogenous Ca^{2+}-dependent phosphatase, *Nature*, 369 (1994) 235–239.
20. Lieberman, D.N. and Mody, I., Kindling-induced long-lasting prolongation of single NMDA channel openings occludes the effect of phosphatase inhibition, *Soc. Neurosci. Abstr.*, 21 (1995) 1113 (Abstract).
21. Löscher, W. and Hönack, D., High doses of memantine (1-amino-3, 5-dimethyladamantane) induce seizures in kindled but not in non-kindled rats, *Naunyn Schmiedebergs Arch. Pharmacol.*, 341 (1990) 476–481.
22. Löscher, W. and Hönack, D., Effects of the competitive NMDA receptor antagonist, CGP 37849, on anticonvulsant activity and adverse effects of valproate in amygdala-kindled rats, *Eur. J. Pharmacol.*, 234 (1993) 237–245.
23. Masukawa, L.M., Higashima, M., Hart, G.J., Spencer, D.D. and O'Connor, M.J., NMDA receptor activation during epileptiform responses in the dentate gyrus of epileptic patients, *Brain Res.*, 562 (1991) 176–180.
24. McBain, C.J. and Mayer, M.L., N-methyl-D-aspartic acid receptor structure and function, *Physiol. Rev.*, 74 (1994) 723–760.
25. McNamara, J.O., Yeh, G., Bonhaus, D.W., Okazaki, M.M. and Nadler, J.V., NMDA receptor plasticity in the kindling model, *Adv. Exp. Med. Biol.*, 268 (1990) 451–459.
26. McNamara, J.O., Excitatory amino acid receptors and epilepsy, *Curr. Opin. Neurol. Neurosurg.*, 6 (1993) 583–587.
27. McNamara, J., Cellular and molecular basis of epilepsy, *J. Neurosci.*, 14 (1994) 3413–3425.
28. McNamara, J., Analyses of the molecular basis of kindling development, *Psychiatry. and Clin. Neurosci.*, 49 (1995) S175–8.
29. Meldrum, B.S., The role of glutamate in epilepsy and other CNS disorders, *Neurology*, 44 (1994) S14–23.
30. Mody, I. and Miller, JJ, Levels of hippocampal calcium and zinc following kindling-induced epilepsy, *Can. J. Physiol. Pharmacol.*, 63 (1985) 159–161.
31. Mody, I. and Heinemann, U., NMDA receptors of dentate gyrus granule cells participate in synaptic transmission following kindling, *Nature*, 326 (1987) 701–704.
32. Mody, I., Stanton, P.K. and Heinemann, U., Activation of *N*-methyl-D-aspartate receptors parallels changes in cellular and synaptic properties of dentate gyrus granule cells after kindling, *J. Neurophysiol.* 59 (1988) 1033–1054.
33. Mody, I., The molecular basis of kindling, *Brain Pathol.,* 3 (1993) 395–403.
34. Momiyama, A., Feldmeyer, D. and Cull-Candy, S.G., Identification of a native low-conductance NMDA channel with reduced sensitivity to Mg^{2+} in rat central neurones, *J. Physiol. (Lond)*, 494 (1996) 479–492.
35. Peters, S., Koh, J. and Choi, D.W., Zinc selectivity blocks the action of *N*-methyl-D-aspartate on cortical neurons., *Science*, 236 (1987) 589–593.
36. Pratt, G.D., Kokaia, M., Bengzon, J., Kokaia, Z, Fritschy, J.-M., Mohler, H. and Lindvall, O., Differential regulation of *N*-methyl-D-aspartate receptor subunit messenger RNAs in kindling-induced epileptogenesis, *Neuroscience*, 57 (1993) 307–318.
37. Raman, I.M., Tong, G. and Jahr, C.E., B-adrenergic regulation of synaptic NMDA receptors by cAMP-dependent protein kinase, *Neuron*, 16 (1996) 415–421.

38. Rassendren, F.A., Lory, P., Pin, J.P. and Nargeot, J., Zinc has opposite effects on NMDA and non-NMDA receptors expressed in Xenopus oocytes, *Neuron*, 4 (1990) 733–740.
39. Roche, K., Tingley, W.G. and Huganir, R.L., Glutamate receptor phosphorylation and synaptic plasticity, *Curr. Opin. Neurobiol.*, 4 (1994) 383–388.
40. Sakurada, K., Masu, M. and Nadanishi, S., Alteration of Ca^{2+} permeability and sensitivity to Mg^{2+} and channel blockers by a single amino acid substitution in the *N*-methyl-D-aspartate receptor, *J. Biol. Chem.*, 268 (1993) 410–415.
41. Schoepfer, R., Monyer, H., Sommer, B., Wisden, W., Sprengel, R., Kuner, T., Lomeli, H., Herb, A., Köhler, M., Burnashev, N., Gunther, W., Ruppersberg, P. and Seeburg, P., Molecular biology of glutamate receptors, *Prog. Neurobiol.*, 42 (1994) 353–357.
42. Schwartzkroin, P.A., Epilepsy: Models, mechanisms, and concepts. Cambridge, UK: Cambridge University Press, (1993).
43. Seeburg, P. H., Burnashev, N., Köhr, G., Kuner, T., Sprengel, R., and Monyer, H., The NMDA receptor channel: molecular design of a coincidence detector, *Rec. Prog. Horm. Res.*, 50 (1995) 19–34.
44. Soltesz, I., Zhou, Z., Smith, G.M. and Mody, I., Rapid turnover rate of the hippocampal synaptic NMDA-R1 receptor subunits, *Neurosci. Lett.*, 181 (1994) 5–8.
45. Stern, P., Cik, M., Colquhoun, D. and Stephenson, F.A., Single channel properties of cloned NMDA receptors in a human cell line: comparison with results from Xenopus oocytes, *J. Physiol. (Lond)*, 476 (1994) 391–397.
46. Tong, G., Shepherd, D. and Jahr, C.A., Synaptic desensitization of NMDA receptors by calcineurin, *Science*, 267 (1995) 1510–1512.
47. Urban, L., Aitken, P.G., Friedman, A. and Somjen, G.G., An NMDA-mediated component of excitatory synaptic input to dentate granule cells in 'epileptic' human hippocampus studied in vitro, *Brain Res.*, 515 (1990) 319–322.
48. Vezzani, A., Speciale, C., Della Vedova, F., Tamburin, M. and Benatti, L., NMDAR1 mRNA splice variants at the C-terminal but not at the N-terminal domain are altered in the kindled hippocampus, *Soc. Neurosci. Abstr.*, 21 (1995) 1475 (Abstract).
49. Wahlestedt, C., Golanov, E., Yamamoto, S., Yee, F., Ericson, H., Yoo, H., Inturrisi, C.E. and Reis, D.J., Antisense oligodeoxynucleotides to NMDA-R1 receptor channel protect cortical neurons from excitotoxicity and reduce focal ischaemic infarctions, *Nature*, 363 (1993) 260–263.
50. Wang, L.Y., Orser, B.A., Brautigan, D.L. and MacDonald, J.F., Regulation of NMDA receptors in cultured hippocampal neurons by protein phosphatases 1 and 2A, *Nature*, 369 (1994) 230–232.
51. Wang, Y.T. and Salter, M.W., Regulation of NMDA receptors by tyrosine kinases and phosphatases, *Nature*, 369 (1994) 233–235.
52. Wang, X.T., Culotta, V.C. and Klee, C.B., Superoxide dismutase protects calcineurin from inactivation, *Nature*, 383 (1996) 434–437.
53. Wlaz, P., Ebert, U. and Löscher, W., Low doses of the glycine/NMDA receptor antagonist R-(+)-HA-966 but not D-cycloserine induce paroxysmal activity in limbic brain regions of kindled rats, *Eur. J. Neurosci.*, 6 (1994) 1710–1719.
54. Yeh, G.C, Bonhaus, D.W., Nadler, J.V. and McNamara, J.O., *N*-methyl-D-aspartate receptor plasticity in kindling: quantitative and qualitative alterations in the *N*-methyl-D-aspartate receptor-channel complex., *Proc. Natl. Acad. Sci. U S A*, 86 (1989) 8157–8160.
55. Zukin, R.S. and Bennett, M.V., Alternatively spliced isoforms of the NMDARI receptor subunit, *TINS*, 18 (1995) 306–313.

DISCUSSION OF ISTVAN MODY'S PAPER

J. McNamara: Is there an effect of okadaic acid on the NMDA channel openings of human TLE granule cells?

I. Mody: In the few cells we hae examined, it appears that just like in kindled neurons, okadaic acid or FK-506 is ineffective in prolonging the NMDA channel openings in human epileptic granule cells.

J. Stringer: How rapidly do these changes occur during kindling?

I. Mody: This is an important point, but we haven't done a study on the progression of these changes during the early stages of kindling.

J. Stringer: Do you think such changes in NMDA channel properties could be induced by epileptiform activity in a slice preparation?

I. Mody: It is possible that the regulation of the NMDA channel function may change with a sufficiently fast time course to be monitored in a slice, but we have no experimental evidence for this.

F. Lopes Da Silva: Have you looked at the degree of hippocampal sclerosis in these patients, and if so, is there any correlation of the NMDA channel activity with the different morphological alterations?

I. Mody: We are planning to do a more thorough analysis of this and to correlate all the measurements such as in vivo recordings, slice physiology, morphology, and single channel recordings. At this time, it appears that all the granule cells we have recorded from come from considerably sclerotic hippocampi.

F. Lopes Da Silva: Does the calcium change or phosphorylation have any effect on GABA receptors?

I. Mody: We have not yet examined GABA receptor function in the human TLE cells. All we know in rat granule cells is that calcium has a biphasic effect on synaptic $GABA_A$ receptors. A moderate rise in calcium seems to have a potentiating effect, whereas at concentrations in excess of 1 μM it seems to reduce the function of synaptic $GABA_A$ channels.

7

LONG-LASTING CHANGES IN THE PHARMACOLOGY AND ELECTROPHYSIOLOGY OF AMINO ACID RECEPTORS IN AMYGDALA KINDLED NEURONS

Patricia Shinnick-Gallagher, N. Bradley Keele, and Volker Neugebauer

Department of Pharmacology and Toxicology
University of Texas Medical Branch
301 University Boulevard
Galveston, Texas 77555-1031

1. INTRODUCTION

The amygdala, an almond-shaped area of the limbic brain, is particularly sensitive to kindling.[10,29,66] One nucleus of the amygdala, the basolateral nucleus, is most often used to induce kindling.[9,20,28,47] Basolateral amygdala (BLA) neurons are divided morphologically[31,32] and electrophysiologically[51,63] into two major classes of neurons: the principal class is comprised of pyramidal and stellate cells, and the smaller proportion of cells are interneurons. Glutamatergic cells are found throughout the nucleus[34] and the stria terminalis (ST), a major bidirectional pathway of the amygdala, contains glutamatergic afferent fibers projecting to the BLA.[42] The BLA also receives input from the lateral amygdala (LA) and is reported to have recurrent projections.[26,58] The BLA contains moderate amounts of γ-aminobutyric acid (GABA)[8] and GABA immunoreactivity.[11,43] Morphologically, interneurons comprising ~ 5% of the cells[31] have been classified as GABAergic[33] and form synapses with the principal cell types. Lesioning the afferent ST pathway did not reduce GABA content, suggesting GABA neurons in the BLA are intrinsic.[8]

Glutamate, the major excitatory neurotransmitter in the brain, activates two classes of receptors: 1) ionotropic receptors which are linked directly to ion channels and 2) metabotropic glutamate receptors (mGluRs) which are coupled to second messenger systems via G-proteins.[17,45] Ionotropic receptors can be further divided into N-methyl-D-aspartate (NMDA) receptors, and non-NMDA types comprised of α-amino-3-hydroxy-5-methyl-4-isoxazolepropionic acid (AMPA) and kainate (KA) subtypes.[17] Similarly, mGluRs, of which there are eight subtypes, are further divided into three subgroups based on their signal transduction, sequence homology, and pharmacological properties.[45]

Kindling 5, edited by Corcoran and Moshé.
Plenum Press, New York, 1998.

GABA, an inhibitory neurotransmitter in the central nervous system, activates two classes of receptors: ionotropic $GABA_A$ receptors which are linked to chloride channels, and metabotropic $GABA_B$ receptors coupled ion channels through G-proteins.[24,36,46]

2. ELECTROPHYSIOLOGY AND KINDLING PARADIGMS

In all our studies we recorded using sharp or whole-cell patch electrodes with current and voltage clamp from BLA neurons in a submerged brain slice preparation.[5,14,38,52] In our early studies[4,5,11,14,52] animals with electrodes in the amygdala were kindled using the classical Goddard[16] paradigm of applying a train (60Hz, 500μA) of stimuli (1 sec) once a day and monitoring seizure severity using the ranking scale of Racine.[48] Amygdala slices contralateral to the stimulation site were then prepared 28 days after the last kindled seizure. In more recent studies,[19,38] stimuli were applied twice daily and slices prepared 5 to 14 days after the last kindled seizure. In our later studies we used ipsilateral and contralateral amygdalae for recording.

3. SYNAPTIC TRANSMISSION IN THE AMYGDALA: IONOTROPIC GLUTAMATE RECEPTORS AND KINDLING

Synaptic potentials can be elicited in the BLA through stimulating afferents contained in the stria terminalis (ST) or lateral amygdala (LA). We analyzed the contribution of ionotropic glutamatergic receptor subtypes to excitatory transmission in the BLA in neurons from control[49] and kindled[14,52] animals. Stimulating the ST or LA evoked an excitatory postsynaptic potential (EPSP) followed either by a fast inhibitory postsynaptic potential (fast-IPSP) or by a fast- and subsequent slow-IPSP. The EPSP increased in amplitude over a several volt range (Fig. 1)[5,38] and consisted of fast and slow glutamatergic components.[49] The fast-EPSP was mediated through non-NMDA receptors and blocked by 6-cyano-7-nitroquinoxaline-2,3-dione (CNQX), a AMPA/KA receptor antagonist; the slow EPSP was sensitive to 2-amino-5-phosphonovaleric acid (APV), an NMDA receptor antagonist.[49]

In kindled neurons, stimulating either the ST or LA pathways evoked epileptiform activity consisting of primary and secondary bursts elicited at lower stimulus intensities than control synaptic potentials (Fig. 1).[5,14,38,52] The EPSP amplitude in kindled neurons

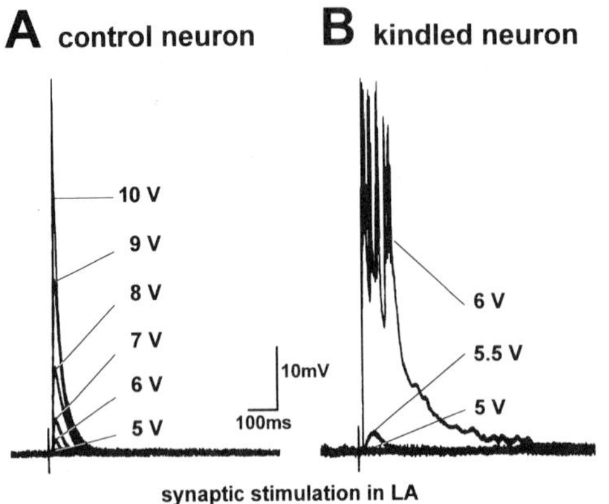

Figure 1. Epileptiform bursting and a steep input-output relationship for synaptic responses are characteristics of amygdala-kindled BLA neurons. A, Monosynaptic responses of a control BLA neuron to electrical stimulation (5–10 V; 150 μs) in the lateral amygdala (LA). EPSP threshold was 6 V while 10 V were required to elicit an action potential. B, Epileptiform bursting induced in a kindled BLA neuron by stimulating the LA. The input-output relationship of the kindled neuron is steeper than that of the control neuron; increasing the stimulus intensity by only 0.5 V above the EPSP threshold elicits bursting. In A and B are superimposed single traces. Membrane potential = –60 mV; recorded under whole cell patch conditions.

increased from threshold to action potential firing over a one volt range.[5,38] These data suggested that synaptic transmission was dramatically affected in kindled neurons whereas basic electrophysiological membrane properties were not affected.[4,14,52]

Superfusing APV attenuated secondary[14,52] but did not block primary epileptiform bursting. In contrast, adding CNQX completely blocked epileptiform activity and unmasked the presence of an NMDA receptor mediated slow-EPSP. The amplitude of the NMDA receptor mediated EPSP was greater in kindled than control neurons,[52] suggesting that epileptiform bursting is mediated through non-NMDA receptors and that NMDA and non-NMDA receptor mediated synaptic transmission is enhanced in amygdala kindled neurons.

4. GABAERGIC SYNAPTIC TRANSMISSION IN CONTROL AND KINDLED AMYGDALA NEURONS

4.1. $GABA_A$ Receptors

Stimulating the ST afferents to BLA neurons evokes two IPSPs: a fast-IPSP and a slow-IPSP. Both IPSPs can be reduced by APV and blocked by CNQX, suggesting polysynaptic transmission in IPSP circuitry and the presence of feed-forward inhibition onto BLA neurons.[50] The fast-IPSP is mediated through $GABA_A$ receptors linked to a chloride channel and is blocked by bicuculline,[50] a $GABA_A$ receptor antagonist. The slow-IPSP is due to activation of postsynaptic $GABA_B$ receptors and depressed by the $GABA_B$ receptor antagonist, 2-hydroxysaclofen.[50] In contrast, stimulating the lateral nucleus elicits in some cells, a CNQX-resistant fast-IPSP[52,65] which is subsequently blocked by bicuculline,[52] suggesting direct inhibition of BLA neurons by GABAergic LA interneurons.

In kindled BLA neurons there are also differences in the two afferent pathways to the BLA. When the ST afferent pathway is stimulated, epileptiform bursting is recorded but no fast- or slow-IPSPs (Fig. 1,2); spontaneous IPSPs are also not observed.[14,52] This reduction in GABAergic transmission was reflected in a decrease of GABA-immunoreactive neurons in the amygdala 2 to 6 months after the last kindled seizure.[11] In contrast, stimulating the LA afferent to the BLA in kindled neurons elicits epileptiform bursting which is blocked by CNQX but unmasks a fast-IPSP followed by a slow-EPSP (Fig 2).[52] Blocking the slow-EPSP reveals a pure fast-IPSP, suggesting that the loss of GABAergic IPSP in kindled neurons is pathway specific.[52]

A pervasive question in studying mechanisms of epileptogenesis is whether epileptiform activity is due to enhanced excitation, disinhibition, or both. We compared NMDA-mediated slow-EPSPs in BLA neurons from control and kindled animals in the presence of bicuculline and CNQX. Kindling caused a significant increase in the slow-EPSP amplitude compared to control, suggesting that disinhibition in kindled neurons is not sufficient enough to account for the increased excitatory transmission.[52]

4.2. $GABA_B$ Receptors

$GABA_B$ receptors are reported to mediate slow IPSPs and to negatively regulate excitatory and inhibitory transmission. Presynaptic $GABA_B$ receptors located on glutamatergic afferents or GABAergic neurons can be activated by endogenous GABA.[24,36] Baclofen, a $GABA_B$ receptor agonist, has a postsynaptic hyperpolarizing action and reduces excitatory and inhibitory synaptic transmission by a presynaptic action on nerve terminals.[24,36] Baclofen has been used in different models of epilepsy with mixed results.

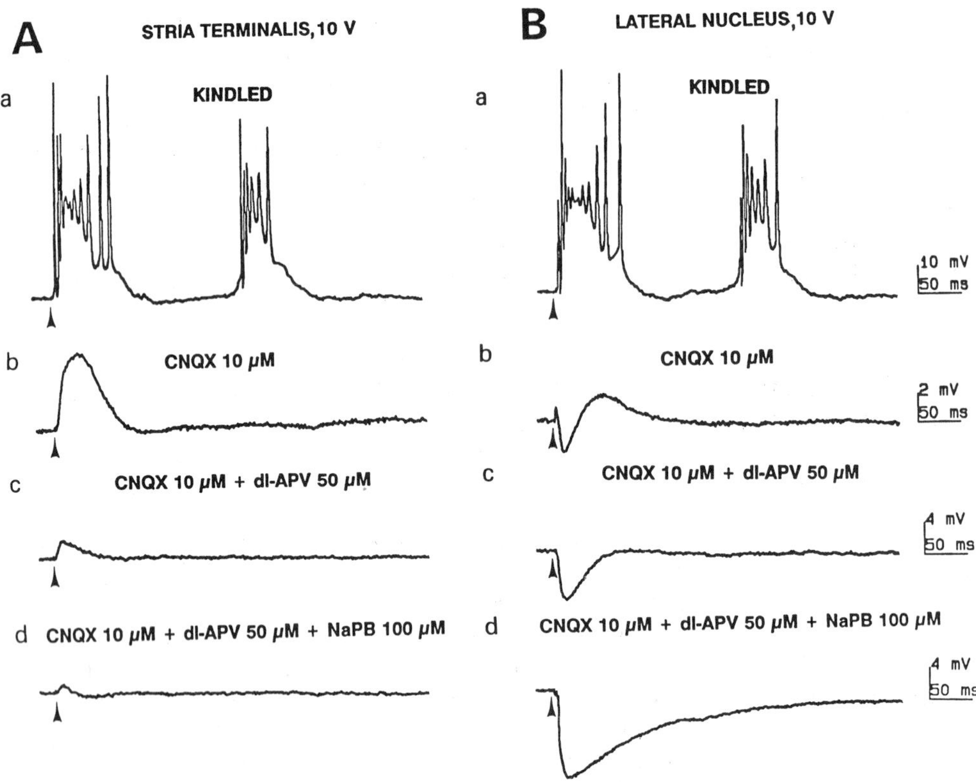

Figure 2. Kindling abolishes feedforward inhibition in BLA neurons. Aa: ST stimulation (10 V, ↑) evoked burst firing in BLA neuron from a kindled animal. Ba: in the same neuron LA stimulation (10 V, ↑) also evoked burst firing. Ab: in the presence of (CNQX) (10 μM), ST stimulation evoked an s-EPSP. Bb: in contrast, LA stimulation evoked a biphasic potential, consisting of an f-IPSP and subsequent s-EPSP. Ac: superfusion of CNQX (10 μM) and APV (50 μM) abolished the s-EPSP. Bc: f-IPSP evoked by LA stimulation was resistant to both CNQX and APV. Ad: in the presence of CNQX, APV, and sodium pentobarbital (NaPB, 100 μM), no IPSP component was recorded on stimulation of the ST pathway. Bd: IPSP evoked by LA stimulation was increased in both amplitude and duration in the presence of NaPB. Note the RMP was −65 mV throughout. Reprinted with permission.[52]

In the BLA balcofen depressed EPSPs in control and kindled neurons, but the EC_{50} was shifted 100 fold from 5nM in control to 500 nM in kindled neurons (Fig. 3B).[5] When these data were fitted to a two site model, the high affinity component was reduced and converted to a low affinity site.[5] The reduced sensitivity of presynaptic $GABA_B$ receptors was also observed when postsynaptic $GABA_A$ and $GABA_B$ receptors were blocked, suggesting that this effect could not be due to a loss of GABAergic inhibition in kindled neurons.

Baclofen also hyperpolarized control and kindled amygdala neurons, an effect accompanied by an increase in conductance. Current-voltage relationships obtained in control and kindled neurons showed that the reversal potential for the baclofen hyperpolarization was not changed. The concentration-response relationship for baclofen was only shifted slightly to the right and there was no change in the EC_{50} for both populations of animals (Fig. 3A). The pre- and postsynaptic actions of baclofen were pharmacologically distinct, the latter but not the former being blocked by 2-hydroxysaclofen and pertussis toxin (PTX) pretreatment. These data show that kindling-induced epileptogenesis reduces the sensitivity of presynaptic $GABA_B$ receptors, an effect which may contribute to

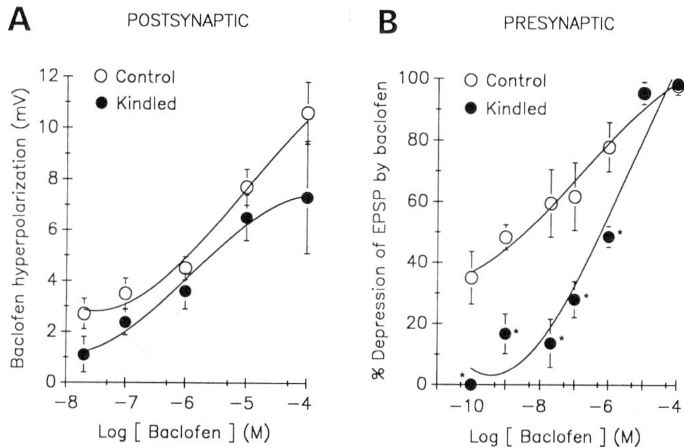

Figure 3. Kindling reduces the sensitivity of pre- but not postsynaptic $GABA_B$ receptors. A, Concentration-response curves for the baclofen-induced hyperpolarization are not significantly different in neurons from control (○) and kindled (●) animals. Amplitude of the baclofen hyperpolarizations is plotted as a function of concentration of baclofen (log scale). The curve was fitted to mean values by a least-squares routine; B, percentage of reduction in EPSP amplitude (mean ± S.E.M.) is plotted as a function of baclofen concentration (log scale). ○ and ●, experimental data from four to seven cells for each concentration applied (control: n = 27, 17 animals; kindled: n = 26, 12 animals). Data were analyzed using an analysis of variance test for repeated measures. *Points of significance for P <.01. Reprinted with permission.[5]

the enhancement of excitatory transmission in kindled animals. The distinct pharmacology of the pre- and postsynaptic $GABA_B$ receptors suggest that there may be two different populations of $GABA_B$ receptors in the amygdala whose long-lasting modification in kindling-induced seizures is different.[5]

5. METABOTROPIC GLUTAMATE RECEPTORS (mGluRS) IN KINDLING

mGluRs are activated by quisqualate (QUIS), glutamate and selective analogues for mGluRs, (1S,3R)-1-aminocyclopentane-1,3-dicarboxylic acid (1S,3R-ACPD),[44] (2S,3S,4S)-α-carboxycyclopropyl-glycine (L-CCG),[22] and L-aminophosphonobutyric acid (L-AP4)[37]. As mentioned previously, mGluRs are currently divided into three subgroups. Group I subtypes consist of mGluR1 and mGluR5 and their splice variants and have relative agonist potencies of: QUIS > L-CCG > 1S,3R-ACPD. Group II is comprised of mGluR2 and mGluR3 and exhibits different agonist potencies (L-CCG > 1S,3R-ACPD > QUIS) while group III, consisting of mGluRs 4, 6, 7 and 8, is activated by L-AP4.[44,54] In general, the first group is coupled to phospholipase C, resulting in phosphoinositide (PI) hydrolysis and subsequent intracellular Ca mobilization and activation of protein kinase C (PKC); the latter two are coupled to inhibition of adenosine-3′,5′-cyclicmonophosphate (cAMP) formation, although mGluRs have been found to be coupled to other second messenger systems.[44]

Of the eight cloned mGluRs to date, mRNA for mGluR2[39], mGluR3[40] and mGluR7[24,38] in moderate densities, together with mGluR1[59] and mGluR4[26] in lower densities, is expressed within the BLA; moderate levels of immunoreactivity for mGluR1α[7,29] and mGluR5[55] are also observed in the BLA.

Metabotropic glutamate receptors are altered in kindling. Excitatory amino acid (EAA)-stimulated PI hydrolysis is increased in the amygdala after kindling.[3,20] The kindling-induced increase in EAA-stimulated PI hydrolysis persisted up to 4 weeks in the amygdala regardless of the site of stimulation[2] and these effects could be reproduced with 1S,3R-ACPD.[1,63]

Studies *in vivo* have shown that mGluR agonists and antagonists can elicit convulsant and anticonvulsant activity. Intrahippocampal injection of 1S,3R-ACPD can produce delayed seizures and neuronal injury in adult rats,[34] In mice, intracerebral[61] or intrathalamic[60] injection of 1S,3R-ACPD or L-CCG induces limbic seizures; 1S,3R-ACPD-induced seizures can be attenuated by low doses of L-CCG or L-AP4.[60,61] Injecting 1S,3R-ACPD into the amygdala of rats produced immediate but transient limbic seizures. This effect was not observed in kindled animals.[59] In amygdala kindled rats, intra-amygdala injection of 1S,3R-ACPD or L-AP4 resulted in marked suppression of kindled seizures.[59] Intracerebral injection of a presynaptic agonist 1S,3S-ACPD, a congener of 1S,3R-ACPD, prevented kindling development and increased seizure threshold in kindled animals.[6]

5.1. Amygdala Postsynaptic mGluRs in Control and Kindled Animals

5.1.1. mGluR-Mediated Hyperpolarizations and outward Currents. BLA neurons can be divided on the basis of their repetitive firing properties into accommodating and non-accommodating cells.[50] Accommodating neurons cease firing in response to a long depolarizing current injection of 400–500 ms. Control and kindled BLA neurons do not differ in their accommodation properties.[4]

Activation of postsynaptic mGluRs by 1S,3R-ACPD results in a membrane hyperpolarization associated with a decrease in membrane resistance or a hyperpolarization followed by a membrane depolarization[53] in ~ 90% of accommodating BLA neurons.[18]

This mGluR agonist-induced hyperpolarization is insensitive to tetrodotoxin, dependent on extracellular K^+ concentrations, sensitive to tetraethylammonium (TEA, 1mM), a potassium channel blocker, and has a reversal potential close to the equilibrium potential for K^+, E_K.[18,53] The hyperpolarization is mediated through G-proteins and is sensitive to intracellular and extracellular calcium concentrations.[53] 1S,3R-ACPD induces membrane hyperpolarizations or outward currents in a concentration-dependent manner. The rank order of potency for mGluR agonists is consistent with a group II-like mGluR.[18] Further experiments showed that the mGluR-induced response was blocked by iberiotoxin, a selective blocker of large conductance (BK) calcium-dependent K channels, and by pretreatment with PTX. These data suggest that the mGluR-induced outward current is due to activation of BK channels mediated through a group II-like mGluR linked to a PTX-sensitive G-protein in BLA neurons.[18] Furthermore, the mGluR-induced hyperpolarization is observed in the different morphological classes of BLA neurons,[53] but is primarily recorded in neurons which accommodated, suggesting that non-accommodating interneurons do not possess this group II-like mGluR.

In amygdala kindled neurons, the incidence of mGluR-induced hyperpolarization was reduced significantly (Fig. 4). L-CCG, which evokes a hyperpolarization or outward current in accommodating control BLA neurons, has no significant postsynaptic action in kindled BLA neurons.[19] 1S,3R-ACPD induced membrane hyperpolarizations or outward currents in accommodating control BLA neurons but only depolarized accommodating kindled neurons (Fig 4).[19]

5.1.2. mGluR-Induced Depolarizations and Inward Currents. 1S,3R-ACPD depolarized non-accommodating BLA neurons and produced a membrane depolarization followed by a hyperpolarization in the majority of accommodating neurons.[18,19] The 1S,3R-ACPD-

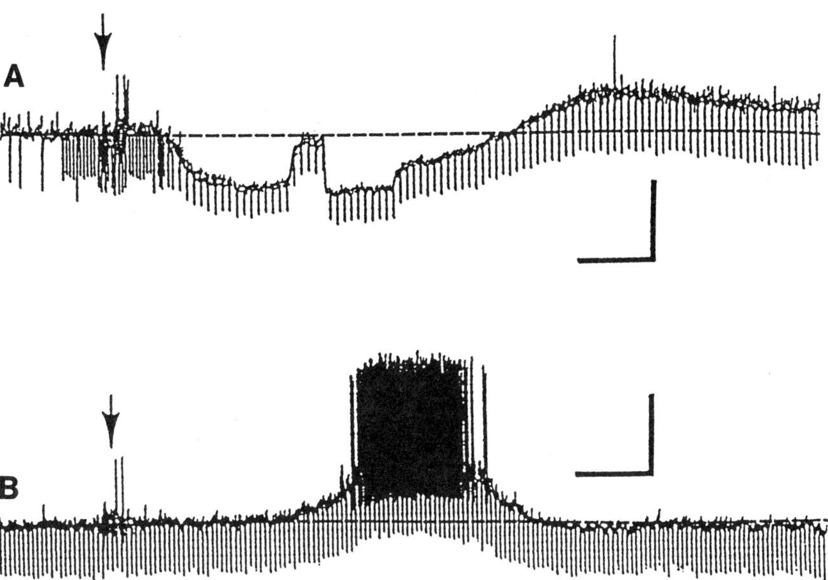

Figure 4. Response to trans-ACPD in control and kindled neurons of the basolateral amygdala. A, Membrane hyperpolarization induced by drop application of 1S,3R-ACPD (arrow; equivalent to 40 μM bath concentration) accompanied by an increase in conductance. During the hyperpolarization, the membrane was returned to control levels to ensure that the conductance change was not due to membrane rectification. A membrane depolarization associated with a decrease in conductance followed the membrane hyperpolarization. RMP = –63 mV. B, In a neuron from a kindled animal, drop application of trans-ACPD (arrow) cause a delayed membrane depolarization. The membrane conductance was decreased in individual electrotonic potentials although obscured by cell firing in the record. RMP = –61 mV. Downward deflections represent electronic potentials generated in response to injecting 200-ms, 0.1-nA current pulses across the membrane as a measure of membrane resistance. Calibration: 10 mV × 20 s. Reprinted with permission.[13]

induced inward current recorded with sharp electrodes is associated with two types of current-voltage (I-V) relationship showing: 1) a decreased conductance in about one half of the neurons. In ≈ 30% of those neurons, the I-V curves intersected around –87mV, which is close to E_K; the remaining neurons had extrapolated reversal potentials more negative than –120mV, suggesting activation of a mixed response; and 2) a parallel shift with no intersection and no change in conductance (Arvanov, Keele and Shinnick-Gallagher, unpublished observations).

Under whole cell patch recording condition, QUIS (50μM) produced an inward current in the presence of D-APV (50μM), CNQX (30μM) and TTX (1μM) not associated with a change in membrane slope conductance (G_M) between –110 and –50mV. In contrast, the 1S,3R-ACPD-induced inward current was accompanied by a decrease in conductance. Adding Ba^{2+} (2mM) and Cs^+ (2mM) to block K^+ conductances did not alter the QUIS (50μM)-induced inward current, I_{QUIS}, but almost completely blocked the current evoked by 1S,3R-ACPD (50μM) while the current evoked by higher concentrations (100–200μM) was enhanced. Like I_{QUIS}, the 1S,3R-ACPD-evoked current remaining in Ba/Cs solution was not associated with a conductance change. This current was activated more potently by QUIS than by 1S,3R-ACPD.[23] Inclusion of the Na^+–Ca^{2+} exchange inhibitory peptide (XIP) in the recording electrode reduced or abolished I_{QUIS} but not the

1S,3R-ACPD inward current associated with a decrease in conductance.[23] These data suggest that I_{QUIS} is due to activation of the electrogenic Na^+–Ca^{2+} exchange current.

Concentration-response relationships for the 1S,3R-ACPD-induced inward current were analyzed in control and kindled non-accommodating BLA neurons. The EC_{50} for 1S,3R-ACPD was shifted to the left in kindled neurons and the maximum response was increased.[19] The 1S,3R-ACPD-elicited inward current recorded in kindled neurons was associated with a conductance decrease. A similar response has been reported to be mediated through group I mGluRs.[12,15]

These studies have shown that the incidence of mGluR-evoked hyperpolarization or outward current is reduced in kindled neurons and the mGluR activated inward current is enhanced. The receptor mediating the membrane hyperpolarization is similar to a group II-like mGluR, while the receptor underlying the membrane depolarization has electrophysiological characteristics of a group I mGluR. These data suggest that in kindled neurons postsynaptic group II-like mGluRs may be downregulated while group I mGluRs are upregulated.[19]

5.2. Presynaptic mGluRs and Kindling

In BLA neurons, mGluR agonists 1S,3R-ACPD and L-AP4, depress excitatory synaptic transmission through a presynaptic mechanism.[54] The group II mGluR agonist, L-CCG, potently depressed monosynaptic excitatory post-synaptic currents (EPSCs) elicited on stimulating the LA, a concentration-dependent effect, whereas the group III specific agonist, L-AP4, was less potent in depressing EPSCs (Fig 5). Although L-CCG can activate group I and II mGluRs, the concentrations used are selective for group II mGluRs.[37,45] The agonist potency of L-CCG and L-AP4 for the two presynaptic mGluRs is dramatically increased in kindled neurons (Fig 5).[38] In control neurons, EPSC amplitudes were depressed ≈ 80% by L-CCG or L-AP4 at the highest concentrations tested (100 μM) whereas, in kindled neurons, complete inhibition of EPSC amplitude occurred at lower concentrations. These agonists also suppressed synaptically-induced bursting in kindled

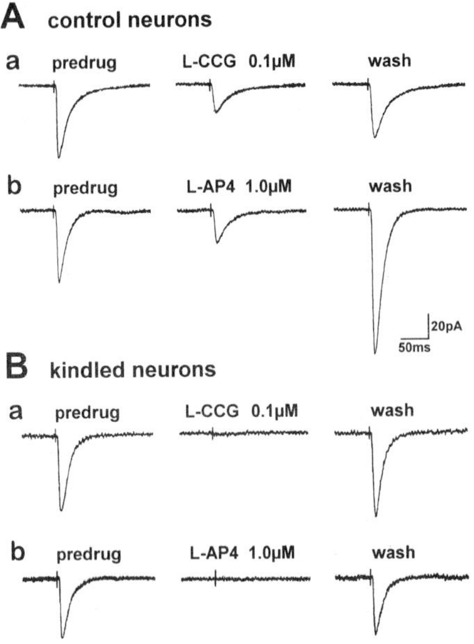

Figure 5. The group II mGluR agonist L-CCG (Aa and Ba) and the group III mGluR agonist L-AP4 (Ab and Bb) completely block synaptic transmission in kindled neurons (B) whereas in control neurons (A) the same concentrations only reduce EPSC amplitude. The traces show EPSCs recorded in different BLA neurons elicited by stimulating the LA (Aa: 10 V, Ab: 12 V, Ba: 7 Vm, Bb: 6 V; 150 μs). Each trace is an average of 6–9 EPSCs recorded immediately before drug addition (predrug), after 10 min in L-CCG (0.1 μM) or L-AP4 (1.0 μM), and after 15 min of washing with control ACSF (wash). A, In control neurons, L-CCG (1.0 μM) and a 10 fold higher concentration of L-AP4 reduced the EPSCs by more than 50%. The depression by L-CCG was slowly reversible whereas a long-lasting (> 55 min) potentiation was typically observed after superfusion with L-AP4. B, In amygdala-kindled neurons, L-CCG (0.1 μM) and L-AP4 (1.0 μM) completely and reversibly blocked EPSCs. Calibration as in Ab; V_{HOLD} = –60 mV.

neurons.[38] Neither L-CCG (up to 10μM) nor L-AP4 (up to 50μM) induced changes in postsynaptic membrane conductance or membrane current. mGluR antagonists specific for group II and group III mGluRs themselves did not significantly affect transmission, suggesting that these presynaptic mGluRs are not activated endogenously under the stimulation conditions used in these experiments. The enhanced depression of synaptic activity in kindling and the lack of intrinsic activation suggest that presynaptic group II and group III mGluRs might be targets for treatment of excessive synaptic activation in epilepsy.[38]

In conclusion, our laboratory has shown that in amygdala neurons from kindled animals:

1. Epileptiform bursting is mediated by non-NMDA receptors.
2. The amplitude of the NMDA component of the EPSP is enhanced.
3. The threshold for action potential firing is lowered resulting in (or contributing to) an increase in the input-output relationship.
4. There is a pathway specific loss of GABAergic IPSPs.
5. Postsynaptic $GABA_B$ receptors are not significantly affected.
6. Presynaptic $GABA_B$ receptor mediated responses are decreased in affinity and efficacy.
7. This decrease in tonic presynaptic inhibition could contribute to epileptiform bursting in kindled neurons.
8. Outward currents mediated by a group II mGluR are lost in kindled neurons.
9. mGluR-mediated inward currents most likely mediated through a group I mGluR are enhanced.
10. These data suggest that postsynaptic group II mGluRs are down regulated and group I mGluRs are up regulated in kindled neurons.
11. This loss of mGluR outward current and mGluR inward current could contribute to epileptiform bursting in kindled animals.
12. Group II and group III mGluR agonists depress synaptic transmission in control amygdala neurons.
13. In kindled neurons there is an increase in the affinity of group II and group III mGluR agonists for their receptors in kindled animals.
14. These data suggest that the changes in pre- and postsynaptic group II. mGluRs are different in kindled neurons.
15. Finally, the exquisite sensitivity of the presynaptic mGluR receptors for their agonists may offer a new therapeutic avenue in the treatment of temporal lobe epilepsy.

ACKNOWLEDGMENTS

Supported by NIH Grant NS 24643 and The Deutsche Forschungsgemeinschaft.

REFERENCES

1. Akiyama, K., Daigen, A., Yamada, N., Itoh, T., Kohira, Il, Ujike, H. and Otsuki, S. Long-lasting enhancement of metabotropic excitatory amino acid receptor-mediated polyphosphoinositide hydrolysis in the amygdala/piriform cortex of deep piriform cortical kindled rats. *Brain Res.*, 569 (1992) 71–77.
2. Akiyama, K., Yamada, N. and Otsuki, S. Lasting increase in excitatory amino acid receptor-mediated polyphosphoinositide hydrolysis in the amygdala/piriform cortex of amygdala-kindled rats. *Brain Res.*, 485 (1989) 95–101.

3. Akiyama, K., Yamada, N. and Sato, M. Increase in ibotenate-stimulated phosphotidylinositol hydrolysis in slices of the amygdala/pyriform cortex and hippocampus of rat by amygdala kindling. *Exp. Neurol.*, 98 (1987) 499–508.
4. Asprodini, E., Rainnie, D.G., Anderson, A.C. and Shinnick-Gallagher, P. *In vivo* kindling does not alter afterhyperpolarizations (AHPs) following action potential firing *in vitro* in basolateral amygdala neurons. *Brain Res.*, 588 (1992) 329–334.
5. Asprodini, E.K., Rainnie, D.G. and Shinnick-Gallagher, P. Epileptogenesis reduces the sensitivity of presynaptic $GABA_B$ receptors on glutamatergic afferents in the amygdala. *J. Pharmacol. Exp. Ther.*, 262 (1992) 1011–1021.
6. Attwell, P.J.E., Kaura, S., Sigala, G., Gradford, H.F., Croucher, M.J., Jane, D.E. and Watkins, J.C. Blockade of both epileptogenesis and glutamate release by (1S,3S)-ACPD, a presynaptic glutamate receptor agonist. *Brain Res.*, 698 (1995) 155–162.
7. Baude, A., Nusser, Z., Roberts, J.D.B., Mulvihill, E., McIlhinney R.A.J., and Olney, J.W. Distribution of metabotropic glutamate receptor mGluR5 immunoreactivity in rat brain. *J. Comp. Neurol.*, 355 (1995) 455–469.
8. Ben-Ari, Y., Kanazawa, I. and Zigmond, R.E. Regional distribution of glutamate decarboxylase and GABA within the amygdaloid complex and stria terminalis system of the rat. *J. Neurochem.*, 26 (1976) 1279–1283.
9. Burnham, W.M. Primary and transfer seizure development in the kindled rat. *Can. J. Neurol. Sci.*, 2 (1975) 417–429.
10. Cain, D.P., Desborough, K.A. and McKitrick, D.J. Retardation of amygdala kindling by antagonism of NMD-aspartate and muscarinic cholinergic receptors: evidence for the summation of excitatory mechanisms in kindling. *Exp. Neurol.*, 100 (1988) 179–187.
11. Callahan, P.M., Paris, J.M., Cunningham, K.A. and Shinnick-Gallagher, P. Decrease of amygdaloid GABA-immunoreactive neurons after kindling. *Brain Res.* 555 (1991) 335–339.
12. Davies, C.H., Clarke, V.R., Jane, D.E. and Collingridge, G.L. Pharmacology of postsynaptic metabotropic glutamate receptors in rat hippocampal CA1 pyramidal neurones. *Br. J. Pharmacol.*, 116 (1995) 1859–1869.
13. Gallagher, J.P., Zheng, F. and Shinnick-Gallagher, P. Long-lasting modulation of synaptic transmission by metabotropic glutamate receptors. In *Metabotropic Glutamate Receptors*, P.J. Conn and J. Patel (Eds.) Humana Press, Totowa, NJ.
14. Gean, P., Shinnick-Gallagher, P. and Anderson, A.C. Spontaneous epileptiform activity and alteration of GABA- and NMDA-mediated neurotransmission in amygdala neurons kindled *in vivo*. *Brain Res.* 494 (1989) 177–181.
15. Gereau, R.W. and Conn, P.J. Roles of specific metabotropic glutamate receptor subtypes in regulation of hippocampal CA1 pyramidal cell excitability. *J. Neurophysiol.*, 74 (1995) 122–129.
16. Goddard, G.V., McIntyre, D.C. and Leech, C.K. A permanent change in brain function resulting from daily electrical stimulation. *Exp. Neurol.*, 25 (1969) 295–330.
17. Hollmann, M. and Heinemann, S. Cloned glutamate receptors. *Ann. Rev. Neurosci.*, 17 (1994) 31–108.
18. Holmes, K.H., Keele, N.B., Arvanov,V.L. and Shinnick-Gallagher, P. Metabotropic glutamate receptor agonist-induced hyperpolarizations in rat basolateral amygdala neurons: Receptor characterization and ion channels. *J. Neurophysiol.*, In Press.
19. Holmes, K.H., Keele, N.B. and Shinnick-Gallagher, P. Loss of metabotropic glutamate receptor (mGluR)-mediated hyperpolarizations and increase in mGluR depolarizations in basolateral amygdala neurons in kindling-induced epilepsy. *J. Neurophysiol.*, In Press.
20. Hosford, D.A. Simonato, M., Cao, Z., Garcia-Carrasco, N., Silver, J.M., Butler, L., Shin, C. and McNamara, J.O. Differences in the anatomic distribution of immediate-early gene expression in amygdala and angular bundle kindling development. *J. Neurosci.*, 15 (1995) 2513–2523.
21. Iadorola, M.J., Nicoletti, F., Naranjo, J.R., Putnam, F. and Costa, E. Kindling enhances the stimulation of inositol phospholipid hydrolysis elicited by ibotenic acid in rat hippocampal slices. *Brain Res.*, 374 (1986) 174–178.
22. Ishida, M., Akagi, H., Shimamoto, K., Ohfune, Y. and Shinozaki, H. A potent metabotropic glutamate receptor agonist: electrophysiological actions of a conformationally restricted glutamate analogue in the rat spinal cord and Xenopus oocytes. *Brain Res.*, 537 (1990) 311–314.
23. Keele, N.B., Arvanov, V.L. and Shinnick-Gallagher, P. Quisqualate-preferring metabotropic glutamate receptor activates Na^+-Ca^{2+} exchange in rat basolateral amygdala neurons. Submitted.
24. Kerr, D.K. and Ong, J. $GABA_B$ receptors. *Pharmacol. and Therapeutics*, 67(2) (1995) 187–246.
25. Kinzie, J.M., Saugstad, J.A., Westbrook, G.L. and Segerson, T.P. Distribution of metabotropic glutamate receptor 7 messenger RNA in the developing and adult rat brain. *Neuroscience*, 69 (1995) 167–176.

26. Krettek, J.E. and Price, J.L. A description of the amygdaloid complex in the rat and cat with observations on intra-amygdaloid axonal connections. *J. Comp. Neurol.*, 178 (1978) 255–279.
27. Kristensen, P., Suzdak, P.D. and Thomsen, C. Expression pattern and pharmacology of the rat type IV metabotropic glutamate receptor. *Neurosci. Lett.*, 155 (1993) 159–162.
28. LeGal LaSalle, G. Amygdaloid kindling in the rat: regional differences and general properties. In *Kindling 2*, J.A. Wada (Ed.), Raven Press: New York, 1981, pp. 31–44.
29. Loscher, W., Ebert, V., Wahnschaffe, U. and Rundfeldt, C. Susceptibility of different cell layers of the anterior and posterior part of the piriform cortex to electrical stimulation and kindling: comparison with the basolateral amygdala and "area tempestas". *Neuroscience*, 66 (1995) 265–276.
30. Martin, L.J., Blackstone, C.D., Huganir, R.L. and Price, D.L. Cellular localization of a metabotropic glutamate receptor in rat brain. *Neuron*, 9 (1992) 259–270.
31. McDonald, A.J. Neurons of the lateral and basolateral amygdaloid nuclei: a Golgi study in the rat. *J. Comp. Neurol.*, 212 (1982) 293–312.
32. McDonald, A.J. Neuronal organization of the lateral and basolateral amygdaloid nuclei in the rat. *J. Comp. Neurol.*, 222 (1984) 589–606.
33. McDonald, A.J. Immunohistochemical identification of γ-aminobutyric acid-containing neurons in the rat basolateral amygdala. *Neurosci. Lett.*, 53 (1985a) 203–207.
34. McDonald, A.J., Beitz, A.J., Larson, A.A., Kuriyama, R., Sellitto, C. and Madl, J.E. Co-localization of glutamate and tubulin in putative excitatory neurons of the hippocampus and amygdala: an immuno-histochemical study using monoclonal antibodies. *Neuroscience,* 30 (1989) 405–421.
35. McDonald, J.W., Fix, A.S., Tizzano, J.P. and Schoepp, D.D. Seizures and brain injury in neonatal rats induced by 1S,3R-ACPD, a metabotropic glutamate receptor agonist. *J. Neurosci.*, 13 (1993) 4445–4455.
36. Misgeld, U., Bijak, M. and Jarolimek, W. A physiological role for $GABA_B$ receptors and the effects of baclofen in the mammalian central nervous system. *Progress in Neurobiol.*, 46 (1995) 423–462.
37. Nakanishi, S. Molecular diversity of glutamate receptors and implications for brain function. *Science*, 258 (1992) 597–603.
38. Neugebauer, V., Keele, N.B. and Shinnick-Gallagher, P. Increase in sensitivity of Group II and Group III metabotropic glutamate receptors (mGluRs) in epileptic neurons. Submitted.
39. Ohishi, H., Akazawa, C., Shigemoto, R., Nakanishi, S. and Mizuno, N. Distributions of the mRNAs for L-2-amino-4-phosphonobutyrate-sensitive metabotropic glutamate receptors, mGluR4 and mGluR7, in the rat brain. *J. Comp. Neurol.* 360 (1995) 555–570.
40. Ohishi, H., Shigemoto, R., Nakanishi, S. and Mizuno, N. Distribution of the messenger RNA for a metabotropic glutamate receptor, mGluR2, in the central nervous system of the rat. *Neuroscience*, 53 (1993a) 1009–1018.
41. Ohishi, H., Shigemoto, R., Nakanishi, S. and Mizuno, N. Distribution of the mRNA for a metabotropic glutamate receptor (mGluR3) in the rat brain: an in situ hybridization study. J. Comp. Neurol., 335 (1993b) 252–266.
42. Ottersen, O.P. and Storm-Mathisen, D.T. Excitatory amino acid pathways in the brain. In *Excitatory Amino Acids and Epilepsy*, R. Schwarcz and Y. Ben-Ari (Eds.) New York: Plenum, 1986, pp. 263–284.
43. Ottersen, O.P., Fischer, B.O., Rinvik, E. and Storm-Mathisen, D.T. Putative amino acids transmitters in the amygdala. In: *Excitatory Amino Acids and Epilepsy*, R. Schwartz and Y. Ben-Ari (Eds.), New York; Plenum, 1986, pp. 53–66.
44. Palmer, E., Monaghan, D.T. and Cotman, C.W. Trans-ACPD, a selective agonist of the phosphoinositide-coupled excitatory amino acid receptor. *Eur. J. Pharmacol.*, 166 (1989) 585–587.
45. Pin, J.-P. and Duvoisin, R. Review: neurotransmitter receptors I. The metabotropic glutamate receptors: structure and functions. *Neuropharmacology*, 34 (1995) 1–26.
46. Rabow, L.E., Russek, S.J. and Farb, D.H. From ion currents to genomic analysis: recent advances in $GABA_A$ receptor research. *Synapse*, 21 (1995) 189–274.
47. Racine, R. and McIntyre, D. Mechanisms of kindling: a current view. In *The Limbic System: Functional Organization and Clinical Disorder*, Anonymous (Ed.), Raven Press: New York, 1986, pp. 109–121.
48. Racine, R.J. Modification of seizure activity by electrical stimulation. Afterdischarge threshold. *Electroencephalogr. Clin. Neurophysiol.* 32 (1972) 269–279.
49. Rainnie, D.G., Asprodini, E.K. and Shinnick-Gallagher, P. Excitatory transmission in the basolateral amygdala. *J. Neurophysiol.*, 66 (1991a) 986–998.
50. Rainnie, D.G., Asprodini, E.K. and Shinnick-Gallagher, P. Inhibitory transmission in the basolateral amygdala. *J. Neurophysiol.*, 66 (1991b) 999–1009.
51. Rainnie, D.G., Asprodini, E.K. and Shinnick-Gallagher, P. Intracellular recording from morphologically identified neurons of the basolateral amygdala. *J. Neurophysiol.*, 69 (1993) 1350–1362.
52. Rainnie, D.G., Asprodini, E.K. and Shinnick-Gallagher, P. Kindling-induced long-lasting changes in synaptic transmission in the basolateral amygdala. *J. Neurophysiol.*, 67 (1992) 443–454.

53. Rainnie, D.G., Holmes, K.H. and Shinnick-Gallagher, P. Activation of postsynaptic metabotropic glutamate receptors by trans-ACPD hyperpolarizes neurons of the basolateral amygdala. *J. Neurosci.*, 14 (1994) 7208–7220.
54. Rainnie, D.G. and Shinnick-Gallagher, P. Trans-ACPD and L-APB presynaptically inhibit excitatory glutamatergic transmission in the basolateral amygdala (BLA). *Neurosci. Lett.*, 139 (1992) 87–91.
55. Roberts, P.J. Pharmacological tools for the investigation of metabotropic glutamate receptors (mGluRs): phenylglycine derivatives and other selective antagonists—an update. *Neuropharmacology*, 34 (1995) 813–819.
56. Romano, C., Sesma, M.A., McDonald, C.T., O'Malley, K., VanDenPol, A.N. and Olney, J.W. Distribution of metabotropic glutamate receptor mGluR5 immunoreactivity in rat brain. *J. Comp. Neurol.* 355 (1995) 455–469.
57. Sacaan, A.I. and Schoepp, D.D. Activation of hippocampal metabotropic excitatory amino acid receptors leads to seizures and neuronal damage. *Neurosci. Lett.*, 139 (1992) 77–82.
58. Savander, V. Go, C.G., LeDoux, J.E. and Pitkanen, A. Intrinsic connections of the rat amygdaloid complex: projections originating in the basal nucleus. *J. Comp. Neurol.*, 361(2) (1995) 345–368.
59. Shigemoto, R., Nakanishi, S. and Mizuno, N. Distribution of the mRNA for metabotropic glutamate receptor (mGluR1) in the central nervous system: An *in situ* hybridization study in adult and developing rat. *J. Comp. Neurol.* 322 (1992) 121–135.
60. Suzuki, K., Mori, N., Kittaka, H., Iwata, Y., Yamada, Y., Osonoe, K. and Niwa, S-I. Anticonvulsant action of metabotropic glutamate receptor agonists in kindled amygdala of rats. *Neurosci. Lett.*, 204 (1996) 41–44.
61. Tizzano, J.P., Griffey, K.I., Johnson, J.A., Fix, A.S., Helton, D.R. and Schoepp, D.D. Intracerebral 1S,3R-1-aminocyclopentane-1,3-dicarboxylic (1S,3R-ACPD) produces limbic seizures that are not blocked by ionotropic glutamate receptor antagonists. *Neurosci. Lett.*, 162 (1993) 12–16.
62. Tizzano, J.P., Griffey, K.I., Schoepp, D.D. Induction or protection of limbic seizures in mice by mGluR subtype selective agonists. *Neuropharmacology*, 34 (1995) 1063–1067.
63. Washburn, M.S. and Moises, H.C. Electrophysiological and morphological properties of rat basolateral amygdaloid neurons *in vitro*. *J. Neurosci.*, 12 (1992) 4066–4079.
64. Yamada, N., Akiyama, K. and Otsuki, S. Hippocampal kindling enhances excitatory amino acid receptor-mediated poly-phosphoinositide hydrolysis in the hippocampus and amydala/pyriform cortex. *Brain Res.*, 490 (1989) 126–132.
65. Yu, B. and Shinnick-Gallagher, P. Interleukin 1-β inhibits synaptic transmission and induces membrane hyperpolarization in amygdala neurons. *J. Pharmacol. Exp. Ther.*, 217 (1994) 590–623.
66. Zhao, D.Y. and Moshe, S.L. Deep prepiriform cortex kindling and amygdala interactions. *Epilepsy Res.*, 1 (1987) 94–101.

DISCUSSION OF PATRICIA SHINNICK-GALLAGHER'S PAPER

K. Morimoto: We examined the nonselective metabotropic glutamate receptor antagonist MCPG in amygdala kindling in vivo and we found very little effect. Kindling was facilitated. Did you find an antagonistic effect?

P. Shinnick-Gallagher: We studied MCPG in three experimental paradigms. In one we analyzed the effect of superfusing MCPG on synaptic transmission in control slices to test whether MCPG could block endogenous activation of a metabotropic glutamate receptor involved in synaptic transmission in the amygdala. We found that by itself MCPG depressed synaptic potentials. We concluded that this effect of MCPG could be due to a nonselective effect or to a block of an endogenously active metabotropic glutamate receptor which is tonically excitatory.

We have also analyzed the effect of MCPG in two epilepsy models. In the 4-aminopyridine (4-AP) in vitro seizure model we found that MCPG blocked the induction of 4-AP seizures but did not affect the maintenance phase of the established seizure activity. Finally, when we studied the effect of the antagonist in vitro on bursting induced by kindling in vivo, MCPG had no effect on epileptiform activity.

I. Mody: You mostly studied excitatory events. Have you looked at inhibitory events?

P. Shinnick-Gallagher: Studying inhibitory events in kindled amygdala neurons is difficult to do. There are only a small number of GABAergic neurons in the lateral amygdala that project to the basolateral amygdala. This pathway is the only one we can study in kindled slices since the inhibitory events elicited by stimulating other pathways in control neurons are not present in kindled neurons.

R. Adamec: How long did you after kindling did you record in slices from kindled animals?

P. Shinnick-Gallagher: In our early experiments we recorded 28 days after the last kindled seizure; in our more recent studies with metabotropic glutamate receptors we analyzed the slices 7 to 14 days after the last kindled seizure. In our most recent studies with whole cell patch recorded synaptic currents, we evaluated the slices 5 to 7 days after three to five stage 5 seizures.

R. Adamec: Your data look like there is an increase in affinity for groups 2 and 3 metabotropic glutamate receptors. What are the consequences of this effect for a group 2 or 3?

P. Shinnick-Gallagher: We tested the effect of antagonists of the group 2 and 3 mGluRs to assess whether these receptors were activated endogenously under our normal stimulating conditions. Neither the group 2 (MCCG) nor the group 3 (MAP-4) antagonists affected synaptic transmission, suggesting that the group 2 or 3 mGluRs are not activated under these conditions. These antagonists also did not affect synaptic transmission or epileptiform bursting in kindled neurons. These data suggest that these mGluRs do not play a role in synaptic transmission in these experimental paradigms.

R. Adamec: What would be the physiological consequences of the changes in the presynaptic mGluRs in kindling?

P. Shinnick-Gallagher: Physiologically it may be possible that the effector linked to the presynaptic mGluR, the calcium channel, may perhaps be upregulated. An upregulation of the calcium current may be reflected in an increased transmitter release and an increase in the agonist affinity for the mGluRs linked to the calcium channels. The exquisite sensitivity of the presynaptic mGluRs for their respective agonists could be utilized therapeutically in the treatment of human complex partial seizures.

8

ROLE OF THE DENTATE GYRUS IN THE SPREAD OF SEIZURES WITHIN THE HIPPOCAMPAL-PARAHIPPOCAMPAL CIRCUIT

Janet L. Stringer and Enhui Pan

Baylor College of Medicine
Department of Pharmacology and Division of Neuroscience
One Baylor Plaza, Houston, Texas 77030

1. INTRODUCTION AND MAXIMAL DENTATE ACTIVATION

Recent studies have begun to provide an anatomic framework for seizures that begin in limbic circuits[7,13,14,18,19]. The major pathway of neuronal activity into and through the hippocampus follows the trisynaptic circuit. The entorhinal cortex activates the granule cells of the dentate gyrus via the perforant pathway, the dentate gyrus activates the CA3 pyramidal cells via the mossy fibers, and finally CA3 activates the CA1 pyramidal cells via the Schaffer collaterals. As can be seen from this circuitry, the dentate gyrus (DG) is in a position to act as a regulator of normal and epileptic activity passing into the hippocampus proper from the entorhinal cortex[2,11,29].

Several years ago, to explore mechanisms of epileptogenesis in the hippocampus, we characterized responses to stimulus trains administered to either the CA3 region of the dorsal hippocampus or to the angular bundle[23,25,29]. Patterns of activation in response to trains of electrical stimulation were described in both CA1 and the dentate gyrus. Maximal activation in the dentate gyrus was demarcated by the appearance of bursts of large amplitude population spikes, an abrupt secondary rise in the extracellular potassium concentration, and a sustained negative shift of the extracellularly recorded DC-coupled potential (Figure 1). Maximal activation of CA1 is demarcated by a prompt and rapid rise in the extracellular potassium to around 10 mM together with an increase in amplitude of the population spikes to 10–15 mV with doubling and tripling.

A number of observations support the hypothesis that the dentate gyrus acts as a gate for the passage of epileptiform activity from the entorhinal cortex into the hippocampus proper. First, stimulation of the angular bundle produces maximal activation in both CA1 and the dentate gyrus, but the stimulus intensity needed to produce maximal activation in CA1 is always higher than that needed to produce maximal activation in the dentate gyrus. Also CA1 activation does not appear until after dentate activation has occurred during the

Kindling 5, edited by Corcoran and Moshé.
Plenum Press, New York, 1998.

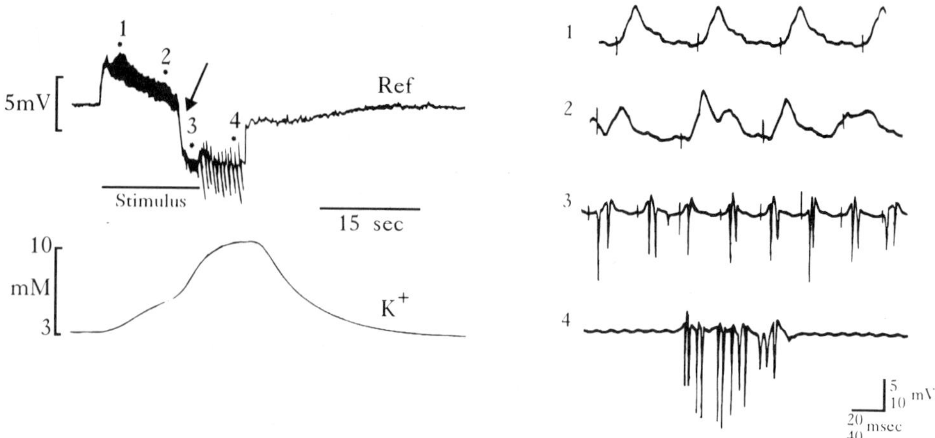

Figure 1. Maximal dentate activation. This figure presents the chart recordings and oscilloscope tracings during and after a stimulus train that evoked maximal dentate activation. On the left side are the chart recordings of the DC-coupled potential (top) and the extracellular potassium concentration (bottom) in the dentate gyrus during and after a 20 Hz stimulus train to the opposite CA3 region. The onset of maximal dentate activation is indicated by the arrow. Oscilloscope tracings taken at the times indicated are presented on the right. The top two tracings use the 5 mV by 20 msec calibration and the bottom two tracings use the 10 mV by 40 msec calibration. Notice the onset of maximal dentate activation is demarcated by a negative shift of the DC-coupled potential and a secondary rise in the extracellular potassium. Maximal dentate activation is also characterized by the appearance of bursts of large amplitude population spikes.

stimulus train. Second, maximal activation of the dentate gyrus is best elicited by stimuli within a limited range of frequencies with both angular bundle and CA3 stimulation. Maximal CA1 activation is elicited by stimuli up to 100 Hz with CA3 stimulation. However, maximal CA1 activation after stimulation of the angular bundle shows the same frequency dependence as dentate activation, suggesting that activity from the angular bundle is relayed through the dentate gyrus before maximal activation in CA1 occurs. Third, unilateral colchicine lesions of the dentate gyrus do not block activation in CA1 from contralateral CA3 stimulation, but the response is not sustained. In fact, the response in CA1 fades when the dentate gyrus would have been predicted to become maximally activated. Presumably maximal dentate activation sustains (or drives) the CA1 discharges. Together, this evidence suggests that before the onset of maximal dentate activation, the dentate gyrus resists propagation of seizure activity into the hippocampus proper. After the onset of maximal dentate activation, seizure activity is amplified as it passes into the hippocampus. This suggests that maximal dentate activation may subserve the "gate" function of the dentate gyrus.

In the normal animal, bilateral maximal dentate activation is necessary before an afterdischarge (epileptiform activity continuing after the end of the stimulus train) occurs[26]. In the intact rat, maximal dentate activation in the dentate gyrus is always associated with epileptiform activity in CA1, CA3 and the entorhinal cortex, suggesting that maximal dentate activation is an indicator of reverberatory activity throughout the hippocampal-parahippocampal circuit[27]. In other words, when maximal dentate activation is present there is always seizure activity in the entorhinal cortex and hippocampus proper. Maximal dentate activation is also elicited by the chemical convulsants, kainic acid, bicuculline, pentylenetetrazol and pilocarpine[28]. The data indicate that maximal dentate activation represents the final seizure expressed after administration of stimulus trains or chemical convulsants and is independent of the mechanism by which the seizure is initiated.

The experiments described thus far were conducted in urethane anesthetized animals. Experiments in awake animals demonstrated that maximal dentate activation can be readily produced without urethane and that it is identical in appearance when elicited in anesthetized and unanesthetized rats[30]. Additionally, maximal dentate activation can be elicited by amygdala stimulation of the same frequency and duration commonly used for kindling. Lengthening of the afterdischarge in the amygdala does not appear until maximal dentate activation was initiated in the dentate gyrus. Once afterdischarges are present in both the amygdala and dentate gyrus, behavioral seizures (immobility, facial twitching, chewing and wet dog shakes) begin.

2. MDA-LIKE EVENTS *IN VITRO*

Bursts of population spikes have been recorded in the dentate gyrus of the hippocampal slice that are similar to maximal dentate activation *in vivo*[15,17,21]. These bursts of large amplitude population spikes are produced by raising the extracellular potassium concentration to 10–12 mM and lowering the extracellular calcium concentration to 0.5 mM. These values of extracellular potassium and calcium are at the extreme range of the levels of these ions that have been recorded during seizure discharges. Trains of electrical stimulation produce epileptiform activity in the dentate gyrus when the extracellular potassium is raised to 5–7 mM and the calcium is lowered to 0.5 mM. This epileptiform activity is not eliminated by blocking synaptic transmission with 0 calcium, or with excitatory amino-acid antagonists 6,7-dinitroquinoxaline-2,3-dione (DNQX) and D,L-2-amino-5-phosphonopentanoate (AP-5). These data demonstrate that the bursts of population spikes generated *in vitro* do not require synaptic transmission. For convenience we will call these bursts of synchronous activity recorded *in vitro*, MDA-like events.

To begin to determine the cellular basis of these MDA-like events, we have recorded intracellularly from the dentate gyrus granule cells during the epileptiform discharge. Intracellular recordings have been obtained from 30 granule cells while simultaneously recording the extracellular field potentials in the dentate gyrus (Figure 2). MDA-like events were produced by perfusing the slices in 0-added calcium and 8 mM potassium artificial

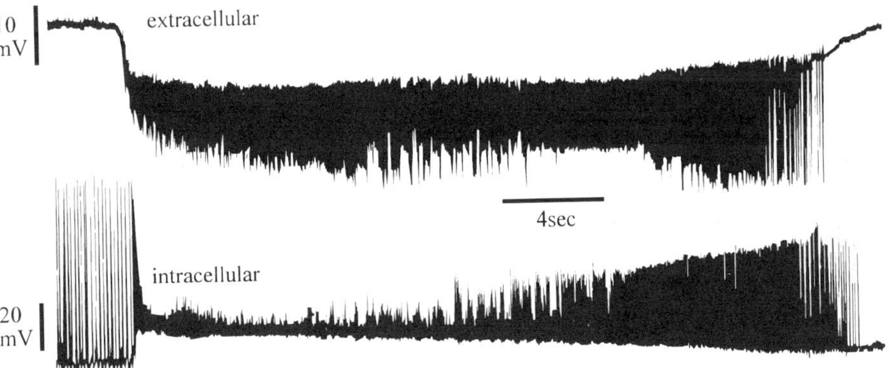

Figure 2. MDA-like events *in vitro*. This figure presents simultaneous extracellular (top) and intracellular recording (bottom) from a granule cell in a hippocampal slice perfused in 8 mM potassium and 0-added calcium. One MDA-like event is shown. Notice the negative DC shift of the extracellular potential associated with the onset of the synchronized activity. On the intracellular recording, notice that the cell is firing action potentials before the onset of the synchronized activity. Calibrations are indicated on the figure.

cerebrospinal fluid. During the MDA-like events, the individual granule cells exhibited a sustained depolarization that matched the duration of the negative extracellular DC shift. At the onset of the MDA-like event, all the granule cells had an initial burst of action potentials associated with a depolarization of around 10 mV. This initial burst of activity was followed by a reduced rate of firing (n=11) or a cessation of firing (n=3) while the depolarization was maintained. During the MDA-like events, action potentials were of reduced amplitude in all cells recorded. Towards the end of the MDA-like event the rate of action potential firing increased. In no cell was there a decrease in the firing rate (spike accommodation) of the action potentials through the MDA-like event. The effect of depolarizing and hyperpolarizing current injections on the amplitude and frequency of the MDA-like events was tested. Current injections had no effect on the frequency of the activity during the MDA-like events, indicating that they were mediated by activity extrinsic to the recorded neuron. Surprisingly, spontaneous epileptiform activity was recorded intracellularly before the appearance of the MDA-like events and between events at a time when the extracellular recording was quiet.

2.1. Cellular Bursts

Epileptiform bursting has been divided into endogenous bursts that are generated within a single cell and network bursts that are dependent on synaptic interactions[9]. The generation of endogenous bursts is dependent on specialized membrane properties of individual neurons. Data supporting the endogenous nature of spontaneous bursts in CA3 hippocampal neurons was reported by Hablitz and Johnston[8]. They demonstrated that in CA3 the burst frequency is a function of the membrane potential, that bursts can be triggered, that bursts are seen in the absence of propagated synaptic input, and that burst currents are absent when voltage clamp is applied to the soma. These results and those of others[32–34] support the hypothesis that hippocampal pyramidal neurons are capable of displaying endogenous bursting behavior. However, there is also evidence that the spontaneous bursts recorded in the CA3 region of the hippocampus are network-driven[9].

Much less is known about the granule cells of the dentate gyrus and their role in burst generation and epileptogenesis in general. There have been several reports describing the characteristics of the granule cells with intracellular recording[3,5,6,12]. Based on intracellular recordings in the presence of penicillin, pentylenetetrazol (PTZ), picrotoxin and lowered chloride, Fricke and Prince concluded that dentate gyrus granule cells are not actively involved in spontaneous or evoked epileptogenesis *in vitro* or *in vivo*[6]. They never observed the granule cells to generate depolarization shifts or prolonged spike bursts[6]. In support of their conclusion, others have observed that stimulation of perforant path fibers could cause up to 3–5 action potentials, but only at high stimulus intensities[3]. In contrast to hippocampal pyramidal cells, bursts of action potentials in the dentate granule cells were never followed by a prolonged afterhyperpolarization[5]. However, a depolarizing afterpotential has been recorded following single action potentials[1,5]. (In CA3 neurons, the depolarizing afterpotential is felt to be an important factor in sustaining burst firing[34].) Some studies describe the presence of small amplitude (4–15 mV) all-or none spikes[1] that have been shown to be due to electrotonic coupling between adjacent granule cells[12]. From these studies it would appear that the dentate gyrus does not express endogenous bursting and is very resistant to the expression of synchronized epileptiform activity.

However, we have recorded spontaneous bursts in the granule cells of the dentate gyrus before and between MDA-like events that may represent endogenous bursting. This spontaneous cellular activity consisted of single action potentials and bursts of action po-

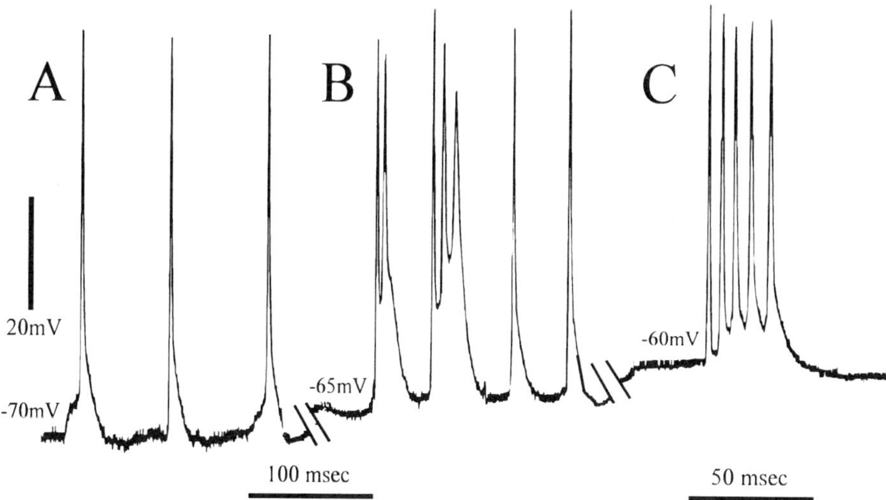

Figure 3. Cellular bursts recorded in dentate gyrus granule cells. Intracellular recording from a granule cell was obtained and then the slice was perfused with 0-added calcium and 8 mM potassium. Spontaneous action potentials appeared (A) after 10–15 minutes. After 15–25 minutes, bursts appeared along with the single action potentials (B). In most cells, the bursts became the predominant activity (C). The membrane potential at each time point is indicated. Calibrations are indicated on the figure.

tentials on a depolarizing envelope (Figure 3). In addition, depolarizing potentials, up to 13 mV, were recorded, primarily before the onset of the MDA-like events. There were no extracellular field potentials associated with these intracellularly recorded potentials, indicating that this activity is not synchronized within the cell layer. To emphasize the cellular nature of the bursts of action potentials that are recorded intracellularly, they have been termed cellular bursts. The effect of depolarizing and hyperpolarizing current injections on the amplitude and frequency of the cellular bursts was also tested. The frequency of the cellular bursts between episodes of MDA-like events was very sensitive to current injection. Depolarizing current increased the frequency and hyperpolarizing current decreased the frequency of the cellular activity.

These data suggest that the cellular bursts are generated intrinsically within the granule cells.

With the results from this study, together with previously published reports, a hypothesis about the role of the dentate gyrus in the propagation of seizures *in vivo* can be proposed. Under normal conditions the dentate gyrus has a very high threshold for the onset of seizure discharges. When an epileptogenic insult to the brain occurs, input to the dentate gyrus increases, resulting in a local increase in the extracellular potassium and decrease in the extracellular calcium.[10] These factors initiate endogenous bursting properties latent in the granule cells. By some non-synaptic mechanism(s), synchronized burst discharges begin.

2.1.1. Role of Extracellular Potassium and Calcium in the Generation of Cellular Bursts. This hypothesis about the role of the dentate gyrus in the propagation of seizure activity into the hippocampus suggests that the onset of cellular bursts in the granule cells is a precursor to the onset of maximal dentate activation (synchronized activity). It is postulated that an increase in activity coming into the dentate gyrus increases $[K^+]_o$ and decreases $[Ca^{++}]_o$[10,22,24,29] sufficiently to initiate bursting in the granule cells. To test this hypothesis the role of increases in extracellular potassium and decreases in extracellular calcium in the onset of cellular bursting in the granule cells of the dentate gyrus *in vitro* was examined. Hippocampal slices were prepared from anesthetized adult Sprague-Dawley rats, and intra- and extracellular recording was carried out in the dentate gyrus. Increasing the extracellular potassium or decreasing the extracellular calcium caused three forms of spontaneous activity to appear: depolarizing potentials, action potentials and cellular bursts (Figure 4). Thus, changing either potassium or calcium can induce the cellular bursts. At no time was any extracellular field activity recorded, confirming the lack of synchronization noted earlier. The shape of the cellular bursts was different in high potassium compared to low calcium (see Figure 4). Increasing potassium or decreasing calcium also caused the granule cells to depolarize and reduced their input resistance (Table 1).

Before the onset of maximal dentate activation *in vivo*, $[K^+]_o$ increases and $[Ca^{++}]_o$ decreases. To test the hypothesis that changes in the extracellular ion concentration may initiate cellular bursts in the granule cells, it was necessary to determine the effect of changing both $[K^+]_o$ and $[Ca^{++}]_o$ on the appearance of the cellular bursts. To do this, the $[Ca^{++}]_o$ was decreased to 1.5 mM and then a granule cell was impaled. After a stable

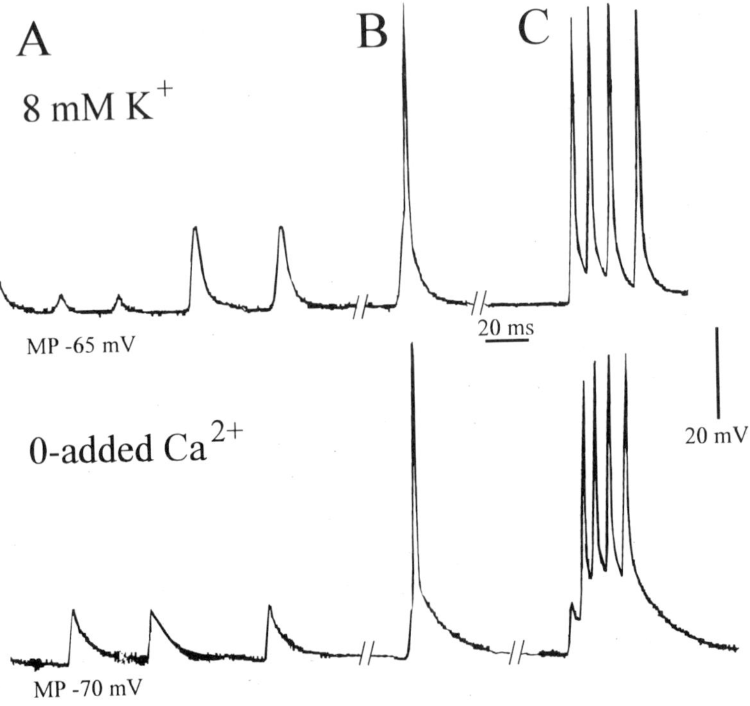

Figure 4. Spontaneous activity recorded in dentate granule cells in 8 mM $[K^+]_o$ or 0-added calcium solutions. The spontaneous activity recorded in 2 different granule cells is shown. The top row illustrates activity in a slice equilibrated in 8 mM $[K^+]_o$ and the bottom row illustrates activity in a slice equilibrated in 0-added calcium. In A, depolarizing potentials are shown and in B typical spontaneous action potentials. Notice that the repolarization phase of both types of activity is faster in the high potassium solution relative to the same potentials recorded in 0-added calcium. In C, examples of the cellular bursts that were recorded from dentate gyrus granule cells are shown. Notice that in 0-added calcium there is a depolarizing envelope with the action potentials riding on this envelope. In 8 mM $[K^+]_o$ the action potentials within the burst actually rise off of the repolarizing phase of the previous action potential. Calibrations and membrane potential (MP) are indicated on the figure.

Table 1. Effect of 8 mM $[K^+]_o$ or 0-added $[Ca^{++}]_o$ on the cellular properties of the dentate granule cells

Condition (n)	Input resistance (MΩ)	Membrane potential (mV)
Control (5)	55.0 ± 2.2	−84.0 ± 1.0
0-added $[Ca^{++}]_o$ (6)	29.3 ± 6.1*	−68.0 ± 4.9*
8 mM $[K^+]_o$ (4)	41.3 ± 1.3*	−60.8 ± 2.2*

*Indicates a significant difference compared to control ($p<0.05$). In addition, the $[K^+]_o$ group was significantly different from the $[Ca^{++}]_o$ group for both parameters.

recording was achieved (n=15), the $[K^+]_o$ was increased from 3 to 7 mM in 1 mM steps and the $[K^+]_o$ at which the cellular bursts appeared was determined. The procedure was repeated using 1.2 and 1.0 mM $[Ca^{++}]_o$ (Fig. 5A). The same procedure was repeated with another set of cells (n=14), but this time the $[K^+]_o$ was fixed and the $[Ca^{++}]_o$ was varied. The $[Ca^{++}]_o$ at which each cell began bursting was determined (Figure 5B). The results indicate that combining an increase in $[K^+]_o$ and a decrease in $[Ca^{++}]_o$ produces cellular bursting in the granule cells with less drastic changes than needed if either ion is the only one changed. Levels of $[K^+]_o$ and $[Ca^{++}]_o$ that initiate cellular bursts (when changed together) are within the range of extracellular potassium and calcium that has been recorded *in vivo* before the onset of maximal dentate activation.

2.1.2. Ability of Chemical Convulsants to Generate Cellular Bursts. We tested the ability of 4 chemical convulsants (bicuculline, picrotoxin, pentylenetetrazol, and penicillin) to generate cellular bursts and synchronized field activity. Slices were perfused with each of the convulsants for 30 minutes and the presence or absence of spontaneous epileptiform activity was determined. Stimuli were administered every minute to the perforant path to test for stimulus-evoked bursts, which were defined as at least 3 action potentials on one depolarizing potential. Field activity and cellular activity were monitored extracel-

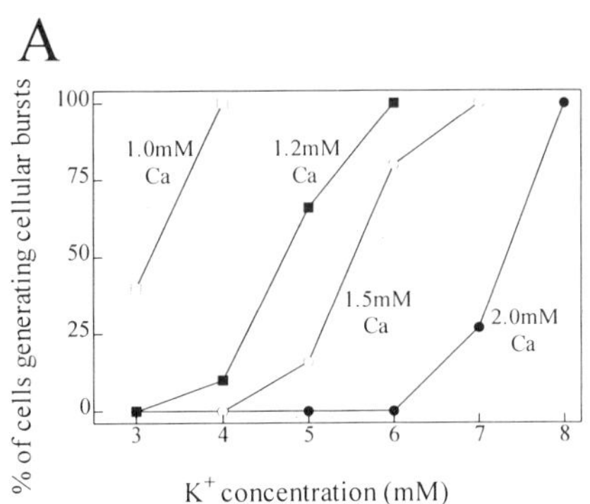

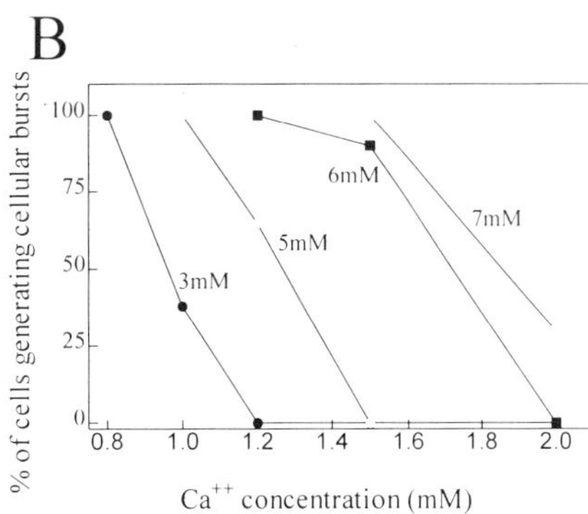

Figure 5. Role of $[K^+]_o$ and $[Ca^{++}]_o$ in the generation of cellular bursts in granule cells of the dentate gyrus. The $[K^+]_o$ and $[Ca^{++}]_o$ levels necessary for the appearance of cellular bursts were determined. In A, the $[Ca^{++}]_o$ was fixed at 2.0 (filled circles), 1.5 (open circles), 1.2 (filled boxes) or 1.0 mM (open boxes) and the $[K^+]_o$ was increased from 3 to 8 in 1 mM steps. The percentage of cells with cellular bursts at each ion concentration is graphed. Decreasing the $[Ca^{++}]_o$, decreased the amount of $[K^+]_o$ needed to initiate the cellular bursts. In B, the $[K^+]_o$ was fixed at 3 (filled circles), 5 (open circles), 6 (filled squares), or 7 (open squares) mM and the $[Ca^{++}]_o$ was decreased in steps and the results are graphed as in A. As the $[K^+]_o$ was increased, the change in the level of $[Ca^{++}]_o$ needed to initiate the cellular bursts was smaller.

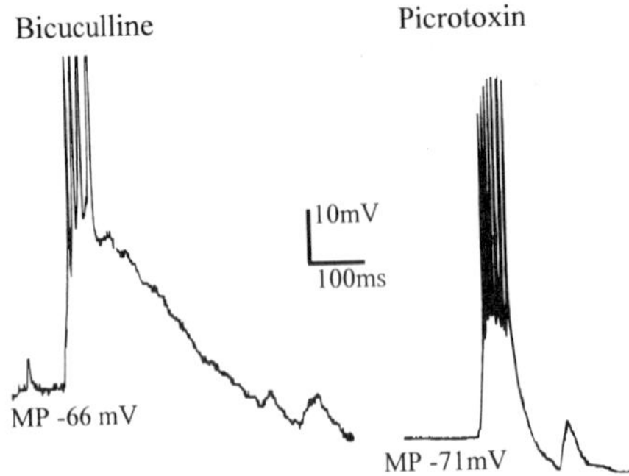

Figure 6. Spontaneous bursts in the granule cells of the dentate gyrus in the presence of chemical convulsants. Intracellular recording from 2 different granule cells are shown, both 15–20 minutes after beginning perfusion with either 20 μM bicuculline (left) or 60 μM picrotoxin (right). Calibrations and pre-burst membrane potentials (MP) are indicated on the figure. Bicuculline did depolarize the membrane potential to a greater extent than picrotoxin. The action potentials on the left have been truncated.

lularly and intracellularly, respectively. After addition of any of the 4 convulsants, the membrane potential of the granule cells depolarized. Picrotoxin (60 μM, n=8), pentylenetetrazol (10 mM, n=9), and penicillin (4 mM, n=9) significantly depolarized the membrane by 6–10 mV. Bicuculline (20 μM, n=8) significantly depolarized the membrane by 20–24 mV.

Stimulus-evoked bursts were recorded in 67% and 87% of the slices perfused with picrotoxin and bicuculline, respectively. However, in only 1 slice perfused with either penicillin or pentylenetetrazol was a stimulus-evoked burst recorded. Spontaneous cellular bursts were also significantly more common in picrotoxin (33%) and bicuculline (75%, Figure 6), than in penicillin (17%) and pentylenetetrazol (0%). At no time were extracellular field events detected in the dentate gyrus during these experiments. These data suggest that some convulsants can induce the intrinsic bursting ability of the granule cells, but, as before, some other mechanisms are involved in the synchronization of the activity.

3. ROLE OF EXTRACELLULAR SPACE IN SYNCHRONIZATION OF CELLULAR ACTIVITY IN THE DENTATE GYRUS

Because the MDA-like events represent synchronization of the granule cells and this occurs in the absence of synaptic transmission, the mechanisms that synchronize the neurons must be non-synaptic. A number of mechanisms have been proposed to enhance synchronization of epileptic discharges. The types of non-synaptic mechanisms that may be involved in the initiation and synchronization of epileptiform activity include changes in extracellular space[20,31], which influence ephaptic interactions, changes in electrotonic coupling through gap junctions[12], and changes in extracellular ions. These non-synaptic interactions have been fairly well described in CA3 and CA1, but less is known about the dentate gyrus.

To date, we have tested the role of changes in extracellular space on synchronization and propagation of epileptiform activity in the dentate gyrus *in vitro* by manipulating the osmolality of the perfusing solution[16]. Using tissue resistance measurements, it has been shown that hyperosmotic solutions expand the extracellular space and that hyposmotic solutions shrink the extracellular space[31]. The reduction in extracellular space associated with hypo-osmolar solutions has been shown to lead to increased seizure susceptibility[20,31], possibly due to an increase in the relative role of nonsynaptic mechanisms of synchronization, particularly ephaptic interactions, or electrical field effects.[4] When a group of neurons fire synchronously they generate an electrical field that causes a transmembrane

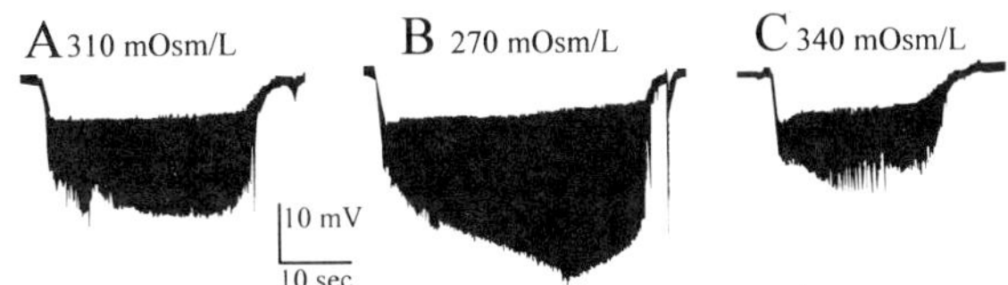

Figure 7. Effect of osmolality on the amplitude of the population spikes within the MDA-like events. Episodic epileptiform bursts were induced by perfusing a slice with 8 mM potassium and 0-added calcium (310 mOsm/l, A). The osmolality was then decreased to 270 mOsm/l (B), increased to 340 mOsm/l (C), and then returned to 310 mOsm/l (not shown). Decreasing the osmolality increased the amplitude of the population spikes within the MDA-like event and increasing the osmolality decreased the amplitude. These changes were reversible upon returning the slice to a solution of normal osmolality. The data shown are all from the same slice. Calibrations are indicated on the figure.

potential difference in neighboring neurons that did not fire. This potential change can depolarize these neurons sufficiently to fire an action potential. It has been hypothesized that the synchronized bursts recorded in the dentate gyrus are mediated by ephaptic interactions[21]. In our experiments, increasing the osmolality reduced the amplitude of the population spikes (Figure 7) and slowed the propagation of the epileptiform activity. Decreasing the osmolality had the opposite effect. These results confirm and extend the results of Roper et al.[20] Assuming there were significant changes in the size of the extracellular space, and therefore the ease with which ephaptic interactions can occur, these results support the hypothesis that ephaptic interactions play a role in the synchronization and propagation of epileptic activity in the dentate gyrus.

4. CONCLUSIONS

Together with previously published reports these data can be used to modify our hypothesis about the role of the dentate gyrus in the propagation of seizures *in vivo* can be proposed. Under normal conditions the dentate gyrus has a very high threshold for the onset of seizure discharges. When an epileptogenic insult to the brain occurs, input to the dentate gyrus increases, resulting in a local increase in the extracellular potassium and decrease in the extracellular calcium[10]. These factors initiate endogenous bursting properties latent in the granule cells, resulting in the appearance of the cellular bursts. By some non-synaptic mechanism(s), these cellular bursts then synchronize into the MDA-like events. Ephaptic interactions probably play a role in the extent of synchronization and propagation of the MDA-like activity, but are less likely to play a role in the initiation of these regularly occurring events.

REFERENCES

1. Assaf SY, Crunelli V, and Kelly JS, Electrophysiology of the rat dentate gyrus *in vitro*, In: *Electrophysiology of isolated CNS preparations*, GA Kerkut and HV Wheal, Eds., Academic Press, 1981, p.153–187.
2. Collins RC, Tearse RG and Lothman EW, Functional anatomy of limbic seizures: Focal discharges from entorhinal cortex in rat. *Brain Res.* 280 (1983) 25–40.
3. Dudek FE, Deadwyler SA, Cotman CW and Lynch G, Intracellular responses from granule cell layer in slices of rat hippocampus: Perforant path synapse, *J. Neurophysiol.* 39 (1976) 384–393.
4. Dudek, F.E., Obenaus, A. and Tasker, J.G., Osmolality-induced changes in extracellular volume alter epileptiform bursts independent of chemical synapses in the rat: Importance of non-synaptic mechanisms in hippocampal epileptogenesis, *Neurosci. Lett.*, 120 (1990) 267–270.

5. Fournier E and Crepel F, Electrophysiological properties of dentate granule cells in mouse hippocampal slices maintained *in vitro*, *Brain Res.* 311 (1984) 75–86.
6. Fricke RA and Prince DA, Electrophysiology of dentate gyrus granule cells, *J. Neurophysiol.* 51 (1984) 195–209.
7. Goddard GV, Dragunow M, Maru E and MacLeod EK, Kindling and the forces that oppose it. In: *The Limbic System: Functional Organization and Clinical Disorders*, (Eds. BK Doane and KE Livingston) pp. 95–108, Raven Press, 1986.
8. Hablitz JJ and Johnston D, Endogenous nature of spontaneous bursting in hippocampal pyramidal neurons, *Cell Molec. Neurobiol.* 1 (1981) 325–334.
9. Johnston D and Brown TH, Mechanisms of neuronal burst generation, pp. 277–301 In: *Electrophysiology of Epilepsy* (Ed. PA Schwartzkroin), Academic Press, 1984.
10. Krnjevic K, Morris ME and Reiffenstein RJ, Changes in extracellular Ca^{++} and K^{+} activity accompanying hippocampal discharges, *Can J. Physiol. Pharmacol.* 58 (1980) 579–583.
11. Lothman EW and Collins RC, Kainic acid-induced limbic seizures: metabolic, behavioural, electroencephalographic and neuropathological correlates. *Brain Res.* 218 (1981) 299–318.
12. MacVicar BA and Dudek FE, Electrotonic coupling between granule cells of rat dentate gyrus: Physiological and anatomical evidence, *J. Neurophysiol.* 47 (1982) 579–592.
13. McNamara JO, Kindling model of epilepsy, *Adv. Neurol.* 44 (1986) 303–318.
14. McNamara JO Pursuit of the mechanisms of kindling *TINS* 11 (1988) 33–36.
15. Pan E and Stringer JL, Burst characteristics of dentate gyrus granule cells: Evidence for endogenous and non-synaptic properties, *J. Neurophysiol.* 75 (1996) 124–132.
16. Pan E and Stringer JL, Influence of osmolality on seizure amplitude and propagation in the dentate gyrus, *Neurosci. Lett.* 207 (1996) 9–12.
17. Patrylo PR, Schweitzer JS and Dudek FE, Potassium-dependent prolonged field bursts in the dentate gyrus: Effects of extracellular calcium and amino acid receptor antagonists, *Neuroscience* 61 (1994) 13–19.
18. Racine RJ, Modifications of seizure activity by electrical stimulation II. Motor seizure. *Electroencephalogr. Clin. Neurophysiol.* 32 (1972) 281–294.
19. Racine RJ and McIntyre D, Mechanisms of kindling: a current view. In: *The Limbic System: Functional Organization and Clinical Disorders*, (Eds. BK Doane and KE Livingston) pp.109–121, Raven Press, New York, 1986.
20. Roper SN, Obenaus A and Dudek FE, Osmolality and nonsynaptic epileptiform bursts in rat CA1 and dentate gyrus, *Ann. Neurology* 31 (1992) 81–85.
21. Schweitzer JS, Patrylo PR and Dudek FE, Prolonged field bursts in the dentate gyrus: Dependence on low calcium, high potassium and nonsynaptic mechanisms. *J. Neurophysiol.* 68 (1992) 2016–2025.
22. Schweitzer JS and Williamson A, Relationship between synaptic activity and prolonged field bursts in the dentate gyrus of the rat hippocampal slice, *J. Neurophysiol.* 74 (1995) 1947–1952.
23. Somjen GG, Aitken PG, Giacchino JL and McNamara JO, Sustained potential shifts and paroxysmal discharges in hippocampal formation, *J. Neurophysiol.* 53 (1985) 1079–1097.
24. Stringer J.L and Lothman E.W. Model of spontaneous hippocampal epilepsy in the anesthetized rat: Electrographic, $[K^{+}]_{o}$ and $[Ca^{++}]_{o}$ response patterns. *Epilepsy Res.* 4 (1989) 177–186.
25. Stringer JL and Lothman EW, Maximal dentate activation: characteristics and alterations after repeated seizures, *J. Neurophysiol.* 62 (1989) 136–143.
26. Stringer JL and Lothman EW, Bilateral maximal dentate activation is critical for the appearance of an afterdischarge in the dentate gyrus, *Neurosci.* 46 (1992) 309–314.
27. Stringer JL and Lothman EW, Reverberatory seizures discharges in hippocampal-parahippocampal circuits, *Exp. Neurol.* 116 (1992) 198–203.
28. Stringer JL and Sowell KL, Kainic acid, bicuculline, pentylenetetrazol and pilocarpine elicit maximal dentate activation in the anesthetized rat, *Epilepsy Res.* 18 (1994) 11–21.
29. Stringer JL, Williamson JM and Lothman EW, Induction of paroxysmal discharge in the dentate gyrus: frequency dependence and relationship to afterdischarge production, *J. Neurophysiol.* 62 (1989) 126–135.
30. Stringer JL, Williamson JM, and Lothman EW, Maximal dentate activation is produced by amygdala stimulation in unanesthetized rats, *Brain Res.* 542 (1991) 336–342.
31. Traynelis, S.F. and Dingledine, R., Role of extracellular space in hyperosmotic suppression of potassium-induced electrogenic seizures, *J. Neurophysiol.*, 61 (1989) 927–938.
32. Wong RKS and Prince DA, Participation of calcium spikes during intrinsic burst firing in hippocampal neurons, *Brain Res.* 159 (1978) 385–390.
33. Wong RKS and Prince DA, Afterpotential generation in hippocampal pyramidal cells, *J. Neurophysiol.* 45 (1981) 86–97.
34. Wong RKS and Schwartzkroin PA, Pacemaker neurons in the mammalian brain: Mechanisms and function, In: *Cellular Pacemakers*, Vol.1 (DO Carpenter, ed.) pp.237–254, Wiley, New York, 1982.

DISCUSSION OF JANET STRINGER'S PAPER

J. McNamara: Why does the seizure stop?

J. Stringer: This is an excellent question. There are a number of theories, but no direct evidence for mechanisms.

J. McNamara: What are the possibilities? Is there synaptic plasticity?

J. Stringer: This is a difficult question, because these seizure-like events occur in the absence of synaptic transmission. Certainly, in vivo, synaptic events probably play a role in seizure termination. We have shown that adenosine and GABA systems may play a role in seizure termination in vivo.

D. McIntyre: Synchronization has been associated with gap junctions. Could they be involved in seizure termination?

J. Stringer: Nonsynaptic mechanisms that have been proposed to mediate synchronization of seizure activity include gap junctions, ephaptic interactions (field effects), and changes in extracellular environment. Gap junction blockers are not soluble in artificial CSF, and therefore we have not been able to use them to test the role of gap junctions in either seizure onset or termination. Changes in ephaptic interactions are usually tested by altering the osmolality of the extracellular solution. In our experiments, extreme changes in osmolality are needed to see an effect on seizure initiation or termination. I doubt that changes to this extent occur in vivo. Finally, changes in extracellular potassium seem to follow the neuronal activity and not anticipate it. In vitro, the potassium goes up with each MDA-like event and then falls. Each of these mechanisms may play a role in seizure onset and synchronization, but are less likely to be involved in seizure termination.

J. McNamara: The potassium does not fall before the end?

J. Stringer: No, the changes in potassium in vitro are the same as we have recorded in vivo. The potassium only falls after the termination of the MDA-like event.

S. Leung: After seizures there is generally no synaptic transmission. Is there any information about synaptic transmission in the period after the MDA-like event?

J. Stinger: In the in vitro experiments, it is possible to elicit a synaptic response immediately after the MDA-like event unless spreading depression occurs. It is necessary to do DC recordings in order to detect spreading depression. Since most of the awake recordings are done with AC recording, spreading depression will not be detectable in those experiments.

J. McNamara: Has MDA been recorded in slices from human tissue?

J. Stringer: No, not yet. Jeff Schweitzer looked for this while he was at Yale. As far as I know, no one has tried to record this type of seizure event in vivo.

9

QUENCHING

Persistent Alterations in Seizure and Afterdischarge Threshold following Low-Frequency Stimulation

Susan R. B. Weiss,* Xiu-Li Li, E. Christian Noguera,* Terri Heynen,* He Li,* Jeffrey B. Rosen, and Robert M. Post

Biological Psychiatry Branch, NIMH
9000 Rockville Pike, Building 10/3N212
Bethesda, Maryland 20892

1. INTRODUCTION

1.1. Kindling

Kindling is the progressive development of seizures to a previously subconvulsant stimulus administered in a repeated and intermittent fashion[31]. Kindled seizures evolve through stages: 1) *development*—afterdischarges increase in duration and spread throughout the brain ultimately culminating in generalized motor seizures; 2) *completed*—seizures can be reliably elicited by the previously subconvulsant stimulation; and 3) *spontaneous*—seizures occur in the absence of exogenous stimulation[31,54,55]. Kindling may be a useful model of epileptogenesis, but its progressive nature and emergent autonomy have led us and others to consider it as a model for the evolution of psychiatric illness as well (e.g., [2,49,52]). Several important practical and theoretical implications have emerged from this conceptualization and have been discussed in detail elsewhere[50,53].

Kindling is also long-lasting. Once kindled seizures develop, animals can be left unstimulated for extended periods of time without a loss of kindled seizure susceptibility. For this reason kindling has been proposed as a model of long-term neural plasticity and memory[30,40,56]. Mechanisms that account for the permanence of the kindled substrate are still being investigated (e.g., [10,26,62]). Thus, the challenge of preventing kindled seizure development or, more importantly, of reversing the kindled substrate, remains an important area of exploration. A number of effective anticonvulsant drugs can modify kindled sei-

* Supported by the Stanley Foundation.

Kindling 5, edited by Corcoran and Moshé.
Plenum Press, New York, 1998.

zure occurrence or progression; however, tolerance develops to the effects of many of these drugs when given repeatedly[34,35,48,66,68], and most are only partially successful in suppressing kindled seizure development. That is, they slow but do not halt its progression, and fail to produce long-lasting effects when treatment is discontinued. For the past several years we have been thinking about potential non-pharmacological strategies to attempt to interfere with kindled seizure development and maintainence of the kindled state.

1.2. Long-Term Potentiation (LTP) and Long-Term Depression (LTD)

LTP is another model of neuroplasticity in which an increase in synaptic efficacy occurs following high frequency electrical stimulation[7,8,36]. LTP can be induced in a variety of brain regions and has been demonstrated both *in vitro* and *in vivo*, where it can last for days to weeks[6,7]. The relationship between LTP and kindling is speculative; clearly, differences exist between these two forms of plasticity[11]; however, LTP may nevertheless be a component of the kindling process[39,57].

Recently, an opposing phenomenon, termed long-term depression, has been described[13,33,37]. Using different stimulation parameters from those that induce LTP or kindling, a decrease in synaptic responsivity can be demonstrated. LTD has been observed in several regions of the brain, including hippocampus, cerebellum, and neocortex, each with slightly different inducing or maintaining characteristics and pharmacology[33,64]. Homosynaptic LTD in the hippocampus occurs when low frequency stimulation (e.g., 1 Hz for 15 min) applied to one neuron decreases responsivity in its target neuron[13,33]. LTD has not previously been demonstrated *in vivo* and was originally described in brain tissue from young, but not adult animals[17]. For this reason, it was thought to be involved more in early development of the nervous system rather than in plasticity in adult animals. However, LTD has since been demonstrated in slices from adult animals[1], and a similar phenomenon, termed depotentiation, has been produced *in vivo*[3,61] and in hippocampal slices from adult animals[5,45]. The parameters for inducing depotentiation resemble those of LTD; the pharmacology is similar but not identical. The main distinction is that the diminished synaptic response of depotentiation requires the prior induction of LTP, and is not readily elicited under baseline conditions. LTP and LTD have also been shown to reverse each other[13,33,37], and it was this observation that prompted us to attempt to alter kindling development using LTD-like stimulation *in vivo*. We termed this procedure quenching, and while we do not know if LTD or depotentiation are actually induced in the amygdala, the term functionally describes the effect on the kindling process.

1.3. Quenching

In this chapter, we describe our recent findings that low frequency stimulation of the amygdala (1 Hz, for 15 min) can block the development of amygdala kindled seizures, and inhibit their expression in fully kindled animals.[67] These effects appear to result from a change in the afterdischarge and/or seizure threshold which persists for weeks to months after quenching is discontinued. While the optimal and critical parameters for quenching require further investigation, frequency, at least, is one important parameter for raising the seizure thresholds in kindled animals. N-methyl-d-aspartic acid (NMDA) glutamate receptors are not critical for quenching, and this differs from the findings for LTD or depotentiation in the hippocampus. The mechanisms of quenching are just beginning to be investigated and its potential utility as a treatment modality for epileptic patients remains to be explored.

2. METHODS

2.1. Kindling

Male Sprague Dawley rats were surgically implanted with a bipolar platinum-iridium electrode in the left amygdala at the stereotactic coordinates A-P 5.7, L 4.5, V 2.0, using interaural zero[47]. Following at least one week of recovery, electrical stimulation was begun using stimulus parameters of 60 Hz biphasic square waves, 1 msec pulsewidth, and 1 second total duration. For some studies, the stimulation intensity was suprathreshold at 800 μA peak to peak; however, for most we used the minimum current required to induce an afterdischarge (AD) in each animal (typically, ~100 to 300μA). The kindling procedure was conducted once daily, 5–7 days per week, and the measures recorded were the afterdischarge duration, seizure intensity (using the rating scale developed by Racine[55]), and seizure duration if a major motor seizure was observed (≥ stage 3).

2.2. Quenching

Quenching stimulation was delivered through the same amygdala electrode used for kindling. The stimulation parameters initially selected were based on the literature for inducing homosynaptic LTD in hippocampal slices *in vitro*. These were 1 Hz (biphasic square waves), 0.1 msec pulsewidth, and 15 min total duration (i.e., 900 pulses). We chose to administer an intensity of 100 μA over the AD (or seizure) threshold. In general, during the quenching procedure the rats' behavior appeared normal, i.e., they were either exploratory or sleeping. However, we were unable to obtain EEG recordings during this 15 min stimulation procedure due to technical limitations.

2.3. Threshold Measurement

To determine the AD threshold, electrical stimulation was applied in 50 μA incrementing steps beginning at 50 μA, with each test stimulus separated by at least 20 min. Using electroencephalographic assessment, ADs were observed as repetitive spike and wave actvity occurring at a frequency of ≥ 1/sec. In kindled animals, seizure thresholds were determined in the same manner with the endpoint being a seizure ≥ Stage 3. In fully-kindled animals, the AD and seizure thresholds were usually the same; however occasionally, animals would show a 50 μA difference between these indices. In all determinations, the maximum intensity tested was 800 μA, to avoid tissue damage.

3. RESULTS AND DISCUSSION

3.1. Quenching Inhibits Amygdala Kindled Seizure Development and Increases AD Thresholds

We initially attempted to alter amygdala kindled seizure development since this seemed the most easily accessible endpoint at which to intervene. In two separate studies, we evaluated the effects of quenching administered daily after each kindling stimulation. All animals were kindled at their AD threshold once daily. Quenching was begun immediately after the cessation of afterdischarge or seizure activity. Three conditions were tested: kindling plus quenching (1 Hz for 15 min; N=8); kindling plus sham (i.e., rats remained in the recording chamber for 15 minutes with no further stimulation; N=8); and kindling plus

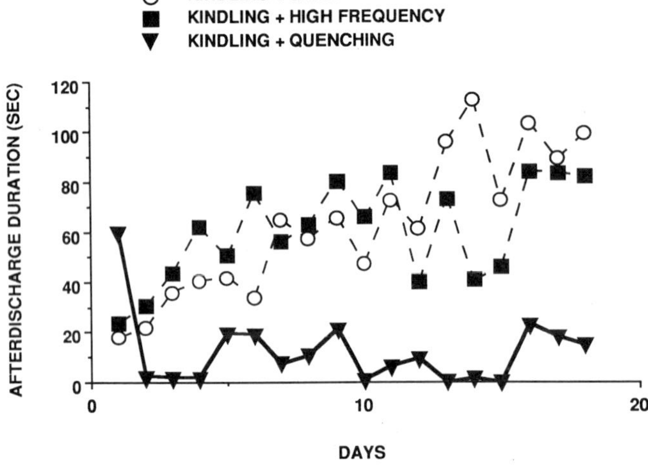

Figure 1a. Quenching inhibits amygdala-kindled seizure development. The group mean afterdischarge duration is plotted over days. Quenching completely suppressed the development of afterdischarges and seizures (not shown) in 7 of the 8 animals. Note, however, that ADs were elicited in these animals on day 1 prior to their first quenching stimulation. Both control groups (sham and high-frequency stimulated) showed typical AD and kindled seizure development.

high frequency stimulation (100 Hz, .01 msec pulsewidth for 15 minutes at 100 μA over the AD threshold; N=4). The latter group was a control for non-specific "interference" effects produced by the additional stimulation after kindling. These studies were conducted until the sham group demonstrated reliable generalized seizures (21 and 18 days in studies I and II, respectively).

The data from the two studies were combined and are presented in Figs. 1a and b. Quenching inhibited the increase in afterdischarge duration and completely blocked seizure development in 7 of the 8 animals tested (Fig. 1a). No significant effects, compared to sham, were produced by the high frequency stimulation.

Following the completion of kindling in the control animals, afterdischarge thresholds were re-determined (days 22 and 19; Fig. 1b). The sham and high frequency groups

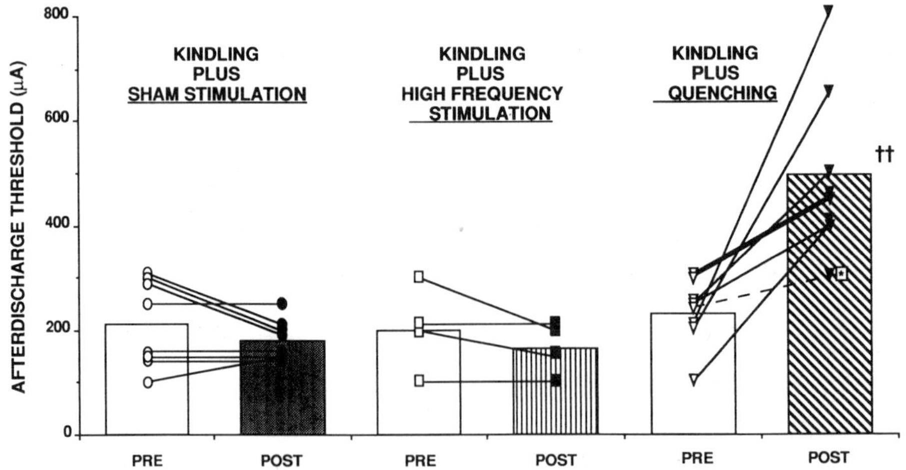

Figure 1b. Quenching increases afterdischarge thresholds. AD thresholds are plotted before kindling was initiated and after seizures developed in the control animals. Group mean (bars) and individual (lines) afterdischarge thresholds are illustrated. Kindling followed by quenching resulted in a large increase in the AD thresholds, which was not observed in either control group. The threshold for one rat that developed seizures during the quenching procedure is indicated by the asterisk; note that this animal did not show a robust elevation in AD threshold. (Reprinted from[67]).

showed no change or a slight nonsignificant decrease in their AD threshold. By contrast, the quenching group showed markedly increased AD thresholds ($p<.01$). Interestingly, the only animal from the quenching group that developed intermittent kindled seizures was also the only rat that failed to markedly increase its AD threshold (indicated on Fig. 1b by the asterisk). Thus, the suppression of amygdala kindled seizure development probably resulted, at least in part, from the quenching-induced increase in afterdischarge thresholds.

After the 22 days of kindling plus quenching stimulation and threshold testing, we discontinued the quenching and continued to kindle the rats from the first study (N=4) to determine whether there was a persistent effect of prior quenching. In one animal, ADs began to occur intermittently after day 42 and seizures began after day 49. The other two did not develop kindled seizures even after 5 months of continued stimulation, although they did occasionally show ADs. The fourth animal continued to have seizures inconsistently, similar to what had been observed during the quenching protocol. All electrode placements were verified to be in the amygdala in these animals[67]. Thus, the quenching-induced suppression of ADs and seizures appears relatively long-lasting and persists to some extent despite the resumption of kindling stimulation.

3.2. Quenching Inhibits Seizures and Increases Thresholds in Fully-Kindled Animals

To answer the question of whether quenching could also inhibit fully-kindled seizures, we used the control animals from the second study (N=7), which were experiencing generalized seizures with most or all kindled stimulations. They were divided into two groups matched for seizure thresholds, and received either daily 15 min of 1 Hz quenching stimulation (at 100 μA over their seizure threshold) or 15 min of sham stimulation for 7–8 days. Following this procedure, their thresholds were re-determined and daily 1 sec kindling stimulation (at the parameters previously used) was resumed.

As Figure 2 illustrates, quenching stimulation inhibited kindled seizures for many weeks. Seizure thresholds increased following quenching (from 212±37 to 337±24 μA;

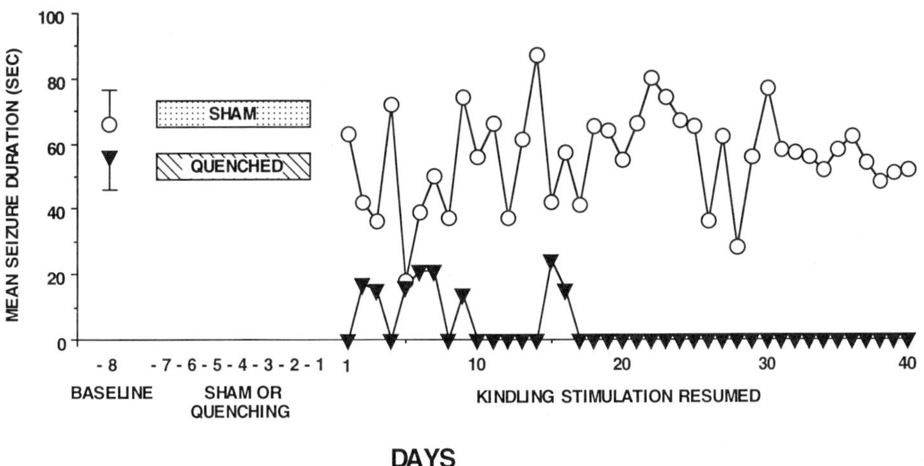

Figure 2. Quenching inhibits seizures in fully-kindled rats. The group mean seizure duration is plotted in kindled rats before (left symbols) and after one week of quenching or sham stimulation. Kindling stimulation was applied at the same intensity used to elicit generalized seizures before treatment. Quenching suppressed kindled seizures for several weeks, while sham stimulation had no effect.

p<.01), but not following sham stimulaton (from 233±44 to 116±16.7 μA). These results suggest that the seizure inhibition produced by quenching was again attributable to an increase in threshold; in this case seizure threshold, compared to afterdischarge threshold in the development studies.

We continued to monitor seizure thresholds every 3–4 weeks in these animals and several others from the first study that also received one week of quenching stimulation after generalized seizures had developed (N=7). Daily kindling continued at the same parameters used to elicit seizures in these rats prior to quenching; however, in most instances, seizures were not evoked. The kindled rats that had not been quenched (sham-stimulated controls) were evaluated concurrently, but these animals experienced seizures between threshold determinations.

Figure 3 illustrates the significant elevation in thresholds that persisted for at least 7 weeks after quenching had been discontinued. Thus, 7 daily exposures to quenching stimulation were sufficient to alter seizure thresholds in fully kindled animals, despite continued application of kindling stimulation. Nevertheless, the kindled state itself was

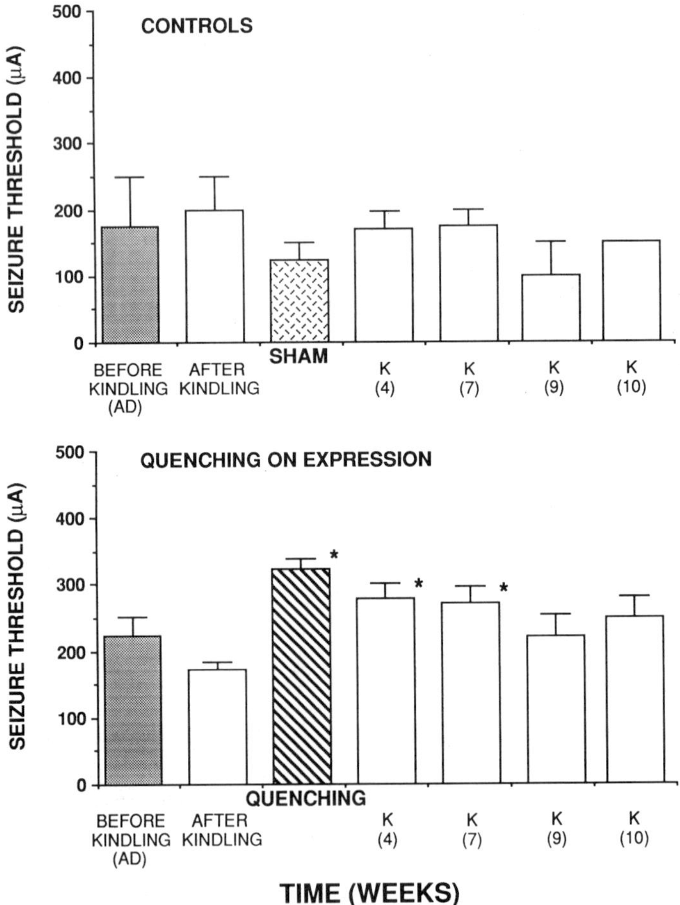

Figure 3. Quenching persistently increases seizure thresholds in fully-kindled animals. Group mean± s.e.m. seizure thresholds are illustrated at various timepoints: before and after kindling; after quenching; and at 3–4 week intervals thereafter. The quenching-induced elevations in threshold were significant for 7 weeks following treatment. Sham-stimulated animals did not show this effect.

not reversed, since with sufficiently high intensity stimulation, as occurred at the time of threshold determinations, a generalized seizure could still be induced.

Whether quenching of fully kindled animals can be further enhanced (with greater numbers of quenching stimulations, intermittent re-exposure to quenching, or different quenching parameters) remains an important question (see section 3.4 below), particularly in relation to the therapeutic potential of this procedure. In one group of rats that initially had kindling blocked by quenching and then were kindled with suprathreshold stimulation (800 μA), high-intensity quenching (800 μA, and 1 Hz for 15 min daily for 1 week) resulted in sustained high mean seizure thresholds of 662±55 μA (this value artificially underestimates the actual threshold value since one rat did not have a seizure at 800 μA, the maximal intensity tested). This effect persisted for during 4 months of periodic re-evaluation; the group mean threshold hovered at approximately 500 μA, a value twice that typically seen in kindled animals. Although the interpretation of these data is clouded by the multiple exposures to quenching and higher intensity stimulation, further manipulation of some of these quenching variables may yield an even more robust and/or long-lasting effect.

3.3. Quenching Prior to Kindling Initiation Retards Seizure Development, i.e., Could Such a Procedure Be Applicable to Primary Prevention?

Two questions that we addressed in these studies were: 1) Does quenching in naive animals slow the development of subsequent kindling; and 2) Is quenching more like depotentiation than LTD, i.e., does it require an already potentiated system to be effective? Amygdala afterdischarge thresholds were determined in experimentally naive rats that were then divided into two balanced groups. Ten days elapsed before beginning the study in order to minimize any residual effects of the threshold determination. Rats then received daily, 15 min quenching (N=5) or sham (N=6) stimulation for 7 days and their afterdischarge thresholds were re-determined. Kindling began on the following day using the stimulation intensity determined in the first threshold test.

Quenching markedly increased the afterdischarge thresholds in these rats (Fig. 4a), indicating that concurrent kindling was not necessary for quenching to be effective in altering baseline AD thresholds. However, when kindling was begun, the quenched animals showed only a transient delay in seizure progression. They were slower to develop afterdischarges (Fig. 4b). Moreover, all of the rats in the sham group had ADs on the first day of stimulation, while none of the quenched animals did. In the quenched group, the mean number of days until an AD was elicited was 4.5 with a range of 2–8 stimulations. Once elicited, the rate and pattern of kindled seizure development were similar to controls (the mean ± s.e.m. number of days of afterdischarges until the first stage 5 seizure was observed was 8.3±1.5 in the sham group vs. 8.0±1.8 in the quenched group). When thresholds were re-determined after seizures developed in both groups, no difference in seizure thresholds was observed.

These results suggest that whereas low frequency stimulation in naive animals can profoundly increase afterdischarge thresholds, this effect was more transient than in the kindling development and maintainence studies described previously. Several procedural differences could account for this. For example, when kindling stimulation preceded quenching during development, an interaction between these two forms of stimulation may have occurred that is similar to that required for depotentiation. Alternatively, in the development studies where quenching was administered for approximately 20 days, longer lasting effects may have occurred because of the greater number of exposures. However,

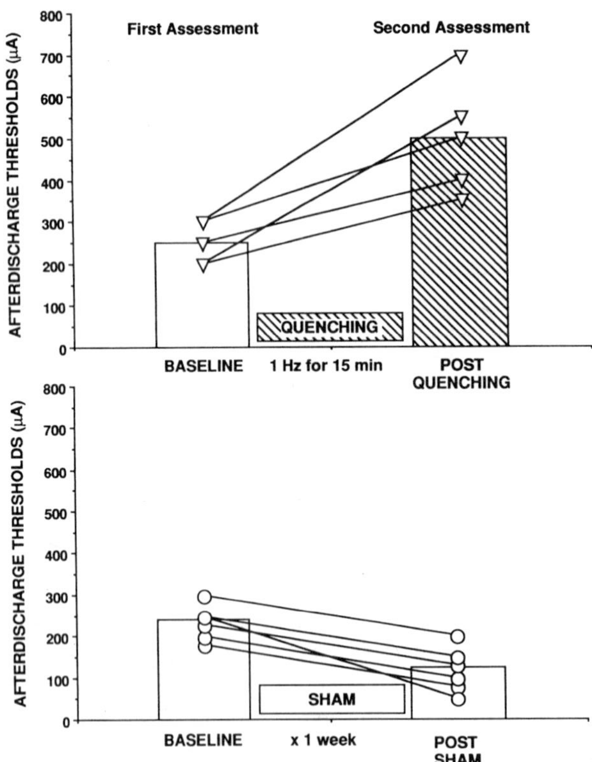

Figure 4a. Quenching prior to kindling intiation increases AD thresholds. Group mean (bars) and individual (lines) afterdischarge thresholds are illustrated before and after one week of quenching or sham stimulation (no kindling occurred). The AD thresholds markedly increased in the quenched animals and decreased in the sham stimulated controls.

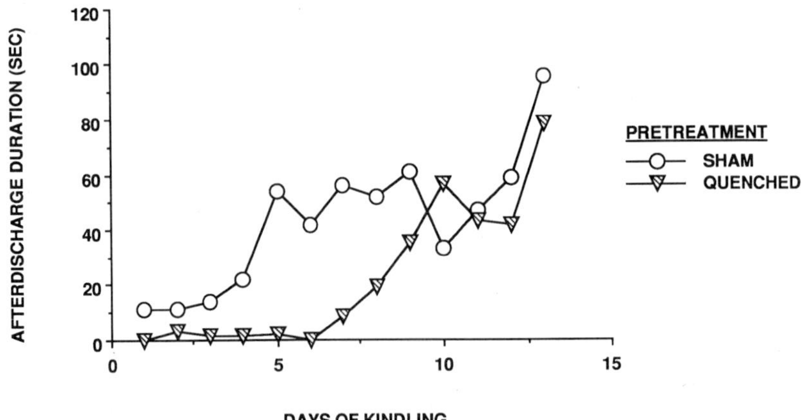

Figure 4b. Quenching in naive (unkindled) animals slows subsequent kindling development. Naive animals that received either quenching or sham stimulation for one week were kindled at their original AD threshold intensity. Quenching modestly slowed the development of ADs ($F=5.64$, d.f.(1,9), $p<.05$ between groups, $p<.001$ for days, no significant interaction). However, this effect was not significant after day 8. A trend in the same direction was observed for seizure duration (not illustrated; $F=3.71$, d.f. (1,9) $p<.10$ between groups, $p<.05$ for days, no significant interaction).

in the fully kindled animals, seven days of quenching were sufficient to elevate seizure thresholds for a long period of time, even after kindling was resumed. Therefore, it is possible that quenching is more persistent in a system that has been prevously activated, either by kindling immediately prior to quenching or by the chronic alterations in excitability occurring in the kindled state.

There was one exception to this lack of persistence—a single rat that showed a large increase in threshold from 300 to 700 μA after quenching, which was maintained even after 40 days of electrical stimulation. This animal failed to develop afterdischarges or kindled seizures until we increased the stimulation current to suprathreshold intensity (800 μA) which then, upon repetition, produced typical kindled seizure development. Histological analysis of the electrode position in this animal revealed the placement to be just outside of the amygdala in the perirhinal cortex adjacent to the external capsule. Though stimulation in this area should indirectly affect the amygdala, the enhanced response to the quenching stimulation may be related to the unique placement of the electrode in this animal. (Note that the data from this animal were not included in the above analyses.)

From the clinical standpoint, a small change in threshold could be sufficient to keep epileptogenic stimuli below that required for AD generation and seizure progression. Moreover, the observation that one animal showed a persistent effect of quenching on subsequent kindled seizure development suggests that the technique might yet be useful when appropriate neuroanatomic or parametric data become available. As greater numbers of genetic markers of illness susceptibility emerge, primary prophylactic therapeutics may become more viable and crucial health care tools.

3.4. Frequency of Quenching Stimulation Is an Important Parameter for Elevations in Thresholds

The design of the quenching studies was based on *in vitro* observations related to LTD induction in the hippocampus. However, since we have not proven that LTD is even induced *in vivo* in the amygdala by our procedure, we began a series of studies to determine whether frequency of stimulation was in fact important to the quenching effect on thresholds. Fully-kindled animals that had been stimulated with suprathreshold current intensity (800 μA), and matched for seizure threshold and number of prior seizures, received one week of quenching stimulation at different test frequencies: 0 (sham), 1, 10, 20, and 60 Hz, using the same pulsewidth (0.1 msec), intensity (100 μA over threshold) and duration (15 min) of stimulation. Seizure thresholds were determined prior to and after quenching stimulation. We did not go higher than 60 Hz since several other animals that had previously been exposed to 100 Hz stimulation at these parameters developed status epilepticus (in the study in which we used 100 Hz stimulation, the pulsewidth was shortened to 0.01 msec to avoid this problem).

The optimal effect observed in all animals was achieved at 1 Hz ($p<.01$); 10 Hz was more variable but still produced a significant elevation of seizure threshold ($p<.05$); 20 Hz increased the threshold in a few animals but this effect was not significant; and no effect was observed at 60 Hz (Fig 5). Thus, in combination with the other parameters used previously for quenching (i.e., stimulus intensity, pulsewidth, and duration), low frequencies appear to be more effective than higher frequencies in raising the seizure threshold of fully-kindled animals.

The sham-stimulated controls showed a significant decrease in their seizure threshold ($p<.05$). This observation is consistent with previous work from our laboratory. Briefly, kindled animals that do not experience seizures for 4 days or longer, show a de-

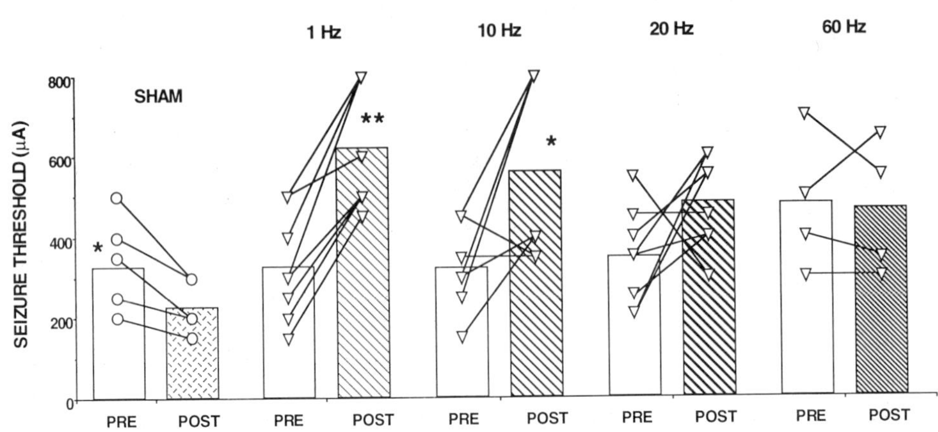

Figure 5. Frequency of stimulation alters the effectiveness of quenching. Seizure thresholds are plotted in kindled rats before and after 1 week of stimulation using different frequencies (0, 1, 10, 20, and 60 Hz). The other stimulation parameters of quenching were unchanged (1 Hz, 0.1 msec pulsewidth, 15 min). Group mean (bars) and individual (lines) seizure thresholds are illustrated. Only stimulation at the lower frequencies of stimulation (1 and 10 Hz) significantly increased the seizure thresholds. The optimal frequency of quenching stimulation for raising seizure thresholds is 1 Hz. * $p < .05$; ** $p < .01$.

crease in their seizure thresholds and in their response to the anticonvulsant carbamazepine,[66] suggesting that the seizures themselves induce transient anticonvulsant adaptations[43] that can facilitate exogenous drug effects. This also implies that the quenching effect is even more profound than the paired comparisions with baseline would suggest. The thresholds should be shifting downward in animals not experiencing a seizure, not upward as observed in quenched animals.

Frequencies lower than 1 Hz, and many other parameters for optimal quenching remain to be studied. Preliminary data mentioned above suggest that intensity may also be an important variable, with greater intensities likely producing a more robust and long-lasting effect on threshold. This may have to be balanced against the potential of greater currents inducing damage to the nervous system. All these issues require further exploration.

3.5. NMDA Glutamate Receptors Are Not Critical for Quenching

Homosynaptic LTD (in the hippocampus) and depotentiation involve NMDA receptor mechanisms, i.e., both can be blocked using competive or non-competitive NMDA antagonists[16,44]. Similarly, LTP in certain regions of the hippocampus (but not others) and amygdala kindled seizure development also require intact NMDA receptor function[7,29,38,41]. Thus, this system seemed a good target to explore potential mechanisms of quenching. Two studies were conducted to examine the possible role of NMDA receptors in quenching of: (1) completed kindled seizures; and (2) kindled seizure development.

3.5.1. We first tested the ability of the noncompetitive NMDA receptor antagonist MK-801 to block the quenching-induced increases in seizure threshold in fully-kindled animals. A series of rats were kindled using suprathreshold stimulation (800 μA). When seizures developed, the rats were divided into three groups (n=6/group) matched on the

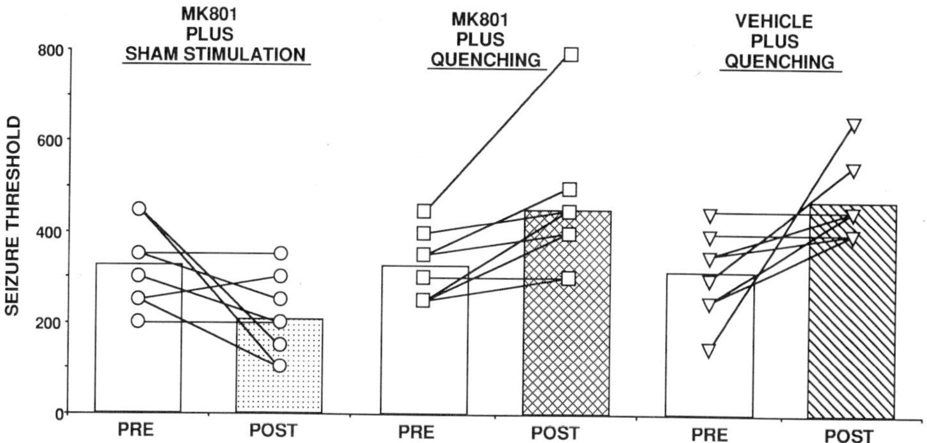

Figure 6. NMDA receptor blockade does not interfere with the quenching-induced elevation of seizure thresholds in fully kindled rats. Seizure thresholds are plotted in kindled rats before and after 1 week of quenching or sham stimulation plus vehicle or MK-801 (0.5 mg/kg) treatment. Group mean (bars) and individual (lines) seizure thresholds are illustrated. Both groups that received quenching stimulation (with and without MK-801) showed a comparable and significant increase in their seizure thresholds, indicating that NMDA receptors are not critical to this effect. The rats that received sham stimulation (plus MK-801) showed a decrease in their seizure threshold comparable to what is typically observed in untreated kindled rats given a week-long seizure-free interval.

basis of seizure threshold and number of prior seizures. The treatments were: MK-801 (0.5 mg/kg) plus sham stimulation; MK-801 (0.5 mg/kg) plus quenching; and vehicle (saline) plus quenching. The drug or vehicle injections were administered 1 hour prior to stimulation; this procedure was repeated for 7 days. Following this, seizure thresholds were re-determined.

MK-801 did not block the increases in seizure thresholds produced by quenching (Fig. 6). The increase in seizure thresholds produced by quenching was significant in both groups. The rats that received MK-801 and sham stimulation demonstrated a decrease in seizure threshold, similar to what we typically observe with time-off from seizures, as described above (section 3.4;[66]). Thus, MK-801 adminstered to kindled animals with no other stimulation does not appear to raise seizure thresholds. Although other doses of MK-801 have not yet been tested, we purposely chose a high dose for this study that produced marked locomotor activating and stereotypic behaviors in all of the rats. The quenching procedure alone did not alter these behaviors.

3.5.2. In a second study, we tested the possible role of NMDA receptors in quenching by determining whether MK-801 could modulate the quenching inhibition of kindled seizure development. Three groups of rats (N=6/group) were matched for their AD thresholds. All rats were kindled at threshold stimulation intensitiy followed by: MK-801 (0.5 mg/kg) plus sham stimulation; MK-801 (0.5 mg/kg) plus quenching; or vehicle (saline) plus quenching. Since MK-801 given prior to kindling stimulation can block seizure development, we administered the drug (or vehicle) 5 min after the kindling stimulation and began the quenching (or sham stimulation) 30 min later. The longer interval between kindling and quenching was necessary since the drug could not be given prior to kindling and it requires time to be absorbed and reach peak concentration.

Two results are notable from this study: 1) MK-801 did not alter the suppressive effect of quenching on AD and seizure development (Fig. 7a) and did not block the quenching-induced increase in AD thresholds (Fig. 7b); and 2) the quenching effect in both groups was somewhat less absolute during the first two weeks of stimulation than in the earlier studies of quenching on kindling development.

We presume that the less robust initial effect of quenching was attributable to the 30-min delay between kindling and quenching. When quenching was applied immediately after the kindling stimulus, ADs were suppressed in most rats beginning on day 2 of stimulation (Fig. 1). In the current study, afterdischarges were observed in most quenched animals (with or without MK-801) for the first several days, but tended to disappear or occur erratically as the study continued (Fig. 7a). Half the rats in each quenched group also had occasional seizures that did not increase in duration or intensity, or become reliably evokable. These occurred within the first 14 days of stimulation and not afterwards in all but one animal. Thus, in both groups of rats that received kindling plus quenching stimulation (with or without MK-801), we observed an almost complete regression in the AD duration and seizure development.

Moreover, in five of the quenched rats (from both groups) that continued to receive threshold kindling stimulation without further quenching, we observed a persistent suppressive effect lasting between 1 week and 2 months. At this point suprathreshold stimulation was applied and kindling developed normally in these rats. Therefore, although the interval between kindling and quenching has not yet been studied systematically, it appears that a delay of 30 minutes, while slowing the onset of the quenching effect, did not prevent the complete inhibition of seizures and ADs in 11 of the 12 animals tested.

On days 28–30, AD thresholds were re-determined (Fig. 7b). Rats in both quenched groups showed markedly elevated AD thresholds compared to sham-treated rats that

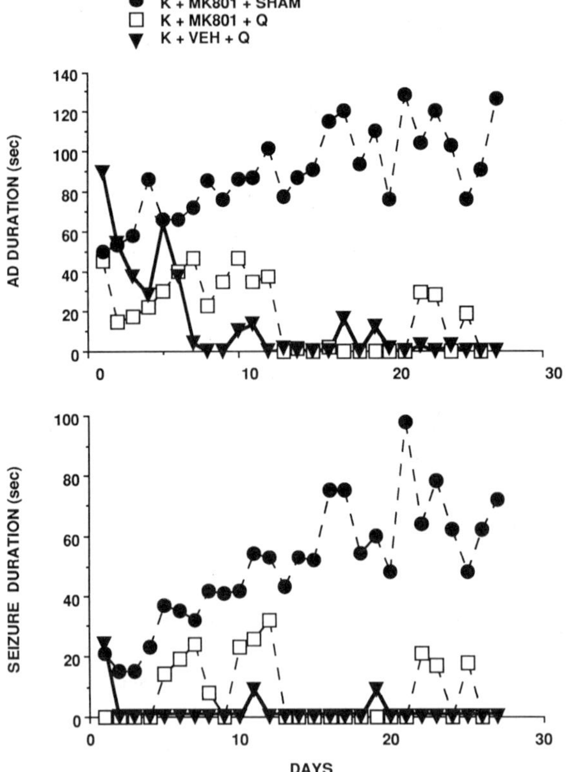

Figure 7a. NMDA receptor blockade did not interfere with the quenching-induced suppression of amygdala-kindled seizure development. The group mean afterdischarge (top) and seizure (bottom) duration are plotted over days in rats that received kindling plus: vehicle and quenching; MK-801 (0.5 mg/kg) and quenching; MK-801 (0.5 mg/kg) and sham stimulation. Drug or vehicle injections were administered 5 min after kindling, and quenching or sham stimulation occurred 30 minutes later. Quenching-suppressed kindling development was not altered by MK-801. MK-801 alone (after kindling stimulation) did not affect the rate of kindling development.

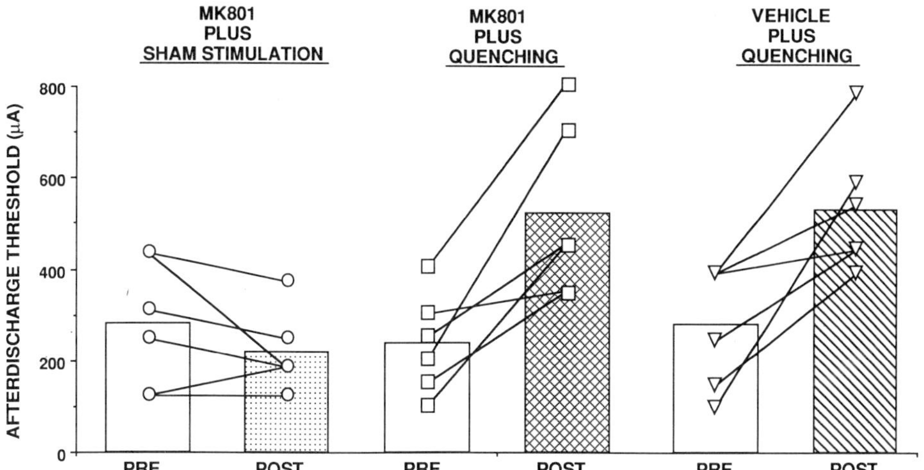

Figure 7b. NMDA receptor blockade did not alter the quenching-induced increase in afterdischarge thresholds. Afterdischarge thresholds are plotted before kindling was initiated and after the control group (non-quenched) developed seizures. Quenching stimulation significantly increased the AD thresholds in both groups; the sham-stimulated (MK-801-treated) group showed no change (or a slight decrease) in their AD threshold, as is typically observed following kindling with no drug treatment.

showed no change or a slight decrease. The kindled rats that received MK-801 plus sham stimulation for 15 min developed amygdala kindled seizures at a rate and pattern similar to that we have observed in previous studies when no drug was given. This suggests that no residual effects of the drug were evident 24 hours after its administration, since MK-801 given more immediately prior to stimulation blocks kindling development robustly[28,41].

Taken together, the results of the two studies suggest that NMDA receptor blockade does not inhibit the quenching effects on kindled seizure development, expression, or thresholds. Other glutamate receptors, however, may be more important to this phenomenon since recent work suggests a role for metabotropic glutamate receptors in LTD and LTP[4,5,46,65]. While these studies did not implicate NMDA mechanisms, they did provide further replication of the magnitude and reliability of the quenching effect.

4. CONCLUSIONS AND GENERAL DISCUSSION

The duality, or balance, between excitation and inhibition leading ultimately to seizures or quiescence has been of interest since the earliest descriptions of kindling by Goddard and associates[31]. They realized that inhibitory processes must develop concurrently with the facilitatory events leading to seizures. For example, when electrical stimulation was repeated at very brief intervals (e.g., 10–20 min) kindling did not result, and seizures were not elicited, even in fully kindled animals[31]. Additionally, stimulation of a secondary site can alter excitability in the primary site and vice versa[9,15,31]. Thus, both focal and transynaptic alterations in seizure susceptibility have been noted for a number of years. The conditions that promote inhibition of seizures have been examined systematically by a number of investigators[18,32,43,51,58,59] and typically, the results indicate that seizures inhibit subsequent seizures, even when totally different brain regions or methods of seizure induction are involved (e.g., [32,51]). Subthreshold stimulation sufficient to induce an afterdischarge can also be inhibitory, although these effects are less robust and shorter-lived[43].

Therefore, the issue of whether non-convulsive, non-pharmacological methods can be developed to block epileptic events has been of interest for both theoretical and clinical reasons. At least three groups have addressed this question previously. Shao and Valenstein[60], using one or several series of 20 1-sec subthreshold stimulations spaced 6.5 sec apart, induced seizure suppression in amygdala kindled rats that lasted up to one week. Shorter interstimulus intervals (< 6.5 sec) were less effective, and the suppression was dependent on testing the animals with an incrementing stimulation paradigm (i.e., if suprathreshold stimulation was attempted first, then the increase in seizure resistance was not observed). Thus, while promising, further work is necessary to characterize this effect.

Tanaka and Naquet[63] used low-frequency stimulation (10 Hz) of subcortical regions (the ventral lateral nucleus of the thalamus and central gray) to inhibit amygdala kindled seizures in cats. They found an increase in seizure latency and sometimes a suppression of the seizure itself; this effect did not last longer than 24 hours, however.

Finally, Gaito and associates conducted an extensive series of studies using low frequency stimulation (usually 1 or 3 Hz) and reported a suppression of amygdala kindled seizures and an increase in seizure thresholds[19–25]. A number of different parameters were examined including frequency[20], interstimulation interval[24], and duration of stimulation[23]. Although Gaito described a long-lasting effect on seizure threshold when low frequency stimulation was applied for 10 min or more[23], he focused instead on the more transient and reversible effects of this method for altering seizure thresholds, which usually did not last more than 2 weeks. This occurred when the low frequency stimulus was applied for ~30 sec to 2 min. In addition, Gaito usually administered the low frequency stimulation both before and after kindling with an hour separating each trial[22]. Nevertheless, Gaito's findings are similar to those presented in this paper. The main drawback to Gaito's work, which makes comparison with the current studies difficult, is that he did not clarify certain aspects of the stimulation methodology and did not provide any electrographic or histological data. Of particular concern is the use of sine wave stimulation, which, if applied for long durations, could result in very large current densities and tissue damage. Gaito evaluated the brains of the short-duration low-frequency stimulated rats histologically, and did not observe any unusual effects[21]. However, it is unclear what might have occurred following the long duration application of this low-frequency stimulation.

In addition to quenching, low frequency stimulation can produce a rapid form of kindling in both rats and cats[12,14,42]. However, the stimulus requirements for rapid kindling have notable differences from quenching. These are high intensities in the range of 6–24 mA for 1 Hz stimulation of the amygdala (in rats), a pulsewidth of at least 1 msec, and a shorter stimulation duration (60 sec). When rats are kindled using these parameters, they develop seizures more rapidly than with conventional kindling but show complete transfer to 60-Hz kindling stimulation. Interestingly, Cain and Corcoran[12] noted that low-frequency kindling did not show transfer to the contralateral amygdala. Thus, this might be an important variable to evaluate in the quenching paradigm.

Whether quenching can be considered another form of long-term neural plasticity will require investigation of a number of variables that have been shown to be important in kindling, LTP, or LTD. Some of these include: 1) regional specificity—can quenching be evoked in regions outside of the amygdala? 2) transfer—can quenching in one structure suppress kindling in another, i.e., is a transynaptic inhibitory process involved? 3) temporal parameters—are there interval requirements for quenching relative to kindling, or to quenching itself? 4) other parameters—of the parameters already implicated; pulsewidth, intensity, and frequency, which are most important? 5) permanence—can quenching be reversed and when? 6) structural or functional changes in the brain—since seizure and afterdischarge thresholds are increased in a profound and long-lasting manner, what anatomical and neurochemical alterations in brain are evident?

In summary, we found that low-frequency (1 Hz) stimulation of the amygdala for 15 min (i.e., a phenomenon we have called quenching) inhibits the development of amygdala kindled seizures and suppresses the expression of generalized kindled seizures in threshold-stimulated rats. These robust results are likely due to the effect of quenching to elevate the AD and seizure thresholds. Furthermore, these effects appear to be long-lasting, even under conditions of continued kindling stimulation. Quenching prior to kindling initiation also elevates the AD threshold and modestly slows subsequent seizure development, although this primary preventive effect is not as persistent as quenching administered concurrently with kindling stimulation or after seizures have developed. Frequency of stimulation is one important parameter: seizure threshold increases were larger and more consistent at 1 Hz and diminished progressively at 10, 20, and 60 Hz. Many other parameters for optimizing the quenching phenomenon remain to be explored. NMDA glutamate receptors do not appear to be involved in quenching and the mechanisms underlying the large and long-lasting effects on threshold remain to be determined. Nonetheless, these preliminary but highly robust data strongly support the possibility of extending these findings to clinical therapeutics. Clinical applications could utilize depth or surface electrodes, or make use of repetitive transcranial magnetic stimulation (rTMS), a rapidly emerging technique for noninvasively stimulating discrete brain regions for the treatment of other neurological and psychiatric illnesses[27].

REFERENCES

1. Abraham, W. C. and Kerr, D. S., Voltage-sensitive calcium channels in the induction of homosynaptic and heterosynaptic LTD in the hippocampus, Fourth IBRO World Conference of Neuroscience, (1995) 22.
2. Adamec, R. E., Does kindling model anything clinically relevant?, *Biol Psych*, 27 (1990) 249–279.
3. Barrionuevo, G., Schottler, F. and Lynch, G., The effects of repetitive low frequency stimulation on control and potentiated synaptics responses in the hippocampus, *Life Sci*, 27 (1980) 2385–2389.
4. Bashir, Z. I., Bortolotto, Z. A., Davies, C. H., Berrett, N., Irving, A. J., Seal, A. J., Henley, J. M., Jane, D. E., Watkins, J. C. and Collingridge, G. L., Induction of LTP in the hippocampus needs synaptic activation of glutamate metabotropic receptors, *Nature*, 363 (1993) 347–350.
5. Bashir, Z. I. and Collingridge, G. L., An investigation of depotentiation of long-term potentiation in the Ca1 region of the hippocampus, *Exp Br Res*, 100 (1994) 437–443.
6. Bear, M. F. and Malenka, R. C., Synaptic plasticity: LTP and LTD, *Cur Opinion Neurobiology*, 4 (1994) 389–399.
7. Bliss, T. and Collingridge, A synaptic model of memory: long-term potentiation in the hippocampus, *Nature*, 361 (1993) 31–39.
8. Bliss, T. and Lomo, T., Long-lasting potentiation of synaptic transmission in the dentate area of the anaesthetized rabbit following stimulation of the perforant path, *J Physiol*, 232 (1973) 331–356.
9. Burchfiel, J. L. and Applegate, C. D., Forebrain and brainstem mechanisms governing kindled seizure development: a hypothesis. In J. A. Wada, *Kindling 4, 37*, Plenum Press, New York, 1990, 93–112.
10. Burnham, W. M. and Cottrell, G. A., The GABA hypothesis of kindling. In J. A. Wada, *Kindling 4*, Plenum Press, New York, 1990, 127–139.
11. Cain, D., Long-term potentiation and kindling: how similar are the mechanisms?, *TINS*, 12 (1989) 6–10.
12. Cain, D. P. and Corcoran, M. E., Kindling with low-frequency stimulation: Generality, transfer, and recruiting effects, *Exp Neurol*, 73 (1981) 219–232.
13. Christie, B. R., Kerr, D. S. and Abraham, W. C., Flip side of synaptic plasticity: Long-term depression mechanisms in the hippocampus, *Hippocampus*, 4 (1994) 127–135.
14. Corcoran, M. E. and Cain, D. P., Kindling of seizures with low frequency electrical stimulation, *Brain Res*, 196 (1980) 262–265.
15. Duchowny, M. S. and Burchfiel, J. L., Facilitation and antagonism of kindled seizure development in the limbic system of the rat, *Electroenceph Clin Neurophysiol*, 51 (1981) 403–416.

16. Dudek, S. M. and Bear, M. F., Homosynaptic long-term depression in area CA1 of hippocampus and effects of N-methyl-D-aspartate receptor blockade, *Proc. Natl. Acad. Sci. USA*, 89 (1992) 4363–4367.
17. Dudek, S. M. and Bear, M. F., Bidirectional long-term modification of synaptic effectiveness in adult and immature hippocampus, *J. Neurosci.*, 13 (1993) 2910–2918.
18. Essig, C. F. and Flanary, H. G., The importance of the convulsion in the occurrence and rate of development of electroconvulsive threshold elevation, *Exp Neurol*, 14 (1966) 448–452.
19. Gaito, J., Suppresion of 60-Hz induced convulsive behavior by 3-Hz brain stimulation, *Bull Psychonomic Soc*, 13 (1979) 223–226.
20. Gaito, J., Gradient of interference by various frequencies on 60 Hz kindling behavior, *Canadian Journal of Neurological Sciences*, 7 (1980) 223–226.
21. Gaito, J., The effect of low frequency and direct current stimulation on the kindling phenomenon in rats, *Canadian Journal of Neurological Sciences*, 8 (1981) 249–253.
22. Gaito, J., Suppression of kindling behavior, *J Psych*, 118 (1984) 113–125.
23. Gaito, J. and ., The effect of variable duration one hertz interference on kindling, *Canadian Journal of Neurological Sciences*, 7 (1980) 59–64.
24. Gaito, J. and Gaito, S. T., The effect of several intertrial intervals on the 1 Hz interference effect, *Canadian Journal of Neurological Sciences*, 8 (1981) 61–65.
25. Gaito, J., Nobrega, J. N. and Gaito, S. T., Interference effect of 3 Hz brain stimulation on kindling behavior in duced by 60 Hz stimulation, *Epilepsia*, 21 (1980) 73–84.
26. Geinisman, Y., Morrell, F. and deToledo-Morrell, L., Alterations of synaptic ultrastructure induced by hippocampal kindling. In J. A. Wada, *Kindling 4,* Plenum Press, New York, 1990, 75–92.
27. George, M. S., Wasserman, E. M., Williams, W. A., Callahan, A., Ketter, T. A., Basser, P., Hallett, M. and Post, R. M., Daily repetitive transcranial magnetic stimulation (rTMS) improves mood in depression, *NeuroReport*, 6 (1995) 1853–1856.
28. Gilbert, M. E., The NMDA-receptor antagonist, MK-801, suppresses limbic kindling and kindled seizures, *Brain Res*, 463 (1988) 90–99.
29. Gilbert, M. E. and Mack, C. M., The NMDA antagonist, MK-801, suppresses long-term potentiation, kindling, and kindling-induced potentiation in the perforant path of the unanesthetized rat, *Brain Res*, 519 (1990) 89–96.
30. Goddard, G. V. and Douglas, R. M., Does the engram of kindling model the engram of normal long term memory, *Can J Neurological Sci*, (1975) 385–398.
31. Goddard, L. S., McIntyre, D. C. and Leech, C. K., A permanent change in brain function resulting from daily electrical stimulation, *Exp. Neurol.*, 25 (1969) 295–330.
32. Herberg, L. J., Tress, K. H. and Blundell, J. E., Raising the threshold in experimental epilepsy by hypothalamic and septal stimulation and by audiogenic seizures, *Brain*, 92 (1969) 313–328.
33. Linden, D. J., Long-term synaptic depression in the mammalian brain, *Neuron*, 12 (1994) 457–472.
34. Loscher, W., Development of tolerance to anticonvulsant effects of GABA-mimetic drugs in animal models of seizure states. In W. P. Koella, *Tolerance to beneficial and adverse effects of antiepileptic drugs,* Raven Press, New York, 1986,
35. Loscher, W. and Schwark, W. S., Development of tolerance to the anticonvulsant effect of diazepam in amygdala-kindled rats, *Exp Neurology*, 90 (1985) 373–384.
36. Madison, D., Malenka, R. and Nicoll, R., Mechanisms underlying long-term potentiation of synaptic transmission, *Annu Rev Neurosci*, 14 (1991) 379–397.
37. Malenka, R. C., Synaptic plasticity in the hippocampus: LTP and LTD, *Cell*, 78 (1994) 535–538.
38. Malenka, R. C. and Nicoll, R. A., NMDA-receptor-dependent synaptic plasticity: multiple forms and mechanisms, *TINS*, 16 (1993) 521–527.
39. Matsuura, S., Hirayama, K. and Murata, R., Enhancement of synaptic facilitation during the progression of kindling epilepsy by amygdala stimulations, *J Neurophys*, 70 (1993) 602–609.
40. McNamara, J. O., Byrne, M. C., Dashieff, R. M. and Fritz, J. G., The kindling model of epilepsy: a review, *Prog Neurobiol*, 15 (1980) 139–159.
41. McNamara, J. O., Russell, R. D., Rigsbee, L. and Bonhaus, D. W., Anticonvulsant and antiepileptogenic actions of MK-801 in the kindling and electroshock models, *Neuropharm.*, 27 (1988) 563–568.
42. Minabe, Y., Tanii, Y., Kadono, Y., Tsutsumi, M. and Nakamura, I., Low-frequency kindling as a new experimental model of epilepsy, *Exp Neurol*, 94 (1986) 317–323.
43. Mucha, R. F. and Pinel, J. P. J., Postseizure inhibition of kindled seizures, *Exp Neurol*, 54 (1977) 266–282.
44. Mulkey, R. M. and Malenka, R. C., Mechanisms underlying induction of homosynaptic long-term depression in area CA1 of the hippocampus, *Neuron*, 9 (1992) 967–975.
45. O'Dell, T. J. and Kandel, E. R., Low-frequency stimulation erases LTP through an NMDA receptor-mediated activation of protein phosphatases, *Learning and Memory*, 1 (1994) 129–139.

46. O'Mara, S. M., Rowan, M. J. and Anwyl, R., Metabotropic glutamate receptor-induced homosynaptic long-term depression and depotentiation in the dentate gyrus of the rat hippocampus in vitro, *Neuropharm*, 34 (1995) 983–989.
47. Paxinos, G. and Watson, C., *The Rat Brain in Stereotaxic Coordinates,* Academic Press, Sydney, 1982,
48. Pinel, J. P. J. and Mana, M. J., Kindled seizures and drug tolerance. In J. A. Wada, *Kindling 3,* Raven Press, New York, 1986, 393–407.
49. Post, R., Transduction of psychosocial stress into the neurobiology of recurrent affective disorder, *Am J Psychiatry*, 149 (1992) 999–1010.
50. Post, R. and Weiss, S., Kindling: implications for the course of treatment of affective disorders. In K. Modigh, O. Robak and P. Vestergaard, *Anticonvulsants in Psychiatry,* Wrightson Biomedical, Hampshire, UK, 1994, 113–137.
51. Post, R. M., Putnam, F., Uhde, T. W. and Weiss, S. R. B., ECT as an anticonvulsant: implications for its mechanism of action in affective illness, *Ann. N.Y. Acad. Sci.*, 462 (1986) 376–388.
52. Post, R. M. and Weiss, S. R. B., Sensitization and kindling: implications for the evolution of psychiatric symptomatology. In P. W. Kalivas and C. D. Barnes, *Sensitization of the Nervous System,* Telford Press, Caldwell, New Jersey, 1988, 257–291.
53. Post, R. M., Weiss, S. R. B. and Smith, M. A., Sensitization and kindling: implications for the evolving neural substrate of PTSD. In M. J. Friedman, D. S. Charney and A. Y. Deutch, *Neurobiological and clinical consequences of stress: From normal adaptation to PTSD,* Raven Press, New York, New York, 1994, in press.
54. Racine, R., Modification of seizure activity by electrical stimulation. I. Afterdischarge threshold, *Electroencephalogr. Clin. Neurophysiol.*, 32 (1972) 269–279.
55. Racine, R., Modification of seizure activity by electrical stimulation. II. Motor seizure, *Electroencephalogr. Clin. Neurophysiol.*, 32 (1972) 281–294.
56. Racine, R., Modification of seizure activity by electrical stimulation. III. Mechanisms, *Electroencephalogr. Clin. Neurophysiol.*, 32 (1972) 295–299.
57. Racine, R. J., Moore, K. A. and Evans, C., Kindling-induced potentiation in the piriform cortex, *Brain Res*, 556 (1991) 218–225.
58. Sackheim, H. A., Decina, P., Portnoy, S., Neeley, P. and Malitz, S., Studies of dosage, seizure threshold, and seizure duration in ECT, *Biol Psych*, 22 (1987) 249–268.
59. Sainsbury, R. S., Bland, B. H. and Buchan, D. H., Electrically induced seizure activity in the hippocampus: time course for postseizure inhibition of subsequent kindled seizures, *Behav Biol*, 22 (1978) 479–488.
60. Shao, J. and Valenstein, E. S., Long-term inhibition of kindled seizures by brain stimulation, *Exp Neurol*, 76 (1982) 376–392.
61. Staubli, U. and Lynch, G., Stable depression of potentiated synaptic responses in the hippocampus with 1–5 Hz stimulation, *Brain Res*, 513 (1990) 113–117.
62. Sutula, T., Reactive changes in epilepsy: cell death and axon sprouting induced by kindling, *Epilepsy Res*, 10 (1991) 62–70.
63. Tanaka, T. and Naquet, R., Influence of subcortical stimulation on amygdaloid kindled cats, *Appl Neurophysiol*, 39 (1976/77) 302–305.
64. Tsumoto, T., Long-term potentiation and long-term depression in the neocortex, *Prog. Neurobiology*, 39 (1992) 209–228.
65. Wang, Y., Rowan, M. J. and Anwyl, R., (RS)-alpha-Methyl-4-carboxyphenylglucine inhibits long-term potentiation only following the application of low frequency stimulation in the rat dentate gyrus in vitro, *Neuro Letters*, 197 (1995) 207–210.
66. Weiss, S. R. B., Clark, M., Rosen, J. B., Smith, M. A. and Post, R. M., Contingent tolerance to the anticonvulsant effects of carbamazepine: relationship to loss of endogenous adaptive mechanisms, *Br Res Rev*, 20 (1995) 305–325.
67. Weiss, S. R. B., Li, X. L., Rosen, J. B., Li, H., Heynen, T. and Post, R. M., Quenching: inhibition of development and expression of amygdala kindled seizures with low frequency stimulation, *NeuroReport*, 4 (1995) 2171–2176.
68. Weiss, S. R. B. and Post, R. M., Development and reversal of contingent inefficacy and tolerance to the anticonvulsant effects of carbamazepine, *Epilepsia*, 32 (1991) 140–145.

DISCUSSION OF SUSAN WEISS'S PAPER

C. Teskey: Have you tried quenching in other structures?

S. Weiss: We are currently testing the hippocampus. We are also looking to see if there is transfer between structures by stimulating one amygdala and quenching the other. These studies are currently in progress, and it's too soon to say what the results are. In the hippocampus we are using much lower intensities since the afterdischarge threshold is much lower in this structure.

C. Teskey: Are you recording evoked response in those animals?

S. Weiss: No, we are not currently recording at sites other than where we are stimulating. We would like to record during the quenching procedure but have not yet resolved the methodological problems of recording while stimulating.

J. McNamara: Given the permanence of the quenching effect, what evidence do you have in regard to damage or killing of neurons?

S. Weiss: Presently we are looking at DNA markers of apoptosis. We have not observed damage using gross histology, but do plan to use silver stain techniques to further examine this question. However, recall that the total amount of stimulation is quite low, given the narrow pulsewidth of 0.1 msec used in these studies. It is unlikely that neuronal loss or damage would occur following the amount of overall current applied in these experiments. In addition, in the naive animals, the effect of quenching is not long lasting. Thus, the permanence of the effect appears dependent on the experimental procedure used. This also argues against a permanent "lesion" produced by the quenching stimulation.

J. McNamara: Others have looked for cell death with kindling and found that loss gets more intense with the progression of kindling.

S. Weiss: So far, we have not found any changes, but we cannot rule it out at the present time.

R. Racine: I was wondering whether quenching may have the same effect as LTP or LTD. To my knowledge there are regional differences in the role of NMDA receptors in the slice preparation as well. Therefore, your findings with MK-801 do not necessarily rule out LTD as a mechanism for the quenching effect. Maybe you should look at LTD and depotentiation in the slice as well.

S. Weiss: There are regional differences in LTP even within the hippocampus, and nothing is known right now about LTD in the amygdala. Thus, we do not yet know whether LTD or LTP is occurring following quenching, and we are presently looking at these effects in an amygdala slice preparation.

J. Wada: In your quenching data, the afterdischarge threshold is elevated. In our experience with inhibition of seizures these is no change in threshold; therefore there may be differences in mechanisms. For example, in those animals that were quenched during development—could they be kindled from the hippocampus? Or was this a pervasive effect?

S. Weiss: We don't know yet about kindling from another area. These animals could still be kindled using suprathreshold stimulation in the amygdala, which we did to make sure the quenched animal were capable of kindling.

J. Engel: Did you examine other parameters with respect to timing requirements relative to kindling—that is, did you compare quenching before vs. after kindling?

S. Weiss: No, we have not tried this yet. Moreover, in the fully kindled animals, we administer one week of quenching alone without concurrent kindling stimulation, and this procedure is also highly effective in increasing seizure and afterdischarge thresholds. Thus we do not yet know the timing requirements for quenching.

J. Engel: The idea of blocking seizures with electrical stimulation has been used clinically by groups in Mexico and in Russia. It is not clear when it is done. Perhaps we can use your model to determine if it would be more effective if done before, during, or after the seizure.

10

KINDLING-LIKE EFFECTS OF ELECTROCONVULSIVE SHOCK SEIZURES

W. McIntyre Burnham,[1] Z. Gombos,[1] J. Nobrega,[2] and G. A. Cottrell[1]

[1]Bloorview Epilepsy Program
Department of Pharmacology, University of Toronto
Toronto, Ontario
[2]Neuroimaging Research Section
Clarke Institute of Psychiatry
Toronto, Ontario

1. ELECTROCONVULSIVE THERAPY (ECT)

Electroconvulsive therapy (ECT) was introduced into clinical practice in 1938[1]. From 1940 to 1950 it was a mainstay of psychiatric inpatient therapy[1,30,32]. Its use declined in the 1950s due to the introduction of psychotropic drugs and to allegations of risk and abuse[33]. Since the 1980s, however, there has been a rebirth of interest in ECT, partly due to economic considerations, and partly to disenchantment with the tricyclic antidepressants[1,33]. In Canada, ECT is administered to about 11% of the hospitalized psychiatric population[22].

ECT has been employed in a variety of disorders, including schizophrenia and mania[1,6,32]. Its major use, however, is in the treatment of depression[1]. It is the treatment of choice for drug-resistant depressives—about 30% of the depressive population[1]. It is also used as first-line therapy in cases of delusional depression.[6] ECT is considered to be the most potent agent available for treating depression, and it is also one of the quickest to act[33,82].

During ECT, electrical current is passed through the patient's brain to induce a generalized, convulsive seizure. It is the seizure *itself* which is the therapeutic agent; the current acts only as a trigger[1,34]. When it was first introduced, ECT was given to conscious patients (without anaesthesia), and high-intensity sine-wave current was used to trigger the seizures[1]. This procedure is now called "unmodified" ECT. In modern practice, ECT is usually given with short-acting anaesthesia, a muscle relaxant, oxygen and near-threshold square-wave current[1,35]. This is called "modified" ECT. The "modified" procedure prevents hypoxia, and decreases the amount of electricity which passes through the brain[1].

Kindling 5, edited by Corcoran and Moshé.
Plenum Press, New York, 1998.

2. SEIZURES AND THE BRAIN—THE TRADITIONAL VIEW

Despite its effectiveness, there have always been questions about the safety of ECT. Almost from the start, there have been suggestions that—in addition to its therapeutic effects—ECT might be causing long-lasting, *non-therapeutic* changes in brain and behaviour[30]. Advocates of ECT deny this, and argue that—in "modified" form—ECT is one of the safest procedures in medicine[82].

Evidence to support this position has been drawn from the older clinical and animal studies, which searched for gross structural damage following ECT.

2.1. Clinical Studies

The clinical literature on ECT was reviewed by Weiner[84] in 1984. Weiner admits that subtle changes might have been missed, but concludes that, "For the typical individual receiving ECT, no detectable correlates of irreversible brain damage appear to occur." (See also [1,32]).

2.2. Animal Studies

Animal studies in the ECT field have involved electroconvulsive shock (ECS) seizures. ECS is the animal analog of ECT. The experimental literature on ECS was summarized by Meldrum[55] in 1986 (see also [1,84]). In agreement with the influential findings of Dam and colleagues[25,26], Meldrum concludes that ECS does not cause brain damage, at least in adult animals. (Effects on the *developing* brain have been reported by Wasterlain and collaborators[83]).

Thus, both clinical and animal studies suggest that ECT/ECS does not cause gross structural damage to the brain.

3. SEIZURES AND THE BRAIN—RECENT EVIDENCE

Recent work in the epilepsy field, however—and, in particular, in the area of kindling research—has shown that repeated seizures may cause long-lasting and functionally significant brain changes in the absence of gross structural damage.

3.1. Clinical Studies

For many years, clinicians taught that—except for status epilepticus—seizures had no lasting effects on brain or behaviour. Recent studies have begun to question this traditional teaching. Anatomical studies have shown neuron loss[24,25] and sprouting[76] in human epileptic brains, and behavioral studies have shown long-lasting seizure-induced changes in both cognition[27,40,45,80] and personality[3,7,13]. In the 19th century—when unchecked seizures were common—"mental disabilities" were frequently reported in epileptic patients[80].

In clinical studies, however, it is hard to distinguish the effects of seizures from the effects of head injury, prior brain abnormalities, social isolation and anticonvulsant therapy[80]. Clearer evidence concerning the long-lasting effects of seizures has come from animal studies.

3.2. Animal Studies

Seizure-induced changes in brain and behaviour have been reported in a variety of animal models, including the "mirror focus" model[58], the kainic acid model[57] and in genetically epilepsy-prone rats[41].

The most extensive evidence, however, has come from studies involving the "kindling" model[38]. Among the *neural* changes reported after kindling have been changes in intracranial evoked potentials[66], cell firing[50,51,78], GABAergic and glutamatergic neurotransmission[36,43,52,56] (for summaries see [15,16,18]), neural growth and sprouting[37,75,81], cell number[20,21,71], gliosis[67], and gene expression[28,79]. Among the *behavioral* changes which have been reported after kindling have been changes in locomotory behaviour[29], learning[14,49,53], predatory attack[2,3,9,48], "aggressiveness"[62], "anxiety"[4,85] and alcohol consumption[47]. These behavioral changes have been reported after 5–10 generalized seizures, and in some cases[2,47] have been shown to last for at least a month.

Thus, both clinical and animal studies suggest that repeated seizure activity changes both brain and behaviour. Many workers now subscribe to the position originally formulated by Pinel[61]—that the "kindling effect" is seen with all types of seizures; that they all leave subtle, but incremental and enduring, changes in the brain.

4. OUR OWN RECENT STUDIES WITH "UNMODIFIED" ECS

Our own recent work with ECS is an extension of our earlier studies on kindling. We had found long-lasting changes in the brains and behaviour of kindled animals, and we suspected that similar changes must occur after ECS/ECT. This was particularly true since a "kindling like" intensification of seizures had already been reported following repeated ECS[63,68,70]. We therefore began a re-assessment of the long-term effects of ECS, applying the techniques and assays that had revealed long-lasting changes in kindling and other repeated-seizure models.

4.1. Technique for "Unmodified" ECS

Our first studies involved "unmodified" ECS—ECS without anesthesia or muscle relaxant. This is similar to the ECT given to psychiatric patients when the technique was first introduced.

The same basic design was used in all experiments. Adult, Long-Evans rats (Charles River) were given 8 "unmodified" ECS trials (number chosen to match clinical practice) or 8 sham "unmodified" ECS trials. ECS was elicited using the stimulus traditionally used in drug-development studies[77]: a 0.2-second train of 60 Hz sine-wave pulses administered at an intensity of 150 mA peak-to-peak through corneal electrodes. Following the eighth ECS, subjects were rested for a seizure-free period—often 24 hours (short-term effects) or 28 days (long-term effects). Biochemical, electrophysiological or behavioral tests were then performed.

These studies have revealed a number of previously unsuspected, long-term effects of ECS.

4.2. Gliosis

When the brain is stressed or damaged, astrocytes respond with a process of gliotic hypertrophy.[69] This may be measured using either the GFAP assay, a semi-quantitative immunoassay[31], or the [^{3}H]PK 11195 assay, a radioligand assay which allows full quantification via autoradiography and densitometry[5]. Studies utilizing the GFAP immunoassay had already shown astrocyte hypertrophy after kindling[67] and following repeated ECS[46,60]. Our own recent [^{3}H]PK 11195 studies have now confirmed and fully quantitated the ECS effect, revealing gliosis in a number of brain areas, including the amygdala and hippocampus, 24 hours after 8 "unmodified" seizures. The same trends are seen at one month, but the effects are no longer significant (Burnham *et al.* in preparation).

4.3. Neuronal Sprouting

Neuronal sprouting has been reported in the hippocampi of both kindled rats[75] and human epileptics[76]. The connections formed by sprouting are aberrant and recurrent, and may contribute to the development of epileptiform excitability[54]. Using the Timm stain, we have found neuronal sprouting, but no cell loss, in the hippocampi of rats sacrificed two weeks after 8 "unmodified" ECS seizures (Burnham *et al.*, in preparation).

4.4. Changes in Oxidative Metabolism

Cytochrome oxidase, the last enzyme in the electron transport chain involved in oxidative metabolism, up- or down-regulates in response to long-term, steady-state changes in neuronal activity[86]. The cytochrome oxidase assay, therefore, offers a biochemical index of chronic, sustained alterations in brain function. One month after 8 "unmodified" ECS seizures, we have found increased cytochrome oxidase activity in 94/96 brain areas. Some of the largest changes are in limbic structures, e.g., the amygdala/pyriform area[59].

4.5. Receptor Binding Changes

In a series of autoradiographic assays, we have looked for post-ECS changes in binding to the GABA-A complex, the glutamate complex, dopamine D_1 and D_2 and 5 HT_2 receptors. No major changes in GABA or glutamate binding have been found (Nobrega *et al.*, in preparation). As previously reported by Barkai *et al.*[8], however, we have found increased binding to both D-1 and D-2 receptors, and, as previously reported by Biegon and Israeli[11], we have found both increased and decreased binding to 5 HT_2 receptors (Burnham *et al.*, in preparation). At present, only short-term studies have been completed (48 hours post-ECS). Long-term studies are now in progress.

4.6. Intracranial Evoked Potentials

Evoked potentials are super-normal in a number of brain pathways following kindled seizures[17,66]. We have recently completed a study of evoked potentials in the entorhinal-dentate pathway following repeated "unmodified" ECS. We have found a significant increase in the amplitude of the population spike, which lasts for at least 3 months, and which may be permanent[19]. Similar effects have been reported by Stewart and collaborators working in Scotland[72–74].

4.7. Post-ECS Behavioral Changes

Anatomical, biochemical and electrophysiological changes are of particular concern when they express themselves as behavioural abnormalities. Recently, Holmes *et al.*[41]

evolved a battery of behavioural tests, which they have used to show long-lasting changes in learning and emotional behaviour following repeated convulsions in genetically epilepsy-prone rats. We have applied a modification of Holmes' test battery following 8 "unmodified" ECS seizures. During the first week following ECS, we found changes in social interactions, response to handling and open-field behaviour. Water-maze learning was not affected. One month after ECS, we found that subjects were still more submissive in social interactions and more "emotional" in open-field tests. Three months after ECS, only the open-field test still showed significant differences (Cottrell *et al.*, in preparation).

5. OUR OWN RECENT ECS STUDIES: "MODIFIED" ECS

Our findings show that ECS seizures can cause long-term changes in brain and behaviour. It is quite possible that ECT can cause similar changes. Our studies, however, utilized "unmodified" ECS, whereas, in modern practice, ECT is usually given in "modified" form (with anaesthesia, muscle relaxant and oxygen, and low-intensity square-wave current). It has been argued that the "modified" procedure protects against any long-term brain changes[34].

We have therefore begun a series of studies with "modified" ECS, the animal analog of "modified" ECT.

5.1. Technique for "Modified" ECS

Our technique for "modified" ECS was designed to match the "modified" ECT procedure used at the Toronto Hospital. ECS is administered following pre-administration of atropine (0.05 mg/kg, s.c.), methohexital (10 mg/kg, i.v.), and, following loss of consciousness, succinylcholine (0.1 mg/kg, i.v.). Injections are done via chronically implanted catheters. After the muscle relaxant has taken effect, the rat's head is cleaned with alcohol and current is passed through electrodes placed on the skin over the right and left "temporal" areas. A one-second train of positive- and negative-going square-wave pulses is used (1 ms, 70 Hz). Current intensity is adjusted to threshold plus 20%. Oxygen is administered throughout the procedure. As in clinical practice, eight seizures are administered on a 3/week schedule. Control subjects receive atropine, methohexital, succinylcholine, oxygen and handling, but no electrical stimulation.

5.2. Intracranial Evoked Potentials after "Modified" ECS

Only one study has been completed with the "modified" procedure so far—a study of evoked-potential enhancement. The data indicate that enhanced evoked potentials occur after "modified" ECS, just as they do after "unmodified" ECS (Gombos *et al.*, in preparation).

These data suggest that the "modified" procedure may *not* protect experimental animals against the "kindling like" effects of ECS, and, by extension, that modern ECT procedures may *not* be protecting patients against long-term effects of ECT.

6. CLINICAL IMPLICATIONS/FUTURE STUDIES

Some of the long-term changes we have found may relate to the therapeutic effects of ECT. It has been suggested, for instance, that changes in monaminergic receptor function may mediate the therapeutic effects of both ECT and antidepressant drugs[8,12,23,39]. It is also possible that long-lasting increases in brain metabolism might be beneficial. Human depressives show *decreased* brain metabolism—as indicated by PET studies of glucose utilization and cerebral blood flow[10,42,44].

Other changes after ECS/ECT are probably non-therapeutic and possibly pathological. Gliosis, for instance, is often associated with neural death or damage[69], and hippocampal sprouting—which results in the formation of aberrant connections—is unlikely to be associated with therapeutic effects. Stewart and Reid[73] have proposed that evoked-potential enhancement may relate to memory loss following ECT. In the future, it will be important for psychiatrists to realize that ECT has "costs" in addition to its very real "benefits".

Ideally, we would like to maintain the therapeutic effects of ECS/ECT, while eliminating unnecessary or undesirable "kindling-like" effects. A recent study by Stewart and Reid suggests that this may be possible. Stewart and Reid[73] administered repeated ECS in the presence of ketamine, a dissociative anaesthetic and neuroprotective agent. They found that—although seizures continued to occur—post-ECS enhancement of evoked potentials was no longer seen. At present, ketamine is the only neuroprotective drug which has been tested, and evoked-potential enhancement is the only long-term effect it has been tested on. We are now engaged in experiments designed to determine whether ketamine—or other neuroprotectants—can eliminate the other long-term changes seen after ECS, and whether this can be accomplished without losing ECS's "therapeutic" effects, as modelled by the Porsolt test[64,65].

REFERENCES

1. Abrams, R., *Electroconvulsive Therapy*, Oxford University Press, New York, 1992.
2. Adamec, R., Behavioral and epileptic determinants of predatory attack behaviour in the cat, *Canad. J. Neurol. Sci.*, 2 (1975) 457–466.
3. Adamec, R., Kindling, anxiety and limbic epilepsy: human and animal perspectives. In: J.A.Wada (Ed.), *Kindling 4*, Plenum Press, New York, 1990.
4. Adamec, R.E. and Morgan, H.D., The effect of kindling of different nuclei in the left and right amygdala on anxiety in the rat, *Phys. Behav.*, 55 (1994) 1–12.
5. Altar, C.A. and Baudry, M., Systemic injection of kainic acid: gliosis in olfactory and limbic brain regions quantified with [^{3}H]PK 11195 binding autoradiography, *Exp. Neurol.*, 109 (1990) 333–341.
6. APA Task Force on ECT. The practice of ECT: recommendations for treatment, training and privileging, *Convulsive Ther.*, 6 (1990) 85–120.
7. Baer, D.M. and Fedio, P., Quantitative analysis of interictal behaviour in temporal lobe epilepsy, *Arch. Neurol.*, 43 (1977) 454–467.
8. Barkai, A.I, Durkin, M. and Nelson, H.D., Localized alterations of dopamine receptor binding in rat brain by repeated electroconvulsive shock: an autoradiographic study, *Brain Res.*, 529 (1990) 208–213.
9. Bawden, H. and Racine, R.J., Effects of bilateral kindling or bilateral sub-threshold stimulation of the amygdala or septum on muricide, ranacide, intraspecific aggression and passive avoidance in the rat, *Physiol. and Behav.*, 22 (1979) 115–123.
10. Baxter, L.R., Schwartz, J.M., Phelps, M.E., Mazziotta, J.C., Guze, B.H., Selin, C.E., Gerner, R.H., and Sumida, R.M., Reduction of prefrontal cortex glucose metabolism common to three types of depression, *Arch. Gen. Psychiat.*, 46 (1989) 243–250.
11. Biegon, A. and Israeli, M., Quantitative autoradiographic analysis of the effects of electroconvulsive shock on serotonin-2 receptors in male and female rats, *J. Neurochem.*, 48 (1987) 1386–1391.
12. Blier, P. and de Montigny, C., Current advances and trends in the treatment of depression, *TIPS*, 5 (1994) 220–226.
13. Blumer, D., Temporal lobe epilepsy and its psychiatric significance. In D. Blumer and D.F Benson (Eds.), *Psychiatric Aspects of Neurologic Disease*, Grun and Stratton, New York,1975.
14. Boast, C.A. and McIntyre, D.C., Bilateral kindled amygdala foci and inhibitory avoidance behaviour in rats: a functional lesion effect, *Physiol. Behav.*, 18 (1977) 25–28.

15. Burnham, W.M., Receptor binding in the kindling model of epilepsy. In A.K. Sen, and T. Lee (Eds.), *Receptors and Ligands in Neurological Disorders,* Cambridge University Press, Cambridge, 1988.
16. Burnham, W.M., The GABA hypothesis of kindling: recent assay studies, *Neurosci. & Behav. Rev.,* 13 (1989) 281–288.
17. Burnham, W.M., Racine, R.J., Milgram, N.W. and Albright, P. S., Effects of phenytoin, carbamazepine, and clonazepam on cortex- and amygdala-evoked potentials in partially kindled rats, *Exp. Neurol.,* 106 (1989) 150–155.
18. Burnham, W.M. and Cottrell, G.A., The GABA hypothesis of kindling. In *Kindling 4*, J.A Wada (Ed.), Plenum Press, New York, 1990.
19. Burnham, W.M., Cottrell, G.A., Diosy, D. and Racine, R.J., Long-term changes in entorhinal-dentate evoked potentials induced by electroconvulsive shock seizures in rats, *Brain Res.,* 698 (1995) 180–184.
20. Cavazos, J.E. and Sutula, T.P., Progressive neuronal loss induced by kindling: a possible mechanism for mossy fibre synaptic reorganization and hippocampal sclerosis, *Brain Res.*, 527 (1990) 1–6.
21. Cavazos, J.E., Das, I. and Sutula, T.P., Neuronal loss induced in limbic pathways by kindling: Evidence for induction of hippocampal schlerosis by repeated brief seizures, *J. Neurosci.*, 14 (1994) 3106–3121.
22. Chandrasena, R., Electroconvulsive therapy: a consensus on contemporary issues, *Psychiat. J. Univ. Ottawa,* 14 (1989) 418–420.
23. Charney, D.S., Menkes, D.B., Phil, M. and Heninger, G.R., Receptor sensitivity and the mechanism of action of antidepressant treatment. Implication for the etiology and therapy of depression, *Arch. Gen. Psych.*, 38 (1981) 1160–1180.
24. Dam, A.M., Epilepsy and neuron loss in the hippocampus, *Epilepsia*, 21 (1980) 617–629.
25. Dam, A.M., Hippocampal neuron loss in epilepsy and after experimental seizures, *Acta Neurol. Scand.*, 66 (1982) 601–642.
26. Dam, M., Hertz, M., Bolwig, T., and Dam, A.M., The number of hippocampal neurons and Purkinje cells in rats after electrically-induced seizures. In M. Dam, L. Gram, and J.K. Penry (Eds.), *Advances in Epileptology XII. Epilepsy International Symposium*, Raven Press, New York, 1981.
27. Dodrill, C.B. and Troupin, A.S., Seizures and adaptive abilities, *Arch. Neurol.*, 33 (1976) 604–607.
28. Dragunow, M. and Robertson, H.A., Kindling stimulation induces c-*fos* protein(s) in granule cells of the rat dentate gyrus, *Nature*, 329 (1987) 441–442.
29. Ehlers, C.L. and Koob, G.F., Locomotor behaviour following kindling in three different brain sites, *Brain Res.*, 326 (1985) 71–79.
30. Endler, N.S. and Persad, E., *Electroconvulsive Therapy: The Myths and Realities*, Hans Huber, Toronto, 1988.
31. Eng, L.F., Regulation of glial intermediate filaments in astrogliosis. In M.D. Norenberg, I. Hertz, and A. Schousboe (Eds.), *The Biochemical Pathology of Astrocytes*, Alan R. Liss, New York, 1988.
32. Fink, M., *Convulsive Therapy: Theory and Practice*, Raven Press, New York, 1979.
33. Fink, M., Fifty years of electroconvulsive therapy, *Convulsive Ther.*, 4 (1988) 2–3.
34. Fink, M., Convulsive therapy and kindling. In T.G. Bolwig, and M.R. Trimble (Eds.), *The Clinical Relevance of Kindling*, John Wiley and Sons, New York, 1989, pp. 195–208.
35. Fink, M., Optimizing ECT, *L'Encephale*, 20 (1994) 297–302.
36. Gean, P., Shinnick-Gallagher, P. and Anderson, A.C., Spontaneous epileptiform activity and alteration of GABA- and of NMDA-mediated neurotransmission in amygdala neurons kindled in vivo, *Brain Res.*, 494 (1989) 177–181.
37. Geinesman, Y., Morrell, F. and deToledo-Morrell, L., Remodelling of synaptic architecture during hippocampal "kindling", *Proc. Natl. Acad. Sci., USA*, 85 (1988) 3260–3264.
38. Goddard, G.V., McIntyre, D.C. and Leech, C., A permanent change in brain function resulting from daily electrical stimulation, *Exp. Neurol.*, 25 (1969) 295–330.
39. Green, A.R., Evolving concepts on the interactions between antidepressant treatments and monamine neurotransmitters, *Neuropharmacology*, 26 (1987) 815–822.
40. Herman, B.P., Wyler, A.R., Richey, E.T. and Rea, J.M., Memory function and verbal learning ability in patients with complex partial seizures of temporal lobe origin, *Epilepsia*, 5 (1987) 547–544.
41. Holmes, G.L., Thompson, J.L., Marchi, T.A., Gabriel, P.S., Hogan, M.A., Carl, F.G., and Feldman, D.S., Effects of seizures on learning, memory, and behavior in the genetically epilepsy-prone rat, *Ann. Neurol.*, 27 (1990) 24–32.
42. Hurwitz, T.A., Clark, C., Murphy,E., Klonoff, H., Martin, W.R and Pate, B.D., Regional brain glucose metabolism in major depressive disorder, *Can. J. Psychiatry*, 35 (1990) 684–688.
43. Jarvie, P.A., Logan, T.C., Geula, C. and Slevin, J.T., Entorhinal kindling permanently enhances Ca^{2+}-dependent l-glutamate release in region inferior of rat hippocampus, *Brain Res.*, 508 (1990) 188–193.
44. Kanaya, T. and Yonekawa, M. Regional cerebral blood flow in depression, *Japan. J. Psychiat. Neurol.*, 44 (1990) 571–576.

45. Kimura, D., Cognitive deficit related to seizure pattern in centrencephalic epilepsy, *J. Neurol. Neurosurg. Psychiat.*, 27 (1964) 291–295.
46. Kragh, J., Bolwig, T.G., Woldbye, D.P.D. and Jorgensen, O.S., Electroconvulsive shock and lidocaine-induced seizures in the rat activate astrocytes as measured by glial fibrillary acidic protein, *Bio. Psychiatry*, 33 (1993) 794–800.
47. Linseman, M.A., Cottrell, G.A. and Burnham, W.M., Decreased voluntary ethanol consumption in amygdala-kindled rats, *Pharmacol., Biochem, & Behavior*, 48 (1994) 31–36.
48. McIntyre, D.C., Amygdala kindling and muricide in rats, *Physiol. and Behav.*, 21 (1978) 49–56.
49. McIntyre, D.C. and Molino, A., Amygdala lesions and CER learning: long term effect of kindling, *Physiol. Behav.* , 8 (1972) 1055–1058.
50. McIntyre, D.C. and Wong, R.K.S., Modification of local neuronal interactions by amygdala kindling *in vitro*, *Exp. Neurol.*, 88 (1985) 529.
51. McIntyre, D.C. and Wong, R.K.S., Cellular and synaptic properties of amygdala-kindled pyriform cortex *in vitro*, *J. Neurophysiol.*, 59 (1986) 1033.
52. McNamara, J.O., Bonhaus, D.W., Nadler, J.V. and Yeh, G.C., N-methyl-D-aspartate (NMDA) receptors and the kindling model. In J.A. Wada (Ed.), *Kindling 4*, Plenum Press, New York, 1990.
53. McNamara, R.K., Kirkby, R.D., dePape, G.E. and Corcoran, M.E., Limbic seizures, but not kindling, reversibly impair place learning in the Morris water maze, *Behav. Brain Res.*, 50 (1992) 167–175.
54. McNamara, J.O., Cellular and molecular basis of epilepsy, *J. Neurosci.*, 14 (1994) 3413–3425.
55. Meldrum, B.S., Neuropathological consequences of chemically and electrically induced seizures, *Ann. N.Y. Acad. Sci.*, 462 (1986) 186–193.
56. Mody, I. and Heinemann, U., NMDA receptors of dentate gyrus granule cells participate in synaptic transmission following kindling, *Nature*, 326 (1987) 701–704.
57. Moore, W., Milgram, N.W., Khurgel, M. and Ivy G.O., Time course and brain distribution of seizure-induced astrocyte hypertrophy in rats, *Neurosci. Abstr.*, 14 (1988) 881.
58. Morrell, F., Physiology and histochemistry of the mirror focus. In H. Jasper, A. Ward, and A. Pope (Eds.), *Basic Mechanisms of the Epilepsies*, Little and Brown, Boston, 1969.
59. Nobrega, J.N., Raymond, R., DiStefano, L. and Burnham, W.M., Long-term changes in regional brain cytochrome oxidase activity induced by electroconvulsive treatment in rats, *Brain Res.*, 605 (1993) 1–8.
60. Orzi, F., Zoli, M., Passarelli, F., Ferraguti, F., Fieschi, C. and Agnati, L.F., Repeated electroconvulsive shock increases glial fibrillary acidic protein, ornithine decarboxylase, somatostatin and cholecystokinin immunoreactivities in the hippocampal formation of the rat, *Brain Res.*, 533 (1990) 223–231.
61. Pinel, J.P.J. and Van Oot, P.H. Generality of the kindling phenomenon: some clinical implications. In J.A. Wada (Ed.), *Kindling*, Raven Press, New York, 1976.
62. Pinel, J.P.J., Treit, D. and Rovner, L.I., Temporal lobe aggression in rats, *Science*, 197 (1977) 1088–1089.
63. Pinel, J.P.J. and Van Oot, P.H., Increased susceptibility to the epileptic effects of alcohol withdrawal following periodic electroconvulsive shocks, *Biol. Psychiat.*, 3(1978) 353–368.
64. Porsolt, R.D., LePichon, M. and Jalfre, M., Depression: a new animal model sensitive to antidepressant treatments, *Nature*, 266 (1977) 730–732.
65. Porsolt, R.D., Anton, G. Blavet, N. and Jalfre, M., Behavioral despair in rats: a new model sensitive to antidepressant treatments, *Eur. J. Pharmacol.*, 47 (1978) 379–391.
66. Racine, R.J., Gartner, J.G. and Burnham, W.M., Epileptiform activity and neural plasticity in limbic structures, *Brain Res.*, 47 (1972) 262–268.
67. Racine, R.J., Milgram, N.W. and Ivy, G.O., The kindling phenomenon: neuropathology and normal function. In T.F. Bolwig, and M.R. Trimble (Eds.), *The Clinical Relevance of Kindling*, John Wiley and Sons, Chichester, 1989, pp. 15–34.
68. Ramer, D. and Pinel, J.P.J., Progressive intensification of motor seizures produced by periodic electroconvulsive shock, *Exp. Neurol.*, 51 (1976) 421–433.
69. Robbins, S.L., Cotran, R.S. and Kumar, V., *Pathologic Basis of Disease*, W.B. Saunders Co., Philadelphia, 1984.
70. Sangdee, P., Turkanis, S.A. and Karler, R., Kindling-like effect induced by repeated corneal electroshock in mice, *Epilepsia*, 23 (1982) 471–479.
71. Spiller, A.E. and Racine, R.J., The effect of kindling beyond the 'stage 5' criterion on paired-pulse depression and hilar cell counts in the dentate gyrus, *Brain Res.*, 635 (1994) 139–147.
72. Stewart, C. and Reid, I.C., Electroconvulsive stimulation and synaptic plasticity in the rat, *Brain Res.*, 620 (1993) 139–41.
73. Stewart, C. and Reid, I.C., Ketamine prevents ECS-induced synaptic enhancement in rat hippocampus, *Neurosci. Lett.*, 178 (1994) 11–14.
74. Stewart, C., Jeffery, K. and Reid, I.C., LTP-like synaptic efficacy changes following electroconvulsive stimulation, *Neuroreport*, 5 (1994) 1041–1044.

75. Sutula, T., He, X.X., Cavazos, J. and Scott, G., Synaptic reorganization in the hippocampus induced by abnormal functional activity, *Science*, 239 (1988) 1147–1150.
76. Sutula, T., Cascino, G., Cavazos, J., Parada, I., Ramirez, L., Mossy fibre synaptic reorganization in the epileptic human temporal lobe, *Ann. Neurol.*, 26 (1989) 321–330.
77. Swinyard, E.A., Electrically induced convulsion. In D.P. Purpura, J.K. Penry, D.M. Woodbury, D.B. Tower, and R.D. Walter (Eds.), *Experimental Models of Epilepsy*, Raven Press, New York, 1972.
78. Teskey, G.C. and Racine, R.J., Kindling-induced hyper-responsiveness of neurons *in vivo*, *Soc. for Neurosci. Abst.*, 17 (1991) 1400.
79. Teskey, G.C., Atkinson, B.G. and Cain, D.P., Expression of the proto-oncogen c-*fos* following electrical kindling in the rat, *Mol. Brain Res.*, 11 (1991) 1–10.
80. Trimble, M.R., Cognitive hazards of seizure disorders, *Epilepsia* , 29 (1988) S19–24.
81. Vanderzee, C.E.E., Rashid, K., Le, K., Moore, K.A., Stanisz, J., Diamond, J., Racine, R.J., Fahneshock, M., Intraventricular administration of antibodies to nerve growth factor retards kindling and blocks mossy fibre sprouting in adult rats, *J. Neurosci.*, 15 (1995) 5316–5323.
82. Varghese, F.T.N. and Singh, B.S., Electroconvulsive therapy in 1985—a review, *Med. J. Australia* , 143 (1985) 192–196.
83. Wasterlain, C.G. and Plum, F., Vulnerability of developing rat brain to electroconvulsive seizures, *Arch. Neurol.*, 29 (1973) 38–45.
84. Weiner, R.D., Does electroconvulsive therapy cause brain damage?, *Behav. and Brain Sci.*, 7 (1984) 1–54.
85. Witkin, J.M., Lee, M.A. and Walczak, D.D., Anxiolytic properties of amygdaloid kindling unrelated to benzodiazepine receptors, *Psychopharmacology*, 96 (1988) 296–301.
86. Wong-Riley, M.T., Cytochrome oxidase: an endogenous metabolic marker for neuronal activity, *Trends in Neurosci.*, 12 (1989) 94–101.

DISCUSSION OF W. M. BURNHAM'S PAPER

F. Lopes Da Silva: Have you tested paired-pulse depression?

M. Burnham: No, we haven't done that yet.

C. Applegate: What type of seizures were the animals having?

M. Burnham: "Unmodified" subjects showed tonic forelimb extension, and often himdlimb tonic extension as well. In "modified" subjects, with muscle relaxant, the convulsion was very mild, often only forelimb clonus. We monitored the electrographic seizures in "modified" subjects.

K. Gale: You referred to markers of glial cells and called it "gliosis." There is a very rapid response of glia, which is probably a normal response and perhaps a response to trophic factors. It is very good, therefore, to refer to "glial hypertrophy" and not "gliosis," which implies damage.

GENERAL DISCUSSION 3

J. Stripling: I was struck by the duration of the effects with the quenching stimulation. I was wondering how you could relate such large effects to minimal manipulations.

S.Weiss: We were as well, and we don't currently know yet how these effects occur.

S. Leung: Did you use the same electrode for quenching and kindling? Have you tried using a different electrode, because, as you know LTP, is presumably presynaptic?

S. Weiss: We used the same electrode and have not yet tried using different electrodes. We plan to begin to do this by kindling in one amygdala and quenching from the other. Hopefully, this will be informative in that regard and also in determining if quenching is a transsynaptic phenomenon.

G. Ronduin: Have you tried this in a different species, for example in the rabbit or cat?

S. Weiss: No, we haven't.

C. Applegate: In studies that applied striatal stimulation prior to amygdala or septal kindling, a delayed effect was found, which was not associated with a change in the afterdischarge threshold. If you stimulate another site do you think that you could get analogous effects?

S. Weiss: We don't know yet. It is an important question to test.

J. Wada: There is good evidence that kindling induces gliosis. We have kindled seizures in macaque monkeys and looked at how the gliosis was distributed, but we could not find any difference after 180 stimulations. Therefore I was wondering if it is transient. Perhaps Dr. Racine could reply.

R. Racine: In collaboration with Gwen Ivy's group at Scarborough, we have found extensive proliferation of astrocytes in the piriform, amygdala, and entorhinal cortex after amygdala kindling. The effect appeared to be long lasting, and we have replicated it probably 3 times. So it is real, and I think that in the rat it is clear that kindling produces astrocyte hypertrophy.

11

THE ROLE OF RHINENCEPHALIC NETWORKS IN EARLY STAGE KINDLING

James L. Burchfiel, Craig D. Applegate, Gary M. Samoriski, and Jay Nierenberg

Department of Neurology, The Program in Neuroscience and the Comprehensive Epilepsy Program
University of Rochester School of Medicine and Dentistry
Rochester, New York 14642

1. INTRODUCTION

Kindling is a powerful model of epilepsy.[11,29] It is the best model we have of mesial temporal lobe epilepsy (MTLE), which is the most devastating type of human epilepsy, accounting for the vast majority of people with medically intractable epilepsy. More than 0.5 million people in the USA are afflicted with MTLE and continue to have seizures despite the best available medical treatment. It has been the hope of investigators that understanding the mechanisms underlying kindling will provide insight into treatment for MTLE. In nearly thirty years of research, however, kindling has yet to give up its most fundamental secrets.

We believe that one reason kindling has been so resistant to elucidation is the lack of a valid conceptual framework to guide investigation. How one conceives of the kindling process will have a profound effect on how one designs and interprets experiments. For example, if one considers the kindling process to be *general* and involve essentially the same neuronal mechanisms throughout the limbic system (or even throughout the brain), then the site of kindling and the site of mechanistic investigation become immaterial. One could design an experiment to kindle from any expedient structure, such as the amygdala, and investigate the neuronal processes altered by this kindling in any other convenient structure, for example the hippocampus. On the other hand, if one considers kindling to involve *specific* structures and neuronal connections, then the design of experiments becomes more exacting. To use the previous example, investigating mechanisms in the hippocampus following amygdala kindling would make sense only if one knew that the hippocampus were part of the specific neuronal network recruited during the process of amygdala kindling.

These considerations become particularly important if one considers the circuit specificity of kindling to involve directionality. Thus, kindling from a specific limbic system

Kindling 5, edited by Corcoran and Moshé.
Plenum Press, New York, 1998.

structure would be expected to alter neuronal processes "downstream" but not "upstream." Obviously, in designing an experiment within such a conceptual framework one would investigate neuronal mechanisms only in the circuitry downstream from the kindling site.

2. HYPOTHESIS

Is the process of kindling general or specific? Does kindling involve the progressive recruitment of neuronal structures into an epileptic network utilizing all possible neuronal pathways simultaneously and equally, like ripples radiating out from a rock thrown into a pond, or does kindling involve particular preferential pathways of recruitment, like a car following a well-marked roadmap?

To resolve this dichotomy concerning the nature of kindling, we have been exploring the hypothesis that kindling is a specific process with the following characteristics[3–6,8]:

- Kindling from a given limbic structure involves a specific preferential pathway of recruitment that establishes a unique kindled network. Afterdischarges (ADs) generated at a limbic structure, such as the amygdala, may be transmitted along many different synaptic pathways, but only specific synaptic connections will be functionally altered by the AD and recruited into the seizure generating network.
- The individual, preferential kindling pathways from different limbic system structures converge upon a common neuronal network that is responsible for generating stage 3 seizure behavior. This common stage 3 network involves areas of the ipsilateral piriform and insular cortices. Thus, the requirement for kindling from any limbic site to progress from stages 1–2 to stage 3 is that a functional connection be established between that site and the common stage 3 network such that an AD generated at the former activates the latter.
- Further progression of kindled seizure development from stage 3 to stages 4–5 generalized seizures requires the additional recruitment of a common network consisting of the bilateral perirhinal cortex.

In this paper and the following one (Applegate, et al., this volume), we will review data from our laboratory, and other laboratories, that test and support this hypothesis. The present paper focuses on the networks involved in the early stages of kindling with particular emphasis on the recruitment of the piriform/insular region at the transition from stages 1–2 to stage 3. The following paper focuses on the recruitment of perirhinal cortex at the transition from stage 3 to stages 4–5.

3. THE EARLY STAGE KINDLING TRANSITION (STAGES 1–2 TO STAGE 3): PERSPECTIVES FROM KINDLING ANTAGONISM AND KINDLING RATES

We have argued previously that the transition from stages 1–2 to stage 3 represents a critical step in the kindling process.[3,4] Several lines of evidence suggest that this early stage transition involves a unique stepwise change in seizure susceptibility, rather than a small advance along a continuum of kindled seizure development.

Our first insight into the special nature of the transition to stage 3 during kindling came from the kindling antagonism model.[6,8] Kindling antagonism describes the outcome from the attempt to kindle from two different limbic sites concurrently. The paradigm consists of the following. Rats or mice are implanted with bipolar stimulating/recording electrodes into two limbic structures, for example, the septal nucleus and the entorhinal cortex. Then, the two sites are stimulated in alternation: on the first trial, the septum is stimulated; on the second trial, the entorhinal cortex is stimulated; on the third trial, stimulation returns to the septum; and so on.

The consistent result of this alternating stimulation paradigm is a dramatic difference in kindled seizure development from the two sites. One site shows a typical kindling progression culminating in stage 5 generalized seizures. By contrast, kindling from the other site is incomplete; kindled seizure development proceeds to a certain stage, but then it fails to progress any further, despite continued stimulation. We have continued the alternating stimulation paradigm so that the site which fails to kindle receives several times the number of stimulations that would normally be required to elicit fully generalized seizures if the site were stimulated alone. Thus, kindling does not fail for lack of adequate stimulation. We refer to the site that exhibits complete kindling as the "dominant" site and the site that exhibits incomplete kindling as the "suppressed" site.

The most significant feature of kindling antagonism is that the block of kindled seizure development from the suppressed site is not random. Kindling always stops at one of two transitions between kindling stages. One of these critical transitions is from stages 1–2 to stage 3. The other critical transition is from stage 3 to stages 4–5. (We address this latter transition in the following paper.) When kindling from the suppressed site halts at the transition to stage 3, we call this condition "absolute antagonism."

We have discovered two important characteristics about absolute antagonism. First, the failure of kindled seizure development from the suppressed site is not due to suppression of local excitability. Stimulation of the suppressed site elicits afterdischarge (AD) activity that is indistinguishable from that of the dominant site: the two sites have the same AD threshold and AD duration consistent with the particular kindling stage. Second, absolute antagonism represents an *arrest* of kindling from the suppressed site. It is not the *expression* of seizure behavior that is suppressed in the antagonism paradigm; it is the kindling process itself that is suppressed. We have demonstrated that kindling from the suppressed site is arrested by stopping the alternating stimulation paradigm, and then stimulating the suppressed site alone in a traditional kindling paradigm. When stimulated alone following the antagonism paradigm, the suppressed site required the same number of trials to reach stage 3 as did the same site stimulated in a completely naive animal.

Thus, despite numerous stimulations, the absolutely antagonized site never appears to really "kindle." This result provided us with the first suggestion that the mechanism of kindling does not involve major neural changes at the site of stimulation. Rather, the antagonism data suggested to us that the significant changes underlying kindling occur in neural populations beyond the stimulation site. We reasoned that the ADs generated from the two sites during alternate stimulation compete in some way to recruit a distant neural population into a "kindled network." This competition is won by the dominant site, and the first sign of the development of a new kindled network is the transition to stage 3 behavior.

The significance of the early stage transition also comes to light if one examines kindling rates from different limbic structures. It is well known that kindling rates vary considerably within the limbic system. What is less well appreciated, but has been pointed out by some investigators[21,36] is that this variability is not reflected uniformly across all stages of kindled seizure development. This is illustrated in Figure 1, which shows average kindling rates in Sprague-Dawley rats from 6 different sites. The rates are displayed as the number of trials spent in each of three blocks of kindling stages: combined stages 1 and 2, stage 3, and combined stages 4 and 5. The most striking aspect of the kindling rate

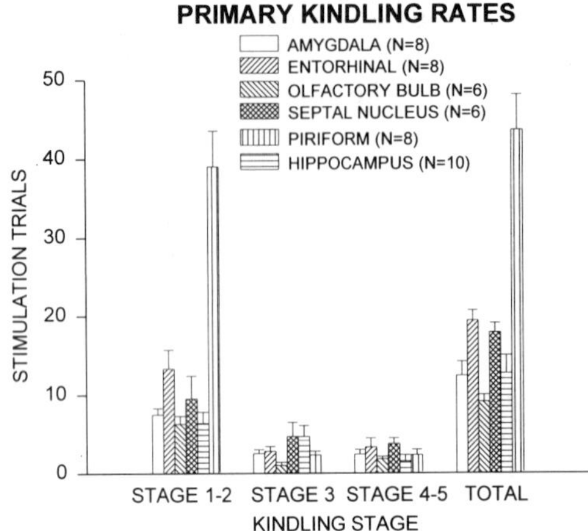

Figure 1. Primary kindling rates for six different limbic system sites. Note that the difference in rates among these sites is almost entirely a function of the number of trials spent in stages 1–2. By contrast, the number of trials spent in stage 3 or stages 4–5 is approximately the same for each site.

data, when they are expressed in this way, is the major distinction between stages 1–2 and the later stages of kindling. The number of trials spent in stages 1–2 varies widely among the different sites, while the kindling rates from stage 3 on are nearly identical. Indeed, nearly all the differences in overall kindling rates among limbic system structures can be accounted for by the number of trials required to reach the first stage 3 seizure. From then on the rate of kindled seizure development is essentially uniform throughout the limbic system.

This sudden change from highly variable kindling rates to a uniform rate suggests a major change in the conditions governing the kindling process. As we will develop later in this paper, our explanation for the abrupt change of kindling characteristics at the transition from stages 1–2 to stage 3 is that ADs generated from different limbic sites converge on and activate a common neural network that expresses stage 3 behavior. Thus, prior to stage 3, the development of kindling from each limbic structure depends on individual factors of local neuronal excitability and AD propagation in specific and unique pathways; whereas, from stage 3 on, individual differences disappear within a common neural substrate.

4. RECRUITMENT OF A COMMON STAGE 3 NETWORK IN THE PIRIFORM AND INSULAR CORTICES DURING LIMBIC KINDLING

4.1. Evidence from Transfer Kindling

The so-called "transfer effect" is a well-known phenomenon associated with kindling.[7,11] Transfer describes the experimental finding that kindling from one brain site facilitates subsequent kindling from another site. Transfer occurs among all limbic sites that are susceptible to kindling and implies a high degree of interdependence among these brain structures. Moreover, the presence of the transfer phenomenon suggests that kindling sites share a common neural system whose seizure susceptibility can be altered by kindling from any of them.

The hypothesis that limbic kindling sites converge upon a common neural system in the piriform and insular cortices makes very specific predictions about the outcome of transfer experiments. The first prediction is that there should be a high degree of transfer from any limbic site to the piriform cortex (PC). If kindling from any limbic site acts via alteration of PC circuitry, then it follows that there should be nearly immediate transfer of kindled seizure development to the PC, since the PC lies "downstream" from these other sites.

We tested this prediction in the following experiments: Groups of adult Sprague-Dawley rats were implanted with pairs of bipolar stimulating/recording electrodes. In all groups, one electrode was placed in the PC. The other electrode varied among the groups as follows: amygdala, olfactory bulb, entorhinal cortex, hippocampus, and septal nucleus. All electrodes were in the same hemisphere. After recovery from surgery, animals in each group were first kindled from the non-PC site to a criterion of 3 consecutive stage 5 seizures. Then, 2 days after completion of this primary kindling, secondary transfer kindling was commenced from the PC.

The results of these transfer experiments to the PC are shown in Figure 2A. Following primary kindling from the entorhinal cortex, amygdala, olfactory bulb, hippocampus and septal nucleus, the transfer to the PC was essentially immediate. Almost all animals receiving primary kindling from the olfactory bulb or septal nucleus emitted a stage 5 seizure with the first stimulation of the PC. For primary kindling from the amygdala or hip-

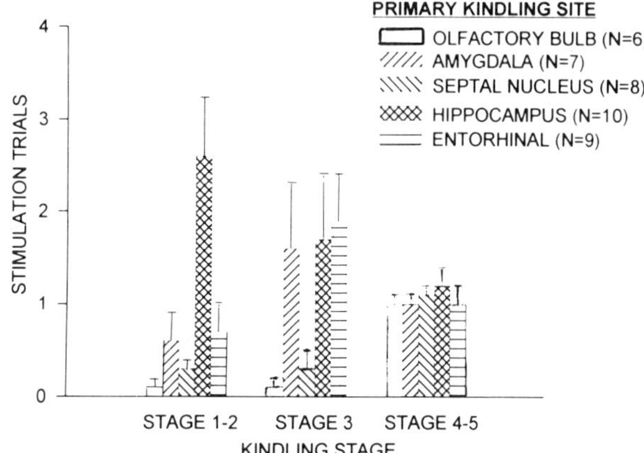

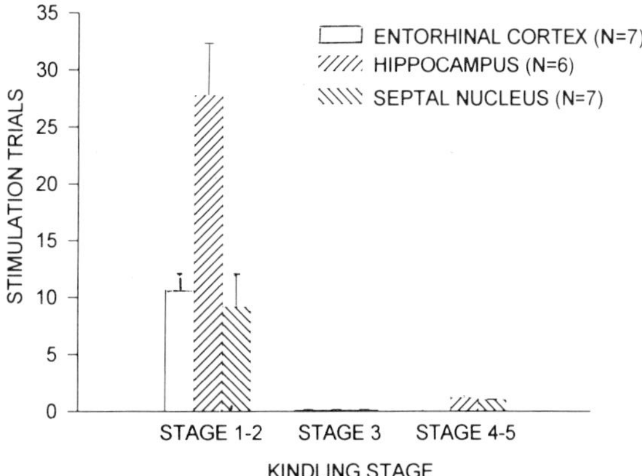

Figure 2. Transfer kindling involving the piriform cortex (PC). **A**. Transfer *to* the PC, i.e., secondary kindling from the PC following primary kindling from five different limbic system sites. Note that following primary kindling from each of these sites, transfer to the PC was essentially complete, suggesting that the PC is "downstream" from each of these sites. **B**. Transfer *from* the PC, i.e., secondary kindling from three different limbic system sites following primary kindling from the PC. Note that following primary kindling from the PC, transfer to each of these sites was incomplete. Comparison with Figure 1 indicates that the number of secondary stage 1–2 trials for each site was the same as if that site were naive, suggesting that these sites are "upstream" from the PC. Note also that all animals jumped from a stage 2 seizure directly to a stage 5 generalized seizure, suggesting that each limbic site propagated to the already fully kindled PC.

pocampus, the average number of PC stimulations to the first stage 5 seizure was 3 and 5, respectively.[5] Thus, these results strongly support the hypothesis that kindling from each of these limbic sites involves functional alterations within a network that includes the PC.

A second prediction of the hypothesis that the PC functions as a specific "downstream" structure for limbic kindling is that transfer to the PC will be more complete than to any other limbic structure. One could argue that the above results of nearly complete kindling transfer to the PC from other limbic sites is simply a reflection of general, nonspecific transfer among limbic sites. If the mechanism of kindling involves the nonspecific strengthening of connections among *all* limbic structures, then complete transfer to the PC would not be unique; one would expect to see a similar degree of transfer between any pair of limbic structures. That such general, nonspecific transfer between limbic structures does not occur is shown by the results of the following experiment.

Two groups of adult Sprague-Dawley rats were implanted with pairs of bipolar stimulating/recording electrodes. In one group, electrodes were implanted in the septal nucleus and ipsilateral amygdala. In the other group, electrodes were implanted in the septal nucleus and ipsilateral PC. Both groups first received primary kindling from the septal nucleus. Then the degree of transfer was assessed to the secondary site, amygdala or PC. As can be seen in Figure 3B, transfer to the PC was complete—all animals emitted a stage 5 seizure on the first stimulation. By contrast, transfer to the amygdala was decidedly incomplete—the animals required an average of 5 trials to make the transition from stage 1–2 seizures to stage 3 seizures. Comparing Figures 3B and 3A, one can see that this number of secondary trials is essentially the same as the number of primary kindling trials required to effect the same transition.

Thus, the state of kindled seizure development within the amygdala appears to be affected little, if at all, by prior kindling from the septal nucleus. This result disproves the notion that kindling from any limbic system site involves a general, nonspecific increase of seizure susceptibility among all other limbic structures. Rather, the striking difference between septal nucleus-amygdala transfer and septal nucleus-PC transfer supports the hypothesis that the PC occupies a specific, nodal position in limbic system kindling.

A third prediction of the hypothesis is that once kindled seizure development crosses the transition from stage 1–2 seizures to stage 3 seizures, transfer to any limbic site will be complete. This prediction is confirmed also by results illustrated in Figure 3B. In contrast to the marked difference in early stage 1–2 trials between secondary amygdala kindling and secondary PC kindling, these two sites show essentially the same number of later stage 3 and 4–5 trials. Moreover, transfer to either the amygdala or the PC during these later stages is essentially complete—nearly all animals jump directly from a stage 2 seizure on one trial to a stage 5 seizure on the next trial. This jump is consistent with the hypothesis of the PC as a convergent, nodal structure for limbic system kindling. If one postulates that the PC occupies a downstream position in septal nucleus kindled seizure development, then primary kindling from the septal nucleus will increase the seizure susceptibility of the PC. It follows that this enhanced excitability of the PC will be evident during direct PC secondary kindling. The postulate also predicts that the enhanced PC excitability will be evident indirectly during secondary amygdala kindling. Our hypothesis states that kindling from the amygdala also converges on the PC, and that recruitment of the PC into the amygdala kindling network occurs at the transition to stage 3. Thus, once secondary amygdala kindling progresses to stage 3, there is recruitment of a preconditioned PC whose excitability has already been enhanced by prior septal nucleus kindling. Hence, at this point, kindling is complete, and the hypothesis predicts an immediate generalization to a stage 5 seizure—the experimentally observed result.

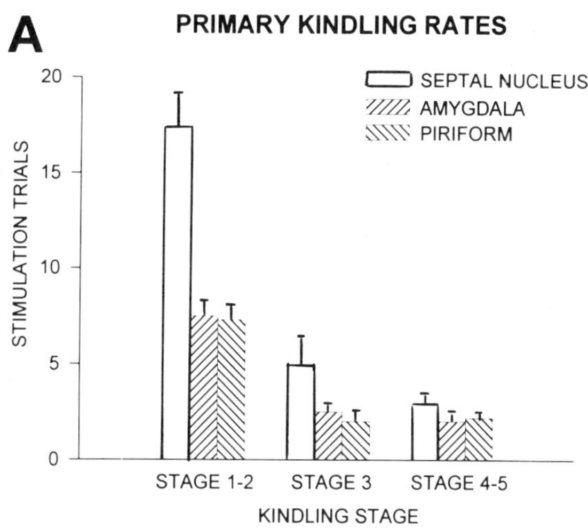

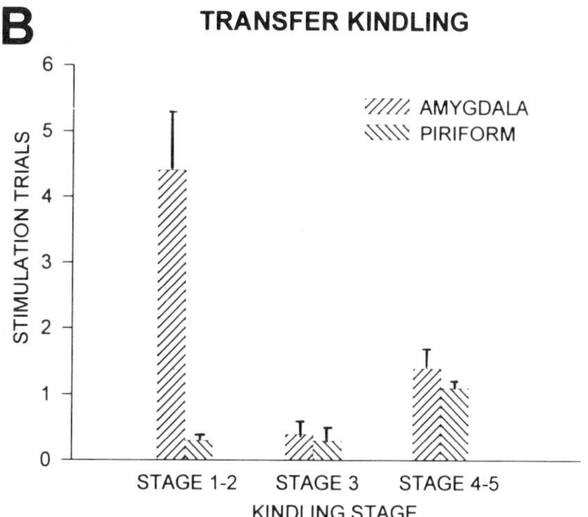

Figure 3. Comparison of transfer kindling between the septal nucleus and the amygdala with transfer kindling between the septal nucleus and the piriform cortex (PC). **A**. Primary kindling rates. Note that the rates are similar for the amygdala and the PC. **B**. Secondary kindling rates from the amygdala or PC following primary kindling from the septal nucleus. Note that transfer to the PC was complete, suggesting that the PC is "downstream" from the septal nucleus. By contrast, transfer to the amygdala was incomplete. The number of secondary stage 1–2 trials exhibited by the amygdala was the same as if the site were naive. This result suggests that kindling from the septal nucleus involves recruitment of a *specific* network that includes the PC but not the amygdala. Note also that once secondary kindling from the amygdala progressed beyond stage 2, there was virtually immediate expression of generalized stage 5 seizures, suggesting that the kindling network recruited from the amygdala also included the preconditioned PC.

A final prediction of the hypothesis is that primary kindling from the PC should have little, if any, effect on secondary kindling from other limbic system structures. If the PC is a convergent, "downstream" structure for limbic system kindling, then it follows that other limbic system sites are "upstream" from the PC. Thus, kindling from the PC should recruit further downstream structures, but should not significantly affect the seizure susceptibility of the upstream sites. We tested this prediction by the following experiments.

Groups of adult Sprague-Dawley rats were implanted with bipolar stimulating/recording electrodes. In all groups, one electrode was implanted in the PC. The other electrode varied among the groups as follows: entorhinal cortex, septum and hippocampus. All electrodes were in the same hemisphere. After recovery from surgery, animals in each group were first kindled from the PC to a criterion of 3 consecutive stage 5 seizures. Then, secondary transfer kindling was initiated from the non-PC site.

The results of these "upstream" transfer experiments are shown in Figure 2B. These results are consistent with the prediction. The seizure susceptibilities of the other limbic system sites were not significantly enhanced following primary kindling of the PC. Secondary kindling from each of the other sites initially progressed as if the site were naive. That is, each site exhibited approximately the same number of stage 1–2 trials as the site would have if it had never experienced any prior kindling (compare transfer rates in Figure 2B with primary rates in Figure 1). Furthermore, once kindling from each site progressed beyond stage 1–2, seizure development was essentially complete; most animals progressed directly from a stage 2 seizure on one trial to a fully generalized stage 5 seizure on the next trial. This result also is consistent with the theory that the PC is a convergent, downstream node for limbic system kindling. Prior kindling from the PC has already altered this structure and the network beyond it responsible for eliciting generalized seizures. Thus, once an unmodified upstream structure (e.g., the hippocampus) has been sufficiently transformed to recruit the PC node into its kindling network, the total kindling process is complete and a generalized seizure ensues.

4.2. Electrophysiological Evidence

We have postulated that kindling from different limbic system structures converges upon a common network involving areas of the ipsilateral piriform and insular cortices, and that activation of these areas is responsible for generating stage 3 seizure behavior. A prediction of this hypothesis is that during limbic system kindling there should be some electrophysiological sign of the recruitment of the PC at the transition from stage 1–2 to stage 3. We have discovered such an electrophysiological sign during kindling from the septal nucleus.[5]

This electrophysiological change within the PC is illustrated in Figure 4. Part A of this figure shows the ADs elicited in the septal nucleus and PC, respectively, following septal stimulation on the first kindling trial. As can be seen, the two ADs exhibit very similar morphology and duration. A reasonable explanation for this similarity of electrophysiological characteristics is that the PC is being passively driven by the septal-generated AD. This relationship between the septal and PC ADs changes dramatically at the transition from stage 1–2 seizures to stage 3 seizures (Figure 4B). Following the transition, the AD recorded from the PC differs dramatically from the septal-generated AD. Furthermore, the new morphology of the AD recorded from the PC shows a remarkable

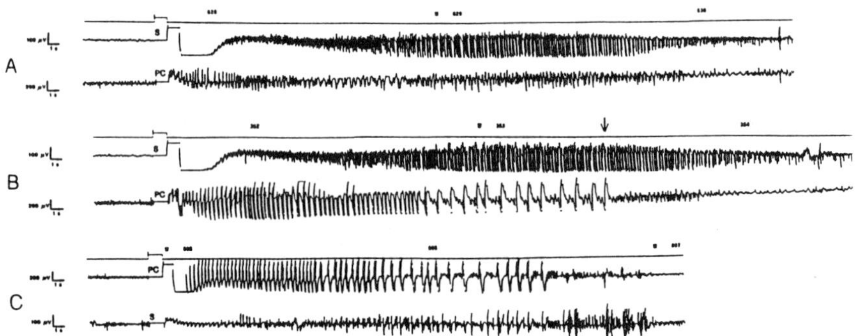

Figure 4. Electrophysiological evidence of active recruitment of the piriform cortex (PC) into a kindling network at the transition from stage 2 seizures to stage 3 seizures. Kindling stimulation was applied to the septal nucleus and afterdischarges (ADs) were recorded simultaneously from both the septum and the PC. **A**. Stage 2 seizure. Note the similarity of the PC and septal ADs, suggesting that the AD elicited in the septum passively drives the AD recorded in the PC. **B**. First stage 3 seizure. Note the sudden change in the morphology of the PC AD, suggesting that the AD in this structure is independently generated and no longer passively driven by the septal nucleus AD. **C**. AD elicited by direct stimulation of the PC in a naive animal. Note the remarkable similarity in morphology between this directly elicited PC AD and the AD recorded in the PC during the first stage 3 seizure (see part B). This morphological similarity suggests that at the transition to stage 3 seizure behavior, the PC now actively generates an intrinsic AD.

similarity to the AD elicited by direct stimulation of the PC (Figure 4C). These data suggest that new AD recorded in the PC is no longer the result of passive driving from the septal nucleus; rather, the PC now appears to be generating its own intrinsic AD. In other words, the PC AD now appears to be generated by a newly recruited, independently functioning neuronal population that was not operating during stage 1–2 trials. Thus, at the transition to stage 3 seizures, the PC AD is *triggered* by the septal AD, not driven.

The consistency of this characteristic change in PC AD morphology at the transition to stage 3 seizures is documented in Table 1. This table lists the trial number at which the first stage 3 seizure occurred during kindling from the septal nucleus and the trial number at which the change in morphology of the PC AD occurred. As can be seen, there was a remarkable coincidence between these two events: the change in the PC AD always occurred at the same trial as the first stage 3 seizure or 1–2 trials before this transition. Significantly, the PC AD never changed after the animal began to exhibit stage 3 behavior. Thus, the appearance of stage 3 seizures during limbic system kindling appears to be heralded by the appearance of new, intrinsically-generated AD in the PC.

Taken together, these electrophysiological data suggest that limbic system kindling involves the recruitment of a neuronal network within the PC, and that the activity of this network causes the transition to stage 3 seizure behavior. During the early phase of kindling, this PC network is not active and only stage 1–2 behavior is generated. We suggest that at the beginning of kindled seizure development, ADs elicited locally by stimulation of a limbic system structure passively propagate to the PC and in some way act on a PC network to increase its excitability. Finally, after the action of a number of ADs, the excitability of the PC network reaches threshold for independent activation. At this point, the activity of this newly recruited network generates an independent AD, and the action of this new AD drives the characteristic behavior of stage 3 seizures.

4.3. Evidence from Fos Induction

The recruitment of a common stage 3 neuronal network during limbic system kindling can be visualized and mapped by the expression of the proto-oncogene *c-fos*. A growing body of evidence indicates that focal seizure activity induces the expression of the *c-fos* protein, Fos.[2,15,20,27,28,35,37] Furthermore, Fos induction occurs in structures several synapses away from the focus.[15,20,35] Thus, Fos expression can serve as a marker of the

Table 1. The relationship between the change in piriform cortical afterdischarge (AD) and the expression of Stage 3 seizures kindled from the septal nucleus in a group of seven rats[a]

	First trial to		
Animal #	AD change	Behavioral change	Seizure type
S1	13 to 15	15	Facial clonus
S2	11 to 13	15	Facial clonus
S3	14 to 15	17	Facial clonus
S4	7	7	Head nodding
S5	14	15	Facial clonus
S6	7 to 9	10	Facial clonus
S7	11	11	Facial clonus

[a]Note that for each animal, the change in the AD morphology preceded or was coincident with the expression of seizures characterized by pronounced facial clonus and head nodding (see text for details).

multi-synaptic network activated by a focal seizure. We have exploited this technique to map and compare the neuronal networks activated by stage 1–2 kindled seizures and stage 3 kindled seizures, respectively.[30,31]

Separate groups of animals were kindled from the amygdala, septal nucleus or olfactory bulb. Animals were sacrificed either after a stage 2 seizure or after the first stage 3 seizure. In both cases, the animals were sacrificed 2 hours after the seizure, the brains were fixed, removed, sectioned, and the sections were incubated with the antibody to Fos. Additional groups of control animals were implanted in the same structures and handled in the same way but not stimulated. Careful analysis was made of the spatial pattern of Fos induction elicited during the two different stages of kindled seizure development. The results of these analyses are presented in Table 2 and Figure 5.

Three main conclusions can be derived from these Fos experiments. First, during either a stage 2 or a stage 3 seizure, Fos expression is almost exclusively ipsilateral to the kindling site; Fos expression in any region of the contralateral hemisphere was minimal and qualitatively resembled that seen in non-stimulated, control animals. Second, during a stage 2 seizure, each kindling site displayed a variable spatial pattern of Fos induction (Table 2). Third, at the first stage 3 seizure, the pattern of Fos induction changed significantly (Table 2 and Figure 5), and, most important, this new pattern of Fos induction during stage 3 seizures showed a remarkable convergence of spatial distribution across the different kindling sites. All three kindling sites exhibited robust Fos labeling in a common group of structures that included the posterior piriform cortex, aspects of the amygdala, the posterior agranular insular cortex and the ventral perirhinal cortex. These data suggest that these structures identified by Fos induction during stage 3 seizures constitute a common, nodal network recruited during kindled seizure development.

5. DISCUSSION

The data we have summarized in this paper are consistent with the hypothesis that limbic system kindling involves a process of progressive recruitment of *specific* neuronal

Table 2. The observed patterns of Fos labeling in the ipsilateral hemisphere following the expression of Stage 2 (pre-stage 3) or Stage 3 seizures kindled from the amygdala (¶), septal nucleaus (§), or olfactory bulb (‡)[a]

Rhinencephalic structure	Pre-stage 3			Stage 3		
Amygdala/hippocampal a.	§	¶	‡	§	¶	‡
Cortical n. amygdala	§	¶	‡	§	¶	‡
Ant. olfactory n.	§		‡	§	¶	‡
Dorsal endopiriform n.	§		‡	§	¶	‡
Piriform cortex		¶	‡	§	¶	‡
Basolateral/lateral amyg.		¶		§	¶	‡
Amygdalopiriform trans. a.				§	¶	‡
Agranular insular cortex				§	¶	‡
Ventral perirhinal cortex					¶	‡
Dorsal perirhinal cortex						

Kindling site: septal nucleus (§), amygdala (¶), olfactory bulb (‡).

[a]Prior to Stage 3 seizures, there is site dependent labeling of some, but not all, of the structures listed. Once Stage 3 seizures are elicited, however, all structures exhibit near maximal Fos labeling, independent of the kindling site (see text for details).

structures into an epileptogenic network. Furthermore, the data suggest that most, if not all, limbic sites susceptible to kindling recruit a common network of rhinencephalic structures at the transition from stage 1–2 seizures to stage 3 seizures. This network involves the posterior piriform cortex, aspects of the amygdala, the posterior agranular insular cortex and the ventral perirhinal cortex. We suggest that activation of this network is the *necessary* condition for expression of the characteristic convulsive head nodding and facial clonus that distinguish stage 3 seizure behavior. The agranular insular cortex may be particularly important in driving this behavior. Zhang and Sasamoto[38] have has shown that electrical stimulation of this area produces clonic chewing behavior typical of that exhibited during stage 3 seizures.

Areas within the common nodal network suggested by our data also have been implicated by others as important structures in kindled seizure development. Racine and co-workers[16,34] have reported that during the kindling process, the PC consistently develops spontaneous epileptiform discharges before other forebrain structures, regardless of the site of stimulation. In addition, when interictal discharges appear in other structures, they generally follow the PC burst. Within the PC, Gale and her colleagues[10,32,33] have discovered a localized area (area tempestas) that has the greatest sensitivity of any brain area to injection of chemical convulsant agents, such as bicuculine, kainic acid, or carbachol. Metabolic studies have shown selective activation of the PC during the early phase of amygdala kindling; during stages 1–3 the PC shows selective uptake of radioactive 2-deoxyglucose.[1]

In vitro electrophysiological experiments have provided direct evidence of increased neuronal excitability in the PC during kindling. McIntyre and Wong[25,26] developed a novel slice preparation that contained both the amygdala and adjacent PC with intact synaptic connections between these two structures. These authors found that in slices from control, non-kindled rats, amygdala stimulation frequently elicited epileptiform-like burst responses in layer II PC neurons. Moreover, these bursts could be elicited from all amygdala nuclei tested, suggesting that a large neuronal network in the PC could be recruited from the amygdala. Following amygdala kindling, McIntyre and Wong found a dramatic increase in PC excitability. Not only was increased bursting triggered in the PC by amygdala stimulation, but more than half of the slices exhibited spontaneous epileptiform bursts in the PC. Similar spontaneous epileptiform burst responses have been reported from Shinnick-Gallagher's laboratory[9] in the basolateral amygdala of kindled rats. As Kelly and McIntyre[17] have pointed out, it is important to emphasize that these spontaneous epileptiform events recorded in the PC and amygdala of kindled rats occurred with the slices maintained in normal bathing medium. By contrast, burst responses in the hippocampus can only be observed when the extracellular medium is manipulated to increase neuronal excitation or reduce inhibition.

Significantly enhanced spontaneous and evoked epileptiform bursts in the PC of kindled rats also have been demonstrated in the extensive and elegant studies of Haberly and his colleagues.[12–14,18,19] They have conducted detailed cellular analyses within the PC of both normal afferant activation and kindling-induced epileptiform bursts. These authors have confirmed the propensity for the PC to generate powerful interictal epileptiform events in kindled rats.[12] Using current source density analysis, they have found that these bursts originate primarily in the endopiriform nucleus, a collection of cells deep within the cortex immediately adjacent to the PC.[13,14] Additional contributions to the bursts responses come from the deep part of layer III of the PC and the claustrum. Furthermore, these authors have discovered a powerful association network within the PC.[18,19] One component of this network consists of longitudinal fibers that spread activation throughout the anterior-posterior extent of the PC. A second component of the associational network involves heavy projections to neighboring areas, including the amygdala, entorhinal cortex, and insular and orbitofrontal regions of the neocortex. This latter associational network is similar to the network we have defined by Fos induction during stage 3 kindled seizures. Thus, our studies and Haberly's studies provide independent evidence suggesting that the PC is part of a network that is capable of widespread propagation within the basal forebrain.

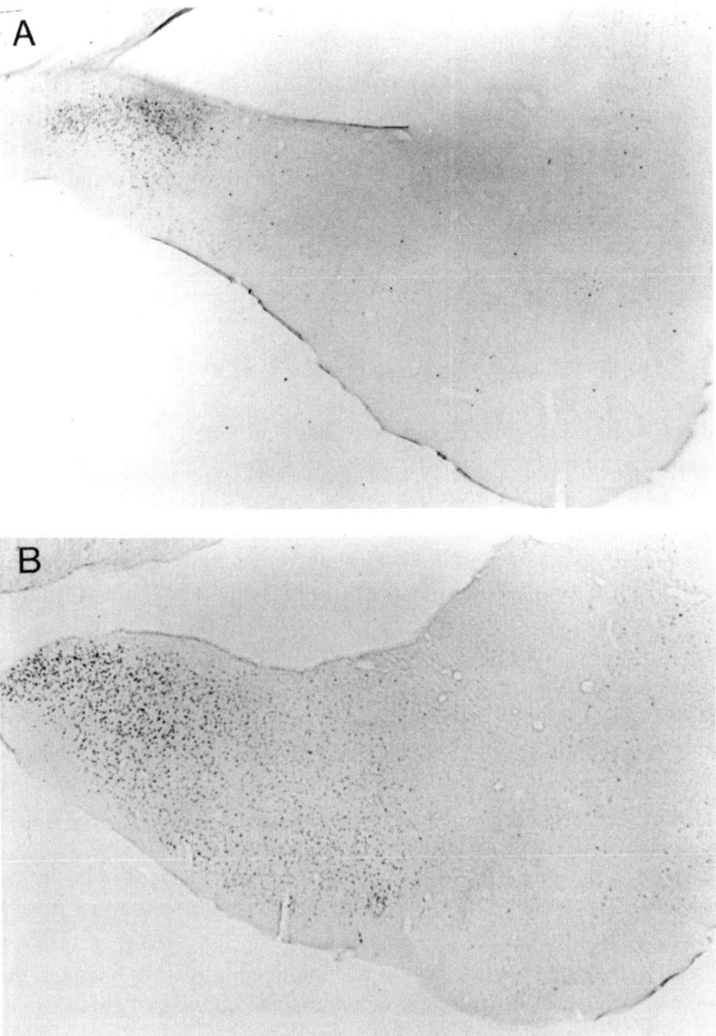

Figure 5. Progressive increase in the spatial distribution of Fos expression during early stage kindling (stages 1–3) from the septal nucleus. **A**. Following a single afterdischarge (AD), prominent Fos labeling is observed in the posteromedial cortical amygdala and the amygdala-hippocampal area of the ipsilateral hemisphere. **B and D**. During stage 2 seizures, Fos labeling spreads to include the posterolateral cortical amygdala and amygdalopiriform transition area. The section in D is anterior to the section in B. **C and E**. With the expression of the first stage 3 seizure, extensive Fos labeling is now observed in the piriform and posterior agranular insular cortices. The section in E is anterior to the section in C. See text and Table 2 for details. Abbreviations: AIP—posterior agranular insular cortex; CL—Claustrum; Den—dorsal endopiriform nucleus; DI—dysgranular insular cortex; ec—external capsule; GI granular insular cortex; Pir—piriform cortex.

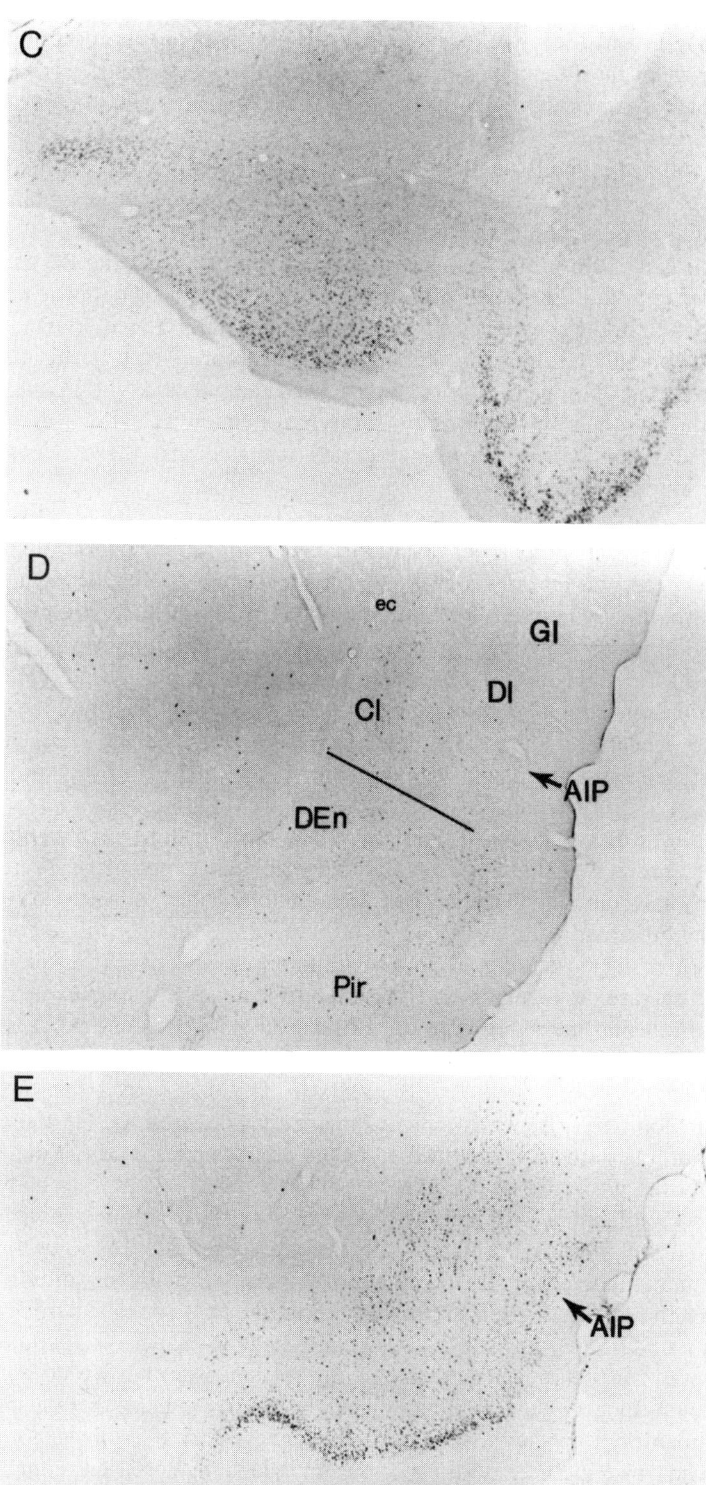
C
D
ec
GI
DI
Cl
AIP
DEn
Pir
E
AIP

Recently, Kelly and McIntyre[17] have suggested that areas of the perirhinal cortex, immediately dorsal to the PC, may function as a critical conduit linking limbic system structures to motor systems involved in kindled seizure development. In particular, the perirhinal cortex has extensive connections to the frontal motor cortex that most likely mediate the generalized convulsive behavior of stage 4–5 seizures. The results of our investigations (Applegate, et al., this volume) of Fos induction during the later stages of limbic system kindling agree with this concept.

In addition, Kelly and McIntyre[17] have reexamined the role of the PC as a critical node in limbic system kindling. They present two pieces of data that appear to diminish the role of the PC. First, they reviewed the experiments of McIntyre and Plant[23,24] who investigated slices containing amygdala, PC and perirhinal cortex in a perfusion medium that was Mg^{++} free. The absence of Mg^{++} in the perfusate augmented NMDA-mediated excitation and produced robust epileptiform burst discharges in the PC. However, simultaneous recording from the PC and perirhinal cortex revealed that these bursts actually originated in the latter structure.

The second set of data presented by Kelly and McIntyre[17] consisted of new experiments assessing the effect of a PC lesion on kindling from the ipsilateral hippocampus. The investigators reasoned that if the PC were a critical node for hippocampal kindling, then a PC lesion should prevent development of kindled seizures. Their experimental paradigm was a rather complicated design involving forebrain commissurotomy and status epilepticus. First, all forebrain commissures were severed, including the corpus callosum, the dorsal and ventral hippocampal commissures, the anterior commissure and the massa intermedia. This procedure lateralizes kindled seizure discharges to the stimulated hemisphere, producing a hemi-convulsion only on the contralateral side of the body. Second, following recovery from the commissurotomy, Kelly and McIntyre induced a type of limbic status epilepticus that is known to destroy either the PC alone or both the PC and perirhinal cortex in one hemisphere. Thus, two experimental preparations were created: both preparations had complete forebrain bisection, but one had a unilateral lesion in only the PC, while the other had a unilateral lesion of both the PC and perirhinal cortex. Both preparations were subjected to hippocampal kindling on the side of the lesion. The result was that kindled seizure development in the ipsilateral hemisphere was disrupted only in animals that had a lesion involving both the PC and the perirhinal cortex. A lesion confined only to the PC did not prevent the propagation of hippocampal discharges through the ipsilateral temporal lobe.

Kelly and McIntyre[17] drew two conclusions from these results: (1) the PC is not critical to the kindling network developed from the hippocampus, and (2) the perirhinal cortex, especially the posterior aspect, is essential for kindled seizure development from the hippocampus. While more work needs to be done, our data seem to be compatible with those of Kelly and McIntyre. Both sets of studies strongly support the concept that kindled seizure development involves specific pathways of AD propagation that recruit a common, nodal rhinencephalic network. We also both agree that the PC is at least part of this common downstream node. Kelly and McIntyre's studies suggest that the PC is not critical to the nodal network. Our data do not speak directly to this issue, but we do not disagree with the conclusion. Indeed, our Fos induction studies clearly indicate that the network recruited at the transition from stage 1–2 seizures to stage 3 seizures involves more than just the PC: the network also includes portions of the amygdala, the posterior agranular insular cortex and the ventral perirhinal cortex. At later stages of kindling, our studies show that there is further recruitment within the perirhinal regions (Applegate, et al, this volume). Thus, our data agree with those of Kelly and McIntyre that the perirhinal cortex is an important part of the nodal network recruited during limbic system. Furthermore, our data suggest that this region is important both during the early transition from stages 1–2 to stage 3 and the late transition from stage 3 to stages 4–5.

The extensive network shown by Fos induction to be recruited during limbic system kindling suggests an alternative explanation for the lesion results of Kelly and McIntyre.[17] We agree with the conclusion that the PC alone is not critical for kindled seizure development within a hemisphere. However, we disagree with the conclusion that the perirhinal cortex is *essential*. Rather, we would argue that the data suggest that what is essential for kindled seizure development is the *whole* network. As long as a substantial portion of the network is present, kindled seizure development can progress. Thus, a lesion of the PC alone is not sufficient to halt the process. We would argue that a lesion of the perirhinal cortex alone also might not be sufficient. What Kelly and McIntyre have demonstrated is that a lesion of *both* the PC and perirhinal cortex is sufficient to halt kindling. Whether a lesion of the perirhinal cortex alone is sufficient remains to be determined. Within the context of our hypothesis, we would predict that a lesion confined to the perirhinal cortex would halt the late transition from stage 3 to stages 4–5, but would have little, if any, effect on the early transition from stages 1–2 to stage 3.

In summary, our data and those of others support the concept that kindled seizure development involves, at least in part, a common anatomical system. We hypothesize that most, if not all, limbic system sites susceptible to kindling converge onto a common rhinencephalic neural network. During the early stages of kindling (stages 1, 2 and 3) this network includes the posterior piriform cortex, the posterior agranular insular cortex, the ventral perirhinal cortex, and portions of the amygdala and peri-amygdalar areas. The implication of this hypothesis is that kindling must be viewed as having a hierarchical and directional organization that involves propagation of AD activity following specific pathways. It follows, then, that the neural reorganization assumed to underlie the enhanced epileptogenicity resulting from kindling also occurs in specific networks. Thus, the experimental search for the cellular and sub-cellular mechanisms of kindling must respect this hierarchical organization. The search only makes sense if conducted within structures that are part of the specific network developed during kindling from a given limbic site and at the appropriate stage of the kindling process when these structures are recruited into the network.

REFERENCES

1. Ackerman, RF, Chugani, HT, Handforth, A, Moshé, S, Caldcott-Hazard, S and Engel, Jr, J. Autoradiographic studies of cerebral metabolism and blood flow in rat amygdala kindling. In: Wada, JA (Ed), *Kindling 3*. New York: Raven Press pp. 73–87, 1986.
2. Applegate, CD, Pretel, S and Piekut, DT. The substantia nigra pars reticulata, seizures and Fos expression. *Epilepsy Research* 20 (1995) 31–39.
3. Burchfiel, JL and Applegate, CD. Forebrain and brainstem mechanisms governing kindled seizure development: An hypothesis. In: Wada, JA (Ed), *Kindling IV*. New York: Plenum Press, pp. 93–112, 1990.
4. Burchfiel, JL and Applegate, CD. Stepwise progression of kindling: Perspectives from the kindling antagonism model. *Neurosci. Biobehav. Rev.* 13 (1990) 289–299.
5. Burchfiel, JL and Applegate, CD. The piriform cortex and kindling: Behavioral and physiological evidence for a common substrate. *Epilepsia* 32 (1991) 632.
6. Burchfiel, JL, Serpa, KA and Duffy, FH. Further studies of antagonism of seizure development between concurrently developing kindled limbic foci in the rat. *Exp. Neurol.* 75 (1982) 476–489.
7. Burnham, WM. Primary and "transfer" seizure development in the kindled rat. In: Wada, JA (Ed), *Kindling*. New York: Raven Press, pp. 61–84, 1976.
8. Duchowny, MS and Burchfiel, JL. Facilitation and antagonism of kindled seizure development in the limbic system of the rat. *Electroenceph. Clin. Neurophysiol.* 51 (1981) 403–416.

9. Gaen, PW, Shinnick-Gallagher, P and Anderson, AC. Spontaneous epileptiform activity and alteration of GABA- and of NMDA-mediated neurotransmission in amygdala neurons kindled in vivo. *Brain Res.* 494 (1989) 177–181.
10. Gale, K. Animal models of generalized convulsive seizures. In: Avoli, M, et al. (Eds), *Generalized Epilepsy*. Birkhauser, pp. 329–343, 1990.
11. Goddard, GV, McIntyre, DC and Leech, CK. A permanent change in brain function resulting from daily electrical stimulation. *Exp. Neurol.* 25 (1969) 294–330.
12. Haberly, LB and Sutula, TP. Neuronal processes that underlie expression of kindled epileptiform events in the piriform cortex in vivo. *J. Neurosci.* 12 (1992) 2211–2224.
13. Hoffman, WH and Haberly, LB. Bursting-induced epileptiform EPSPs in slices of piriform cortex are generated by deep cells. *J. Neurosci.* 11 (1991) 2021–2031.
14. Hoffman, WH and Haberly, LB. Role of synaptic excitation in the generation of bursting-induced epileptiform potentials in the endopiriform nucleus and piriform cortex. *J. Neurophysiol.* 70 (1993) 2550–2561.
15. Hunt, SP, Pini, A and Evans, G. Induction of c-fos-like protein in spinal cord neurons following sensory stimulation. *Nature* 328 (1987) 632–634.
16. Kairiss, EW, Racine, RJ and Smith, GK. The development of the interictal spike during kindling in the rat. *Brain Res.* 322 (1984) 101–110.
17. Kelly, ME and McIntyre, DC. Perirhinal cortex involvement in limbic kindled seizures. *Epilepsy Res.* 26 (1996) 233–243.
18. Ketchum, KL and Haberly, LB. Membrane currents evoked by afferent fiber stimulation in rat piriform cortex. I. Current source-density analysis. *J. Neuropsyiol.* 69 (1993) 248–260.
19. Ketchum, KL and Haberly, LB. Membrane currents evoked by afferent fiber stimulation in rat piriform cortex. II. Analysis with a system model. *J. Neuropsyiol.* 69 (1993) 261–281.
20. Krukoff, TL, Morton, TL, Harris, KM and Jhmandas, JH. Expression of c-fos protein in rat brain elicited by electrical stimulation of the parabrachial nucleus. *J. Neurosci.* 12 (1992) 3582–3590.
21. Le Gal La Salle, G. Amygdaloid kindling in the rat: Regional differences and general properties. In: Wada, JA (Ed), *Kindling 2*. New York: Raven Press. Pp 31–47, 1981.
22. Loscher, W, Ebert, U, Wahnschaffe, U and Rundfeldt, C. Susceptibility of different cell layers of the anterior and posterior part of the piriform cortex to electrical stimulation and kindling: Comparison with the basolateral amygdala and "area tempestas". *Neuroscience* 66 (1995) 265–276.
23. McIntyre, DC and Plant, JR. Pyriform cortex involvement in kindling. *Neurosci. Biobehav. Rev.* 13 (1989) 277–280.
24. McIntyre, DC and Plant, JR. Long-lasting changes in the origin of spontaneous discharges from amygdala-kindled rats: Piriform cortex versus perirhinal cortex in vitro. *Brain Res.* 624 (1993) 268–276.
25. McIntyre, DC and Wong, RKS. Modification of local neuronal interactions by amygdala kindling examined in vitro. *Exp. Neurol.* 88 (1985) 529–537.
26. McIntyre, DC and Wong, RKS. Cellular and synaptic properties of amygdala-kindled pyriform cortex in vitro. *J. Neurophysiol.* 55 (1986) 1295–1307.
27. Morgan, JI, Cohen, DR, Hempstead, JL and Curran, T. Mapping patterns of c-fos expression in the central nervous system after seizure. *Science* 237 (1987) 192–197.
28. Morgan, JI and Curran, T. Stimulus-transcription coupling in the nervous system: Involvement of the inducible proto-oncogenes fos and jun. *Ann. Rev. Neurosci.* 14 (1991) 421–451.
29. McNamara, JO, Byrne, M, Dashieff, R and Fitz, J. The kindling model of epilepsy: A review. *Prog. Neurobiol.* 15 (1980) 139–159.
30. Nierenberg J, Applegate CD, Burchfiel JL and Piekut DT. Fos immunolabeling following kindled seizures elicited from different brain sites. *Soc. Neurosci. Abs.* 19 (1993) 605.
31. Nierenberg J, Applegate CD, Burchfiel JL and Piekut DT. FOS immunolabeling following kindled partial seizures elicited from different brain sites. *Soc Neurosci. Abs.* 20 (1994) 1458.
32. Piredda, S and Gale, K. A crucial epileptogenic site in the deep prepiriform cortex. *Nature* 317 (1985) 623–625.
33. Piredda, S and Gale, K. Role of excitatory amino acid transmission in the genesis of seizures elicited for the deep prepiriform cortex. *Brain Res.* 377 (1986) 205–210.
34. Racine, RJ, Mosher, M and Kairiss, EW. The role of the pyriform cortex in the generation of the interictal spikes in the kindled preparation. *Brain Res.* 454 (1988) 251–263.
35. Sagar, SM, Sharp, FR and Curran T. Expression of c-fos mapping in the brain: Metabolic mapping at the cellular level. *Science* 240 (1988) 1328–1331.
36. Sato, M and Nakashima, T. Kindling: Secondary epileptogenesis, sleep and catecholamines. *Can. J. Neurosci.* 2 (1975) 439–446.
37. White, LE and Price, JL. The functional anatomy of limbic status epilepticus in the rat. I. Patterns of ^{14}C-2-deoxyglucose uptake and fos immunochemistry. *J. Neurosci.* 13 (1993) 4787–4809.

38. Zhang, G and Sasamoto, K. Projections of two separate cortical areas for rhythmical jaw movements in the rat. *Brain Res. Bull.* 24 (1990) 221–230.

DISCUSSION OF JAMES BURCHFIEL'S TALK

Stripling: In your comparison between septal and olfactory bulb kindling in the piriform cortex, it seems that you would expect the piriform to show fos expression immediately, because the olfactory bulb and the entire olfactory cortex are really one tight network. For comparison, you would still need the same number and stage of seizures and the same duration of ADs that you elicited from the olfactory bulb. I thought that you would see piriform fos sooner than stage 3 from the septum.

Burchfiel: So did we. Piriform neurons have a low threshold for fos expression, and express fos in response to many different inputs. Both the piriform and dorsal endopiriform express fos following 1 AD or stage 2 seizures elicited from the olfactory bulb, but at stage 2 aspects of the extended network I showed in the Tables, earlier, are missing. A good example of that is the insular cortex. For the septal nucleus, 1 AD results in fos labelling in the amygdala/hippocampal transition area, and this labelling spreads to include the cortical amygdala at stage 2. At stage 3, however, the piriform and insular cortices and other areas express fos as a unit and relate directly to the expression of the behavioral seizure type. It has been this relatively sudden onset of fos labelling at stage 3 from the septum that has helped us to interpret labelling patterns following bulb and amygdala kindling. I think the key is that the behavioral seizure dictates the spatial pattern of fos expression. At stage 3 a common set of structures express fos independent of the kindling site.

Gale: If you stimulate the olfactory bulb and if you are directly driving the piriform cortex, you would expect to see fos activation independent of whether there has been a seizure.

Burchfiel: That's right. Coulombic stimulation of the bulb promotes fos labelling in the piriform and endopiriform nucleus, but the number of cells expressing fos is far less than that seen after an AD. For fos, triggering intrinsic local networks is a much better stimulus than simply driving those networks noncontingently like with repetitive low frequency stimulation.

Corcoran: Jim, are you characterizing seizure stages according to Racine's scheme or according to your own classification scheme?

Burchfiel: When I refer to stage 3 seizures, I am using the classification scheme that Craig Applegate and I have described. We use Sprague-Dawley rats, and these animals rarely, if ever, exhibit the unilateral forelimb clonus that is Racine's stage 3. Since our rats go from pronounced facial clonus and headnodding right into bilateral forelimb clonus with rearing, we define these behaviors as stage 3. These are also the first really convulsive looking, AD driven behaviors that we see. Prior to headnodding and facial clonus, AD driven behaviors appear integrated, albeit out of context. That is, if you didn't know the animal was experiencing an AD, you wouldn't necessarily say that the behaviors you observe were manifestations of a seizure.

12

THE ROLE OF RHINENCEPHALIC NETWORKS IN THE LATE STAGES OF KINDLING

Craig D. Applegate, James L. Burchfiel, Russell J. Ferland, and Jay Nierenberg

Departments of Neurology and Neurobiology and Anatomy
The Program in Neuroscience and The Comprehensive Epilepsy Program
University of Rochester School of Medicine and Dentistry
Rochester, New York 14642

1. INTRODUCTION

The stereotyped development of kindled seizures from all limbic system structures strongly suggests the recruitment of a common neuronal network for seizure expression. Our own research (see Burchfiel, Applegate, Samoriski and Nierenberg, this volume), as well as that of others, has implicated the involvement of several paleocortical regions including the ipsilateral piriform, ventral perirhinal and insular cortices in the transition from stage 2 to stage 3 kindled seizures, independent of the site of focal afterdischarge initiation.[5,17,19,22,28] Thus, the evolution of afterdischarge driven species typical behaviors such as arrest, grooming and wet dog shakes (stages 1–2) to pronounced facial clonus and headnodding (stage 3) involves the recruitment of the ipsilateral piriform and insular cortices for behavioral seizure expression.

The neural substrates responsible for the continued development of kindling from stage 3 to stages 4–5 are currently undefined. However, it is believed that the expression of bilaterally generalized clonic seizures involves the recruitment of additional structures into the stage 3 neural network. Recent evidence (see McIntyre et al., this volume) has indicated that the perirhinal cortex and the projections of this area to frontal motor cortical areas represent a candidate substrate for mediating the expression of stage 4–5 kindled seizures.[21,23] Together with our own data that define a network involved in the progression of early stage kindling, these data would suggest that the further progression of kindling to secondary generalization, requires the recruitment of the perirhinal cortex by the previously established piriform/insular cortical network.

Hypothetically, the rate of kindled seizure development is dictated by the number of synapses focal afterdischarge must propagate through, and alter, to access and recruit the common stage 3–5 network. This conceptual framework would predict that variance in

Kindling 5, edited by Corcoran and Moshé.
Plenum Press, New York, 1998.

kindling rate among limbic system structures should be accounted for entirely by the number of stage 1–2 seizures required to access the stage 3 network. This framework would further predict that once the common stage 3 network is recruited, the number of trials to progress from stage 3 to stage 5 should be approximately equal across all limbic sites. Both of these predictions are supported by the literature (e.g.,[5–7,15]). An additional prediction of this framework is that the more rapid kindling rates observed for secondary kindling sites in the transfer paradigm should be accounted for almost entirely by a reduction in the number of stage 3–5 trials. Our data (see Burchfiel, Applegate, et al. this volume) support this prediction.

The anterior perirhinal cortex exhibits the fastest reported kindling rates in the brain with stimulation resulting in short latency bilateral forelimb clonus (stage 5 seizures) within 3 to 4 trials.[21] The fact that the perirhinal has a robust projection to the ipsilateral frontal cortex and that short latency bilateral forelimb clonus can be elicited from the frontal cortex following a single stimulation, suggests that the perirhinal and frontal motor cortices may represent a final common pathway for the expression of generalized clonic seizures. Support for this concept comes from recent observations indicating that the induction of spreading depression through the infusion of 3 mM KCl onto the ipsilateral frontal cortex eliminates the expression of generalized clonic seizures in animals fully kindled from the amygdala.[12]

In this paper, we report convergent experimental evidence that supports a role for the perirhinal cortex as a final common pathway for the expression of generalized clonic seizures. Our data suggest that the expression of generalized clonic seizures whether evoked from a naive, or a kindled state, involves a recruitment of the perirhinal cortex. Our data further suggest that the *bilateral* recruitment of the perirhinal cortex may be a requirement for clonic seizure expression.

2. FOS INDUCTION FOLLOWING PERIRHINAL STIMULATION IN NAIVE RATS

2.1. Introduction

A growing number of studies have used the expression of the proto-oncogene c-fos as a marker of multi-synaptic networks following discrete electrical stimulation of the brain.[11,13,24,25,29] These studies have indicated that following 10–20 minutes of stimulation, the expression of the c-fos protein (Fos) is induced in structures 2 to 3 synapses removed from the site of stimulation.[11,13,29] These observations suggest that the induction of Fos can detail the pattern of connectivity of a structure beyond that available using traditional tracing methods. Thus, the expression of Fos protein following electrical activation of a brain area has the potential to define functionally relevant multi-synaptic networks with resolution at the cellular level.

2.2. Animals and Protocols

Male, Sprague-Dawley rats (N=9) were implanted with unipolar electrodes into the perirhinal cortex (AP –4.0mm; ML +6.6mm; V –4.0mm from dura). The electrodes had a 0.5mm bared tip and were referenced to a skull screw near the midline, ipsilateral and posterior to the stimulation site. All surgery was performed under deep pentobarbital anesthesia under conditions that met or exceeded local, state and federal guidelines.

Rats were allowed to recover for 5 to 7 days, and were then handled daily and attached to the stimulation apparatus daily for an additional 7 days. This habituation is essential. In the absence of habituation, we have observed significant Fos expression in response to handling and exposure to the experimental apparatus in many structures we were interested in studying. Following habituation, the afterdischarge (AD) threshold to our standard kindling stimulus (a 1 second train of 1 ms monophasic square waves delivered at 100 Hz) was established. Two to 4 days following AD determination, animals were stimulated in the perirhinal. Eight rats received stimulation. The last rat in this series was handled identically but did not receive stimulation. Perirhinal stimulation consisted of 3 per second, 50 ms trains of 0.2 ms square waves delivered at 400 Hz. The starting current was 50–100 μA below the AD threshold and animals were continuously stimulated until a generalized clonic seizure was elicited or for 20 minutes. During the stimulation period, the current was increased in some animals to promote behavioral responses to the stimulation.

Ninety minutes following the beginning of stimulation, all animals were injected with a lethal dose of pentobarbital and perfused through the heart with phosphate buffered saline (PBS) followed by 4% paraformadehyde in PBS. Brains were removed, cryoprotected with 30% sucrose in PBS, and sectioned (40 μm) from the frontal pole through the medulla into 6 wells using a freezing microtome.

The tissue was then processed for immunolabeling of Fos protein using standard techniques. Briefly, free floating tissue sections were incubated with: (1) antiserum to Fos (Santa Cruz Biotechnology, Inc.) diluted 1:40,000 in PBS containing 1% normal goat serum and 0.4% Triton X-100 for 48 hours at 4°C, (2) Biotinylated goat anti-rabbit immunoglobulin G in PBS containing 0.04% Triton X-100 for 60 minutes, and (3) ABC reagents (avidin DH and horseradish peroxidase H) from the Vecstain ABC kit (Vector Laboratories) for 60 minutes. Visualization of the antibody-antigen complex was accomplished by reaction with the catalyst 3,3′-diaminobenzidine (7.5mg/10mls in PBS) in the presence of the co-substrate hydrogen peroxide (0.03%). Tissue was reacted until a brown color developed or, in cases in which nickel intensification was used, until a black color developed. Controls for immunocytochemical procedures consisted of eliminating the primary antibody from the first incubation step or pre-absorption of the primary antibody with synthetic antigen for 48 hours prior to application to the tissue. No immunolabeling has been observed under either of these control conditions.

Based on the results of our Fos study (see below), we were interested in documenting whether or not the perirhinal cortices were reciprocally interconnected. Four animals were pressure injected with a 10% solution of the tracer Lucifer yellow into the left perirhinal cortex (25–100 nl over 15 minutes). Seven days following the injection, animals were perfused and the tissue was processed for immuncytochemical localization of transported Lucifer yellow. Immunocytochemical protocols were identical to those described above except that the initial incubation was done with an antiserum to Lucifer yellow (Molecular Probes, Inc.) diluted 1:8000.

2.3. Behavioral Results

Stimulation of the perirhinal cortex resulted in the expression of generalized clonic seizures in 7 of the 8 stimulated animals. The latency to generalized seizures was variable, ranging from 2 to 17 minutes. The seizures were characterized by bilateral forelimb clonus with rearing, and sometimes falling, and were often preceeded by head nodding and facial twitching that was synchronous with the stimulation. In 5 of the 8 animals, the clonic seizure motor manifestations were driven by the stimulation. That is, when the stimulation was stopped after 5–15 seconds of bilateral forelimb clonus and rearing, the behaviors stopped and there was no indication of afterdischarge in the EEG. In addition, the animals were not obviously post-ictal. We will refer to these stimulation driven clonic motor behaviors as 'stimulus-locked' behaviors. In the remaining two animals that exhibited generalized clonic seizures, the seizure behaviors continued after the stimulation was stopped, and self-sustained trains of AD were observed in the EEG. In the last stimulated animal no behavioral response to the stimulation was observed. The AD threshold for this animal was 200 μA and he received stimulation for 20 minutes at 100 μA with no increase in the current during the stimulation period.

2.4. Fos Expression

The pattern of Fos induction in the 5 rats that exhibited 'stimulus-locked' generalized clonic motor manifestations were remarkably similar across animals. An example of these results are shown in Figure 1.

Ipsilateral to the stimulation site, Fos expression was ubiquitous, with dense labeling in many limbic, neocortical and paleocortical areas. While the hippocampus was variably labeled ipsilaterally, the amygdala consistently exhibited robust Fos labeling. In particular, the lateral and basolateral nuclei were densely labeled ipsilateral to the stimulating electrode. The piriform, insular, entorhinal and perirhinal cortices also exhibited dense labeling in all lamina throughout the anterior-posterior extent of these areas. Similarly, neocortex including frontal areas as well as temporal and parietal neocortex were robustly labeled in the ipsilateral hemisphere.

By contast, the pattern of contralateral Fos labeling following 'stimulus-locked' generalized clonic motor behaviors was much more discrete. In the contralateral hemisphere, only three areas exhibited Fos labeling above that seen in controls. The perirhinal cortex, particularly in the dorsal superficial layers, but with significant labeling in the deeper layers; the frontal motor cortex, particularly the superficial and deepest layers of the forelimb and hindlimb regions; and the lateral nucleus of the amygdala. In some animals, the perirhinal labeling extended into the temporal neocortex either in the superficial layers only or including both the superficial and deep layers. Other rhinal cortical areas such as the piriform, insular and entorhinal did not exhibit appreciable Fos labeling in the contralateral hemisphere. In one animal exhibiting 'stimulus-locked' clonic motor behaviors, this contralateral pattern of Fos labeling was only weakly developed.

In the two animals that expressed self-sustained seizures in response to perirhinal stimulation, the ipsilateral pattern of Fos expression described above was present bilaterally. Finally, in the animal that failed to exhibit any motor seizure manifestations, there was labeling above that seen in unstimulated controls (Figure 1) in the ipsi- and contralateral perirhinal cortex and the frontal cortices, but the labeling was only in scattered cells and was by no means as definitive as that seen following stimulation elicited clonic motor behaviors.

2.5. Lucifer Yellow Results

Injections of Lucifer yellow into the left perirhinal resulted in the retrograde labeling of neurons in the perirhinal cortex of the contralateral hemisphere. An example of these results is shown in Figure 1. While not a comprehensive analysis, this outcome suggesting the reciprocol interconnection of the perirhinal cortices is consistent with recent anterograde tracing studies documenting projections from the perirhinal to the homotopic cortex contralaterally.[23] Together with our Fos results, these data suggest that the reciprocol interaction between the perirhinal cortices may be excitatory in nature.[25]

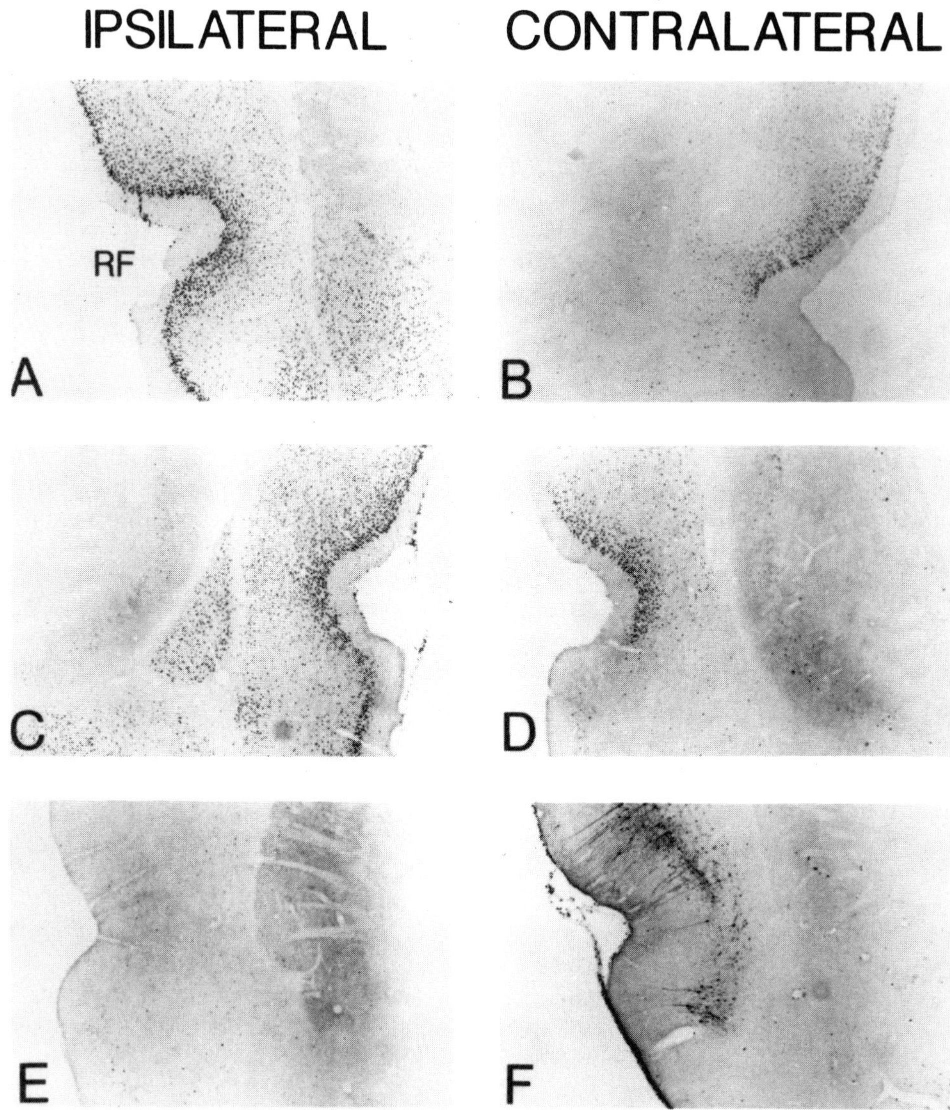

Figure 1. Two examples of the pattern of Fos labeling observed following stimulation of the perirhinal cortex of naive rats. Stimulation in both cases resulted in 'stimulus-locked' generalized clonic motor behaviors. In both cases, Fos labeling in the ipsilateral hemisphere (A,C) was dense and involved many cortical and subcortical areas. By contrast, Fos labeling in the contralateral hemisphere (B,D) was largely confined to the dorsal aspects of the perirhinal cortex. An example of the ipsilateral hemisphere of a handled, unstimulated animal is shown in E. In F, the retrograde labeling of layer V neurons in the perirhinal cortex of a rat injected with Lucifer yellow (50 nl) into the perirhinal on the opposite side. This result indicates that the perirhinal cortices are reciprocally interconnected. In conjunction with our Fos data, this reciprocol pattern of connectivity involves a physiologically excitatory component. See text for details. RF = rhinal fissure. Magnification = 10X.

3. FOS INDUCTION FOLLOWING GENERALIZED CLONIC SEIZURES IN KINDLED RATS

3.1. Introduction

The results of our initial study suggest that the perirhinal cortex can serve as a motor substrate for the expression of generalized clonic seizures. Stimulation of the perirhinal can produce motor manifestations that appear identical to stage 4 or stage 5 kindled seizures. These motor behaviors are directly driven by the stimulus and do not continue in the absence of continued stimulation. Our results further indicate that these clonic behaviors are associated with robust Fos labeling of many neo- and paleocortical areas as well as many subcortical limbic system structures ipsilateral to the site of stimulation. Contralaterally, however, Fos expression is limited to the perirhinal cortex, lateral nucleus of the amygdala and frontal motor cortex. In this study, we examined the pattern of Fos labeling following the first generalized clonic seizure (stage 4 or 5) elicited during the kindling of several limbic system sites.

3.2. Animals and Protocols

Male, Sprague-Dawley rats were stereotaxically implanted with chronically indwelling bipolar electrodes under deep pentobarbital anesthesia. Following a seven day postoperative period during which animals were handled, thresholds for AD were determined and animals received daily, or twice daily, kindling stimulation until either the first stage 3 seizure (characterized by pronounced clonic jaw movements and head-nodding) or the first stage 4 or 5 seizure (minimally characterized by bilateral forelimb clonus with rearing) was elicited.

Animals were kindled to the first generalized clonic seizure from the olfactory bulb (N=2; AP +7.3; ML + 0.6; V –2.5), septal nucleus (N=2; AP +1.8; M +1.0; V –5.0), piriform cortex (N=2; AP –0.3; ML +6.3; V –7.0), amygdala (N=1; AP –0.8; ML +4.8; V – 7.7) or the perirhinal cortex (N=1; AP +0.2; ML +4.0; V –7.0). Similarly, animals were kindled to the first stage 3 seizure from the amygdala, septal nucleus, the olfactory bulb (N=3/site; coordinates as shown above) or the perirhinal cortex (N=2). These stage 3 animals were the same as those described by Burchfiel, Applegate, Samoriski and Nierenberg, this volume.

The kindling stimulation was a 1 second train of 1 millisecond monophasic square wave pulses delivered at 100 Hz. Thresholds were determined by raising the current in 50 μA steps from a starting current of 50 μA every 3 minutes until an AD was elicited. On the day following threshold determination, kindling trials were begun at +50 μA above AD threshold. Ninety minutes following the first trial that the desired seizure stage was observed in, animals were injected with a lethal dose of pentobarbital and perfused through the heart with 4% paraformaldehyde. Perfusion protocols and protocols for processing tissue for Fos immunolabeling were identical to those described above.

3.3. Fos Expression following Stage 3 Seizures

Independent of the kindling site, Fos labeling following stage 3 kindled seizures was *always* confined to the ipsilateral hemisphere (Figure 2 G,H). Structures that exhibited labeling following stage 3 seizures included various amygdala nuclei, the piriform cortex

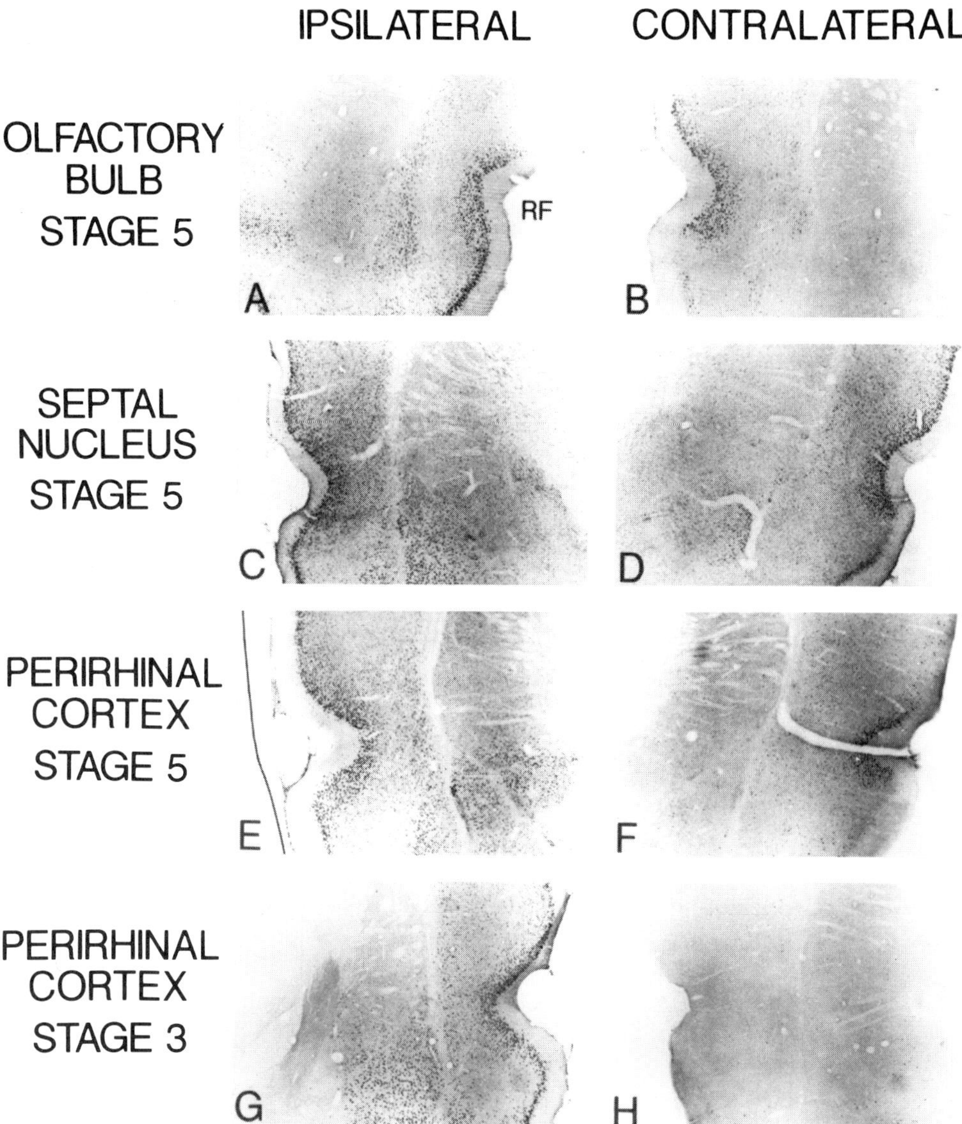

Figure 2. Examples of the pattern of Fos labeling following the first Stage 5 kindled seizure from three limbic system structures. In all cases, Fos labeling in the hemisphere ipsilateral to the kindling site (A,C,E,) was widespread and robust. In the contralateral hemisphere, however, only the perirhinal (B,D,F) and the insular cortices exhibited Fos labeling. The data suggest that the *bilateral* recruitment of the perirhinal cortex is necessary for the expression of generalized clonic seizures. This interpretation is reinforced by the observation that Stage 3 kindled seizures from the perirhinal cortex result in ipsilateral, but not contralateral perirhinal labeling (G,H). See text for details. RF = rhinal fissure. Magnification = 10X.

and the posterior division of the agranular insular cortex (AIP). These areas always exhibited Fos labeling in the hemisphere ipsilateral to the site of kindling following stage 3 seizures regardless of the site of AD initiation. Importantly, Fos labeling in the AIP was never observed following kindling from any site until a stage 3 seizure was expressed. These results are discussed in detail by Burchfiel et al. in this volume.

3.4. Fos Expression Following Generalized Kindled Seizures

The pattern of Fos immunolabeling following the first stage 4 or stage 5 kindled seizure was largely confined to the hemisphere ipsilateral to the kindling electrode from all sites (Figure 2). The ipsilateral insular, piriform (including the dorsal endopiriform area), entorhinal and perirhinal cortices were robustly labeled independent of the kindling site. In addition, many neocortical areas were densely labeled ipsilaterally following a stage 5 seizure from any site including temporal, parietal and frontal cortex. Subcortically, the lateral, basolateral, basomedial and cortical amygdala nuclei exhibited dense Fos labeling ipsilaterally, again independent of the kindling site. Robust labeling of the ipsilateral amygdalo-piriform transition area and the amygdalo-hippocampal area also contributed to this pattern of stage 4–5 Fos labeling in the ipsilateral hemisphere.

With the exception of 2 animals, Fos immunolabeling in the contralateral hemisphere was much more discrete (Figure 2). Independent of the kindling site, the perirhinal cortex showed Fos immunolabeling. In some animals, labeling was confined to the deep layers, and in others, the superficial layers exhibited dense labeling. In these latter animals, labeling was invariably present in deep layers, but either the labeling itself was light or the number of deep layer neurons expressing Fos were scattered. In general, the pattern of perirhinal labeling in the contralateral hemisphere was similar if not identical to that seen following 'stimulus-locked' seizures elicited by perirhinal stimulation described above.

The contralateral frontal cortex exhibited Fos labeling as did the agranular insular cortex on the contralateral side in these animals, independent of the site of seizure initiation. The contralateral piriform cortex and lateral nucleus of the amygdala were labeled in approximately half of the cases. The labeling of these structures was apparently site specific. Following kindled seizures elicited from the amygdala, olfactory bulb or perirhinal cortex, the piriform and amygdala *failed* to show Fos labeling. However, labeling in both the contralateral piriform cortex and lateral amygdala were seen following stage 5 seizures elicited from either the septal nucleus or piriform cortex.

In the remaining 2 animals, one kindled from the olfactory bulb and the other from the piriform cortex, the pattern of labeling was dense and symmetrical in both hemispheres.

In terms of the induction of Fos expression, the results of this analysis indicate that the first generalized kindled seizure predominantly activates the ipsilateral hemisphere. There is robust and widespread Fos expression in most cortical areas and in subcortical limbic structures in the ipsilateral hemisphere independent of the site of seizure initiation. By contrast, the induction of Fos protein in the contralateral hemisphere was confined largely to the agranular insular, perirhinal and the frontal motor cortices. The pattern of Fos induction observed in kindled animals was virtually identical to that seen following the elicitation of clonic motor behaviors with perirhinal cortical stimulation in naive rats, and was strikingly similar to the pattern of fos mRNA induction seen after seizures induced by focal chemical stimulation of the deep prepiriform cortex.[14,18] Thus, bicuculline injections into "area tempestus" promote a rapid increase in fos mRNA that is predominantly ipsilateral to the injection site. Increases in signal in the contralateral hemisphere were confined to the perirhinal cortex on the uninjected side. Together, these data suggest that the expression of generalized clonic seizures with rearing, bilateral forelimb clonus and falling, is associated most closely with the expression of Fos in the perirhinal cortex, bilaterally.

4. EFFECTS OF KCL INJECTIONS IN THE CONTRALATERAL PERIRHINAL CORTEX ON AMYGDALA KINDLED SEIZURE EXPRESSION

4.1. Introduction

The data presented in the two experiments described above suggest the hypothesis that the bilateral recruitment of the perirhinal cortex is a requirement for the expression of generalized clonic seizures whether elicited from the naive or the kindled state. If the bilateral recruitment of the perirhinal cortex is a requirement for the expression of stage 5 kindled seizures, then a lesion of the contralateral perirhinal cortex in a kindled animal should result in a regression of the expressed seizure from a stage 5 to a stage 3 seizure. In the present pilot experiment, we present data that support this prediction.

4.2. Animals and Protocols

Male, Sprague-Dawley rats (N=4) were sterotaxically implanted with a chronically indwelling bipolar stimulating electrode into the left basolateral amygdala and with a chronically indwelling cannula aimed at the right perirhinal cortex under deep pentobarbital anesthesia. Coordinates for the electrode were AP –.03; ML +4.5; V –7.0 and for the cannula were AP –4.0; ML –6.2; V –4.2 from dura.

Following a one week recovery, AD thresholds were established as described previously and animals were kindled (see above) until stimulation elicited a single stage 5 seizure. On the next day, animals were infused with a 3 mM KCl solution in artificial CSF into the right perirhinal cortex through an injection stilette that extended 1.5 mm beyond the tip of the guide cannula. KCl was infused in a volume of 2.0 μL over one minute into the contralateral perirhinal cortex followed 30 seconds later by kindling stimulation to the amygdala. No obvious behavioral effects of the KCl infusion were noted at the time of stimulation. That is, animals did not become hemi-paretic or display any other overt lateralizing behavioral signs at the time of amygdala stimulation (90 seconds following the start of the injection).

4.3. Results of KCL Injections

Prior to injection, all animals displayed normal AD and behavioral kindling characteristics to the first stage 5 seizure, and electrodes were histologically verified to be in the basolateral amygdala. Pretreatment of the contralateral perirhinal cortex with KCl resulted in aborted seizures in 3 of the 4 animals tested. In the 3 animals affected by KCl injections, the cannula were histologically located in the deep layers of the perirhinal cortex, at approximately the middle of the anterior-posterior extent of this area (Figure 37; Paxinos and Watson). In the animal in which KCl failed to influence clonic seizure expression, the cannula was located medially in the ventral hippocampus at the same level.

Behaviorally, the motor seizures consisted of rearing with a brief bout (< 2 s) of forelimb clonus that rapidly resolved into either headnodding or more integrated post-ictal behaviors that included searching, sniffing and escape behaviors.

In 2 of the 3 animals in which the behavioral seizures were arrested, the afterdischarge duration from the contralateral amygdala was attenuated. In one case, the AD was reduced from 57 seconds before KCl to 17 seconds following injection. In a second case,

AD was modestly reduced from 64 to 46 seconds, and in the third case, AD duration was basically unaffected (112 seconds pre- vs. 110 seconds post-injection). While the number of animals tested in this paradigm is small, the effects were robust and were observed in each animal in which cannula placements were found to be in the perirhinal cortex.

These data provide preliminary, functional support for the hypothesis that the expression of stage 4 and stage 5 clonic motor seizures depends on the *bilateral* recruitment of the perirhinal cortex. While our Fos and transfer kindling data suggest that the development of kindled seizures relies predominantly on the recruitment of networks in the ipsilateral hemisphere (see Burchfiel, Applegate, Samoriski and Nierenberg, this volume), the data presented here suggest the *bilateral* involvement of the perirhinal cortex in the network for late kindled seizure stage development.

5. THE ANATOMY OF KINDLED SEIZURES

The rapid, activity dependent induction of the proto-oncogene c-fos has been used as a marker of spatially distributed, multi-synaptic neural networks following exposure of animals to a variety of experimental paradigms.[25] Seizures represent a particularly potent stimulus for inducing the expression of Fos in many brain structures,[24,30] and it is generally assumed that the spatial pattern of Fos observed following seizures represents a map of the neural systems involved in the propagation of seizure activity and in the behavioral expression of seizures. However, the pattern of Fos induction observed following seizure activity may not identify all relevant structures involved in the propagation of seizures, and the observed spatial distribution of Fos undoubtedly includes the labeling of structures secondarily activated as a consequence of the metabolic stress of the ictal event.[1] Thus, the Fos maps observed following seizures can be interpreted only with the aid of convergent evidence from other studies that define the involvement of any given brain area in seizure expression using other approaches. The advantage of generating Fos maps following seizures, however, is that the technique provides a high degree of anatomical and cellular resolution, targeting those neurons specifically activated in a physiologically defined context.

Our data indicate that electrical stimulation of the perirhinal cortex can produce clonic motor manifestations in the absence of triggering self-sustained AD. The motor behaviors elicited in response to 3/second trains of stimulation are virtually identical in topography to those seen following limbic kindling, but are apparently driven by the stimulation rather than stimulation-induced AD. These data suggest that the perirhinal cortex is closely associated with neural systems responsible for the expression of generalized clonic seizures. The kindling rate of the perirhinal cortex has been reported to be the most rapid in the brain,[21] with stimulation-induced seizures evolving into short latency bilateral forelimb clonus in 3–4 trials. This observation suggests that compared to kindling from other limbic system sites, kindling from the perirhinal cortex needs to promote a reorganization in relatively few synapses to gain access to motor substrates for seizure expression.

The direct projections of the perirhinal cortex to the ipsilateral frontal motor cortex have been suggested to represent a substrate for seizure activity to gain access to the motor system for clonic seizure expression.[23] The origin of this projection is from pyramidal cells in layer V, and recent laminar analysis of perirhinal kindling indicates that generalized clonic seizures are "kindled" from this layer in 1–2 trials.[8] In addition, the induction of spreading depression in the frontal cortical projections of layer V perirhinal neurons reduces both the motor expression of seizures and the AD duration in rats kindled from the ipsilateral amygdala.[12] These data suggest that perirhinal efferents to frontal motor cortex represent the final common pathway for generalized clonic seizure expression and that interruption of AD propagation at this endpoint in the ipsilateral hemisphere significantly interferes with the expression of all generalized motor seizure behaviors.[4,9]

One of the few areas that consistently expressed Fos in the contralateral hemisphere, following either perirhinal stimulation that resulted in clonic motor behaviors or generalized clonic kindled seizures from several limbic sites, was the perirhinal cortex. These observations are consistent with the pattern of Fos mRNA induction following generalized clonic seizures elicited in another focal seizure model, chemical activation of the deep prepiriform cortex.[14,18] Bicuculline injections into this area produces generalized clonic seizures and promotes transcription of the c-fos gene in the contralateral hemisphere that is restricted to the perirhinal and posterior piriform cortices. Together, these data have lead us to the hypothesis that the final expression of generalized clonic seizures involves not only the recruitment of the ipsilateral perirhinal cortex but involves the recruitment of the contralateral perirhinal cortex as well. Preliminary support for this hypothesis comes from our observation that KCl injections into the contralateral perirhinal cortex results in a reduction in seizure stage to stage 3, in amygdala kindled rats. In addition, our outcome is consistent with reports that spreading depression in the contralateral frontal cortex lateralizes seizure expression in amygdala kindled rats in a similar manner to that seen in amygdala kindled animals in which the hemispheres have been disconnected.[19]

Our preliminary retrograde tracing study indicates that the perirhinal cortices are reciprocally interconnected. This result is consistent with anterograde tracing studies documenting the robust projections from layer V and more superficial lamina of the perirhinal to all lamina of the perirhinal cortex in the contralateral hemisphere.[23] Since the induction of Fos protein in neurons has been most tightly linked to depolarizing synaptic events, the induction of Fos in the contralateral perirhinal cortex following generalized clonic seizures suggests that the reciprocol pattern of interconnection between the perirhinal cortices possesses an excitatory component, physiologically. Thus, once the ipsilateral perirhinal cortex is recruited by focally elicited AD, the contralateral perirhinal cortex would be recruited simultaneously and participate in the bilateral manifestations of generalized clonic seizures. Within this framework, the network recruited to mediate the expression of late stage kindling (stages 4–5) would involve the perirhinal cortex bilaterally and projections from this cortical area to frontal motor cortex (Figure 3).

Comparisons of the pattern of Fos expression following the elicitation of stage 2 and stage 3 seizures from several limbic structures has led us to the conclusion that the expression of stage 3 seizures involves the recruitment of a common neural network ipsilateral to the kindling site. This network involves the recruitment of the posterior piriform, aspects of the amygdala, the posterior agranular insular cortex and the ventral perirhinal cortex in the ipsilateral hemisphere. Our data suggest that the recruitment of this network is *required* for the expression of convulsive headnodding and pronounced facial clonus (stage 3 behaviors). The data presented here suggest that the continued development of kindling from stage 3 to stages 4–5 seizures involves the further recruitment of the perirhinal cortex and its projections to frontal motor cortex, *bilaterally*. These data suggest the progressive recruitment of a more spatially distributed rhinencephalic network that parallels the progression of kindling, such that the movement from one kindled seizure stage to the next not only recruits additional structures into the network, but reinforces the network previously established for the expression of earlier stage seizure behaviors.

If this conception is correct, then the interruption of propagation through this common network at any point should either block motor seizure expression entirely or reduce

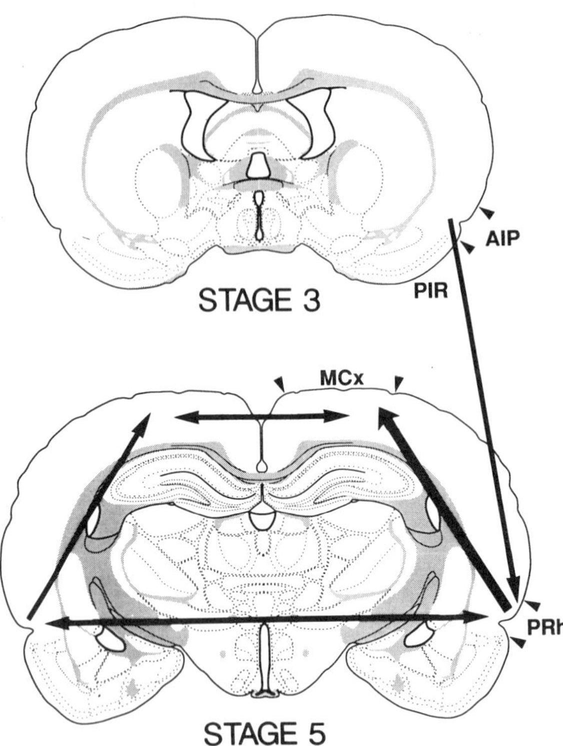

Figure 3. Hypothesized "common neural network" for the expression of Stage 3–Stage 5 kindled seizures. This network is recruited independent of the site of afterdischarge initiation. Based on our Fos experiments, the expression of pronounced facial clonus and head nodding (Stage 3 seizures) involves the recruitment of the piriform cortex, aspects of the amygdala, the ventral perirhinal cortex and the insular cortex in the hemisphere ipsilateral to the site of kindling stimulation. The further progression of kindling to secondarily generalized clonic seizures (Stages 4–5), involves the further recruitment of the perirhinal cortex, bilaterally. Extant data indicate that these structures comprise a facilitated propagation pathway for the expression of Stage 3–5 kindled seizures independent of the site of kindling stimulation. See text for details. See also, McIntyre et al. and Burchfiel et al., this volume. Abbreviations: AIP = agranular insular cortex, posterior division; MCtx = frontal motor cortex; Pir = piriform cortex; Prh = perirhinal cortex.

seizure expression to an earlier stage. The literature provides substantial support for this idea. For example, injections of muscimol into the amygdala-posterior piriform area reliably reduces seizures from stage 5 to stage 2 in animals kindled from the entorhinal cortex, hippocampus, olfactory bulb or insular cortex without affecting focal AD durations.[2,16] Similarly, injections of the NMDA receptor antagonist APV into the agranular insular cortex blocks amygdala kindled convulsions.[10] In addition, muscimol injections into the piriform or perirhinal cortex blocks generalized clonic seizure expression elicited from the deep prepiriform cortex.

A corollary prediction of this conception is that the transfer kindling to any component of this common recruited rhinencephalic network should be extremely rapid, independent of the site of primary kindling. Our data on transfer kindling to the ipsilateral posterior piriform cortex from any limbic structure indicates that secondary kindling of this structure results in stage 5 seizures in 1–3 trials.[6,7] These data not only confirm our observations from Fos immunolabeling suggesting that the piriform cortex is a component of a common propagation network, but also support the hypothesis that once established, AD triggered from any component of this network should rapidly result in generalized clonic seizures. Thus, extant data would indicate that once recruited by focal AD, an extended rhinencephalic network is established, and forms a facilitated propagation network that depends on interactions among the various components for the expression of convulsive behaviors. These networks are predominantly established in the hemisphere ipsilateral to the kindling site.[7] Data presented here, however, would indicate that the progression of kindling to secondary generalization (stages 4–5) involves the bilateral recruitment of the perirhinal cortex into the previously established ipsilateral, stage 3 network.

REFERENCES

1. Applegate, CD, Pretel, S and Piekut, DT. The substantia nigra pars reticulata, seizures and Fos expression. *Epilepsy Research* 20 (1995) 31–39.
2. Applegate, CD and Burchfiel, JL. Microinjections of GABA agonists into the amygdala complex attenuates kindled seizure expression in the rat. *Experimental Neurol.* 102 (1988) 185–189.
3. Battye, RA and McIntyre, DC. Intrinsic responses and morphological features of neurons in the rat perirhinal cortex. *Soc. Neurosci. Abs.* 21 (1995) 1971.
4. Browning, RA, Maggio, R, Sahibzada, N and Gale, K. Role of brainstem structures in seizures initiated from the deep prepiriform cortex in rats. *Epilepsia* 34 (1993) 393–407.
5. Burchfiel, JL and Applegate, CD. Forebrain and brainstem mechanisms governing kindled seizure development: An hypothesis. In: Wada JA, (Ed) *Kindling IV*. New York: Plenum Press, pp. 93–112, 1990.
6. Burchfiel, JL and Applegate, CD. The piriform cortex and kindling: Behavioral and physiological evidence for a common substrate. *Epilepsia* 32 (1991) 632.
7. Burchfiel, JL and Applegate, CD. Evidence suggesting that kindling-induced reorganization is primarily ipsilateral and involves two different systems. *Soc. Neurosci. Abs.* 19 (1993) 605.
8. Felstead, LL, Kelly, ME and McIntyre, DC. Laminar and topographic analysis of perirhinal cortex kindling in the rat. *Soc. Neurosci. Abs.* 21 (1995) 1971.
9. Halonen, T, Tortorella, A, Zrebeet, H and Gale, K. Posterior piriform and perirhinal cortex relay seizures evoked from area tempestas: Role of excitatory and inhibitory amino acid receptors. *Brain Research* 652 (1994) 145–148.
10. Holmes, KH, Bilkey, DK and Laverty, R. The infusion of an NMDA antagonist into the perirhinal cortex suppresses amygdala-kindled seizures. *Brain Research* 587 (1992) 285–290.
11. Hunt, SP, Pini, A and Evans, G. Induction of c-fos-like protein in spinal cord neurons following sensory stimulation. *Nature* 328 (1987) 632–34.
12. Kelly, ME, Battye, RA and McIntyre, DC. Lateralization of amygdala kindled convulsions by unilateral spreading depression. *Soc. Neurosci. Abs.* 21 (1995) 1971.
13. Krukoff, TL, Morton, TL, Harris, KM and Jhmandas, JH. Expression of c-fos protein in rat brainn elicited by electrical stimulation of the parabrachial nucleus. *J. Neurosci.* 12 (1992) 3582–3590.
14. Lanaud, P, Maggio, R, Gale, K, and Grayson, DR. Temporal and spatial patterns of expression of c-fos, zif/268, c-jun and jun-B mRna's in rat brain following seizures evoked focally from the deep prepiriform cortex. *Experimental Neurol.* 119 (1993) 20–31.
15. Le Gal La Salle, G. Amygdaloid kindling in the rat: Regional differences and general properties. In: Wada JA, (Ed.) *Kindling 2*. New York: Raven Press. pp 31–47, 1981.
16. Le Gal La Salle, G and Feldblum, S. Role of the amygdala in development of hippocampal kindling in the rat. *Experimental Neurol.* 82 (1983) 447–455.
17. Loscher, W, Ebert, U, Wahnschaffe, U and Rundfeldt, C. Susceptibility of different cell layers of the anterior and posterior part of the piriform cortex to electrical stimulation and kindling: Comparison with the basolateral amygdala and "area tempestas". *Neuroscience* 66 (1995) 265–276.
18. Maggio, R, Lanaud, P, Grayson, DR and Gale, K. Expression of c-fos mRNA following seizures evoked from an epileptogenic site in the deep prepiriform cortex: Regional distribution in brain as shown by in situ hybridization. *Experimental Neurol.* 119 (1993) 11–19.
19. McIntyre, DC. Split-brain rat: Transfer and interference of kindled amygdala convulsions.In: *Kindling*, J. Wada (Ed). Raven Press, New York, 85–101, 1976.
20. McIntyre, DC and Plant, JR. Long-lasting changes in the origin of spontaneous discharges from amygdala-kindled rats: piriform vs perirhinal cortex *in vitro*. *Brain Research* 624 (1993) 268–276.
21. McIntyre, DC, Kelly, ME and Armstrong, JN. Kindling in the perirhinal cortex. *Brain Research* 615 (1993) 1–6.
22. McIntyre, DC and Kelly, ME. Are differences in dorsal hippocampal kindling related to amygdala piriform area excitability? *Epilepsy Research* 14 (1993) 49–61.
23. McIntyre, DC, Kelly, ME and Staines, WA. Efferent projections of the anterior perirhinal cortex of the rat. *J. Comp. Neurol.* In Press.
24. Morgan, JI, Cohen, DR, Hempstead, JL and Curran, T. Mapping patterns of c-fos expression in the central nervous system after seizure. *Science* 237 (1987) 192–197.
25. Morgan, JI and Curran, T. Stimulus-transcription coupling in the nervous system: Involvement of the inducible proto-oncogenes fos and jun. *Ann. Rev Neurosci.* 14 (1991) 421–451.
26. Nierenberg J, Applegate CD, Burchfiel JL and Piekut DT. Fos immunolabeling following kindled seizures elicited from different brain sites. *Soc. Neurosci. Abs.* 19 (1993) 605.

27. Nierenberg J, Applegate CD, Burchfiel JL and Piekut DT. FOS immunolabeling following kindled partial seizures elicited from different brain sites. *Soc Neurosci. Abs.* 20 (1994) 1458.
28. Racine, RJ, Mosher, M and Kairiss, EW. The role of the piriform cortex in the generation of interictal spikes in the kindled preparation. *Brain Res.* 454 (1988) 251–263.
29. Sagar, SM, Sharp, FR, and Curran, T. Expression of c-fos mapping in the brain: Metabolic mapping at the cellular level. *Science* 240 (1988) 1328–1331.
30. Smeyne, RJ, Schilling, K, Robertson, L, Luk, D, Oberdik, J, Curran, T and Morgan, JI. Fos-lacZ transgenic mice: Mapping sites of gene induction in the nervous system. *Neuron* 8 (1992) 13–23.
31. White, LE and Price, JL. The functional anatomy of limbic status epilepticus in the rat. I. Patterns of ^{14}C-2-deoxyglucose uptake and fos immunochemistry. *J. Neurosci.* 13 (1993) 4787–4809.

DISCUSSION OF CRAIG APPLEGATE'S PAPER

J. McNamara: You said that with this antibody you used to measure c-fos expression, you looked 24 hours after the last seizure?

C. Applegate: Oh no, 90 minutes.

J. McNamara: Well, is this antibody selective for fos, or fos-b, or frod1, or frod2?

C. Applegate: It's selected for fos. It's a Santa Cruz antibody.

J. McNamara: They say that it's selective for fos, but its not clear that it is. The reason I say that is that it could explain some of the discrepancies with in situ hybridization studies, because it's easier to have mislabelling given the antibodies we have.

C. Applegate: The way we're using this, I'm not sure it's critical. It might be more critical for our interpretation once we understand what fos is really doing. The way we're using this is simply as an activational marker—as a way of saying, "This neuron has been turned on, for whatever reason, by this input."

J. McNamara: I understand, but if there turn out to be discrepancies between the fos immunoreactivity and looking for one of the things that that antibody may be seeing, that could explain the discrepancy.

K. Gale: I was intrigued by your attempt to inhibit the perirhinal cortex in the kindling model. You did that on the contralateral side; what happens if you do it on the ipsilateral side?

C. Applegate: I'm going to leave that for Dan McIntyre to describe.

J. McNamara: How do you know that KCl is producing spreading depression and nothing else? I wouldn't be surprised if KCl would activate a seizure.

C. Applegate: Well actually, 30 minutes after that injection, all of those animals had several seizures. At the time we weren't recording from that hemisphere, but in the ipsilateral hemisphere, where we had an electrode, we didn't see seizures in those animals. We also didn't see any lateralizing motor signs in those animals that would suggest other sorts of confoundings.

K. Gale: Did you try a glutamate antagonist?

C. Applegate: Lidocaine also worked in those animals.

J. Wada: According to your last scheme in your slide, are you implying that secondary generalization does not take place in the rodent brain without input from the contralateral limbic system?

C. Applegate: I wasn't trying to imply that, no. The point I was trying to make is that because of the reciprocal pattern of interconnectivity and some special properties which Dr. McIntyre will describe about the perirhinal cortex, bilateral recruitment of the perirhinal seems to be important, at least in so far as these fos maps are telling us something functional about how the system is organized.

13

THE PERIRHINAL CORTEX AND KINDLED MOTOR SEIZURES

Dan C. McIntyre and Mary Ellen Kelly

Institute of Neuroscience
Department of Psychology
Life Sciences Research Building
Carleton University
Ottawa, Ontario K1S 5B6, Canada

1. INTRODUCTION

Complex partial seizures with secondary generalization are an enduring problem for many patients with temporal lobe epilepsy. The often intractible nature of these seizures can bring the patient to the surgeon for therapeutic relief. The problem for the surgeon, in this circumstance, is to identify the exact tissue that needs to be excised to provide that relief. Thus, a thorough understanding of the neurological substrates critical to the propagation of temporal lobe seizures is necessary in that assessment. There are several experimental animal models that could be applied to this problem, each with its own virtues and drawbacks. When applied to temporal lobe epilepsy, the kindling technique nicely models complex partial seizures with secondary generalization, and would appear to be a good model to assess the functional anatomy underlying the syndrome.

Our current interest in the functional anatomy of kindling began a number of years ago when we discovered that status epilepticus could be triggered from a kindled amygdala focus in rats by protracted exposure of that focus to low-intensity electrical stimulation. The long-lived seizures that were triggered by this procedure would spontaneously offset after several hours, and were temporally associated with the loss of the ipsilateral piriform cortex[15]. This suggested an important role for the piriform cortex, or nearby structures, in status epilepticus, and maybe temporal lobe epilepsy. Subsequently, we developed an *in vitro* slice preparation of this area to examine its epileptogenic properties in more detail[16,17]. It was observed that the piriform cortex was capable of independent seizure development, and that previous kindling of the amygdala resulted in permanently enhanced excitability in the piriform cortex[16,17]. During this same period, Racine's group showed[10] that interictal spikes, which often characterize the epileptic state in man, developed early in the piriform cortex during kindling and, regardless of the site of kindling,

Kindling 5, edited by Corcoran and Moshé.
Plenum Press, New York, 1998.

usually anticipated interictal spikes in other areas. Further evidence highlighting a potentially important role for the piriform cortex area in epilepsy was the observation by Piredda and Gale[25] that a small area deep in the anterior piriform cortex (the ventral endopiriform nucleus) exhibited exquisite sensitivity to a variety of convulsive agents. Collectively, these data suggested that the piriform cortex contained cells and/or networks of cells that might be critically important for the development, maintenance and/or generalization of convulsive seizures of temporal lobe origin.

2. PERIRHINAL CORTEX KINDLING EXPERIMENT

While further exploring our amygdala/piriform slice preparation, looking for regional excitability differences in the presence of magnesium free medium, we noticed[20] that an area of cortex dorsal to the piriform cortex, namely the perirhinal cortex, showed depolarizing responses that were more provocative than the piriform cortex, and, in field recordings, appeared like the responses others were observing in the entorhinal cortex (e.g., [26]). Since no other information about the perirhinal cortex was available at that time, we decided to examine its excitability in intact animals using the kindling technique. We compared[22] the kindling profile of the perirhinal cortex to the fastest kindling structures known previously, i.e., the piriform cortex and amygdala, and to the slow kindling dorsal hippocampus. In that assessment, remarkably the perirhinal cortex kindled faster than all of the other limbic structures (Figure 1). In addition, like the piriform cortex and amygdala, the perirhinal seizures provoked strong clonic convulsions. Perhaps more remarkable, the latencies from the onset of the electrical stimulus to the onset of the forelimb clonus in perirhinal cortex kindling were many times faster than the other structures (Figure 2). These results suggested that the perirhinal cortex is extremely well-connected to the motor system(s) controlling forelimb clonus.

The discovery of fast perirhinal kindling with short convulsion latencies begged the question—"what are the projections of the perirhinal cortex that could account for these kindling effects?" Reviewing the anatomical literature provided no answer. A few experiments described posterior perirhinal connections to the entorhinal cortex or hippocampus[12,27,28], but none examined the anterior perirhinal cortex (where we had been kindling) or mentioned connections from the perirhinal cortex to motor systems. Because kindling stimulation of the anterior perirhinal cortex, at intensities below threshold for triggering an afterdischarge, produced stimulus-bound forced clonic movements like low-intensity frontal motor cortex stimulation, we predicted that the convulsive seizures triggered from the perirhinal cortex might involve recruitment of frontal cortex motor mechanisms.

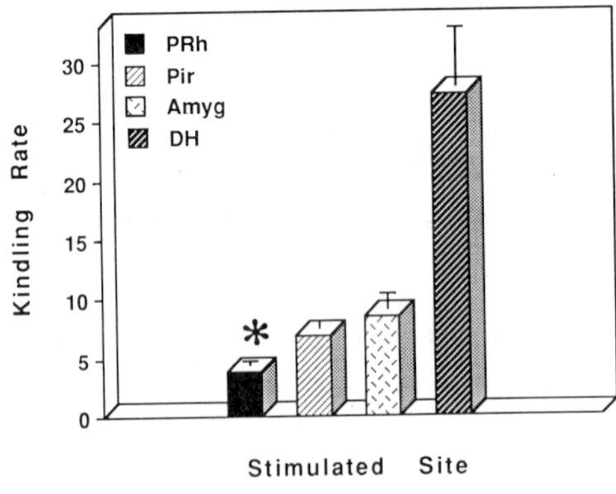

Figure 1. Mean (± S.E.M.) kindling rate to the first stage-5 convulsion in rats kindled from either the anterior perirhinal cortex (PRh), piriform cortex (Pir), basolateral amygdala (Amyg) or dorsal hippocampus (DH). * = Significantly different from all other groups, $P < 0.05$.

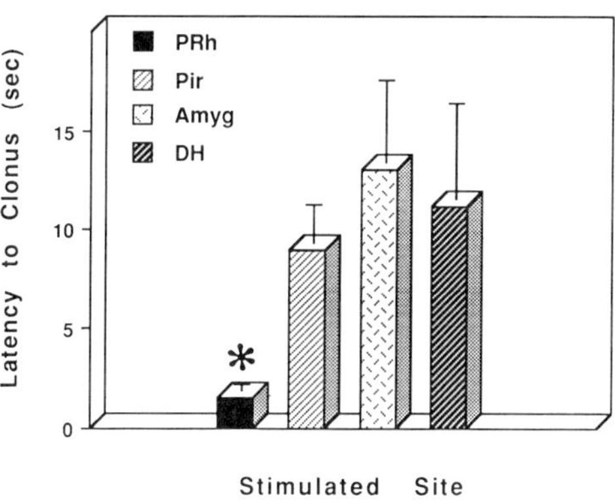

Figure 2. Mean (± S.E.M.) latency to forelimb clonus for the 6 stage-5 convulsions in rats kindled from either the anterior perirhinal cortex (PRh), piriform cortex (Pir), basolateral amygdala (Amyg) or dorsal hippocampus (DH). * = Significantly different from all other groups, P <0.05.

3. PERIRHINAL CORTEX ANATOMICAL EXPERIMENTS

To answer the previous question more directly, we prepared rats for anatomical studies to determine the efferent connections of the anterior perirhinal cortex. To do so, we injected, by iontophoresis, the anterograde tracer *Phaseolus vulgaris* leucoaggulutinin (PhAL) into the anterior perirhinal cortex[23]. The PhAL injections labelled small aggregates of neurons that could be grouped into three different locations. Each location represented pairs of adjacent laminae. One location exclusively labelled neurons in the perirhinal cortex layer VI, the second location involved layers V and VI, and the third location involved layers III and V. As the perirhinal cortex is agranular, no layer IV appears in its cytoarchitecture. These three different injection locations provided strong labelling of varicose fibers in a variety of different forebrain and midbrain structures that could provide important contributions to the kindled motor convulsion. The cortical and subcortical structures with known motor functions that were in receipt of labelled varicose fibers from the three different perirhinal cortex injections sites are indicated in Table 1.

A broader distribution of the efferent structures from those three injection sites is indicated in our recent publication[23]. A composite summary of the PhAL labelling from the three injection sites is presented in Figure 3. As can be seen in Figure 3, many PhAL-labelled fibers were present in known cortical motor structures, including the frontal motor cortex (Fr1-2),[24] parietal (Par1-2), orbital, agranular insular and infralimbic cortices and claustrum. Subcortical projections of interest to motor activities included the ventral striatum, dorsolateral caudate nucleus, globus pallidus, nucleus acccumbens, basolateral amygdala, and several thalamic nuclei (ventral, posterior and dorsomedial), plus the dorsolateral substantia nigra. All of these structures are related directly to motor function or have efferent connections to the frontal motor cortex, as shown below.

The Phal labelling of varicose fibers in the frontal cortex was massive. These fibers could be traced from their respective injection sites through a course anteriorly in layers I and VI of the parietal cortex to the frontal cortex. Large numbers of fibers also passed anteriorly along in the cortex of the rhinal fissure to innervate the insular and orbital cortices and the claustrum. The innervation of the frontal cortex was observed to be extremely divergent, since only a single small injection site provided dense varicose labelling throughout the entire frontal motor cortex. The majority of these cortical projection fibers appeared to originate from perirhinal cells in layer V, while the majority of the subcortical projections described above arose from the cells in layer VI. Additionally, it was exclu-

Table 1. Cortical and subcortical distribution of PhAL-labelled varicose fibers in structures with known motor functions, or structures with direct projections to the frontal motor cortex, following an injection of PhAL into layers III/V, V/VI or VI of the anterior perirhinal cortex[a]

	Layer III/V	Layer V/VI	Layer VI
Cortical region			
Claustrum	++	+++	++
Entorhinal	++	+++	++
Frontal, Fr2,1,3	++	++++	+
Infralimbic	+++	+++	0
Insular, agranular	+++	++++	+++
Parietal, Par2,1	+	++++	++
Orbital			
Medial	+	+	+
Lateral	+	+++	++
Subiculum	+	++	0
Subcortical region			
Accumbens nucleus	++	++++	+
Amygdala			
Central nucleus	0	+	+
Basolateral nucleus	+	+	++++
Dorsolateral caudate putamen	+	++	+
Central grey	++	+++	+
Thalamus			
Mediodorsal nucleus	0	+	++
Posterior nucleus	+	+++	++++
Sub- and parafasiculus	+	++	++
Ventral posteromedial nucleus	0	+	++
Fundus striati	++	++++	+
Parabrachial nucleus	+	++	++
Substantia nigra, reticulata, lateral	+	++	+

[a]Symbols indicate the density of labelled varicose fibers, varying from none to extensive (0 to ++++). Abbreviations taken from Paxinos and Watson[24].

sively layer V that provided efferents to the contralateral perirhinal cortex by way of the anterior commissure and the corpus callosum.

To anatomically confirm the perirhinal cortex efferents to the frontal motor cortex, which we predicted from our behavioural experiments and observed in our anterograde tracing experiments, we performed retrograde tracing studies. Here we injected Fluoro-gold (FG) into one of several different sites in the frontal motor cortex of rats[23]. Such injections labelled a relatively large number of structures, indicating direct projections to the frontal motor cortex. The significant cortical structures projecting to the ipsilateral motor cortex included, the parietal cortex (both Par1, 2),[24] the orbital cortex (medial, ventral and lateral), agranular insular cortex and the claustrum; the latter two structures merged posteriorly with the perirhinal cortex. The retrograde labelling in the perirhinal cortex appeared in all four cell layers in the dorsal half of the area (area 36), while the ventral perirhinal area (area 35) showed projection neurons exclusively in layer V. Indeed, in the caudal part of the brain, except for a small projection from the deep layers of the lateral entorhinal cortex (layer VI), it was only the layer V cells in the perirhinal cortex that showed frontal motor cortex projections. No significant projections were evident from any other cortical structure. These cortical retrograde tracing results are summarized in Figure 4.

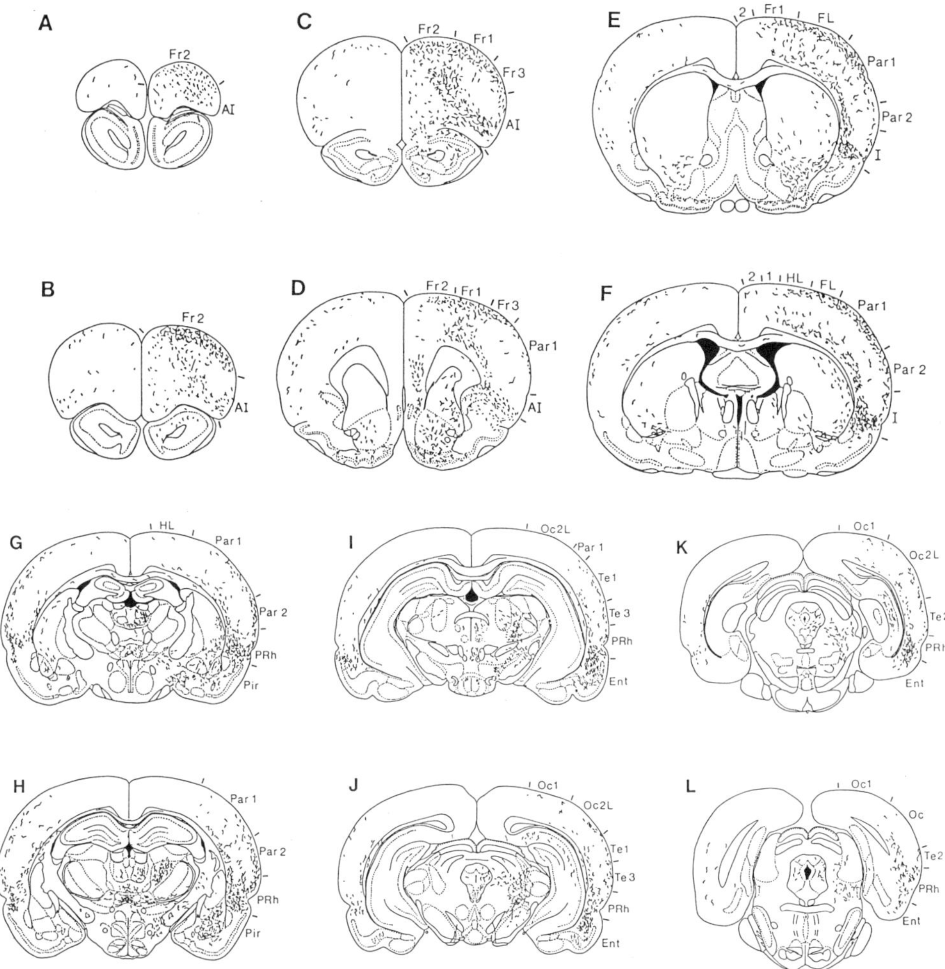

Figure 3. Summary schematic drawing of all the PhAL-labelled efferent fibers evident following an injection into the right anterior perirhinal cortex. Lettered figures and abbreviations are adapted from Paxinos and Watson[24].

There were also several subcortical projections to the frontal motor cortex clearly evident in the FG labelling. The subcortical FG labelled many cells in the basolateral amygdala and thalamus, particularly in the ventral and posterior nuclei. These subcortical projections are indicated in the left half of each brain section schematic drawing in Figure 5. Furthermore, and importantly, many of these subcortical structures and cortical structures were in receipt of extensive variscose terminals from the perirhinal cortex, evidenced in our anterograde tracing PhAL experiments. The remarkable parallel between the retrograde FG labelling (shown in each left hemisection) and the anterograde PhAL labelling (shown in each right hemisection) in several structures is seen also in Figure 5.

Thus, in addition to the direct, dense perirhinofrontal projection, there appears to be an additional vast networks of cells projecting to the frontal motor cortex that also are innervated by the perirhinal cortex. Clearly, the perirhinal cortex is postured to influence the frontal motor cortex directly (a) by its dense *divergent* projections, seen in the PhAL anterograde tracing experiments, and (b) by its concentrated *convergent* projections, seen in

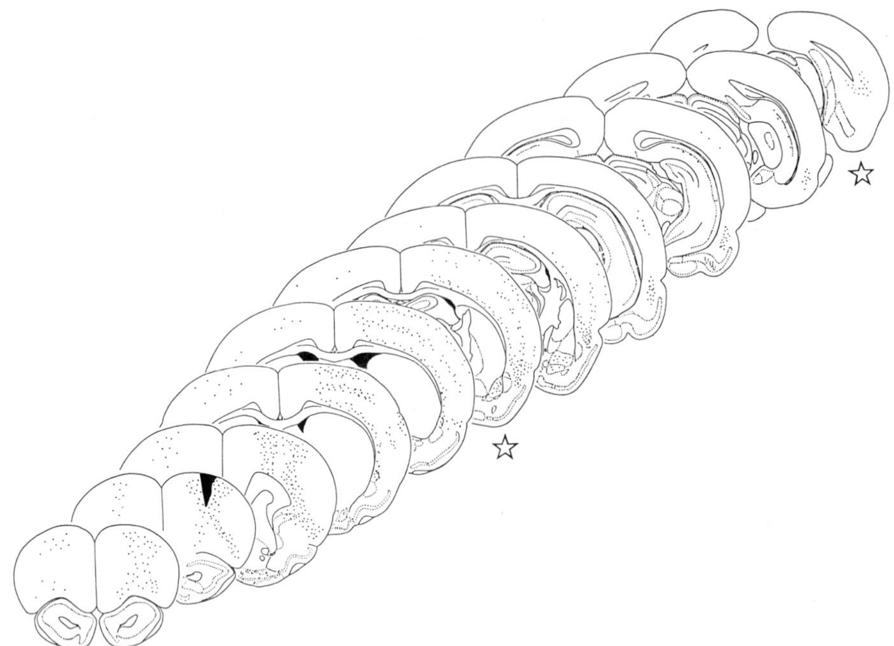

Figure 4. Summary schematic drawing of the neocortical, amygdala and hippocampal-subicular neurons retrogradely labelled following a Fluorogold injection into the Fr2/1 region of the frontal cortex indicated by the blackened injection site in the second section. The perirhinal cortex is located in the rhinal fissure between the starred sections.

the FG retrograde tracing experiments—where a single focal frontal cortex injection of FG retrogradely labelled the entire perirhinal cortex. In addition, the perirhinal cortex must have powerful, indirect influence over the frontal cortex through its innervation of the structures indicated above in the FG experiments, which show direct communication with the frontal cortex. Several of these other FG labelled cortical structures innervated by the perirhinal cortex have been implicated in the development or expression of kindled convulsions. These structures include, the insular cortex[8], orbital cortex[3], and claustrum[13]. The exact physiological nature of these varied connections between the perirhinal and frontral cortex, however, has yet to be determined.

4. CORTICAL SPREADING DEPRESSION EXPERIMENT

If transsynaptic activation of the frontal motor cortex is responsible for the motor expression of kindled limbic convulsions, then interference with the motor cortex should have significant consequences for a convulsive seizure triggered from a limbic structure like the amygdala. We directly tested this proposal by examining the influence of unilateral cortical spreading depression (CSD) on the appearance and form of amygdala kindled convulsions (in preparation). CSD was selected because it could provide a widespread and reversible depression of the frontal cortex, against which a kindled amygdala convulsion could be profiled. After implantation of bipolar stimulating/recording electrodes in both amygdalae and frontal cortices, a cannula guide over one frontal motor cortex was positioned. Patency of the cannula was maintained by daily saline infu-

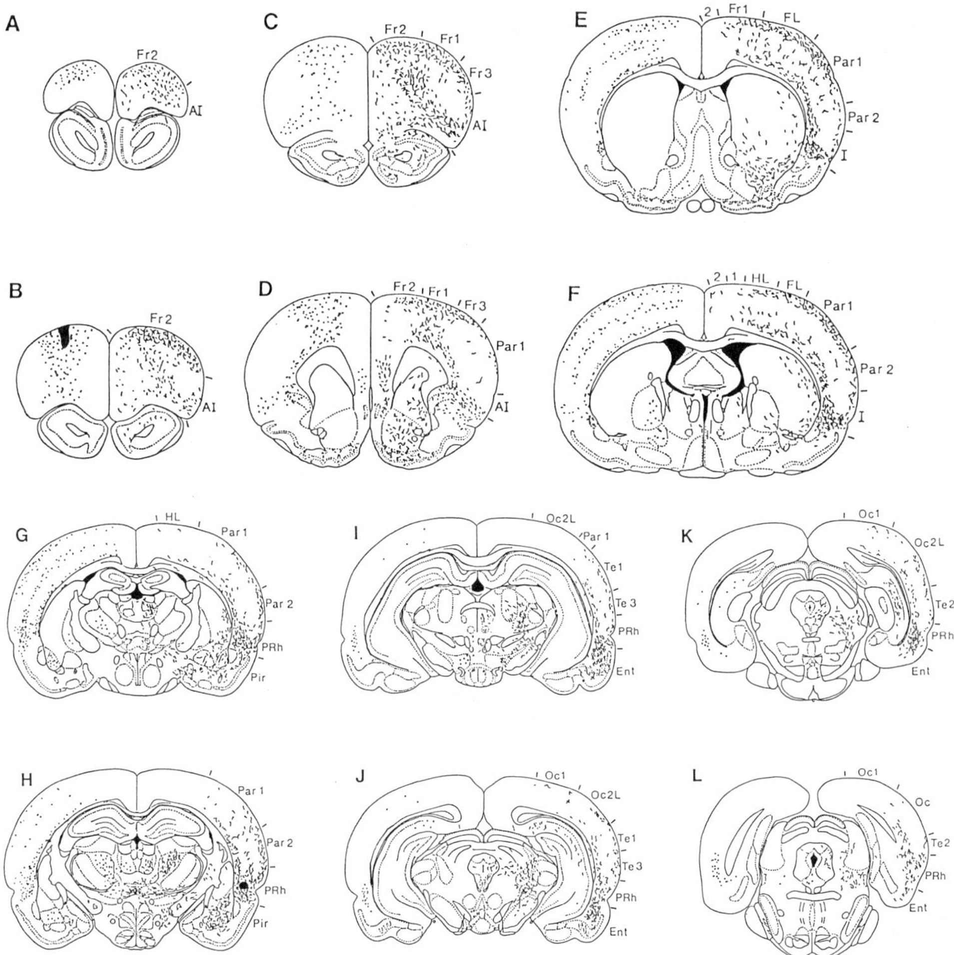

Figure 5. Summary schematic drawing comparing the distribution of neurons retrogradely labelled following a Fluorogold injection into the frontal motor cortex (shown in the **left** hemisphere) to the distribution of anterogradely labelled fibers following an injection of PhAL into the anterior perirhinal cortex (shown in the **right** hemisphere). Notice the remarkable similarity in distribution patterns in the neocortex of neuron (left) and fiber (right) in sections C–F, and in the amygdala and thalamus in H. Also, notice the dissimilarity in neuron and fiber patterns in the accumbens and caudate nucleus in sections D–E, and in the midbrain in sections I–L.

sions. One week after surgery, the rats began a kindling protocol that involved a single daily stimulation of one amygdala, either contralateral or ipsilateral to the cannula; by kindling either contralateral or ipsilateral to the cannula, two groups were formed. After kindling rats to their first stage 5 convulsion, a saline infusion (2 μl) into the cannula was provided, which was followed in 3 min by a triggered amygdala seizure. In all cases, the ensuing seizure and convulsion were normal both in form and duration. On the next trial, the following day, CSD was induced in the rats with a 2 μl injection of 25% KCl via the cannula. Again, 3 minutes later the kindled amygdala was stimulated. In the group that had CSD initiated in the cortex contralateral to the kindled amygdala, the duration of both the electrographic seizure in the two amygdalae and the motor convulsion was similar to that observed during the previous saline trial. On the other hand, the form of that convulsion was dramatically altered. The forelimb clonus was completely unilateral, and appeared superficially the same as the unilateral clonic convulsions witnessed in our earlier split-brain experiments using amygdala kindled rats[14]. By contrast, when the kindled seizure was triggered in rats with CSD of the hemisphere ipsilateral to the kindled amygdala, significant decrements occurred in both the electrographic seizure and the motor convulsion. The electrographic seizure in both amygdalae was greatly shortened, while the clonic convulsive response was completely blocked. These results strongly suggest that amygdala kindled seizures manifest their convulsive form by recruitment of the frontal cortex. More specifically, the results suggest that the amygdala discharge results first in the recruitment of the *ipsilateral* hemisphere, which then likely becomes bilateral through its callosal projections to the contralateral hemisphere[14]. In addition, since the ipsilateral CSD but not the contralateral CSD significantly truncated the primary amygdala electrographic seizure, we suggest, like Holmes et al.[8], that the ipsilateral neocortical networks are part of the network that influences the focal activity in the amygdala. Further, we propose that the perirhinal cortex may be critical to this larger network by serving as the vehicle through which limbic seizures recruit the structures that control stage-5 convulsions.

5. DISCUSSION

Although our original kindling studies suggested[5] that the amygdala might be pivitol in organizing the convulsive seizures that seem to be common to all limbic kindled sites, this view was changed by our discovery[15] of convulsive complex partial status epilepticus (where the ensuing convulsions appeared like protracted kindled seizures) and the obvious correlation between the spontaneous offset of these seizures and the progressive loss of the piriform cortex. Subsequently, *in vitro* studies of the piriform cortex[16,17] confirmed it to be an epileptogenic area, which readily retained the hyperexcitability engendered by previous amygdala kindling. As a result, we proposed[18,19,21] that the seizure discharges in the piriform cortex, by way of its strong association network[6], might be capable of recruiting the entire temporal lobe into the prototypic limbic convulsive response. This view is now being championed by others (e.g., [1,7,9]). Although, based on its intrinsic excitability and connectivity, there can be little doubt that the piriform cortex is an important amplifier of seizure activity, its connections to motor systems are somewhat limited. More importantly, in a recent but complicated study, we showed[11] that near-complete loss of the piriform cortex (following status epilepticus) had no effect on the development or expression of convulsive seizures kindled from the dorsal hippocampus. This result clearly showed that loss of the piriform cortex did not preempt convulsive seizure development from other limbic sites. On the other hand, in that same study, rats with piriform cortex destruction plus additional damage to the perirhinal cortex showed an interference with the normal development and expression of convulsive seizures. Such an observation is consistent the experiments on the perirhinal cortex that we have described in this chapter. These findings collectively highlight several important features of the perirhinal cortex, including a) the fastest kindling rates and shortest convulsion latencies of any forebrain structure, b) efferents that massively innervate the frontal motor cortex both directly via divergent and convergent communication, and indirectly through other cortical and subcortical forebrain structures, and c) the loss of the forelimb clonic response during an amygdala-triggered seizure when the perirhinal projection field in the frontal cortex is suppressed by cortical spreading depression.

Obviously the anterior perirhinal cortex is importantly related to motor systems, while the larger perirhinal cortex probably serves more generally as a broad associative interface between several neocortical structures and the limbic system[2,4]. In future experiments, we will examine in more detail the anatomical organization of the perirhinal cortex, and its intrinsic and extrinsic responses, with particular attention to the perirhinofrontal connection.

REFERENCES

1. Burchfiel, J.L. and Applegate, C.D., Forebrain and brainstem mechanisms governing seizure development: A hypothesis. In J.A. Wada (ed.), *Kindling 4.* Plenum Press, New York, 1990, pp. 93–112.
2. Burwell, R.D., Witter, M.P. and Amaral, D.G. Perirhinal and postrhinal cortices of the rat: A review of the neuroanatomical literature and comparison with findings from the monkey, *Hippocampus*, 5 (1995) 390–408.
3. Corcoran, M.E., Urstad, H., McCaughran, J.A., Jr. and Wada, J.A., Frontal lobe and kindling in the rat. In J.A. Wada (ed.), *Kindling*. Raven Press, New York, 1976, pp. 215–228.
4. Deacon, T.W., Eichenbaum, H., Rosenberg, P. and Eckmann, K.W., Afferent connections of the perirhinal cortex in the rat. *J. Comp. Neurol.*, 220 (1983) 168–190.
5. Goddard, G.V., McIntyre, D.C. and Leech, C.K., A permanent change in brain function resulting from electrical stimulation, *Exp. Neurol.*, 25 (1969) 295–330.
6. Haberly, L.B. and Bower, J.M., Analysis of association fiber system in piriform cortex with intracellular recording and staining techniques, *J. Neurophysiol.*, 51 (1984) 90–112.
7. Haberly, L.B. and Sutula, T.P., Neuronal processes that underlie expression of kindled epileptiform events in the piriform cortex in vivo, *J. Neurosci.*, 12 (1992) 2211–2224.
8. Holmes, K.H., Bilkey, D.K. and Laverty, R., The infusion of an NMDA antagonist in perirhinal cortex suppresses amygdala-kindled seizures, *Brain Res.* , 587 (1992) 285–290.
9. Honack, D., Wahnschaffe, U. and Loscher, W., Kindling from stimulation of a highly sensitive locus in the posterior part of the piriform cortex: comparison with amygdala kindling and effects of antiepileptic drugs, *Brain Res.*, 538 (1991) 196–202.
10. Kairiss, E.W., Racine, R.J. and Smith, G.K., The development of interictal spike during kindling in the rat, Brain Res., 322 (1984) 101–110.
11. Kelly, M.E. and McIntyre, D.C., Perirhinal cortex involvement in limbic kindled seizures, *Epilepsy Res.* (in press).
12. Kosel, K.C., Van Hoesen, G.W. and Rosene D.L., A direction projection from the perirhinal cortex (area 35) to the subiculum in the rat, *Brain Res.*, 269 (1983) 347–351.
13. Kudo, T., and Wada, J.A., Claustrum and amygdaloid kindling. In J.A. Wada, (ed.), *Kindling 4,* Plenum Press, New York, 1990, pp. 397–408.
14. McIntyre, D.C. Split-brain rat: transfer and interference of amygdala kindled convulsions, *Can. J. Neurol. Sci.*, 2 (1975) 429–437.
15. McIntyre, D.C., Nathanson, D. and Edson, N., A new model of partial status epilepticus based on kindling, *Brain Res.*, 250 (1982) 53–64.
16. McIntyre, D.C. and Wong, R.K.S., Modification of local neuronal interactions by amygdala kindling in vitro, *Exp. Neurol.*, 88 (1985) 529–537.
17. McIntyre, D.C. and Wong, R.K.S., Cellular and synaptic properties of amygdala-kindled pyriform cortex in vitro, *J. Neurophysiol.*, 55 (1986) 1295–1307.
18. McIntyre, D.C. (1986) Kindling and the pyriform cortex. In J.A. Wada (ed.), *Kindling 3*, Raven Press, New York, 1986, pp.249–262.
19. McIntyre, D.C. and Racine, R.J., Kindling mechanisms: current progress on an experimental epilepsy model, *Prog. Neurobiol.*, 27 (1986) 1–12.
20. McIntyre, D.C. and Plant, J.R., Pyriform cortex involvement in kindling, *Neurosci. Biobehav. Rev.*, 13 (1989) 277–280.
21. McIntyre, D.C. and Kelly, M.E., Is the pyriform cortex important for limbic kindling? In J.A. Wada (ed.), *Kindling 4*, Plenum Press, New York, 1990, pp. 21–31.
22. McIntyre, D.C., Kelly, M.E. and Armstrong, J.N., Kindling in the perirhinal cortex. *Brain Res.*, 615 (1993) 1–6.
23. McIntyre, D.C., Kelly, M.E. and Staines, W.A., Efferent projections of the anterior perirhinal cortex in the rat, *J. Comp. Neurol.*, 369 (1996) 302–318.
24. Paxinos, G. and Watson, C., *The Rat Brain in Stereotaxic Coordinates*, Academic Press, New York.

25. Piredda, S. and Gale, K., A crucial epileptogenic site in the deep prepiriform cortex. *Nature*, 317 (1985) 623–625.
26. Walther, H., Lambert, J.D.C., Jones, R.S.G., Heinemann, U and Hamon, B., Epileptiform activity in combined slices of the hippocampus, subiculum and entorhinal cortex during perfusion with low magnesium medium, *Neurosci. Lett.*, 69 (1986) 156–161.
27. Witter, M.P. and Groenewegen, H.J., Connections of the parahippocampal cortex in the cat. III. Cortical and thalamic efferents. *J. Comp. Neurol.*, 252 (1986) 1–31.
28. Witter, M.P., Groenewegen, H.J., Lopes da Silva, F.H. and Lohman, A.H.M., Functional organization of the extrinsic and intrinsic circuitry of the parahippocampal region. *Prog. Neurobiol.*, 33 (1989) 161–254.

DISCUSSION OF DAN MCINTYRE'S PAPER

J. Wada: Beautiful data. I agree the motor cortex is very important for two reasons from our own observations. What you saw in rodents, we saw in cats and primates. If you bisect anterior corpus callosum, then you can lateralize kindled convulsions. Secondly, in terms of human temporal lobe epilepsy, most of the problem is not patients who have secondary generalized convulsions, but rather limbic complex-partial seizures, which are nonconvulsive. Unless the patient has convulsive seizures which cannot be controlled by medication, just removing the perirhinal cortex will not offer great relief of symptoms. There are people who have generalized convulsions who never have secondary generalized convulsions.

D. McIntyre: It would be very interesting to know how the perirhinal actually is involved even in partial seizures. In man it may not be carrying powerful communication into the motor systems, and the rat may be a very simple version of that network.

K. Gale: I want the question that I asked Craig to be answered by Dan: If inhibition restricts the perirhinal cortex ipsilateral to the amygdala kindling, what does that do?

D. McIntyre: Yes, the question was, have we done spreading depression on the ipsilateral perirhinal, and the answer is no, we haven't actually done that with the perirhinal. When Craig said I would answer it, it was in the context of doing the neocortical spreading depression. I think the point of that was that in the rat, the neocortical network is seemingly part of the network that the amygdala is using to elaborate its own focal seizures, because its focal seizure went from 60 sec down to 10.

K. Gale: But you don't know that it necessarily has to get there through the perirhinal cortex?

D. McIntyre: No, I don't know necessarily, it could be amygdala, it could be any number of ways; but I can't envision any outcome other than if you were to put the spreading depression ipsilaterally on the perirhinal cortex, it also would truncate that discharge in much the same way. It can hardly get shorter and still have a discharge from an animal who normally has a 60 sec discharge to one who has 10.

K. Gale: So the prediction would be that it could potentially block the seizures...

D. McIntyre: And it did, in this case. Even doing it at the frontal cortex it blocked the convulsive seizure absolutely. You're suggesting that it might also block entirely the focal seizure in the amygdala?

K. Gale: Yes.

D. McIntyre: Well, it's possible, but I think not because we know that this stuff can survive in a slice. I think that there's got to be a threshold at which you can trigger a brief afterdischarge. It may not need all of that network to elaborate.

P. Engel: To get back to the human work. The only large series that I know of amygdalohippocampectomies is Heinz-Gregor Wieser's from Zurich, and he showed that the outcome related not to how much amygdala-hippocampus was removed but how much parahippocampus was also taken. Almost everybody else who does that procedure takes off about 3 cm of the pole, which includes at least piriform cortex.

J. Pinel: I'm very interested in your hypothesis about the fact that the lesions in the rhinal cortex was the critical factor in these temporal lobe surgeries done for epilepsy. I just wanted to point out that for years it was thought that the removal of the hippocampus was responsible for the object recognition deficits that are seen after temporal lobe surgery. Then there was the long debate over whether it was the hippocampus or the amygdala, and now the story has emerged very clearly in the last few years, in both monkeys and rat research, that it's neither and is in fact the perirhinal cortex.

C. Teskey: Have you kindled up the neocortex directly in your studies?

D. McIntyre: We have kindled neocortex many many times. In frontal cortex as you are inducing clonic-tonic-clonic (CTC) seizures, you are probably directly driving the spinal cord, which has all of these mechanisms, and it may well be that as you come at it from the perirhinal, it can access motor cortex and can recruit the clonic limbic form of convulsion. If you kindle an animal long enough, they start to have those good strong CTC seizures or if you do what Mac Burnham does and you simply suspend them so their limbs are free to move, you will see tonic seizures. So it's not like it's something wildly different, it's just slightly different.

14

COMPARISON OF SYNAPSE REMODELING FOLLOWING HIPPOCAMPAL KINDLING AND LONG-TERM POTENTIATION

Yuri Geinisman,[1] Frank Morrell,[2] Leyla deToledo-Morrell,[2] Inna S. Persina,[1] and Eddy A. Van der Zee[1]

[1]Department of Cell and Molecular Biology
Northwestern University Medical School
Chicago, Illinois 60611
[2]Department of Neurological Sciences
Rush Medical College
Chicago, Illinois 60612

1. INTRODUCTION

Hippocampal kindling and long-term potentiation (LTP) are widely regarded as models of synaptic plasticity[2,28,31]. In the kindling paradigm[23,24], a behaviorally ineffective electrical stimulus of a high frequency is delivered daily to a local forebrain area. This leads to progressive intensification of paroxysmal neuronal activity and alterations in motor behavior that culminate eventually in a generalized seizure. Once this response to the constant stimulus has been attained, cessation of stimulation for many months and even years does not result in the loss of the newly acquired abnormal reaction: reintroduction of the original stimulus reliably evokes a generalized seizure[24,25,30,31,33,42]. Thus, kindling involves a virtually permanent augmentation of synaptic responsiveness in the stimulated circuit.

Closely related to kindling is the other, most popular model of synaptic plasticity, hippocampal LTP. The essence of LTP is a persistent increase in the amplitude of synaptic responses resulting from the localized application of brief, high frequency trains of electrical pulses[3,4]. Hippocampal LTP and kindling are strikingly similar in many respects[6]. The stimulation patterns, which are most effective for the induction of LTP, are similar to those that elicit kindling[3,36]. Potentiation of synaptic responses appears to be an early and invariant feature of the kindling process[38], though kindling-induced potentiation has different characteristics compared to those of LTP[34]. Prior induction of LTP in the hippocampal circuit subsequently stimulated to evoke kindling leads to more rapid kindling of that circuit[39]. There is, however a major difference between the two models of synaptic plasticity. As opposed to kindling, hippocampal LTP is characterized by a relatively rapid decay of

Kindling 5, edited by Corcoran and Moshé.
Plenum Press, New York, 1998.

augmented synaptic responses that occurs within a few hours to a few weeks[1,35]. This raises the question of why hippocampal LTP is transient while the effect of kindling is essentially permanent.

One possibility is that the different duration of LTP and kindling may be a consequence of differences in synapse remodeling in the stimulated synaptic field. Although LTP is less enduring than kindling, the time scales of both phenomena are sufficient for structural synaptic modifications to take place. In fact, previous morphological work has shown that hippocampal LTP[10,13,16,21,22,27,41] and kindling[17–20,37,40] are accompanied by a restructuring of synaptic connectivity. The earlier electron microscopic data on LTP were reported with regard to its induction phase, spanning a period of hours following cessation of potentiating stimulation[10,13,16,27,41]. These data, however, could not be compared with those on kindling[17–20] since the latter were obtained weeks after termination of high frequency stimulation that evoked a fully developed kindled state.

Recent studies from our laboratory examined changes in the number of synapses associated not only with the induction phase of hippocampal LTP[22], but also with its maintenance over a period of about two weeks[21]. The results obtained strongly suggest that the process of synapse remodeling, which is initiated during LTP induction, is then modulated during the maintenance phase of LTP to support the decay of synaptic enhancement and its retention at a relatively low level. The present study was designed to determine whether structural synaptic alterations induced by hippocampal kindling are different from those observed during LTP induction and maintenance.

2. EXPERIMENTAL DESIGN

The material obtained in our previous kindling experiment[20] was reanalyzed in this study. The data on LTP were reported by us earlier[21,22] and are presented here for comparison purposes. The experimental procedures and the protocol of tissue preparation for electron microscopy were described in detail elsewhere[16,21].

Briefly, LTP and kindling were induced by stimulation of the same afferent hippocampal pathway. Young adult male F344 rats were implanted chronically with bipolar stimulating electrodes into the right medial perforant path. In the LTP experiments, high frequency stimulation (fifteen 20-millisecond bursts of 400 Hz delivered at 0.2 Hz) was carried out on each of four consecutive days. Potentiated animals were examined morphologically either 1 hour or 13 days following the fourth stimulation to analyze synapse restructuring associated with the induction or maintenance phase of LTP, respectively. In the kindling experiment, animals were stimulated twice a day (with 1 ms pulses at 60 Hz for 2 s at a current level that initially produced an afterdischarge of 10 s or less) to a criterion of 5 generalized seizures. Kindled rats were examined 4 weeks after reaching criterion. Coulombic control rats were stimulated with parameters that do not evoke LTP or kindling. Each coulombic control animal was matched with a corresponding potentiated or kindled rat according to the current level and the total amount of current delivered. Unstimulated but implanted control rats were not examined since our previous studies showed that such animals do not differ significantly from coulombic controls with respect to the number of synapses per neuron[16,18,19].

Synapses were analyzed in the middle molecular layer (MML) of the right dentate gyrus, i.e. in the terminal synaptic field of medial perforant path axons that were stimulated during LTP induction and kindling. The synaptic population of the MML has been morphologically characterized[15]. It includes two major categories of synaptic contacts: axodendritic synapses involving dendritic shafts and axospinous ones involving dendritic spines. The axodendritic synaptic category consists of two morphologically distinct subtypes. Axodendritic synapses of one subtype are referred to as symmetrical synaptic contacts[12] since they have pre- and postsynaptic densities of equal thickness. In axodendritic junctions of the other subtype, the postsynaptic density (PSD) is noticeably thicker than the presynaptic one. This gives such synaptic contacts a marked asymmetry, and they are correspondingly classified as asymmetrical synapses[12]. Axospinous synaptic contacts are also morphologically heterogeneous and can be divided into perforated synapses[7,11,32] that exhibit a discontinuous PSD profile in some serial sections and nonperforated ones showing continuous PSD profiles in all consecutive sections. Perforated axospinous synapses can be subdivided further into several subtypes[15] that are schematically shown in Fig. 5. All these morphological varieties of synaptic contacts were differentially quantified.

Estimates of the number of synapses per postsynaptic granule cell were obtained with the unbiased method of double disector[5,26] as specified by us earlier[16,17,21]. It is necessary to emphasize here that the number of synaptic contacts per postsynaptic neuron, i.e. the synapse-to-neuron ratio, can be used as a measure of changes in the absolute synapse number only when certain requirements are met. One of these is that the number of postsynaptic nerve cells should remain stable under experimental conditions studied so that alterations in the synapse-to-neuron ratio can be attributed to changes in the number of synapses[26]. In our experiments, the numerical density of granule cells was not significantly changed in either potentiated[21] or kindled[18] rats as compared with their respective controls. This observation is consistent with the data obtained by a detailed analysis of changes in the number of dentate granule cells following perforant path kindling[9]. A loss of granule cells was found to develop after 30 class V seizures, but not after 3 episodes of generalized seizures[9]. Another requirement is that principal postsynaptic neurons should be the only source of postsynaptic elements involved in all synaptic contacts counted. Although this is certainly not the case for the MML, the vast majority of its postsynaptic elements are represented by dendritic shafts and spines of granule cells[21]. It is also necessary to mention that synapses were sampled only from the hidden blade of the dorsal part of the dentate gyrus. Being biased towards the area of interest, such sampling does not allow conclusions to be made with regard to the entire dentate gyrus.

3. STRUCTURAL SYNAPTIC ALTERATIONS ASSOCIATED WITH THE INDUCTION PHASE OF LTP

Electrophysiologically, the extent of potentiation was ascertained by the formula $T_1 - T_0/T_0$ where T_1 is the value for a given measure following high frequency stimulation and T_0 is the baseline value. One hour after the fourth high frequency stimulation (i.e., immediately before sacrifice), the slope of the extracellularly recorded field potential (EPSP) was potentiated by 74 ± 23%, the population spike amplitude by 873 ± 261% and the input-output (I-O) function (population spike amplitude/EPSP slope) by 441 ± 103% (mean ± SEM for a group of 7 rats). A paired t-test comparison of baseline values with those at the 1 hr test interval following the fourth high frequency stimulation showed that the extent of potentiation of synaptic responses relative to baseline was highly significant ($t = 5.158$, df = 6, $p < 0.01$ for the EPSP slope, $t = 5.930$, df = 6, $p < 0.001$ for the population spike amplitude and $t = 6.545$, df = 6, $p < 0.001$ for the I-O function). Similar analyses carried out on coulombic control animals (n = 7) at an equivalent time interval following the last low frequency stimulation did not reveal any significant changes in the three measures used as compared to baseline.

The effect of LTP induction on synaptic ultrastructure was assessed by examining potentiated animals electron microscopically 1 hour after the fourth potentiating stimulation[22]. A differential quantitative analysis of various morphological types of synapses showed that a change in number selectively involved only one synaptic subtype. Figure 1 demonstrates a synapse belonging to this subtype in electron micrographs of consecutive serial sections. The presynaptic axon terminal is seen as a single profile in sections where it is contacted by a distal part of the postsynaptic spine head (Fig. 1a, b). At more proximal levels of the postsynaptic element, the axon terminal appears in the form of three profiles separated from each other by bands of spine cytoplasm interconnecting inner surfaces of two opposite walls of the spine head (Fig. 1c-e). The bands of spine cytoplasm border

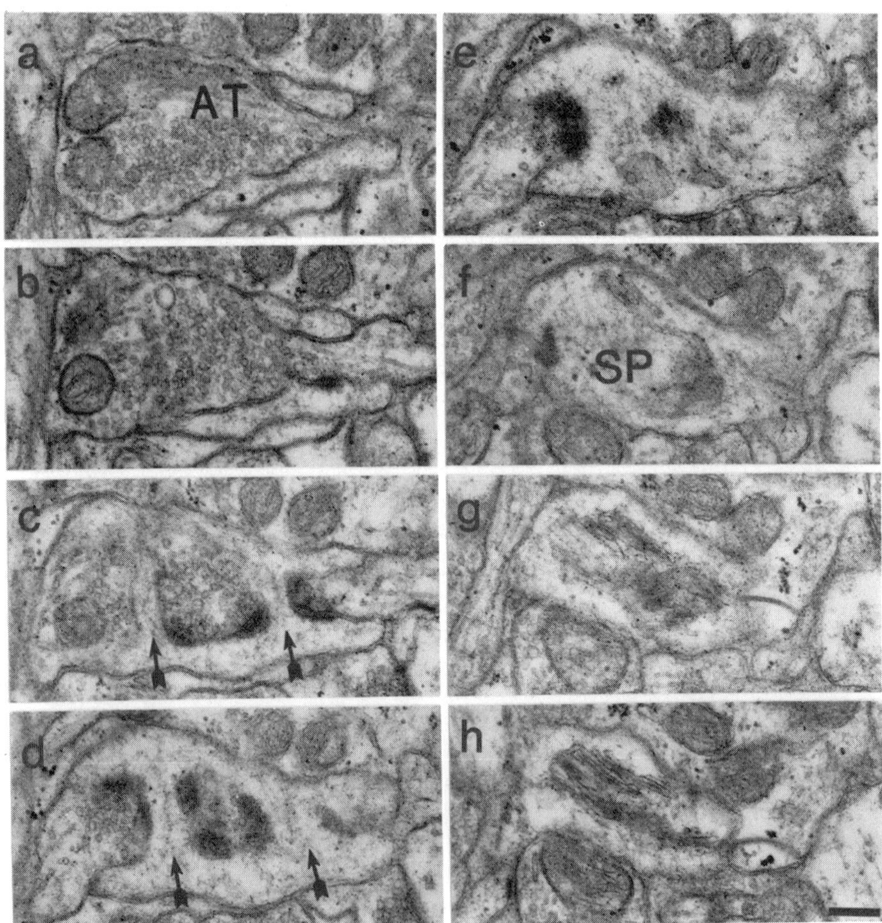

Figure 1. Electron micrographs of serial ultrathin sections (a-h) demonstrating an axospinous synapse with three completely partitioned transmission zones. All profiles of the presynaptic axon terminal in contact with the postsynaptic dendritic spine are shown. The axon terminal (labeled "AT") is seen as a single profile in sections passing through distal levels of the spine head (a, b) and as three separate profiles in the following sections (c, d). The spine head (labeled "SP") is consecutively sectioned from its distal end (a) to the proximal one (h). The proximal portion of the spine head is continuous with a short neck emanating from a parent dendrite (not shown). In some sections containing electron dense PSD profiles (c–e), the spine head exhibits bands of cytoplasm (arrows) interconnecting its opposite walls. On both sides of these bands is a discrete complex of PSD profiles (c–e), each complex being apposed by a separate axon terminal profile (c–e). Bar = 0.25 μm. From Geinisman et al. (1993),[22] with permission.

three distinct complexes of PSD profiles, each one being apposed by a separate presynaptic terminal profile (Fig. 1d).

A three-dimensional reconstruction of this synapse from the micrographs of serial sections shows that its single presynaptic axon terminal has three protrusions at the distal end (Fig. 2a). The cavity of the postsynaptic spine head is divided into three compartments by spine partitions (Fig. 2b). The partitions provide barriers between the presynap-

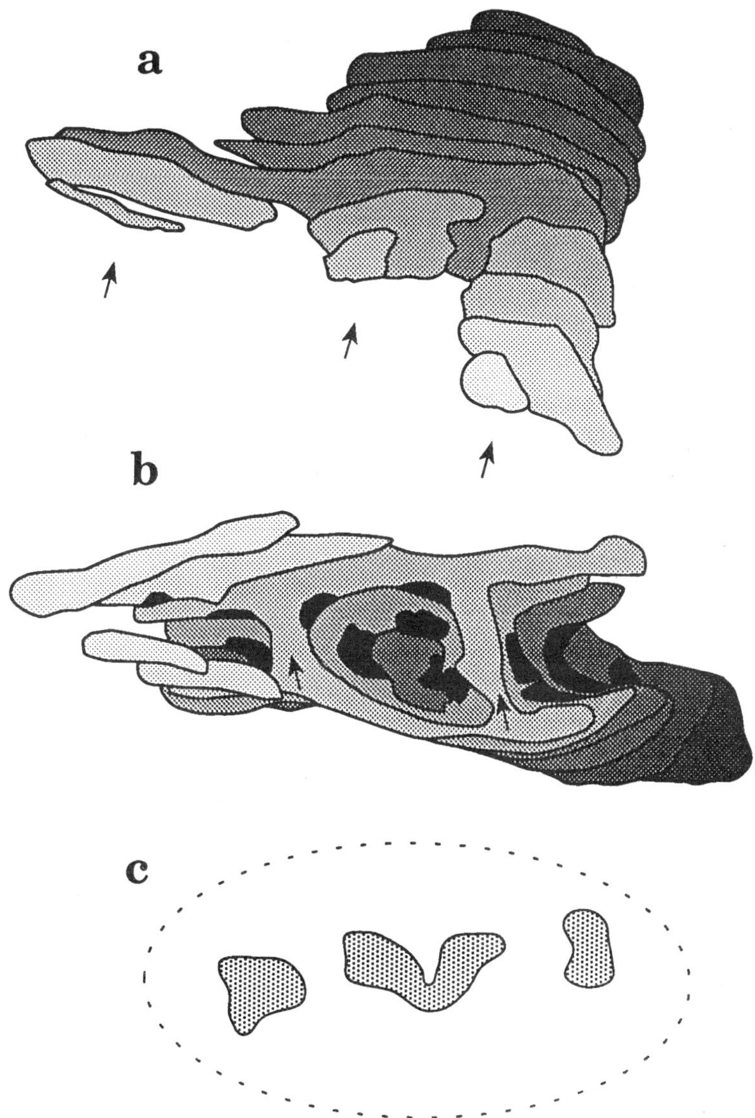

Figure 2. Reconstructions of the axospinous synapse shown in Fig. 1. a: a 3D reconstruction of the presynaptic axon terminal showing three separate protrusions (arrows) which emanate from its distal end. b: a 3D reconstruction of the postsynaptic spine head exhibiting partitions (arrows). These partitions divide a spine head cavity into three compartments, each one being fitted by a corresponding protrusion of the presynaptic axon terminal. PSD segments delineating two separate transmission zones are placed on each side of the partitions. c: a 2D reconstruction of the PSD demonstrating that it consists of three distinct segments. From Geinisman et al. (1993),[22] with permission.

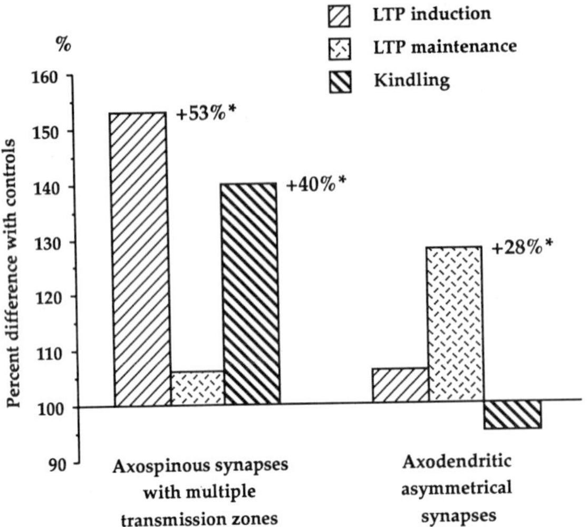

Figure 3. Changes in the number of synapses observed in potentiated and kindled rats relative to respective coulombic controls. Axospinous perforated synapses with multiple, completely partitioned transmission zones were significantly increased in numbers both during the induction phase of LTP (i.e., 1 hour after cessation of potentiating stimulation) and following kindling (4 weeks after a criterion of 5 generalized seizures was reached). The maintenance phase of LTP (examined 13 days after cessation of potentiating stimulation) was accompanied by an increase in the number of axodendritic asymmetrical synapses. $^{**}p < 0.05$, two-tailed randomization test for two independent samples.

tic bouton protrusions which fit into the corresponding compartments of the postsynaptic spine head. Separated by the spine partitions are three distinct transmission zones, each one being formed presynaptically by an axon terminal protrusion and outlined postsynaptically by a PSD segment (Fig. 2b). The PSD segments can be visualized with the aid of two-dimensional reconstructions as three separate plates (Fig. 2c).

Such axospinous perforated synapses with multiple, completely partitioned transmission zones were markedly (by 53%) and selectively increased in number in potentiated rats examined 1 hour after the fourth high frequency stimulation as compared with coulombic controls (Fig. 3). Change of this magnitude is most likely to have functional consequences. Each granule cell acquires 67 synapses of this particular subtype as a result of LTP induction, an addition that is equal to 2.3% of the entire synaptic population of the MML. The additional axospinous synapses are presumed to be especially efficacious relative to other axospinous junctions. Their multiple (2–4) transmission zones may represent functionally independent units, provided that the synaptic cleft contains a barrier for transmitter diffusion between neighboring transmission zones and that each PSD segment incorporates a newly inserted or activated receptor cluster[14,22]. It has been estimated that activation of only 1–5% of the total number of usual synaptic contacts in the MML is sufficient to evoke granule cell discharge[29]. It is reasonable, therefore, to suggest that the observed increase in the number of efficacious axospinous synapses with multiple, completely partitioned transmission zones could underlie the enhancement of synaptic responses during the induction phase of LTP.

4. STRUCTURAL SYNAPTIC ALTERATIONS ASSOCIATED WITH THE MAINTENANCE PHASE OF LTP

Analysis of electrophysiological recordings made 13 days following the fourth high frequency stimulation showed that the EPSP slope was potentiated by 51 ± 9%, the population spike amplitude by 137 ± 73% and the I-O function by 55 ± 44% (mean ± SEM for a group of 9 animals). At the 1 hour test interval after the fourth high frequency stimulation, the extent of potentiation in these animals was, however, significantly higher. It amounted to 111 ± 25% for the EPSP slope, 695 ± 169% for the population spike amplitude, and 263 ± 57% for the I-O function. Although the augmentation of synaptic responses had decayed over the 13 day period following the induction of LTP, there was still significant potentiation relative to baseline. A paired *t*-test comparing baseline values with those at the 13 day test interval revealed statistically significant increases for both the EPSP slope ($t = 6.463$, df = 8, $p < 0.001$) and the population spike amplitude ($t = 3.302$, df = 8, $p < 0.02$). The increase in the I-O function, however, was not significant ($t = 1.163$, df = 8, $p > 0.2$). Coulombic control animals (n = 9) tested 13 days after the last low frequency stimulation did not exhibit any significant change in the electrophysiological measures used relative to baseline.

Quantitation of synaptic contacts in the MML during the maintenance phase of LTP provided an unexpected result[21]. The increase in the number of axospinous perforated synapses with multiple, completely partitioned transmission zones observed 1 hour after the last high frequency stimulation was not found in animals examined 13 days after cessation of potentiating stimulation: the number of these axospinous junctions returned to the control level during LTP maintenance (Fig. 3). The latter LTP phase, however, was accompanied by a selective increase (+28%) in the number of axodendritic asymmetrical synapses in the potentiated synaptic field (Fig. 3). Interestingly enough, such alteration was not associated with the induction phase of LTP (Fig. 3).

The pattern of synaptic plasticity which characterizes the maintenance phase of LTP includes two basic phenomena: a decay of the maximum degree of synaptic enhancement that is observed during LTP induction and, simultaneously, the retention of a lesser degree of synaptic augmentation for a relatively long period of time. These two phenomena may be accounted for by different structural synaptic modifications. The *decay* may be a consequence of those changes in axospinous synapses with multiple, completely partitioned transmission zones that result in the return of their number to the control level.

Support of the *retention of synaptic augmentation* during the maintenance phase of LTP could be mediated by the increase in the number of axodendritic asymmetrical synapses since they are supposed to be excitatory in function and have a relatively high strength due to their strategic location directly on dendritic shafts, rather than on spines. During LTP maintenance, each granule cell of the dentate gyrus was estimated to acquire some 30 additional asymmetrical synapses involving its dendrites in the MML, which translates in a 1% increase in the total number of MML synapses. The change of such magnitude appears to be sufficient to exert a measurable facilitating effect on the amplitude of synaptic responses elicited from the population of dentate granule cells[29].

5. RELATIONSHIP BETWEEN STRUCTURAL SYNAPTIC MODIFICATIONS CHARACTERISTIC OF THE INDUCTION AND MAINTENANCE PHASES OF HIPPOCAMPAL LTP

Although the increases in the number of synapses observed following the induction and during the maintenance phase of LTP involve different synaptic subtypes, these changes may be related to each other. Such a possibility is suggested by the existence of a special type of perforated synaptic junction which appears to be transitional between axospinous and axodendritic ones[21]. In these synapses (Fig. 4), the postsynaptic spine lacks a neck, and the spine head is lowered on one side to the level of the parent dendrite surface. The presynaptic terminal forms a single asymmetrical synaptic contact of the perforated

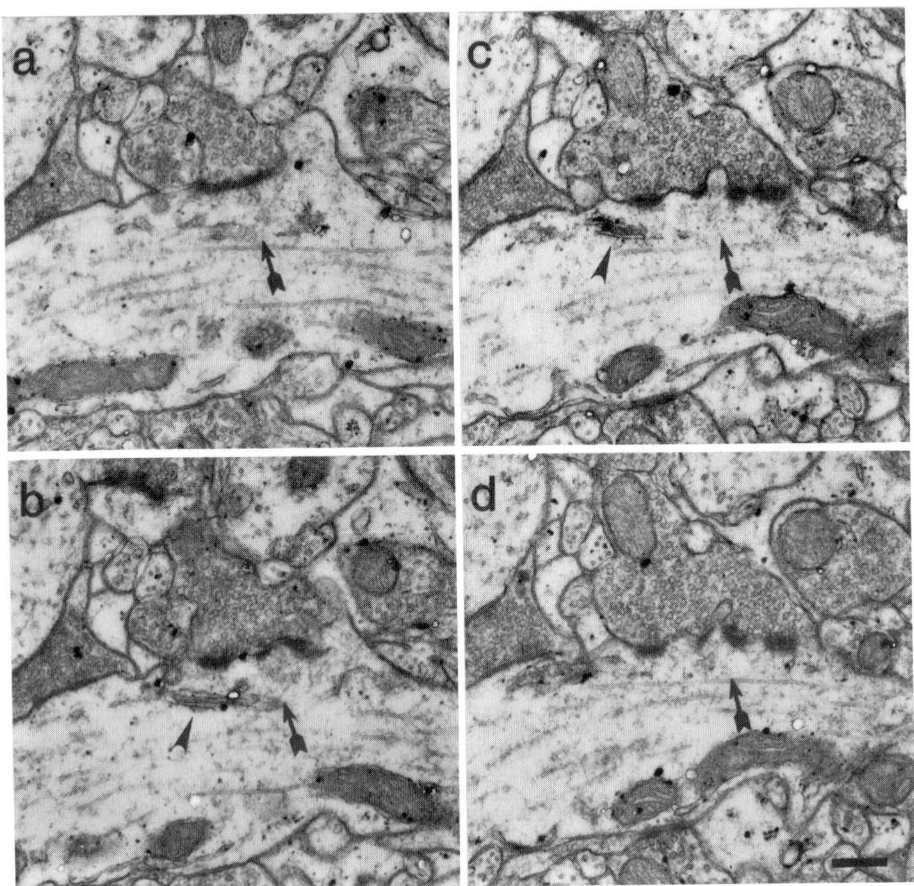

Figure 4. Electron micrographs of consecutive serial sections (a–d) through the middle molecular layer of the rat dentate gyrus demonstrating a special type of perforated synaptic contact (arrows). The postsynaptic element of this synapse can be classified as a dendritic spine which is associated with a spine apparatus (arrowheads). In some serial sections (c and d), however, the spine is retracted into the parent dendrite and levels with its surface. Bar = 0.25 μm. From Geinisman et al. (1993),[21] with permission.

variety which extends from the spine to its parent dendrite. It is conceivable that, under certain conditions, the postsynaptic spine may be completely retracted into the parent dendrite, and the axospinous asymmetrical synapse formerly associated with the spine becomes an axodendritic one.

A remodeling of this kind may represent a mechanism by which the initial increase in the number of axospinous synapses that occurs shortly after LTP induction is transformed into a subsequent increase in the number of axodendritic synapses during LTP maintenance. It is tempting, therefore, to speculate that the transition from the induction to the maintenance phase of LTP may be due to the transformation in the morphological substrate of synaptic plasticity. Such a transformation can be viewed as an efficient form of response conservation within the adaptive system, since a relatively moderate increase in the number of axodendritic asymmetrical synapses during LTP maintenance might serve to sustain an adequate degree of synaptic enhancement to be recorded as a durable electrophysiological change.

6. STRUCTURAL SYNAPTIC ALTERATIONS FOLLOWING HIPPOCAMPAL KINDLING

As indicated above, high frequency stimulation used to elicit a fully developed kindled state was administered twice a day and terminated when a criterion of five class V seizures was reached. The number of stimulations required to reach the criterion was 78 ± 14 (mean ± SEM for a group of 7 rats). To allow possible immediate effects of seizures on brain morphology to dissipate, kindled animals were examined electron microscopically 4 weeks after cessation of stimulation. Coulombic control rats (n = 7) were stimulated with parameters (120 pulses at 2 Hz) that do not evoke kindling. Quantitative ultrastructural analyses demonstrated that the number of axospinous synapses with multiple, completely partitioned transmission zones was markedly (by 40%) and significantly increased in kindled rats relative to their coulombic controls (Fig. 3). This change was selective: no other synaptic subtype, including asymmetrical axodendritic junctions (Fig. 3), exhibited an increase in number following kindling.

Thus, the effect of kindling on synaptic ultrastructure is very similar to that of the induction phase of LTP, but is strikingly different compared with the effect of the maintenance phase of LTP (Fig. 3). The time elapsed between cessation of high frequency stimulation and fixation of tissue for electron microscopy was twice longer in the kindling experiment (4 weeks) than in the experiment with LTP maintenance (about 2 weeks). In spite of this, kindled animals did not show the kind of structural synaptic alterations that were observed during the maintenance phase of LTP. Although kindled animals were not examined at earlier time points following the termination of stimulation, one would expect that the structural synaptic change described above developed early during the kindling process and then was retained over a period of 4 weeks.

It is not surprising, however, that kindling causes, as does LTP induction, in the formation of only those axospinous synapses that may represent specialized synaptic contacts of an unusually high efficacy[14,22]. The selective and substantial increase in the number of such synapses following kindling may provide a structural substrate of the prominent and unceasing augmentation of synaptic responsiveness in the stimulated circuit that characterizes the kindling phenomenon.

7. SIMILARITIES AND DIFFERENCES IN PATTERNS OF SYNAPSE RESTRUCTURING ASSOCIATED WITH HIPPOCAMPAL LTP AND KINDLING

Elucidation of structural characteristics of hippocampal synapses in the stimulated synaptic field has suggested that a restructuring of preexisting synaptic contacts, rather than the formation of new ones, may account for a long-lasting augmentation of synaptic responsiveness which defines both LTP and kindling. A model postulating the consecutive steps of synapse restructuring that underlies synaptic plasticity associated with LTP was proposed in our previous work[16,21,22]. The results of the present study indicate that the model is also applicable to kindling. According to this model (Fig. 5), the sequence of synapse restructuring that may result in a marked augmentation of synaptic responses during the induction of LTP and following kindling is postulated to commence with the conversion of nonperforated axospinous synapses (Fig. 5a) into perforated ones. It involves the consecutive formation of synaptic contacts that have initially a focal spine partition with a fenestrated PSD (Fig. 5b), then a sectional partition with a horseshoe-shaped PSD (Fig.

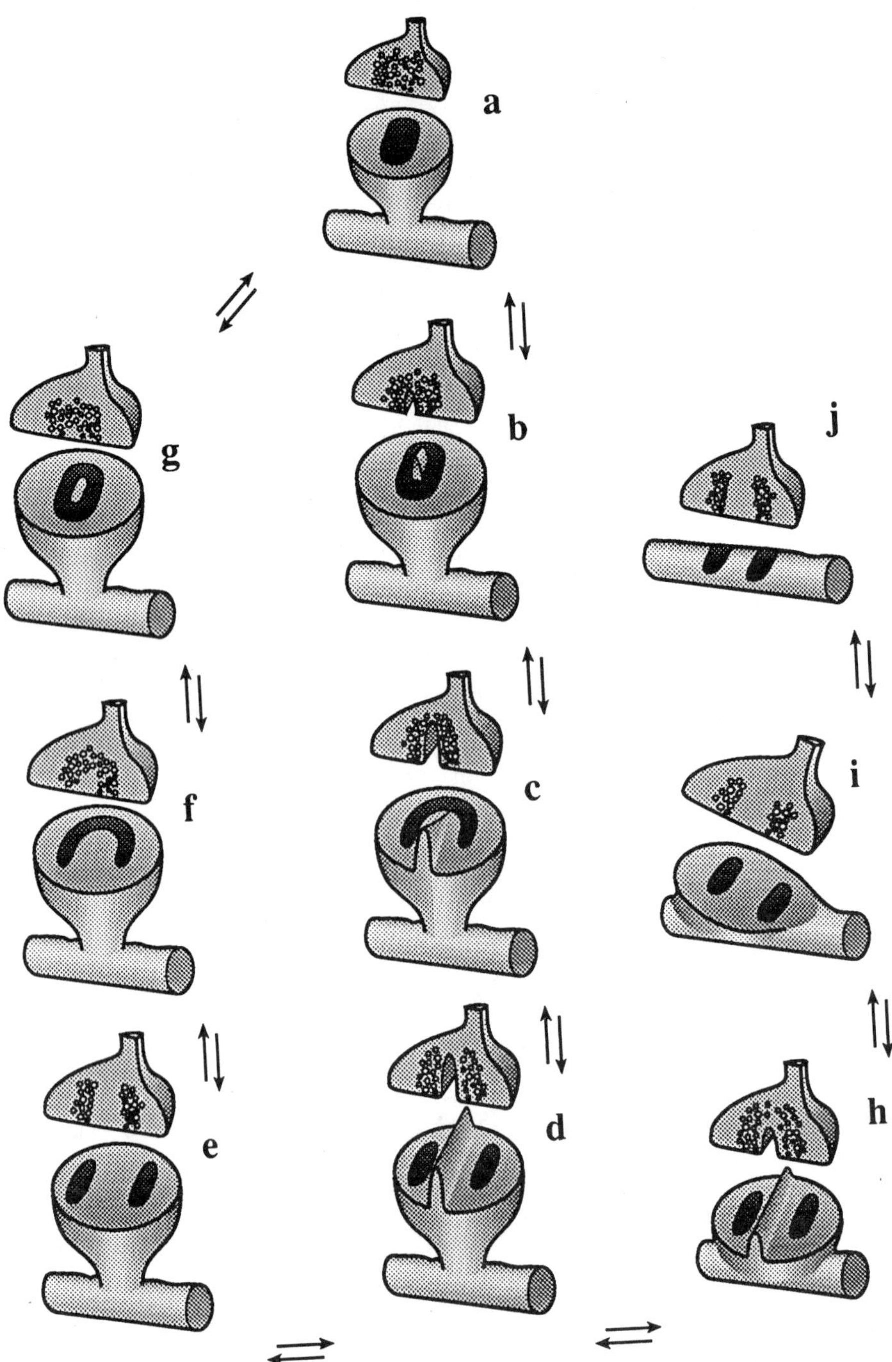

Figure 5. The diagram illustrating the proposed model of structural synaptic plasticity associated with LTP and kindling as described in the text. The schematic shows the various structural intermediates in synaptic plasticity. A remodeling of preexisting synaptic contacts is presumed to result in the observed selective increases in the number of either axospinous synapses with multiple, completely partitioned transmission zones (d) following the induction of LTP and kindling or axodendritic asymmetrical synapses (j) during the maintenance phase of LTP. From Geinisman et al. (1993),[21] with permission.

5c), and finally a complete partition(s) with a segmented PSD (Fig. 5d). Synapses belonging to the latter subtype have multiple (2–4) transmission zones instead of only a single one, as is usual. These synaptic contacts are presumed to be especially efficacious axospinous junctions[14,22], and an increase in their number following the induction of LTP or kindling is supposed to significantly augment synaptic transmission.

During the maintenance phase of LTP, which is accompanied by a decay of synaptic enhancement, the number of these synaptic contacts returns to the control level. The reversal of the morphological change associated with the induction of LTP may reflect a disassembly of complete spine partitions in such synapses and their conversion into other synaptic subtypes. Among these are nonpartitioned axospinous synapses with a segmented (Fig. 5e), horseshoe-shaped (Fig. 5f) and fenestrated (Fig. 5g) PSD. Additionally, some axospinous synapses with multiple, completely partitioned transmission zones are proposed to be remodeled into asymmetrical axodendritic junctions which are increased in numbers during LTP maintenance. In the process of this remodeling, the postsynaptic spine loses its neck (Fig. 5h) and is gradually retracted into the parent dendrite (Fig. 5i) until it levels with the dendritic surface (Fig. 5j). Consequently, the axospinous perforated synaptic contact that was located on the spine becomes an axodendritic asymmetrical synapse. An increase in the number of such synaptic junctions may be responsible for the retention of synaptic enhancement at a relatively low during the maintenance phase of LTP.

In contrast to LTP, kindling does not appear to involve the sequence of structural synaptic modifications that lead to the formation of additional asymmetrical axodendritic synapses from axospinous synaptic contacts that have multiple, completely partitioned transmission zones. This suggests that it is the stabilization of the latter subtype of axospinous junctions that makes kindling, as opposed to LTP, a virtually permanent form of synaptic plasticity. Further studies are necessary to explore the mechanisms (e.g., changes in adhesion molecules) by which the presumably most efficacious axospinous synapses are stabilized.

The authors thank William Goossens for his skillful technical assistance. This work was supported in part by grants AG 08794 from NIA, BNS-8912372 from NSF and RO1 NS34582 from NINDS.

REFERENCES

1. Barnes, C.A., Memory deficits associated with senescence: A neurophysiological and behavioral study in the rat, *J. Comp. Physiol. Psychol.*, 93 (1979) 74–104.
2. Bliss, T.V.P. and Collingridge, G.L., A synaptic model of memory: Long-term potentiation in the hippocampus, *Nature*, 361 (1993) 31–39.
3. Bliss, T.V.P. and Gardner-Medwin, A., Long-lasting potentiation of synaptic transmission in the dentate area of the unanaesthetized rabbit following stimulation of the perforant path, *J. Physiol.*, 232 (1973) 357–374.
4. Bliss, T.V.P. and Lømo, T., Long-lasting potentiation of synaptic transmission in the dentate area of the anaesthetized rabbit following stimulation of the perforant path, *J. Physiol.*, 232, (1973) 331–356.
5. Brændgaard, H. and Gundersen, H.J.G., The impact of recent stereological advances on quantitative studies of the nervous system, *J. Neurosci. Methods*, 18 (1986) 39–78.
6. Cain, D.P., Long-term potentiation and kindling: How similar are the mechanisms?, *Trends Neurosci.*, 12 (1989) 6–10.
7. Calverley, P.K.S. and Jones, D.G., Contribution of dendritic spines and perforated synapses to synaptic plasticity, *Brain Res. Rev.*, 15 (1990) 215–249.
9. Cavazos, J.E., Das, J. and Sutula, T.P., Neuronal loss induced in limbic pathways by kindling: Evidence for induction of hippocampal sclerosis by repeated brief seizures, *J. Neurosci.*, 14 (1994) 3106–3121.
10. Chang, F.-L. and Greenough, W.T., Transient and enduring morphological correlates of synaptic activity and efficacy change in the rat hippocampal slice, *Brain Res.*, 309 (1984) 35–46.

11. Cohen, R.S. and Siekevitz, P., Form of the postsynaptic density. A serial section study, *J. Cell Biol.*, 78 (1978) 36–46.
12. Colonnier, M., Synaptic patterns of different cell types in the different laminae of the cat visual cortex. An electron microscopic study, *Brain Res.*, 9 (1968) 268–287.
13. Desmond, N.L. and Levy, W.B., Changes in the numerical density of synaptic contacts with long-term potentiation in the hippocampal dentate gyrus, *J. Comp. Neurol.*, 253 (1986) 466–475.
14. Edwards, F.A., LTP—a structural model to explain the inconsistencies, *Trends Neurosci.*, 18 (1995) 250–255.
15. Geinisman, Y., Perforated axospinous synapses with multiple, completely partitioned transmission zones: Probable structural intermediates in synaptic plasticity. *Hippocampus*, 3 (1993) 417–434.
16. Geinisman, Y., L. deToledo-Morrell, and F. Morrell, Induction of long-term potentiation is associated with an increase in the number of axospinous synapses with segmented postsynaptic densities, *Brain Res.*, 566 (1991) 77–88.
17. Geinisman, Y., Morrell, F. and deToledo-Morrell, L., Remodeling of synaptic architecture during hippocampal "kindling", *Proc. Natl. Acad. Sci. USA*, 85 (1988) 3260–3264.
18. Geinisman Y., Morrell F. and deToledo-Morrell, L., Increase in the relative proportion of perforated axospinous synapses following hippocampal kindling is specific for the synaptic field of stimulated axons *Brain Res.*, 507 (1990) 325–331.
19. Geinisman, Y., Morrell, F. and deToledo-Morrell, L., Alterations of synaptic ultrastructure induced by hippocampal kindling. In J.A. Wada (Ed.), *Kindling 4*, Plenum, New York, 1990, pp. 75–92.
20. Geinisman, Y., Morrell, F. and deToledo-Morrell, L., Increase in the number of axospinous synapses with segmented postsynaptic densities following hippocampal kindling, *Brain Res.*, 569 (1992) 341–357.
21. Geinisman, Y., deToledo-Morrell, L., Morrell, F., Persina, I.S. and Beatty, M.A., Synapse restructuring associated with the maintenance phase of hippocampal long-term potentiation, *J. Comp. Neurol.*, 368 (1996) 413–423.
22. Geinisman, Y., deToledo-Morrell, L., Morrell, F., Heller, R.E., Rossi, M. and Parshall, R.F., Structural synaptic correlate of long-term potentiation: Formation of axospinous synapses with multiple, completely partitioned transmission zones, *Hippocampus*, 3 (1993) 435–446.
23. Goddard, G.V., The development of epileptic seizures through brain stimulation at low intensity, *Nature*, 214 (1967) 1020–1021.
24. Goddard, G.V., The kindling model of epilepsy, *Trends Neurosci.*, 6 (1983) 275–279.
25. Goddard, G.V., McIntyre, D. and Leech, C., A permanent change in brain function resulting from daily electrical stimulation, *Exp. Neurol.*, 25 (1969) 295–330
26. Gundersen, H.J.G., Bagger, P., Bendtsen, T.F., Evans, S.M., Korbo, L., Marcussen, N., Møller, A., Nielsen, K., Nyengaard, J.R., Pakkenberg, B., Sørensen, F.B., Vesterby, A. and West, M.J., The new stereological tools: Disector, fractionator, nucleator and point sampled intercepts and their use in pathological research and diagnosis, *Acta Pathol. Microbiol. Immunol. Scand.*, 96 (1988) :857–881.
27. Lee, K.S., Schottler F., Oliver, M., and Lynch, G., Brief bursts of high-frequency stimulation produce two types of structural change in rat hippocampus, *J. Neurophysiol.*, 44 (1980) 247–258.
28. Lynch, G., Muller, D., Seubert, P. and Larson, J., Long-term potentiation: Persisting problems and recent results, *Brain Res. Bull.*, 21 (1988) 363–372.
29. McNaughton, B.L., Barnes, C.A. and Anderson, P., Synaptic efficacy and EPSP summation in granule cells of rat fascia dentata studied *in vitro*, *J. Neurophysiol.*, 46 (1981) 952–966.
30. Morrell, F., Goddard's kindling phenomenon. In H.C. Sabelli (Ed.), *Chemical Modulation of Brain Function*, Raven, New York, 1973, pp. 207–223.
31. Morrell, F. and deToledo-Morrell, L., Kindling as a model of neuronal plasticity. In J.A. Wada (Ed.), *Kindling 3*, Raven, New York, 1986, pp. 17–33.
32. Peters, A. and Kaiserman-Abramof, I.R., The small pyramidal neuron of the rat cerebral cortex. The synapses upon dendritic spines, *Z. Zellforsch.*, 100 (1969) 487–506.
33. Racine, R., Kindling: The first decade, *Neurosurgery*, 3 (1978) 234–252
34. Racine, R. J. and Cain, D. P., Kindling-induced potentiation. In F. Morrell (Ed.), *Kindling and Synaptic Plasticity: The Legacy of Graham Goddard*, Birkhäuser, Boston, 1991, pp. 38–53.
35. Racine, R. J., Milgram, N.W. and Hafner, S., Long-term potentiation phenomena in the rat limbic forebrain, *Brain Res.*, 260 (1983) 217–231.
36. Racine R., Newberry, F. and Burnham, W.M., Post-activation potentiation and the kindling phenomenon, *Electoenceph. Clin. Neurophysiol.*, 39 (1975) 261–273.
37. Represa, A., Jorquera, I., Le Gal La Salle, G., Ben-Ari, Y., Epilepsy induced collateral sprouting of hippocampal mossy fibers: Does it induce the development of ectopic synapses with granule cell dendrites?, *Hippocampus*, 3 (1993) 257–268.
38. Sutula, T. and Steward, O., Quantitative analysis of synaptic potentiation during kindling of the perforant path, *J. Neurophysiol.*, 56 (1986) 732–746.

39. Sutula, T. and Steward, O., Facilitation of kindling by prior induction of long-term potentiation in the perforant path, *Brain Res.*, 420 (1987) 109–117.
40. Sutula, T., Xiao-Xian, H., Cavazos, H. and Scott, G., Synaptic reorganization in the hippocampus induced by abnormal functional activity, *Science*, 239 (1988) 1147–1150
41. Trommald, M., Vaaland, J.L., Blackstad, T.W. and Andersen, P., Dendritic spine changes in rat dentate granule cells associated with long-term potentiation, In A. Guidotti (Ed.), *Neurotoxicity of Excitatory Amino Acids*, Raven, New York, 1990, pp. 163–174.
42. Wada, J.A. and Sato, M., Generalized convulsive seizures induced by daily electrical stimulation of the amygdala in cats: Correlative electrographic and behavioral seizures, *Neurology*, 24 (1974) 565–574.

DISCUSSION OF YURI GEINISMAN'S PAPER

M. Burnham: I have a question about how long it take these changes to occur. Years ago Racine and I kindled once an hour or once a half hour and seem to get kindling effect very quickly. Would these restructuring changes take place that quickly?

Y. Geinisman: In this model we have shown to you there are no time constraints. What is required for an access point of a synapse to be remodelled into the presumably most efficacious form is just to construct a complete spine partition, and that depends on the membrane fluidity. So it does not require new protein synthesis.

I. Mody: I was wondering if you could comment on the fact that you are saying that these diffusion barriers on the spine may actually functionally separate two release sites. I can't think how action potentials could depolarize at all presynaptic terminals — the calcium channels would not open at both sides of the release site as they did before.

Y. Geinisman: What I was trying to tell you, rather unsuccessfully, was that the distance of complete partitions might prevent the spillover of transmitter from one transmission zone to another. Does that satisfy you?

I. Mody: Yes, that's fine, but what I'm saying is that you will have two release sites that function together every time an action potential is going to depolarize a terminal. And therefore you are going to insert receptors by dividing them into half, and that is not going to make a more efficacious synapse. What's going to make a more efficacious synapse is to double the number of receptors that have full release sites .

Y. Geinisman: Yes, but it seems to me that I mentioned that another condition for such synapses with multiple transmission zones to be the most efficacious one and the other condition was that each spine segment must contain either an unstructured or activated receptor cluster, exactly as you say.

I. Mody: Which leads me to another question: What do you think actually happens first, do you think that these channels or receptors are basically being inserted and then the synapse splits? Or do you think that actually there are multiple release sites originally on the presynaptic terminal which release transmitter onto the postsynaptic site and then that splits, or invagination or whatever happens there splits and then the receptors start being inserted?

Y. Geinisman: I don't know.

15

NEURONAL GROWTH AND NEURONAL LOSS IN KINDLING EPILEPTOGENESIS

Ronald J. Racine,[1,2] Beth Adams,[1] Philip Osehobo,[1] Norton W. Milgram,[3] and Margaret Fahnestock[2]

[1]Department of Psychology
McMaster University
Hamilton, Ontario L8S 4K1
[2]Department of Biomedical Sciences
McMaster University
Hamilton, Ontario L8N 3Z5
[3]Department of Psychology
University of Toronto
Scarborough College
West Hill, Ontario M1C 1A4

1. KINDLING CORRELATES AND MECHANISMS

Goddard published his first brief description of the kindling phenomenon in 1967[36]. Although we have learned quite a lot about this model of epilepsy in the last 30 years, the underlying mechanisms continue to elude us. Part of the difficulty arises from the fact that various patterns of neural activation, we now know, can trigger a wide variety of long-lasting post-activation effects. Excess neural activation (e.g. epileptiform events) can produce an even greater number of effects, and any of these could contribute to the development of an epileptogenic state.

We can group these effects into three major categories: 1) those that reflect an enhanced connectivity within excitatory systems, 2) those that reflect a decreased (or increased) level of function within inhibitory systems, and 3) those that reflect a change in the intrinsic response properties of neurons, rendering them more susceptible to firing in a burst mode. All of these effects have been implicated in kindling epileptogenesis, but none, thus far, has been shown to be essential. Our research has focused on the first two categories of mechanisms. Although the possibility that the intrinsic response properties of the activated cells is altered has received some support[57,71], we have no recent data to report on this topic. We have directed much of our efforts toward the investigation of the following four mechanisms.

Kindling 5, edited by Corcoran and Moshé.
Plenum Press, New York, 1998.

1.1. Enhanced Connectivity in Preexisting Synapses

We and others have found that kindling produces a strong and long-lasting enhancement in connectivity[25,72–74,77,82]. Kindling-induced potentiation (KIP) is similar in many respects to long-term potentiation (LTP), which can be defined as an increase in synaptic strength produced by brief, high frequency stimulation of excitatory afferents. However, KIP is different from most forms of long-term potentiation (LTP), investigated in parallel experiments, in that it lasts much longer than LTP. It is not known whether KIP can last long enough to account for the longevity of kindling.

1.2. Axonal Sprouting—Growth of New Synapses

More recently, it has been shown that kindling can actually induce axonal growth in excitatory pathways in the hippocampus. Specifically, sprouting is induced in the mossy fibers running from the dentate gyrus granule cells to the pyramidal cells of area CA3. This pathway has been shown to sprout collaterals back into the granule cell layer[91] and into the normal target site of mossy fibers in area CA3[5,80]. It is not yet clear whether this sprouting is an example of an enhanced connectivity in excitatory circuitry leading to epileptogenesis, but this suggestion has been made several times[15,80,91].

1.3. Reduced Inhibition

Several investigators have attempted to link epileptogenesis to a decrease in inhibitory transmission. Using the paired pulse measure of inhibition, which allows levels of inhibition to be monitored over a period of months, we have found that inhibition actually appears to be potentiated in several sites, in much the same way as responses in excitatory systems. We have found this to be the case in the dentate gyrus[94] and in the piriform cortex[75]. These two sites have also shown some of the most dramatic activation-induced alterations in kindling and related experiments (e.g. [28,41,44,48,56,57,76]). We have also found evidence for enhanced inhibition in area CA3[74] and in the entorhinal cortex and perirhinal cortex following kindling (unpublished results). The only site at which we have found reduced inhibition is hippocampal area CA1, confirming results reported by King et al.[47] Rainnie et al.[79], however, have found evidence for reduced inhibition in the amygdala and Zhao and Leung[103] have reported reduced inhibition in area CA3 in slice preparations taken from kindled animals. These results need to be confirmed in intact tissue, but Callahan et al.[12] have reported a long-lasting decrease in the number of GABA-immunoreactive neurons in the amygdala of kindled rats.

1.4. Cell Loss

Clinical findings provided the initial grounds for suggesting a link betwen cell loss and epileptogenesis. Substantial hippocampal degeneration is often a hallmark of temporal lobe epilepsy. If the damaged or lost cells are critical for the normal function of inhibitory systems, then increased epileptogenic reactivity would be a logical outcome. A link to kindling epileptogenesis came from reports that cells are lost in the hilus of the dentate gyrus in kindled animals[17]. This came as something of a surprise, since both Graham Goddard and R. Racine had done cell counts around kindled foci many years ago and found no differences when compared to tissue from control animals. Although it now seems clear that cell loss can occur as a result of the induction of status epilepticus[3,65], the effect remains controversial in the kindling literature. In any case, it has been suggested that some of the cells lost from the hilus in more extreme models of epileptic activation are cells that normally innervate inhibitory interneurons[86]. If so, then this cell loss could shift the balance between excitation and inhibition. This is another potential mechanism that will be explored in this chapter.

2. NEUROTROPHINS, NEURAL GROWTH AND SEIZURES

The remainder of this paper will focus on the possibility that two of the events described above—mossy fiber sprouting and/or hilar cell loss—could serve as kindling mechanisms (and more generally as epilepsy mechanisms). Much of our recent research has utilized the experimental manipulation of neurotrophic factors in an attempt to tease apart the the relationships between neural growth, neural damage and epileptogenesis.

Neuronal cells require specific neurotrophic factors for their development and survival. They are collectively called neurotrophins and include the following members: nerve growth factor (NGF)[10,30,52], brain-derived neurotrophic factor (BDNF)[2,51], neurotrophin-3 (NT-3)[40,53,81], neurotrophin-4/5 (NT-4/5)[8,39,42], and the recently-discovered neurotrophin-6 (NT-6)[38].

Neurotrophins are necessary for the survival, maintenance and regulation of both PNS and CNS neurons in the developing and adult nervous systems[8,40,51,53,81,101]. As mentioned above, they also promote neurite outgrowth. For example, NGF has been shown to be necessary for the damage-induced sprouting response of certain neurons in both PNS and CNS of adult rats[23,96].

In the adult CNS, the highest levels of NGF and BDNF mRNA and/or protein are synthesized in cortex, hippocampus, amygdala, and olfactory bulb. NT-3 mRNA is found primarily in hippocampus, whereas NT-4/5 is widely expressed throughout the adult brain[29,68,93,100].

Recently, it has been demonstrated that seizures can cause alterations in gene expression for a variety of molecules, including neurotrophic factors and their high-affinity receptors. Hippocampal kindling dramatically induces mRNA for NGF and BDNF, while lowering or not affecting the mRNA for NT-3[7,26,28]. This increase in NGF and BDNF mRNA is also reflected by an increase in protein, albeit with a somewhat different time course[6,66]. Kindling also upregulates mRNA levels for trkB and trkC, the high affinity receptors which preferentially bind BDNF and NT-3, respectively[7,59].

The upregulation of NGF and BDNF raises the possibility that neurotrophins are involved in both the progression of kindling and the synaptic plasticity associated with kindling. In support of this hypothesis, we have confirmed a report by Funabashi et al.[32] that intraventricular administration of antiserum to NGF delays the development of amygdaloid kindling[98]. We have also found that anti-NGF inhibits the kindling-induced collateral sprouting of mossy fibers[98]. In addition, we found that an NGF peptide that blocks the biological activity of NGF also delays kindling and blocks mossy fiber sprouting[78].

Neurotrophins have also been shown to protect hippocampal cells from ischemic damage. Even NGF, which has no high affinity trkA receptors in the hippocampus (although see Cellerino[18]), has been shown to rescue hippocampal cells fom ischemic cell death[11,84,102]. These findings raise the possibility that the neurotrophins themselves promote sprouting and reduce cell loss in the hippocampus. If so, then the neurotrophins could provide a useful tool for teasing out the causal relationships among these phenomena and the developing epileptogenesis. Even without such a tool, however, we can begin to dissociate some of these phenomena.

3. CAUSAL RELATIONSHIPS AMONG CELL LOSS, SPROUTING, INHIBITION AND EPILEPTOGENESIS

Although our previous research has shown that the hippocampus is not a particularly reactive structure with respect to kindling epileptogenesis[44,76], we have returned to this system for several reasons: 1) we believe that the mechanisms underlying kindling are expressed in many brain areas, including the hippocampus (albeit, more slowly there), 2) we are interested in the mechanisms underlying growth in forebrain pathways in adult preparations, and 3) the demonstrated phenomena (cell loss and sprouting in the hippocampus) have received wide attention, and appear to have been accepted by several investigators as likely mechanisms of kindling or epilepsy.

Several potential causal relationships are suggested by the findings reviewed above (particularly the mossy fiber sprouting and the hilar cell loss). We will list them here and then address them one by one. 1) Perhaps the first question to address is whether kindling produces a reliable cell loss in the hilus of the dentate gyrus, and, if so, could that cell loss serve as a kindling mechanism? 2) If there is a cell loss, and it contributes to epileptogenesis, then it presumably reflects a failure in inhibitory systems. Can it be shown that such a relationship exists between hilar cell loss and inhibition in the dentate gyrus? 3) It has been argued that mossy fiber sprouting contributes to epileptogenesis. Is such a causal relationship supported by data? 4) It has been argued that mossy fiber sprouting is triggered by the hilar cell loss. Is it possible that the sprouting is purely activation-induced and not dependent upon cell loss? 5) On the other hand, it has also been argued that the sprouting serves to restore the inhibition that is lost as a result of cell degeneration. Can either recovering or potentiated inhibition in the dentate gyrus be accounted for by mossy fiber sprouting? 6) Can reduced inhibition in the dentate gyrus account for any aspect of the developing epileptogenesis from triggered to spontaneous seizures?

3.1. Cell Loss and Epileptogenesis

The demonstrations of cell loss resulting from status epilepticus raised several interesting questions: 1) how much seizure activity is required to produce the first signs of cell loss, 2) which structures are most sensitive to such degenerative effects, and 3) does this cell loss contribute to the developing epileptogenesis?

The hippocampus and the piriform cortex nearly always sustain damage in response to excess activation[45,55,60], but it has been argued that the cells in the hilus of the dentate gyrus are the most sensitive in the brain and are the first to be damaged following seizure activity[86]. However, the amount of seizure activity required to produce such damage and the role of that damage in the developing epileptogenesis have been more difficult to determine. Cavazos and Sutula[17] reported hilar cell loss with kindling, suggesting that even limited, spaced seizure activity can produce hilar damage. The loss was about 12% after kindling to 3 stage 5 convulsions, and increased to 40% after kindling to 30 stage 5 convulsions. We were able to provide a partial replication of these results. Spiller and Racine[89] kindled animals to 4 and 44 stage 5 convulsions and found a significant decrease in cell density in the hilus, but the reductions were much lower than those reported by Cavazos and Sutula.

Bertram and Lothman[9], however, measured cell counts as well as hilar volume in hippocampal tissue from kindled animals. Although cell density did decrease as a result of kindling, this was found to be due entirely to an expansion of hilar volume. This appeared to be the case even in animals that had received as many as 1500 stimulations! Furthermore, E. Bertram (personal communication) pointed out that the hilus in Figure 5 of

Spiller and Racine[89] appeared to be larger in the tissue from kindled animals. However, Cavazos et al.[14] then published another paper that seemed to establish, definitively, a real neuronal loss in the hilus of kindled animals. They reported cell losses not only in the hilus of the dentate gyrus, but also in CA1, CA3, entorhinal cortex and the rostral endopyriform nucleus.

A recent entry in this debate came from Watanabe et al.[99] Using mice carrying a null mutation of c-fos, and a thorough counting procedure, they found a significant kindling-induced increase in hilar volume but no evidence of cell loss. Thus, the weight of data seemed to be shifting back towards our original conclusion of many years ago that kindling does not produce cell loss. This conclusion was also supported by an experiment utilizing a sensitive silver stain for neuronal degeneration, which showed no increase in the incidence of degenerating neurons in kindled tissue[49]. We have also found that kindling of the piriform cortex once per day does not lead to either decreases in neuron density in the hilus or to an increase in hilar volume (A. Spiller and R. Racine, in preparation). We have subsequently found that more severe epileptogenic activations, including repeated electroconvulsive shock (Z. Gombos, A. Spiller, G. Cottrell, R. Racine and W. Burnham, in preparation) and 2–3 hours of kainic acid induced status epilepticus (C. Ikeda-Douglas, E. Head, D. Holsinger, B. Adams, R. Racine and N. Milgram, in preparation), also had no effect on hilar neuronal density (see Figure 1).

In an attempt to manipulate cell loss and kindling more directly, we infused NGF into the ventricles during the course of kindling (B. Adams, P. Osehobo, M. Sazgar, M. Fahnestock, and R. Racine, under review). If hilar cell loss promotes epileptogenesis, and if the NGF provides neuroprotection for hilar cells, then NGF should also retard kindling. This experiment was done before we had confirmed that hilar neurons were not, in fact, lost with our kindling procedures. Nevertheless, we did find that NGF blocked the reductions in hilar cell density (and the corresponding increase in hilar area). Kindling, however, was facilitated rather than retarded by this procedure, providing a reasonably clear dissociation between the measures of hilar cell number and kindling rate. Similar experiments are ongoing in which we have infused BDNF into the dentate gyrus. This manipulation actually retarded kindling, confirming a report by Larmet et al.[50], but it had no effect on cell density, again providing a dissociation between these two measures.

Direct damage to the dentate gyrus with colchicine has no effect on the rate of perforant path kindling[63], yet these are the cells, according to some hypotheses, that are disinhibited by hilar damage to produce an increased epileptic responsivity. Finally, metallic ion deposits in the hilus will trigger seizure discharge, but direct damage to the hilus, caused by direct current delivered through platinum electrodes, will not[33].

In summary, it seems safe to conclude that hilar cell damage cannot be a primary mechanism underlying kindling, and is probably not a primary mechanism underlying temporal lobe epilepsy (except, perhaps, in those cases where an early risk factor has been determined—see O'Connor et al.[67]). Excess neuronal activation can lead to neuron loss, but by the time the activity levels have reached that state, the tissue may have already become severely epileptic. Neuronal damage *can* serve as a focus of epileptic activity. We do not believe, however, that *hilar* damage is particularly epileptogenic, and it clearly cannot serve as a primary mechanism for kindling.

3.2. Cell Loss and Inhibition

Perhaps hilar cell loss cannot account for kindling epileptogenesis, but what about the suggestion that it can account for a loss of inhibition in those cases where inhibition

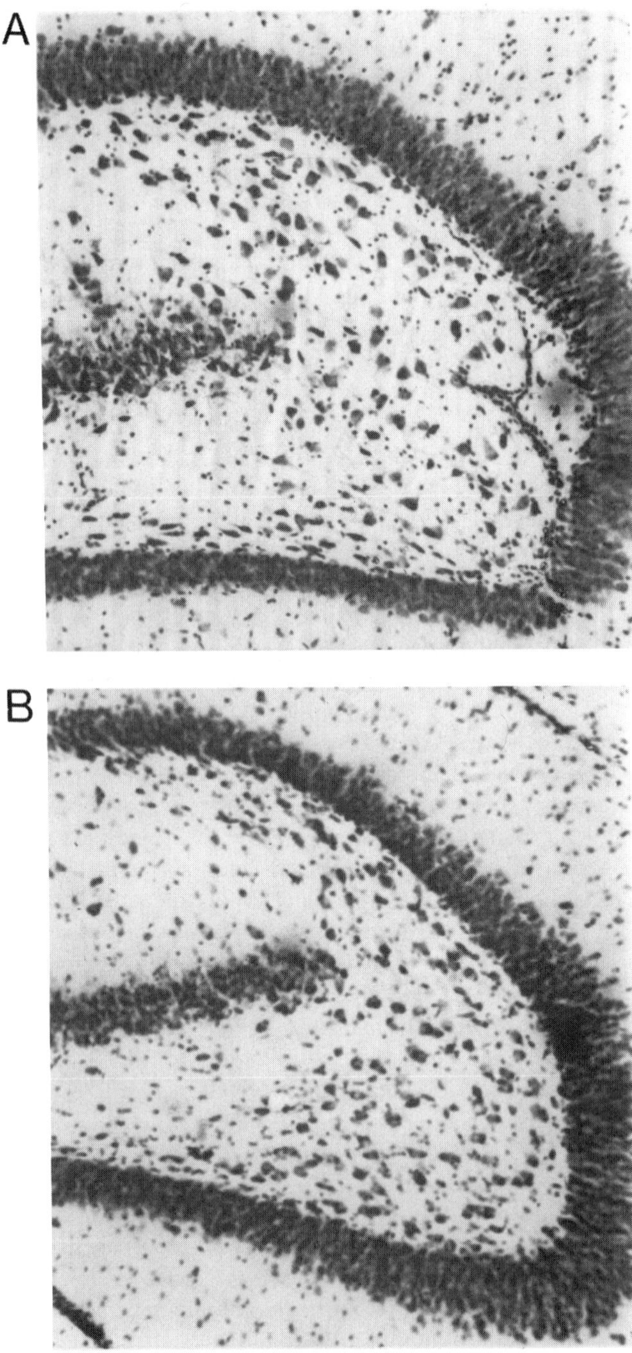

Figure 1. The neuron density is shown in these Nissl stained sections of the hilar region from a non-status animal (A) and an animal that experienced 3 hours of kainic acid-induced status (B). As can be seen, there is little indication of cell loss in this tissue. While kainic acid-induced status *can* lead to cell loss in this region, these results show that it is not inevitable, and the resulting post-status epileptogenesis can occur without measurable cell loss.

has been shown to be reduced? There seems to be little doubt that hilar neurons are lost in some of the status models, including Sloviter's 24 hr stimulation model[86]. Could inhibition be compromised as a result? This question is more difficult to answer definitively. What we can say is that we continue to find *increased* inhibition in the dentate gyrus when we kindle to a standard stage 5 criterion[22,94], when we kindle to 40 stage 5 convulsions beyond that criterion[89], and when we kindle to the point where spontaneous ictal episodes begin to appear (over 200 stimulations)[61]. If damage to the hilar region is to account for epileptogenesis, then it would have been expected to occur at least in the case of the spontaneously convulsing animals who had received hundreds of kindling stimulations. Also, cell loss has been reported in the hippocampus in many cases of temporal lobe epilepsy in humans[1,21,31,35,46,54,64,83], and inhibition may be increased in this tissue, as well[43,95]. Finally, we have found that the levels of inhibition are also elevated following a period of status epilepticus induced by the administration of kainic acid[62]. In this case, the inhibition is often reduced for a period of a few days, but it then recovers to higher than baseline levels. A similar recovery of inhibition was subsequently reported by Sloviter[87]. We believe that the *transient* loss of inhibition is due to the seizure discharge (see Ben-Ari et al.[4]; Tuff et al.[94]) rather than the other way around. It is also possible that the failure of inhibition reported by Sloviter in his 24 hour stimulation model is transient. At least some recovery of inhibition in this model was reported by Shirasaka and Wasterlain[85]. Further work needs to be done to determine how much seizure activity is required to produce actual neuronal loss in the hilus (as opposed to the decreased density discussed above), and how this real cell loss relates to measures of inhibition and measures of ongoing seizure activity.

3.3. Sprouting and Epileptogenesis

If hilar cell loss cannot account for kindling epileptogenesis, (and possibly not for any form of epileptogenesis), what about mossy fiber sprouting? An example of such kindling-induced sprouting, as revealed by the Timm stain, is shown in Figure 2. Here again the evidence is not particularly compelling. For example, Milgram et al.[62] have shown that spontaneous seizure activity can appear very early after a bout of kainic acid-induced status epilepticus. It is possible to see this activity 24 or 48 hours after recovery from status. This is too early to be readily accounted for by sprouting in the mossy fiber system. Whenever the time course for sprouting in hippocampal pathways has been monitored, it has taken 4–6 days to become detectable (although see Ebert and Loscher[27]) and at least 10–14 days to reach near asymptotic levels (Cavazos et al.[15]; Van der zee et al.[96]).

A similar discrepancy in time course has been demonstrated in a very different preparation, the mutant mouse *stargazer*. Qiao and Noebels[69] reported that both hilar cell loss and mossy fiber sprouting appeared long *after* the development of spontaneous seizure activity in this preparation.

Although mossy fiber sprouting has been reported for both amygdalar[15,78,80,97,99] and hippocampal[15,17,91] kindling, we have found a very limited sprouting restricted to the inner molecular layer (IML) of the dentate gyrus in animals kindled in the piriform cortex only once per day. In a related demonstration, Ebert and Loscher[27] reported that mossy fiber sprouting was only reliably induced by a rapid amygdala kindling procedure, whereas kindling with one stimulation per day produced no sprouting. Once again, the timing is inconsistent with a critical role for this form of sprouting. The piriform cortex kindles very rapidly, and spontaneous inter-ictal spikes develop even more quickly[76]. With three Hz stimulation, kindling can apparently be completed within minutes[24] (see also Corcoran et

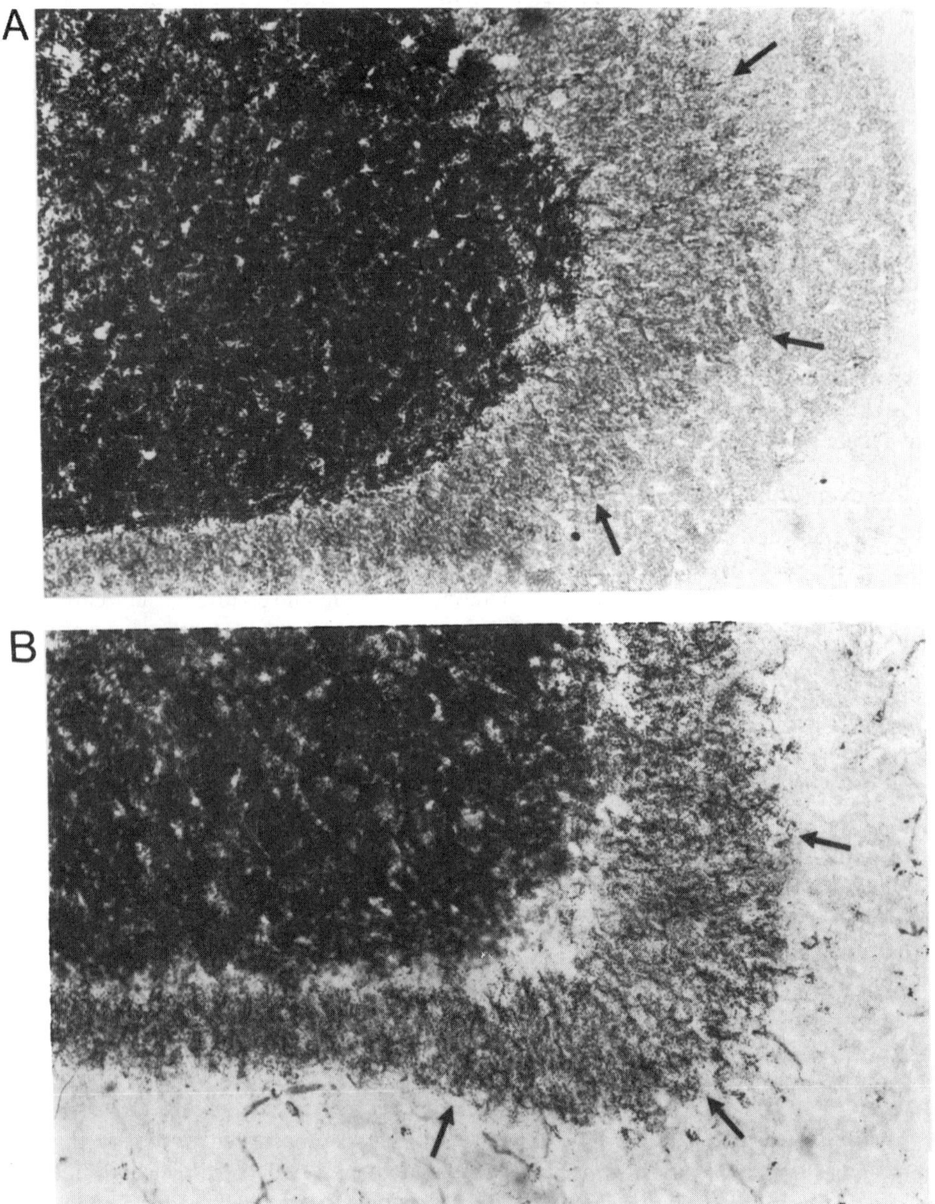

Figure 2. The Timm density in the inner molecular layer of the dentate gyrus is shown for a non-kindled animal (A) and a kindled animal (B). Fingers of Timm granules are often seen extending into this region as well, but nearly all animals show an increased density in this band (arrows) with kindling. This is generally interpreted as evidence for enhanced mossy fiber spouting back into the molecular layer of the dentate gyrus.

al., this volume). These developments in epileptogenesis are too rapid to be accounted for by the usual forms of sprouting. Finally, Sperber[88] reported that kainic acid-induced seizures, which reliably trigger sprouting in adult rats, do not trigger mossy fiber sprouting in immature rats (see also Hass et al., this volume).

Using neurotrophin manipulations, we have found that NGF infusions promote both kindling and sprouting, which is consistent with a sprouting mechanism for kindling. However, BDNF infusions retard kindling without affecting sprouting[50]. In ongoing experiments, we have replicated these effects of BDNF infusion on kindling and have also found a trend towards increased sprouting in the infused animals. If this holds up with further testing, then this will provide another dissociation between mossy fiber sprouting and kindling.

3.4. Sprouting and Inhibition

If mossy fiber sprouting cannot readily account for developing epileptogenesis, perhaps Sloviter[87] is correct when he suggests that sprouting accounts for the recovering inhibition that is often seen in seizure models. Here again, however, the timing doesn't alway fit. The recovering and/or increasing inhibition that we have found in several models of epilepsy can develop quite rapidly. The only thing that slows it down, or rather blocks its appearance, is the presence of spontaneous discharge, which, as we have pointed out, produces a transient failure in inhibition. Sprouting requires more time to appear and to reach asymptotic levels. Also, sprouting appears to be quite long-lasting[15], while the *augmented* inhibition seen in some seizure models decays back to baseline levels with a time-course similar to that of LTP decay[22,88]. In fact, prior attempts to establish the functional significance of sprouting suggest that it affects excitatory rather than inhibitory transmission[20].

3.5. Cell Loss and Sprouting

Perhaps one of the most interesting questions about kindling-induced sprouting is whether it is triggered by cell loss or is purely activity-dependent. If it is activity-dependent, then it becomes an interesting phenomenon in its own right, and one which may prove to be important in the study of CNS plasticity.

Several investigators have assumed that sprouting, in seizure models, is triggered by cell loss, particularly hilar cell loss (e.g. [13,17,92]). It now seems clear, however, that mossy fiber sprouting can occur without hilar cell loss. For example, Spiller and Racine (in preparation) have found that kindling of the piriform cortex can induce mossy fiber sprouting into the inner molecular of the dentate gyrus in the absence of even the altered cell density or hilar volume changes described above. In addition, Adams et al. (submitted) have found that the infusion of nerve growth factor into the ventricles can significantly enhance mossy fiber sprouting into both area CA3 and the inner molecular layer of the dentate gyrus, while *reducing* the hilar cell density (or hilar volume) changes. Similarly, in collaboration with Z. Gombos, A. Spiller and W.M. Burnham (in preparation), we have found that repeated exposure to electroconvulsive shock can induce sprouting into both area CA3 and the inner molecular layer without producing any changes in hilar cell density. Finally, in another work in progress, M. Emonds, R.Racine and B. Adams have found that the induction of LTP in the dentate gyrus by perforant path stimulation is associated with sprouting in the mossy fiber system. We have not yet taken cell counts in the hilus in these sections, but it seems unlikely that there will be any cell loss detected.

Meberg et al.[58] reported that kainic acid aministration, which produced cell damage *and* seizure activity, triggered mRNA expression for the growth protein F1/GAP-43, while ibotenate administration, which produced damage *without* seizure activity, did not.

Chafetz et al.[19] found that the mutant mouse *stargazer* showed aberrant levels of neuropeptide Y in the mossy fibers following the development of seizure activity. There was no evidence of cell injury, suggesting that plasticity in this system is triggered by the bursting pattern of activation during seizure discharge. Whether these measures are related to enhanced mossy fiber sprouting remains to be seen.

Sundstrom et al.[90] found a delayed sprouting, but no damage, in the contralateral hippocampus following a unilateral intracerebroventricular injection of kainic acid. Sprouting was found in both the IML and in area CA3. The authors suggested that the seizure activity, rather than cell loss or denervation, might have triggered the sprouting.

In summary, these experiments all indicate that sprouting can be induced without detectable cell loss in the hilus of the dentate gyrus, and that hilar cell loss does not invariably lead to sprouting. It is possible, of course, that the critical cell losses are very small and not detectable with standard counting procedures. Another possibility is that the sprouting is triggered by a more subtle form of degeneration, such as the loss of synaptic connections into a potential target of the sprouting fibers. This seems unlikely in the case of LTP-induction, where no seizure activity has been induced, but it cannot be ruled out.

3.6. Inhibition and Epileptogenesis

The proposal, discussed above, that cell loss in the hilus of the dentate gyrus results in a reduced level of inhibition, raises the question of the role of dentate gyrus inhibition in epileptogenesis. It is possible that Sloviter's 24 hour stimulation procedure, which appears to produce an extensive and highly selective loss of cells in the hilus, may lead to some compromise in the local inhibitory mechanisms. Without further investigation of that preparation, the question cannot yet be answered. In most other experimental epilepsy preparations, however, the answer seems to be clear. In the kindling model, for example, we have found *increased*, rather than decreased, inhibition in the dentate gyrus whether we kindle to a standard criterion[22,94], to an additional 40 stage 5 convulsions[89], or to the point where spontaneous ictal seizures begin to appear[61] (see Figure 3). We have also found that inhibition can recover to higher than baseline levels, after an initial transient reduction, following the induction of status epilepticus by kainic acid[62].

Evidence for enhanced inhibition in the hippocampus has also been reported for cases of temporal lobe epilepsy in humans[43,95]. Taking all of these results together, it seems extremely unlikely that failure of inhibition in the dentate gyrus could account, even in part, for many cases of temporal lobe epilepsy. It is still possible that a failure of inhibition at other brain sites may account for a developing epileptogenesis. Inhibition does appear to be reduced in area CA1 of the hippocampus, and possibly in the amygdala, as a result of kindling. In our hands, however, most of the areas that we have tested in intact animals have shown enhanced inhibition. Furthermore, this enhancement is, itself, transient and decays back to baseline levels over a period of several weeks. Consequently, it also appears unlikely that the *enhanced* inhibition could account for epileptogenesis (e.g. via an augmentation of phasic activity).

4. CONCLUSIONS AND SUMMARY

We have addressed very specific, though influential, hypotheses in this paper, and our conclusions have largely been negative. We do not believe that the weight of evidence supports a causal role for hilar cell loss or mossy fiber sprouting in epileptogenesis. Nor do we believe that the mossy fiber sprouting is induced by neuronal loss, because we see no evidence of damage in our preparations. Similarly, the evidence does not support a causal role for either cell loss or sprouting in modulating the levels of inhibition in the

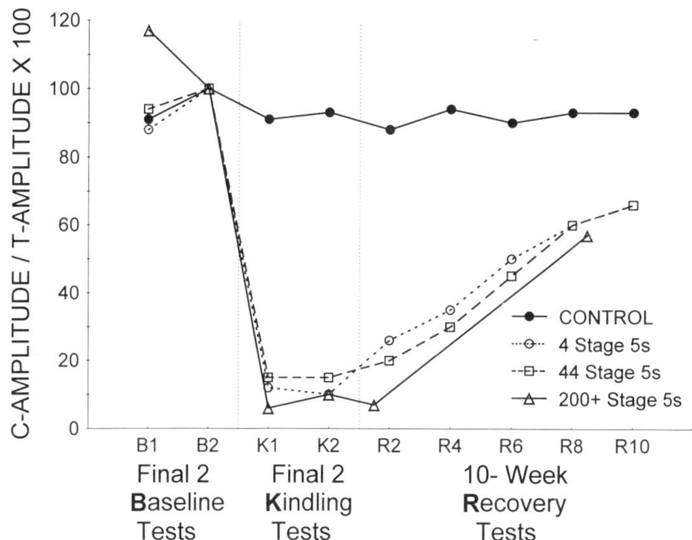

Figure 3. Kindling leads to an enhanced level of paired pulse depression in the dentate gyrus. This figure shows that extended kindling (to 44 stage 5 seizures) and kindling to the point at which the animals exhibit spontaneous seizures produce and maintain the same levels of enhanced inhibition. It also shows that this inhibition recovers at about the same rate back towards baselines levels even though the kindled state itself appears to be permanent. B1 and B2 represent baseline levels and all measures are standardized to the second baseline measure. K1 and K2 represent the final 2 kindling tests. R2-R10 represent paired pulse measures taken during a 10 week recovery period. These points are based primarily on measures taken from the experiments of Spiller and Racine (1994) and Ikeda-Douglas et al. (see text).

dentate gyrus. Finally, the evidence seems rather clear that most cases of increased epileptogenesis are accompanied by enhanced, rather than reduced, dentate gyrus inhibition. While more subtle relationships might still surface, such as a loss of synaptic terminals driving mossy fiber sprouting, such relationships remain to be demonstrated.

Even though mossy fiber sprouting is not likely to serve as a primary kindling mechanism, growth in some other system can not yet be ruled out. However, there is still the problem of timing. Most forms of sprouting develop relatively slowly, over several days. Massed stimulation, in contrast, can lead to an increased epileptogenesis within a few hours. Growth on a more subtle level, such as the restructuring of existing synapses (e.g. [34]), is still a possibility.

In any case, there are a large number of effects triggered by the kindling protocols, and many more are likely to be discovered. There is no compelling evidence in support of a primary role for any of these potential mechanisms, and it seems likely that multiple factors will eventually be found to contribute to epileptogenesis. Even this assertion, however, is purely speculative. This may seem like little progress after 30 years of intensive research on the kindling phenomenon, but the brain is extraordinarily complex, and we are dealing with a procedure that activates almost all of it.

REFERENCES

1. Babb, T.L., Brown, W.J., Pretorious, J., Davenport, C., Lieb, J.P. and Crandall, P.H., Temporal lobe volumetric cell densities in temporal lobe epilepsy, *Epilepsia*, 25 (1984) 729–740.

2. Barde, Y.-A., Edgar, D., and H. Thoenen, Purification of a new neurotrophic factor from mammalian brain, *EMBO J.*, *1* (1982) 549–553.
3. Ben-Ari, Y., Limbic seizure and brain damage produced by kainic acid: mechanisms and relevance to human temporal lobe epilepsy, *Neurosci.*, 14 (1985) 375–403.
4. Ben-Ari, Y., Krnjevic, K., and Reinhardt, W., Hippocampal seizures and failure of inhibition, *Canadian J. Psychol.*, 57 (1979) 1462–1466.
5. Ben-Ari, Y., and Represa, A., Brief seizure episodes induce long-term potentiaiton and mossy fibre sprouting in the hippocampus, *Trends in Neurosci.*, 13 (1990) 312–318.
6. Bengzon, J., Söderström, S., Kokaia, Z., Kokaia, M., Ernfors, P., Persson, H., Ebendal, T. and Lindvall, O., Widespread increase of nerve growth factor protein in the rat forebrain after kindling-induced seizures, *Brain Res.*, 587 (1992) 338–342,
7. Bengzon, J., Kokaia, Z., Ernfors, P., Kokaia, M., Leanza, G., Nilsson, O.G., Persson, H., and Lindvall, O., Regulation of neurotrophin and trkA, trkB and trkC tyrosine kinase receptor messenger RNA expression in kindling, *Neurosci.*, 53 (1993) 433–446.
8. Berkemeier, L.R., Winslow, J.W., Kaplan, D.R., Nikolics, K., Goeddel, D.V., and Rosenthal, A., Neurotrophin-5: a novel neurotrophic factor that activats trk and trkB, *Neuron*, 7 (1991) 857–866.
9. Bertram, E.H. and Lothman, E.W., Morphometric effects of intermittent kindled seizures and limbic status epilepticus in the dentate gyrus of the rat, *Brain Res.*, 603 (1993) 25–31.
10. Bradshaw, R.A., Blundell, T.L., Lapatto, R., McDonald, N.Q., and Murray-Rust, J., Nerve growth factor revisited, *Trends Biochem. Sci.*, 18 (1993) 48–52.
11. Buckan, A.M., Williams, L. And Bruederlin, B., Nerve growth factor: pretreatment ameliorates ischemic hippocampal neuronal injury, *Stroke*, 21 (1990) 177–181.
12. Callahan, P.M., Paris, J.M., Cunningham, K.A. and Shinnick-Gallagher, P., Decrease of GABA-immunoreactive neurons in the amygdala after electrical kindling in the rat, *Brain Res.*, 555 (1991) 335–339.
13. Cantallops, I. and Routtenberg, A., Rapid induction by kainic acid of axonal growth and F1/GAP-43 protein in the adult rat hippocampal granule cells, *J. Comp. Neurol.*, 366 (1996) 303–319.
14. Cavazos, J.E., Das, I. and Sutula, T.P., Neuronal loss induced in limbic pathways by kindling: evidence for induction of hippocampal sclerosis by repeated brief seizures, *J. Neurosci.*, 14 (1994) 3106–3121.
15. Cavazos, J.E., Golarai, G. and Sutula, T.P., Mossy fiber synpatic reorganization induced by kindling: time course of development, progression, and permanence, *J. Neurosci.*, 11 (1991) 2798–2803.
16. Cavazos, J.E., Golarai, G. and Sutula, T.P., Septotemporal variation of the supragranular projection of the mossy fiber pathway in the dentate gyrus of normal and kindled rats, *Hippocampus*, 2 (1992) 363–372.
17. Cavazos, J.E. and Sutula, T.P., Progressive neuronal loss induced by kindling: a possible mechanism for mossy fiber synaptic reorganization and hippocampal sclerosis, *Brain Res.*, 527 (1990) 1–6.
18. Cellerino, A., Expression of messenger RNA coding for the nerve growth factor receptor trkA in the hippocampus of the adult rat, *Neurosci.*, 70, (1995) 613–616.
19. Chafetz, R.S., Nahm, W.K. and Noebels, J.L., Aberrant expression of neuropeptide Y in hippocampal mossy fibers in the absence of local cell injuiry following the onset of spike-wave synchronization, *Mol. Brain Res.*, 31 (1995) 111–121.
20. Cronin, J., Obenaus, A., Houser, C.R. and Dudek, F.E., Electrophysiology of dentate granule cells after kainate-induced synaptic reorganization of mossy fibers, *Brain Res.*, 573 (1992) 305–310.
21. Dam, A.M., Epilepsy and neuron loss in hippocampus, *Epilepsia*, 21 (1980) 617–629.
22. de Jonge, M. and Racine, R.J., The development and decay of kindling-induced increases in paired-pulse depression in the dentate gyrus, *Brain Res.*, 412 (1987) 318–328.
23. Diamond, J., Coughlin, M., Macintyre, L., Holmes, M., and Visheau, B., Evidence that endogenous B-nerve growth factor is responsible for the collateral sprouting but not the regeneration of nociceptive axons in adult rats, *Proc. Natl. Acad. Sci. U.S.A.*, 84 (1987) 6596–6600.
24. Dennison, Z., Teskey, G.C. and Cain, D.P., Persistence of kindling: effect of partial kindling, retention interval, kindling site, and stimulation parameters, *Epilepsy Res.*, 21 (1995) 171–182.
25. Douglas, R.M., and Goddard, G.V., Long-term potentiation of the perforant path-granule cell synapse in the rat hippocampus, *Brain Res.*, 86 (1975) 205–215.
26. Dugich-Djordevic, M.M., Tocco, G., Willoughby, D.A., Najm, I., Pasinetti, G., Thompson, R.F., Baudry, M., Lapchak, P.A. and Hefti, F., BDNF mRNA expression in the developing rat brain following kainic acid-induced seizure activity, *Neuron*, 8 (1992) 1127–1138.
27. Ebert, U. And Loscher, W., Differences in mossy fibre sprouting during conventional and rapid amygdala kindling of the rat, *Neurosci. Lett.*, 190 (1995) 199–202.
28. Ernfors, P., Bengzon, J., Kokaia, Z., Persson, H. and Lindvall, O., Increased levels of messenger RNAs for neurotrophic factors in the brain during kindling epileptogenesis, *Neuron*, 7 (1991) 165–176.

29. Ernfors, P., Wetmore, C., Olson, L., and Persson, H., Identification of cells in rat brain and peripheral tissues experessing mRNA for members of the nerve growth factor family, *Neuron*, 5 (1990) 511–526.
30. Fahnestock, M., Structure and biosynthesis of nerve growth factor, *Current Topics Microbiol. Immunol.*, 165 (1991) 1–26.
31. Falconer, M.A., Mesial temporal (Ammon's horn) sclerosis as a common cause of epilepsy-etiology, treatment and prevention, *Lancet* (1974) September 28 (1974) 767–770.
32. Funabashi, T., Sasaki, H., and Kimura, F., Intraventricular injection of antiserum to nerve growth factor delays the development of amygdaloid kindling, *Brain Res.*, 458 (1988) 132–136.
33. Gall, C.M. and Isackson, P.J., Limbic seizures increase neuronal production of messenger RNA for nerve growth factor, *Science*, 245 (1989) 758–761.
34. Geinisman, Y., Morrell, F. and deToledo-Morrell, L., Increase in the relative proportion of perforated axospinous synapses following hippocampal kindling is specific for the synaptic field of stimulated axons, *Brain Res.*, 507 (1990) 325–331.
35. Gloor, P., Mesial temporal sclerosis: historical background and overview from a modern perspective. In: Luders, H. (ed.) *Epilepsy surgery*, New York, Raven Press, 1991, pp 689–703.
36. Goddard, G.V., Development of epileptic seizures through brain stimulation at low intensity, *Nature*, 214 (1967) 1020–1021.
37. Goddard, G.V., McIntrye, D.C. and Leech, C.K., A permanent change in brain function resulting form daily electrical stimulation, *Exp. Neurol.*, 25 (1969) 295–330.
38. Gotz, R., Koster, R., Winkler, C., Raulf, F., Lottspeich, F., Schartl, M., and Thoenen, H., Neurotrophin-6 is a new member of the nerve growth factor family, *Nature*, 372 (1994) 266–268.
39. Hallbook, F., Ibanez, C. F., and Persson, H., Evolutionaary studies of the nerve growth factor family reveal a novel member abundantly expressed in Xenopus ovary, *Neuron*, 6 (1991) 845.
40. Hohn, A., Leibrock, J., Bailey, K., and Barde, Y.-A., Identification and characterization of a novel member of the nerve growth factor/brain-derived neurotophic factor famil,. *Nature*, 344 (1990) 339–341.
41. Hughes, P. and Dragunow, M., Muscarinic receptor-mediated induction of Fos protein in rat brain, *Neurosci. Lett.*, 150 (1993) 122–126.
42. Ip, N.Y., Ibanez, C.F., Nye, S.H., McClain, J., Jones, P.F., Gies, D.R., Belluscio, L., Le Beau, M.M., Espinosa, R. III, Squinto, S.P., Persson, H., and Yancopoulos, G.D., Mammalian neurotrophin-4, structure, chromosomal localization, tissue distribution, and receptor specificity, *Proc. Natl. Acad. Sci. U.S.A.*, 89 (1992) 3060–3064.
43. Isokawa-Akesson, M., Wilson, C.L, and Babb, T.L., Inhibition in synchronously firing human hippocampal neurons, *Epilepsy Res.*, 3 (1989) 236–247.
44. Kairiss, E.W., Racine, R.J. and Smith, G.K., The development of the interictal spike during kindling in the rat, *Brain Res.*, 322 (1984) 101–110.
45. Kelly, M.E., and McIntyre, D.C., The effects of piriform and perirhinal cortex damage on convulsive seizures in kindled rats. *Epilepsia*, 36, (suppl. 4) (1995) p87.
46. Kim, J.H., Guimaraes, P.O., Shen, M.Y., Masukawa, L.M. and Spencer, D.D., Hippocampal neuronal density in temporal lobe epilepsy with and without gliomas, *Acta Neuropathol.,* 80 (1990) 41–45.
47. King, G.L., Dingledine, R., Giacchino, J.L. and McNamara, J.O., Abnormal neuronal excitability in hippocampal slices from kindled rats, *J. Neurophysiol.*, 54 (1985) 1295–1304.
48. Khurgel, M., Racine, R.J. and Ivy, G.O., Kindling causes changes in the composition of the astrocytic cytoskeleton, *Brain Res.*, 592 (1992) 338–342.
49. Khurgel, M., Ivy, G.O. and Racine, R.J. Seizure-induced activation of astrocytes in the absence of neuronal degeneration. *Neurobiology of Disease,* 2 (1995) 23–35.
50. Larmet, Y., Reibel, S., Carnahan, J., Nawa, H., Marescaux, C. And Depaulis, A., Protective effects of brain-derived neurotrophic factor on the development of hippocampal kindling in the rat, *Neuroreport*, 6 (1995) 1937–1941.
51. Leibrock, J., Lottspeich, F., Hohn, A., Hofer, M., Hengerer, B., Masiakowski, P., Thoenen, H. and Barde, Y.-A., Molecular cloning and expression of brain-derived neurotrophic factor, *Nature*, 341 (1989) 149–152.
52. Levi-Montalcini, R., The nerve growth factor 35 years later, *Science*, 237 (1987) 1154–1162.
53. Maisonpierre, P.C., Belluscio, L., Squinto, S., Ip, N., Furth, M.E., Lindsay, R.M., and Yancopoulos, G.D., Neurotrophin-3: a neurotrophic factor related to NGF and BDNF, *Science,* 247 (1990) 1446–1451.
54. Margerison, J.H. and Corsellis, J., Epilepsy and the temporal lobes, *Brain*, 89 (1966) 499–530.
55. McIntyre, D.C., Nathanson, D. and Edson, N., A new model of partial status epilepticus based on kindling, *Brain Res.*, 250 (1982) 53–63.
56. McIntyre, D.C. and Plant, J.R., Pyriform cortex involvement in kindling, *Neurosci. BioBehav. Rev.*, 13 (1989) 277–280.

57. McIntyre, D.C., and Wong, R.K.S., Cellular and synaptic properties of amygdala-kindled pyriform cortex in vitro, *J. Neurophysiol.*, 55 (1986) 1295–1307.
58. Meberg, P.J., Jarrard, L.E., Routtenberg, A., Is the lack of protein F1/GAP-43 mRNA in granule cells target-dependent? *Brain Res.*, 706 (1996) 217–226.
59. Merlio, J.-P., Ernfors, P., Kokaia, Z, Middlemas, D.S., Bengzon, J., Kokaia, M., Smith, M.-L., Siesjö, B.K., Hunter, T., Lindvall, O., and Persson, H., Increased production of the TrkB protein tyrosine kinase receptro after brain insults, *Neuron*, 10 (1993) 151–164.
60. Milgram, N.W., Green, I., Siberman, M., Riexinger, K. and Petit, T.L., Establishment of status epilepticus by limbic system stimulation in previously unstimulated rats, *Exp. Neurol.*, 88 (1985) 253–264.
61. Milgram, N.W., Michael, M., Cammisuli, S., Head, E., Ferbinteanu, J., Reid, C., Murphy, M.P., and Racine, R., Development of spontaneous seizures over extended electrical kindling. II. Persistence of dentate inhibitory suppression, *Brain Res.*, 670 (1995) 112–120.
62. Milgram, N.W., Yearwood, T., Khurgel, M., Ivy, G.O. and Racine, R., Changes in inhibitory processes in the hippocampus following recurrent seizures induced by systemic administration of kainic acid, *Brain Res.*, 551 (1991) 236–246.
63. Mitchell, C.L., and Barnes, M.I., Effect of destruction of dentate granule cells on kindling induced by stimulation of the perforant path, *Physiol. Behav.*, 53 (1993) 45–49.
64. Mouritzen-Dam, A., Epilepsy and neuron loss in the hippocampus, *Epilepsia*, 21 (1980) 617–629.
65. Nadler, J., Cuthbertson, G., Kainic acid neurotoxicity toward the hippocampal formation: dependence on specific excitatory pathways, *Brain Res.*, 195 (1980) 47–56.
66. Nawa, H., Carnahan, J. and Gall, C., BDNF protein measured by a novel enzyme immunoassay in normal brain and after seizure: partial disagreement with mRNA levels, *Eur. J. Neurosci.*, 7 (1995) 1527–1535.
67. O'Connor, W.M., Masukawa, L., Freese, A., Sperling, M.R., French, J.A. and O'Connor, M.J., Hippocampal cell distributions in temporal lobe epilepsy: a comparison between patients with and without an early risk factor, *Epilepsia*, 37 (1996) 440–449.
68. Phillips, H.S., Hains, J.M., Laramee, G.R., Rosenthal, A., and Winslow, J.W., Widespread expression of BDNF but not NT3 by target areas of basal forebrain cholinergic neurons, *Science*, 250 (1990) 290–294.
69. Qiao, X. and Noebels, J.L., Developmental analysis of hippocampal mossy fiber outgrowth in a mutant mouse with inherited spike-wave seizures, *J. Neurosci.*, 13 (1993) 4622–4635.
70. Racine, R.J., Modification of seizure activity by electrical stimulation: II. Motor seizure, *Electroenceph. Clin. Neurophysiol.*, 32 (1972) 281–294.
71. Racine, R.J., Burnham, W.M., Gilbert, M., and Kairiss, E.W., Kindling mechanisms: I. Electrophysiological studies, In Wada, J.A. (ed.)*Kindling 3*, Raven Press, New York, 1986, pp 263–282.
72. Racine, R.J., Chapman, C.A., Teskey, G.C., and Milgram, N.W., Post-activation potentiation in the neocortex. III. Kindling-induced potentiation in the chronic preparation, *Brain Res.*, 702 (1995) 77–86.
73. Racine, R.J., Gartner, J.G. and Burnham, W.M., Epileptiform activity and neural plasticity in limbic structures, *Brain Res.*, 47 (1972) 262–268.
74. Racine, R.J., Milgram, W.N., and Hafner, S., Long-term potentiation phenomena in the rat limbic forebrain, *Brain Res.*, 260 (1983) 217–231.
75. Racine, R.J., Moore, K.-A., and Evans, C., Kindling-induced potentiation in the piriform cortex, *Brain Res.*, 556 (1991) 218–225.
76. Racine, R.J., Mosher, M., and Kairiss, E.W., The role of the pyriform cortex in the generation of interictal spikes in the kindled preparation, *Brain Res.*, 454 (1988) 251–263.
77. Racine, R.J., Newberry, F., and Burnham, W.M., Post-activation potentiation and the kindling phenomenon, *Electroencephalgr. Clin. Neurophysiol.*, 39 (1975) 261–271.
78. Rashid, K., Van der Zee, C.E.E.M., Ross, G.M., Chapman, C.A., Stanisz, J., Riopelle, R.J., Racine, R.J. and Fahnestock, M., A nerve growth factor peptide retards seizure development and inhibits neuronal sprouting in a rat model of epilepsy, *Proc. Natl. Acad. Sci. USA.*, 92 (1995) 9495–9499.
79. Rainnie, D.G., Asprodini, E.K. and Shinnick-Gallagher, P., Kindling-induced long-lasting changes in synaptic transmission in the basolateral amygdala, *J. Neurophysiol.*, 67 (1992) 443–454.
80. Represa A. and Ben-Ari Y., Kindling is associated with the formation of novel mossy fibre synapses in the CA3 region, *Exp. Brain Res.*, 92 (1992) 69–78.
81. Rosenthal, A., Goeddel, D.V., Nguyen, T., Lewis, M., Shih, A., Laramee, G.R., Nikolics, K., and Winslow, J.W., Primary structure and biological activity of a novel human neurotophic factor, *Neuron*, 4 (1990) 767–773.
82. Russell, R.D., and Stripling, J.S., Effect of olfactory bulb kindling on evoked potentials in the piriform cortex, *Brain Res.*, 361 (1985) 61–69.
83. Sagar, H.J. and Osbury, J.M., Hippocampal neuron loss in temporal lobe epilepsy: correlation with early childhood convulsions, *Ann. Neurol.*, 22 (1987) 334–340.

84. Shigeno, T., Mima, T. Takakura, K., Graham, I., Kato, G., Hashimoto, Y. And Furukawa, S., Amelioration of delayed neuronal death in the hippocampus by nerve growth factor, *J. Neurosci.*, 11 (1991) 2114–2119.
85. Shirasaka, Y., and Wasterlain, C.G., Chronic epileptogenicity following focal status epilepticus, *Brain Res.*, 655 (1994) 33–44.
86. Sloviter, R.S., Permanently altered hippocampal structure, excitability, and inhibition after experimental status epilepticus in the rat: the "dormant basket cell" hypothesis and its possible relevance to temporal lobe epilepsy, *Hippocampus*, 1 (1991) 41–66.
87. Sloviter, R.S., Possible functional consequences of synaptic reorganization in the dentate gyrus of kainate-treated rats, *Neurosci. Lett.*, 137 (1992) 91–96.
88. Sperber, E.F., Age dependency of seizure-induced hippocampal dysfunction, in Wolf, P. (ed.) *Epileptic seizures and syndromes*, Hohan Libbey & Co., 1994, pp 469–480.
89. Spiller, A. E., and Racine, R.J., The effect of kindling beyond the 'stage 5' criterion on paired-pulse depression and hilar cell counts in the dentate gyrus, *Brain Res.*, 635 (1994) 139–147.
90. Sundstrom, L.E., Mitchell, J. And Wheal, H.V., Bilateral reorganization of mossy fibers in the rat hippocampus after a unilateral introcerebroventricular kainic acid injection, *Brain Res.*, 609 (1993) 321–326.
91. Sutula, T., Xiao-Xian, H., Cavazos, J. and Scott, G., Synaptic reorganization in the hippocampus induced by abnormal functional activity, *Science*, 239 (1988) 1147–1150.
92. Tauck, D.L., and Nadler, J.V., Evidence of functional mossy fiber sprouting in hippocampal formation of kainic acid treated rats, *J. Neurosci.*, 5 (1985) 1016–1022.
93. Timmusk, T., Belluardo, N., Metsis, M. And Persson, H., Widespread and developmentally regulated expression of neurotrophin-4 mRNA in rat brain and peripheral tissues, *Eur. J. Neurosci.*, 5 (1993) 605–613.
94. Tuff, L.P., Racine, R.J., and Adamec, R., The effects of kindling on GABA-mediated inhibition in the dentate gyrus of the rat: I. Paired pulse depression, *Brain Res.*, 277 (1983) 79–90.
95. Uruno, K., O'Connor, M.J., and Masukawa, L.M., Effects of bicuculline and baclofen on paired-pulse depression in the dentate gyrus of epileptic patients, *Brain Res.*, 695 (1995) 163–172.
96. Van der Zee, C.E.E.M., Fawcett, J. and Diamond, J., Antibody to NGF inhibitis collateral sprouting of septohippocampal fibers following entorhinal cortex lesion in adult rats, *J. Comp. Neurol.*, 326 (1992) 91–100.
97. Van der Zee, C.E.E.M., Lourenssen, S., Stanisz, J. and Diamond J., NGF-deprivation of adult rat brain results in cholinergic hypofunction and selctive impairment in spatial learning, *Eur. J. Neurosci.*, 7 (1995) 160–168.
98. Van der Zee, C.E.E.M., Rashid, K., Lee, K., Moore, K.-A., Stanisz, J., Diamond, J., Racine, R.J. and Fahnestock, M., Intraventricular administration of antibodies to nerve growth factor retards kindling and blocks mossy fiber sprouting in adult rats, *J. Neurosci.*, 15 (1995) 5316–5323.
99. Watanabe, Y., Johson, R.S., Butler, L.S., Binder, D.K., Spiegelman, B.M., Papaioannou, V.E., McNamara, J.O., Null mutation of c-fos impairs structural and functional plasticities in the kindling model of epilepsy, *J. Neurosci.*, 16 (1996) 3827–3836.
100. Whittemore, S.R., Ebendal, T., Larkfors, L., Olson, L., Seiger, A., Stromberg, I., and Persson, H., Development and regional expression of beta nerve growth factor messenger RNA and protein in the rat central nervous system, *Proc. Natl. Acad. Sci. USA*, 83 (1986) 817–821.
101. Yamamori, T., Molecular mechanisms for generation of neural diversity and specificity: roles of polypeptide factors in development of post-mitotic neurons, *Neurosci. Res.*, 12 (1992) 545–582.
102. Yamamoto, S., Yoshimine, T., Fujita, T., Kuroda, R., Irie, T., Fujioka, K. And Hayakawa, K., Protective effect of NGF ategollagen mini-pellet on hippocampal delayed neuronal death in gerbils, *Neurosci. Lett.*, 141 (1992) 161–165.
103. Zhao, D. And Leung, L.S., Hippocampal kindling induced paired-pulse depression in the dentate gyrus and paired-pulse facilitation in CA3, *Brain Res.*, 582 (1992) 163–167.

DISCUSSION OF RON RACINE'S PAPER

M. Burnham: All these years you've been looking for basic mechanism of kindling and all these years you keep finding that its not anything. Do you have any feelings about what it is?

R. Racine: Yes, well I think that the talk by Patricia Schinnick-Gallagher this morning was one of the ones that interested me most. My own feeling is that there are lots of different mechanisms contributing to kindling. Potentiation is clearly one of them; it is contributing to propagation, it has to, but is not critical. If there is anything that is critical I suspect that it is a change in the intrinsic bursting properties of cells. That is what I suspect is where the mechanism is going to be discovered.

R. Adamec: Could you review your evidence that kindling primarily increases inhibition.

R. Racine: We have looked in the amygdala, piriform cortex, the entorhinal cortex, and several other areas. In our hands, using our kindling procedure, we get increased inhibition in every one of those areas. The only area we have ever found decreased inhibition in is CA1.

P. Shinnick-Gallagher: Could you explain how you measure inhibition in your paired-pulse depression?

R. Racine: We use paired-pulse measures in the standard way, depending upon what the response is. For example, in hippocampus we'd be looking at both the EPSP and the pop-spike ratios. We also use triple pulse measures, so we keep the test pulse constant and we vary the conditioning pulse for example. We often use trains of pulses as well, as Bob Sloviter does. So we use a lot of different field potential measures of inhibition.

P. Shinnick-Gallagher: So you're measuring the amplitude of the first EPSP population spike as a function of the second?

R. Racine: The second as a function of the first.

P. Shinnick-Gallagher: So when you say that paired-pulse depression is enhanced, do you mean that the second pulse is greater?

R. Racine: The second response is smaller than the first response.

F. Lopes da Silva: Do you measure that over time or only at one point?

R. Racine: All of our work is chronic; so we're usually measuring over weeks or months.

F. Lopes da Silva: No, no, at the time that you do it, do you change the interval between the paired-pulses?

R. Racine: Yes, we typically go out to about 1000 msec, sometimes 2000.

F. Lopes da Silva: And do you see suppression throughout the three stages—throughout the whole thing?

R. Racine: When I'm talking about decreased inhibition, I'm usually talking about the early inhibition that is probably recurrent. Sometimes we see an increase in the inhibition in the late phase as well, but not always.

P. Shinnick-Gallagher: Why is it inhibition?

R. Racine: Why isn't it inhibition?

P. Shinnick-Gallagher: It could be just a depletion of transmitter release.

R. Racine: We know it's not a depletion of transmitter release because these things can follow for enormously long periods of time with fairly high rates; so it can't be transmitter depletion. In the few forebrain systems that have been studied, I think the amount of transmitter released at a terminal is actually a very small amount of the pool available. So transmitter depletion is not very likely.

P. Engel: You've used GABA agonists and antagonists to manipulate inhibition?

R. Racine: Yes we have, but that doesn't get directly at the transmitter depletion issue.

O. Lindvall: I had questions related to the role of the neurotrophins. The increases that we see are important to protect cells, and that could be one reason why we don't see more cell loss or cell death than you have seen. We have also counted cells in all our mice and we have never seen any cell loss. Then the role of the neurotrophins is perhaps not to regulate sprouting but to regulate excitability. They can change excitability in a very profound way, which can be important perhaps not for the permanence of the kindling phenomenon but could be important for the establishment of kindling.

R. Racine: There have been transient changes in the excitability demonstrated with neurotrophins. Our infusions are long-term, via osmotic pumps, implanted pumps, so that we infuse NGF, anti-NGF, BDNF, and so on, over a long period of time. That has somewhat different effects, probably, in terms of the direct effects on excitability.

16

DISSOCIATIONS BETWEEN KINDLING AND MOSSY FIBER SPROUTING

Michael E. Corcoran, Lisa L. Armitage, Darren K. Hannesson, Elaine M. Jenkins, and Paul Mohapel

Department of Psychology
University of Victoria
Victoria, British Columbia V8W 3P5, Canada

1. INTRODUCTION

One of the most provocative hypotheses about the mechanisms of kindling has been Sutula's proposal[21] that epileptogenesis involves establishment of aberrant recurrent excitatory circuits in the dentate gyrus (DG). The mossy fibers of dentate granule cells contain zinc, which can be visualized in appropriately prepared sections using the Timm stain. Temporal lobe biopsies from patients with epilepsy and various preparations of experimental epilepsy in animals[21] show evidence of enhanced Timm staining in the inner molecular layer (IML) of the DG, and this is taken as evidence for the sprouting of axon collaterals from the mossy fibers that innervate cells in or near the IML. Sutula's group has shown that kindling from multiple sites is associated with enhanced Timm staining in the IML[4,22], and he has suggested that the sprouted fibers form aberrant excitatory synapses on dendrites of the granule cells[21]. Thus a positive feedback loop would be established that could increase excitatory synaptic drive and lead to the elaboration and propagation of ictal discharge characteristic of kindling.

The evidence that sprouting accompanies kindling is strong: Sutula and colleagues[4,22] found that kindling of three different limbic sites produced aberrantly located Timm granules in the supragranular molecular layer of the DG in rats killed 18 hr after a generalized stage 5 seizure. It was also evident after 10 or 12 perforant path afterdischarges (ADs), well before the development of generalized stage 5 seizures. They[4] demonstrated that the magnitude of aberrant Timm staining in the supragranular DG increased between 1 and 7 days after triggering of 5 ADs, which parallels the time course of sprouting of mossy fibers after hippocampal lesions, and reaches asymptote after about 40 ADs were triggered. Although the density of aberrant Timm staining decayed to control values during a nonstimulation interval following 5 perforant path ADs (presumably reflecting retraction or resorption of sprouted fibers), it persisted over intervals of 3 to 4 months

Kindling 5, edited by Corcoran and Moshé.
Plenum Press, New York, 1998.

after kindling of generalized seizures. Sutula and colleagues concluded that the increased Timm staining is probably due to sprouting of the mossy fibers and reactive synaptogenesis. They cited the correlation between sprouting and the duration of epileptic activity, and the persistence of the changes after completion of kindling, as evidence that sprouting of the mossy fibers or other limbic pathways plays an important role in the establishment and permanence of kindling. Represa and colleagues[17,18] confirmed that limbic kindling produces aberrant bilateral staining of Timm granules in the supragranular DG in Wistar rats. They also found that amygdaloid but not entorhinal kindling produced aberrant Timm granules in the infrapyramidal zone of field CA3. The sprouted fibers formed synapses with the basilar dendrites of CA3 pyramidal neurons that showed the typical features of mossy synapses in stratum lucidum, including complex giant spines[17].

Although the correlation between sprouting and kindling is impressive, there are some gaps in the data that preclude immediate acceptance of Sutula's model. For one, there is uncertainty as to what neurons are innervated by sprouted fibers. Sutula's original report[22] provided ultrastructural data from 4 rats indicated that the aberrantly located Timm granules were located in synaptic terminals, suggesting that sprouting and axonal reorganization were indeed involved, but the data did not indicate what type of cell (granule cells or interneurons) the Timm-labelled terminals were synapsing on. On the other hand, Represa's data[17,18] suggest that sprouted mossy fibers can form synapses with basilar dendrites of CA3 pyramidal neurons. Another possibility is suggested by the results of Ribak and Peterson[19], who examined the intragranular projections of the mossy fibers in seizure-sensitive and seizure-resistant gerbils and in normal Sprague-Dawley rats. They found that rats and both types of gerbil displayed a Timm-stained fiber plexus in the granule cell and IML of the DG. The intragranular fibers were associated with 3 of the 5 types of basket cell located at the hilar-granule cell border. Ultrastructurally, Timm-labelled axon terminals formed synapses with the cell bodies and apical dendrites of basket cells in the granular layer and with the aspiny dendrites of basket cells in the hilus, and there was no evidence of synapses with granule cell bodies. Thus Ribak and Peterson's results indicate that, under normal circumstances, some mossy fiber axons form recurrent circuits with basket cells in the granular layer and possibly in the IML. Because these axons synapse preferentially with basket cells in non-kindled animals, the sprouted mossy fibers described by Sutula et al.[22] after kindling might have formed synapses with basket cells.

There is also uncertainty about whether synapses formed by sprouted mossy fibers are functional. Potentially relevant information comes from a study by Sloviter[20], who examined the time course of changes in excitability and sprouting of the mossy fibers after subcutaneous injection of kainic acid in rats. He found that increased excitability and epileptiform responses were evident in the DG 3 days after kainic acid, at which time there was evidence of degeneration of hilar neurons and denervation of the IML but no sign of sprouting. Rats that failed to display loss of hilar neurons showed normal feedforward and recurrent inhibition, whereas rats with extensive bilateral loss of hilar neurons displayed obvious loss of feedforward and recurrent inhibition. When tested 2 months later, recurrent inhibition had recovered in the rats that had initially displayed loss of inhibition, correlated with dense sprouting of mossy fibers into the IML. Light microscopic analysis suggested that the sprouted mossy fibers were innervating the soma and dendrites of presumed basket cells in the granular layer and interneurons in the inner molecular layer. Sloviter[20] suggested that degeneration of hilar neurons denervates inhibitory neurons, disfacilitating them and leaving them "dormant," which in turn leads to loss of inhibition and development of epileptiform responses. Extensive denervation leads to sprouting of the mossy fibers, resulting in reinnervation of the dormant inhibitory neurons and restoration of recurrent inhibition. Sloviter's data clearly indicate that, in kainate-treated rats, epileptogenesis and decreased inhibition precede sprouting of the mossy fibers.

One approach to understanding the functional significance of sprouting is to examine further the correlation or association between sprouting and kindling, to determine the boundaries of the relation. For example, Racine, Fahnestock, and colleagues have examined the effects of drugs that interfere with the actions of nerve growth factor (NGF) and found that sprouting and kindling are both suppressed by infusions of drugs that block the actions of NGF.[16,23] We have taken a similar tack in our research, and unexpectedly discovered evidence for *dissociations* between sprouting and kindling.

2. SPROUTING AND KINDLING AFTER TRANSECTION OF THE FIMBRIA-FORNIX

Our first series of experiments involved an attempt to examine the effects of transections of the fimbria-fornix (FF) on kindling and kindling-induced sprouting in rats. The experiment was prompted by the observation[3] that interictal discharge (IID) develops in the hippocampal formation within about 3 weeks of transection of the FF. We predicted that FF transection would facilitate kindling and wondered what effect it would have on kindling-induced sprouting.

Bilateral transection of the FF was produced via surgical insertion of a microscalpel[8], and postmortem histological examination indicated that in all cases the transections involved complete severing of the dorsal fornix and extensive damage to the fimbria bilaterally, with occasional sparing of the ventrolateral tips of the fimbria. Control rats received sham insertion of the microscalpel. We implanted electrodes bilaterally into the perforant path (PP) 14 to 18 days after the transections, and postmortem histological examination indicated that electrode placements were distributed in the vicinity of the angular bundle in the subiculum bordering field CA1 and in the entorhinal cortex. Kindling with PP stimulation began about 28 days after the transection, at a time when IID is well established.[3] AD thresholds (ADT) were determined, and then seizures were kindled with once daily application of unilateral stimulation to the PP at stimulation 100 μA above threshold. After kindling of 6 stage 5 seizures from the primary site, stimulation was transferred to the secondary PP until 3 consecutive seizures were kindled. Twenty-four hr later the rats were killed, and horizontal sections of the brains were prepared with the neo-Timm stain to examine the density of sprouting in the IML of the dorsal hippocampus. Electrode placements and the extent of the FF transections were assessed from sections counterstained with cresyl violet. The time course of the effects of FF transection on mossy fiber sprouting was examined in other rats that were killed at various intervals after the transections, but the data will not be reported here.

Transection of the FF resulted in a significant decrease in ADT evoked by stimulation of the PP. As shown in Figure 1A, mean ADT in controls was 415.4 μA and in FF-transected rats was 171.9 μA ($p<0.05$). There were no significant differences in the duration of the first AD (controls, mean of 35.2 sec; transected, mean of 31.8 sec). In contrast to the effects of transections on ADT, significantly more ADs were required to kindle the first stage 5 seizure in FF-transected rats compared to controls (means of 28.2 and 19.3 ADs, respectively, $p<0.05$), as shown in Figure 1B. Significantly more ADs were also required to kindle 6 consecutive stage 5 seizures in transected rats than in controls (means of 31.0 and 20.1 ADs, respectively, $p<0.05$), although the difference in the number of ADs to 6 consecutive stage 5 seizures failed to reach statistical significance (means of 32.1 and

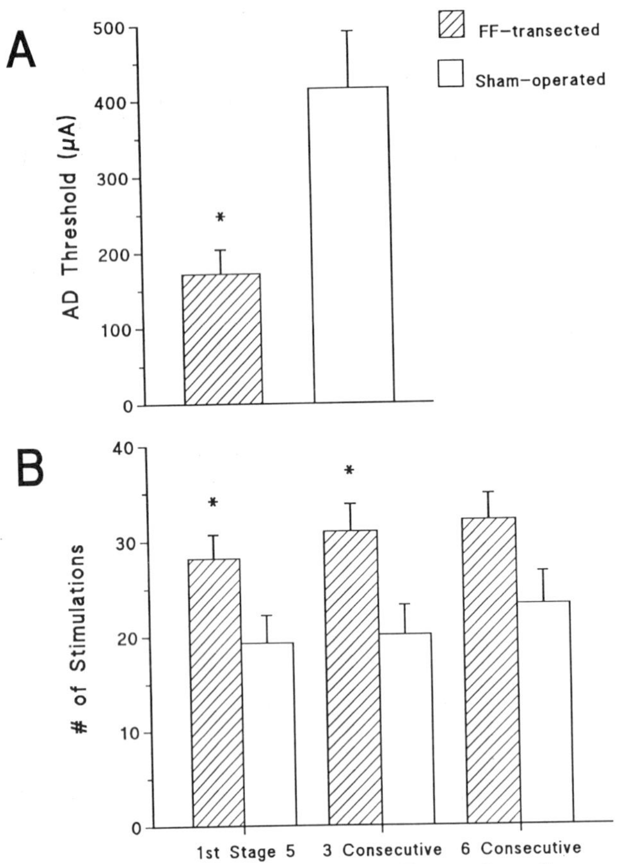

Figure 1. A, Mean (±SEM) ADT of FF-transected rats and sham-operated controls; B, Mean (±SEM) number of ADs required for kindling of stage 5 seizures in FF-transected rats and sham-operated controls. $^*p<0.05$.

23.2, respectively, $p=0.058$). We also measured the latency to and duration of clonus as well as the duration of the AD during the first 6 stage 5 seizures. Although the groups did not differ in latency to clonus, over the first 6 consecutive stage 5 seizures FF-transected rats showed significantly longer clonus (transected, 37.0 sec; controls, 27.4 sec; $p<0.01$) and AD (transected, 98.9 sec; controls, 89.5 sec; $p<0.01$) than controls (data not shown).

Three patterns of distribution of Timm granules were observed in rats in this study. Sham-operated controls (Figure 2A) that were not subjected to kindling displayed minimal levels of sprouting, occasionally appearing as isolated fascicles or patchy aggregations of Timm granules in the IML. Sham-operated controls subjected to kindling (Figure 2B) displayed moderate levels of sprouting, evident as Timm granules in a continuous yet patchy pattern observed in the supragranular region between tips an crests of the DG, distributed fairly evenly throughout the dorsal and ventral hippocampal formation. Unexpectedly, a similarly intermediate level of sprouting was displayed by FF-transected rats that were not subjected to kindling (Figure 2C), although sprouting in transected rats was evident mostly in the dorsal hippocampal formation. FF-transected rats subjected to kindling displayed a continuous and dense band of Timm granules that spanned into the IML and was consistent throughout the entire dorsal and ventral hippocampal formation (Figure 2D).

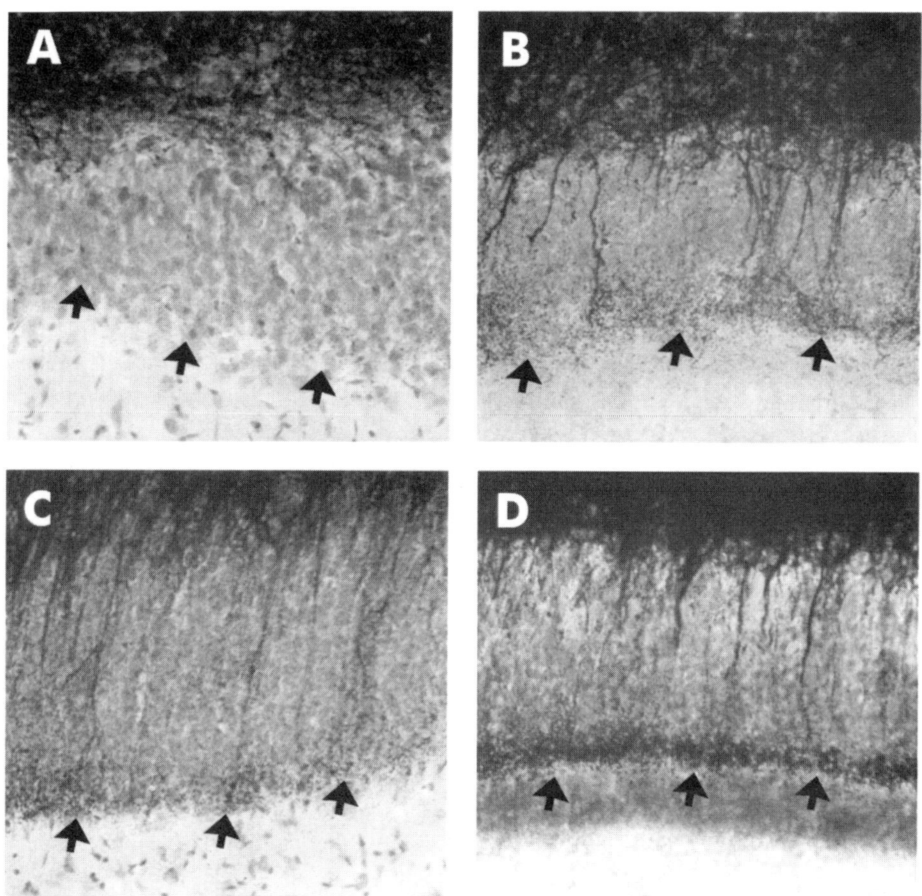

Figure 2. Representative examples of Timm staining in the IML of sham-operated control rats that were not kindled (A), sham-operated control rats that were kindled (B), FF-transected control rats that were not kindled (C), and FF-transected rats that were kindled (D).

Several aspects of the results of this study are worthy of comment. First, transection of the FF results in a moderate degree of sprouting. There is evidence[9,10] that receptors for NGF and other neurotrophins exist on cholinergic terminals in the hippocampus that project through the FF, and it would be reasonable to hypothesize that mossy fiber sprouting depends on NGF acting on these cholinergic terminals. This hypothesis leads to the clear prediction that transection of the FF should reduce or preclude the sprouting associated with kindling. In contrast to the prediction, we found that sprouting in kindled rats with FF transections exceeds sprouting in kindled controls or transected controls. Clearly mossy fiber sprouting does not require the presence of cholinergic or other fibers that project through the FF. Second, transection of the FF had mixed effects on PP kindling. ADTs were lower and ADs and clonus were longer in transected rats, but the kindling of convulsive seizures was delayed. Some fibers in the FF may inhibit AD and clonus, whereas others seem to be important for kindling itself.

Thus, notwithstanding the very dense sprouting seen after kindling in rats with FF transections, kindling was retarded. One interpretation of our results is that the sprouting induced by FF transection contributes to the local regulation of AD but not to the development of convulsive seizures, and it would be interesting to determine whether FF transection would affect AD and clonus provoked by kindling of sites other than the PP. Regardless of their implications for the mechanisms of regulation of AD, our findings seem to contradict Sutula's hypothesis[21] that kindling of convulsive seizures is due to establishment of aberrant excitatory synaptic connections consequent to sprouting of mossy fibers in the IML of the DG, and they highlight an apparent dissociation between kindling and mossy fiber sprouting. Interpretation of the dissociation is not conclusive, however, because it is possible, as noted above, that transection of the FF produces multiple effects that are incompatible: sprouting of the mossy fibers, an effect that could facilitate kindling or exacerbate AD; and interruption of the neural circuitry involved in elaboration of convulsive seizures, an effect that would delay kindling. We therefore turned to another paradigm, rapid amygdaloid kindling with low-frequency stimulation, to examine the relation between sprouting and kindling further.

3. SPROUTING AND RAPID (LOW-FREQUENCY) KINDLING

Seizures can be kindled very rapidly with long trains of low-frequency stimulation at high intensities[5,12,13]. Stimulation of the amygdala with trains at 3 pps results in development of stage 5 seizures after a mean of about 3 to 5 stimulations[5,12,13], well below the mean of ≥12 ADs with conventional stimulation at 60 pps, and in some cases results in first-trial generalized seizures. Because of the short time course of low-frequency kindling, it was not apparent a priori whether sprouting would be evident after this form of kindling. We therefore attempted to determine whether sprouting is associated with rapid kindling.

We implanted electrodes bilaterally into the basolateral amygdala of male Long-Evans rats. Ten days later, ADTs were assessed. Conventionally kindled rats received high-frequency amygdaloid stimulation once/24 hr at an intensity 100 μA above the ADT. Stimulation consisted of a 1-s train of square wave pulses at 60 pps, and rats were killed 24 hr after the first (HF1) or fifth (HF5) stage 5 seizure. The low-frequency group received amygdaloid stimulation once/24 hr at an intensity of 1000 μA. Stimulation consisted of a 60-s train of square-wave pulses at 3 pps, and rats were killed 24 hr after the first stage 5 seizure (LF1). Because of variability in staining, we felt that it was essential to yoke a control rat to each kindled rat. Controls carried electrodes and were handled but did not receive stimulation. Yoked experimental and control rats were killed and perfused together, and sections from yoked pairs of rats were stained together to control for variability in staining. The rats were killed with overdose of pentobarbital and perfused transcardially with sodium sulfide / formaldehyde solutions. We stained horizontal sections of the hippocampus (Bregma −3.60 to −4.10) with the neo-Timm stain for mossy fiber sprouting, and we stained coronal sections of the amygdala with cresyl violet to verify electrode placements.

With few exceptions[7,23], previous research examining mossy fiber sprouting after kindling has employed descriptive or qualitative techniques to characterize the extent of sprouting[4,17,18,22]. Because our pilot work had indicated that the magnitude of kindling-induced sprouting is often very modest, we felt that it was important to quantify sprouting more precisely. We therefore employed a computerized image analyzer to develop a technique for quantification of mossy fiber sprouting in the posterior supragranular layer of the DG, by creating a digitized image of hippocampal sections and comparing the luminance of the inner edge of the IML (proximal to the granular layer), where sprouting was evident, to the luminance of the outer edge of the IML (proximal to the middle molecular layer), which contained few if any Timm granules and was treated as background. The difference in luminance, within each section, was converted to a percentage according to the following formula:

$$\left[\frac{\text{Outer edge IML} - \text{Inner edge IML}}{\text{Outer edge IML}}\right] \times 100 = \%\ \text{difference}$$

Our operational criterion for mossy fiber sprouting was met when the luminance of the inner portion of the IML was lower than the luminance of the outer portion of the IML (i.e., when there were more Timm granules in the inner edge than in the outer edge of the IML).

The mean number of stimulations required to kindle the first stage 5 seizure in each group was: LF1, 4.7; HF1, 14.2; HF5, 13.1. As shown in Figure 3, control groups yoked to groups HF1 and HF5 showed marginal amounts of sprouting, with mean differences in

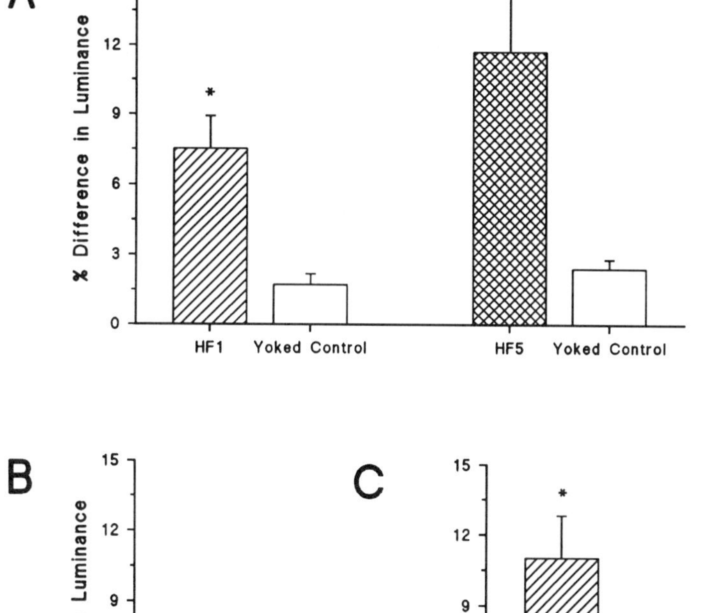

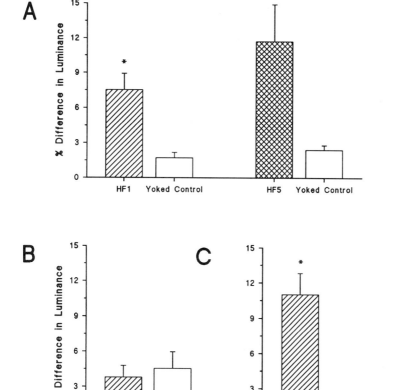

Figure 3. Mean (±SEM) differences in luminance in the IML of rats killed 24 hr after kindling of 1 (HF1) or 5 (HF5) stage 5 seizures with conventional high-frequency stimulation (A), of rats killed 24 hr after kindling of 1 stage 5 seizure (LF1) with low-frequency stimulation (B), or of rats killed approximately 14 days after kindling of 1 stage 5 seizure (LF1 Delay) with low-frequency stimulation (C). $^{*}p \leq 0.01$.

luminance of 1.8 and 2.4 percent, respectively. Both high-frequency groups showed highly significant increases in sprouting in the IML as a consequence of kindling. The HF1 group displayed a mean difference of 7.5 percent (Figure 3A), significantly greater than control ($p<0.01$), indicating that significant sprouting was detectable 24 hr after kindling of a single stage 5 seizure. This is in agreement with previous reports of Sutula and colleagues.[4] The HF5 group displayed a mean difference of 11.7 percent (Figure 3B), significantly greater than control ($p=0.01$), indicating that the amount of sprouting increased with the triggering of increasing numbers of stage 5 seizures.

As shown in Figure 3B, somewhat more sprouting was seen in the control group yoked to the low-frequency kindled group (mean difference in luminance of 4.5 percent) than in the other control groups. In contrast to the groups kindled with high-frequency stimulation, however, the LF1 group failed to display levels of sprouting significantly different from that in yoked controls. Indeed, the LF1 group showed slightly but nonsignificantly *less* sprouting than controls, with a mean difference in luminance of 3.8 percent. The pattern of sprouting seen in controls was minimal, with Timm granules occasionally appearing in the IML of the more dorsal aspects of the DG. We saw a simlar pattern of minimal sprouting in the LF1 group. The HF1 group displayed moderate sprouting, with a patchy but continuous distribution of Timm granules in the IML, between the tip and crest in dorsal aspects of the DG. The HF5 and LF1 Delay groups displayed a distribution of Timm granules between the tip and crest of the DG that was slightly denser than in the HF1 group. The patterns of distribution of Timm granules are shown in Figure 4.

These results indicate that the time course of rapid (low-frequency) kindling and the time course of mossy fiber sprouting are different. Although we detected highly significant increases in the density of Timm granules in the IML of the DG after kindling of 1 or 5 generalized seizures with amygdaloid stimulation, in good agreement with previous demonstrations that conventional kindling is associated with mossy fiber sprouting[4,7,22] in the DG, we saw no evidence of increased Timm granules after rapid kindling with low-frequency amygdaloid stimulation. Because the rapidly kindled rats were killed 24 hr after the first stage 5 seizure, a mean of about 6 days had passed after the first AD. Arguably this interval is too short for significant levels of sprouting to occur. That is, it is conceivable that mossy fiber sprouting would be seen after rapid kindling if the rats were killed at a longer interval after kindling. To address this possibility, we attempted to determine whether significant levels of sprouting are evident in rapidly kindled rats allowed to survive for a longer time after development of the first generalized seizure. We rapidly kindled seizures with low-frequency stimulation of the amygdala and then killed the rats approximately 2 weeks after the first stage 5 seizure. Although there was considerable individual variability, significantly higher levels of Timm granules were seen in the IML of rapidly kindled rats than in yoked controls (Figure 3C). The mean difference in luminance in the rapidly kindled rats was 11.0 percent, as compared to 1.8 percent in yoked controls ($p=0.01$).

4. CONCLUSIONS

We have described several dissociations between kindling and mossy fiber sprouting, in agreement with similar results from other laboratories[7,24]. Collectively these results suggest that the sprouting of mossy fibers into the IML of the DG is neither a prerequisite nor an invariable correlate of limbic kindling. These data may indicate that sprouting is a consequence of the high-frequency ictal discharge that is the hallmark of kindling[14], rather

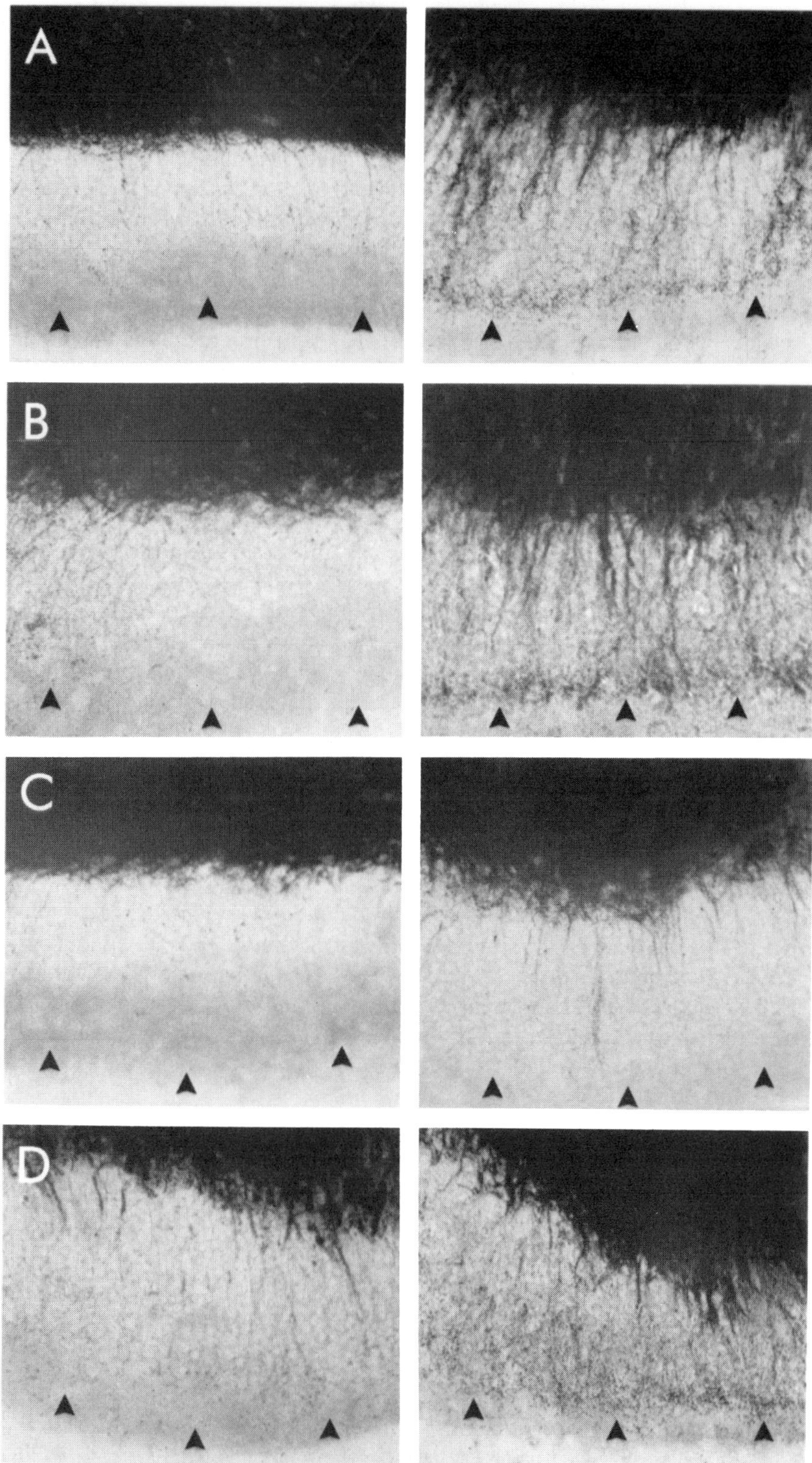

Figure 4. Representative examples of Timm staining the IML of sham-operated control rats (left) and kindled rats (right). A, HF1 group; B, HF5 group; C, LF1 group; D, LF delay group.

than a causal mechanism of kindling. The results and interpretation are not conclusive, however, for several reasons.

First, as noted above, although FF transections produced significant sprouting of the mossy fibers, they also had mixed effects on PP kindling, including both increased excitability (lowered ADTs, longer durations of AD and clonus) and reduced susceptibility to kindling of convulsive seizures. It could be argued that the sprouting consequent to transections was responsible for the increases in excitability reflected in changes in AD and clonus, reminiscent of the increased IID seen after FF transections[3]. If sprouting were an important mechanism of kindling[21], however, one might expect the transections to also accelerate seizure development itself. On the other hand, FF transections interrupt major pathways into and out of the hippocampal formation, which some[6] although not all data[15] suggest is important for kindling, and interfere with induction of long-term potentiation (LTP) in the DG[2], a form of long-lasting synaptic plasticity. Interruption of critical pathways, reduction of synaptic plasticity, or both could have interfered with the progressive recruitment of independent ictal activity in other regions that presumably underlies development of convulsive seizures.

Second, in the case of rapid (low-frequency) kindling, we found that the time course of kindling is uncoupled from the time course of sprouting. Twenty-four hr after triggering of the first generalized seizure, increases over control levels of Timm granules in the IML were not evident in rapidly kindled rats. In rats killed 2 or more weeks after kindling the first generalized seizure, on the other hand, variable but significant increases in Timm granules were detectable. One possible interpretation of this result is that very low levels of mossy fiber sprouting are already present about 6 days after the onset of rapid kindling, the point at which the rats in group LF1 were killed, and that sprouting reaches levels of detectability only within 14 more days, the point at which the rats in the delay group were killed. This argument assumes the fundamental correctness of Sutula's hypothesis[21] that sprouting of the mossy fibers into the IML is an important mechanism of kindling, and hence it must further posit that functionally significant (although undetectable) sprouting occurs in response to the few stimulations delivered during rapid kindling. An alternative interpretation is that sprouting is not involved in the mechanisms of kindling, but rather is a consequence of kindling, seizures, or some associated process. According to this interpretation, the sprouting that accompanies conventional kindling is more readily detected because of the match between the time course of sprouting and the time course of kindling. At this point we know of no data that allow a conclusive discrimination between the two interpretations (but see below).

We also note that our characterization of sprouting was restricted to an examination of Timm granules in the IML of the DG. It is possible that we would have found more reliable correlations between kindling and sprouting if we had looked in other sites, for example hippocampal field CA3[16–18,23]. This possibility can only be addressed empirically. Even if sprouting outside the DG were reliably correlated with kindling, however, one would be forced to conclude that the relation between sprouting and kindling is more complicated than has been appreciated previously. That is, there potentially are multiple patterns of sprouting associated with kindling, only some of which involve the DG. This complexity clearly was not anticipated in Sutula's original hypothesis[21].

It remains to be determined what the functional consequences of mossy fiber sprouting are for kindling. Among the possibilities are that sprouted fibers synapse with the granule cells themselves[21] or with CA3 pyramidal neurons[16–18,23] and increase excitatory synaptic drive; that they synapse with inhibitory interneurons[19] and increase inhibitory synaptic drive[20]; that they release zinc, which produces an antiepileptic effect[11]; that they release zinc, which diminishes GABA-mediated inhibition in the DG[1]; or that they mediate some combination of these effects.

It is also unclear what aspect of the kindling procedure is responsible for mossy fiber sprouting. That is, as noted above, current results do not allow a determination of whether sprouting is a consequence of repetitive AD or some other effect of kindling stimulation (for example, LTP). In their original description of a relation between kindling and sprouting[21], Sutula and colleagues reported that significant levels of sprouting were detected in control rats receiving nonepileptogenic low-frequency stimulation. In preliminary experiments, we have observed an increased density of Timm granules in the IML of rats in which LTP was induced by PP stimulation (unpublished observations), and Racine's group (personal communication) has seen increased Timm staining in field CA3 after induction of LTP with PP stimulation. If reliable, these results suggest that at least some of the mossy fiber sprouting associated with kindling is a consequence of the activation or synaptic modification that is induced by high-frequency stimulation, and is not specifically related to kindling itself.

Finally, we wonder whether the sprouting associated with kindling is to be sought only in the mossy fibers. Perhaps, during kindling, sprouting occurs in other fiber tracts that do not contain zinc and hence cannot be visualized with the Timm stain. It would be useful to measure a less restricted marker for synaptic terminals to address this question.

ACKNOWLEDGMENTS

We thank Trevor Gilbert for establishing an earlier version of the Timm stain in our laboratory and collecting preliminary data. We also thank Greg Armitage for assistance. Supported by a grant from the Medical Research Council of Canada awarded to MEC.

REFERENCES

1. Buhl, E.H., Otis, T.S. and Mody, I., Zinc-induced collapse of augmented inhibition by GABA in a temporal lobe epilepsy model, *Science*, 271 (1996) 369–373.
2. Buzsáki, G. and Gage, F.H., Absence of long-term potentiation in the subcortically deafferented dentate gyrus, *Brain Res.*, 484 (1989) 94–101.
3. Buzsáki, G., Hsu, M., Slamka, C., Gage, F.H. and Horváth, Z., Emergence of propagation of interictal spikes in the subcortically denervated hippocampus, *Hippocampus*, 1 (1991) 163–180.
4. Cavazos, J.E. , Golarai, G. And Sutula, T., Mossy fiber synaptic reorganization induced by kindling: time course of development, progression, and permanence, *J. Neurosci.*, 11 (1991) 2795–2803.
5. Corcoran, M.E. and Cain, D.P., Kindling of seizures with low-frequency electrical stimulation, *Brain Res.*, 196 (1980) 262–265.
6. Dashieff, R. and McNamara, J.O., Intradentate colchicine retards the development of amygdala kindling, *Ann. Neurol.*, 11 (1982) 347–352.
7. Ebert, U. and Löscher, W., Differnces in mossy fibre sprouting during conventional and rapid amygdala kindling of the rat, *Neurosci. Lett.*, 190 (1995) 199–202.
8. Hannesson, D.K. and Skelton, R.W., Recovery of spatial performance in the Morris water maze following bilateral transection of the fimbria/fornix in rats, *Behav. Brain Res.*, submitted.
9. Lapchak, P.A., Araujo, D.M. and Hefti, F., Cholinergic regulation of hippocampal brain-derived neurotrophic factor mRNA expression: evidence from lesion and chronic cholinergic drug treatment studies, *Neuroscience*, 52 (1993) 575–585.
10. Lindefors, N., Renfors, P. Falkenberg, T. and Persson, H., Septal cholinergic afferents regulate expression of brain-derived neurotrophic factor and β-nerve growth factor mRNA in rat hippocampus, *Exp. Brain Res.*, 88 (1992) 78–90.
11. Mitchell, C.L. and Barnes, M.I., Proconvulsant action of diethyldithiocarbamate in stimulation of the perforant path, *Neurotoxicol. Teratol.*, 15 (1993) 165–171.

12. Pelletier, M.R. and Corcoran, M.E., Intra-amygdaloid infusions of clonidine retard kindling, *Brain Res.*, 598 (1992) 51–58.
13. Pelletier, M.R. and Corcoran, M.E., Infusions of alpha-2 adrenergic agonists and antagonists into the amygdala: effects on kindling, *Brain Res.*, 632 (1993) 29–35.
14. Racine, R.J., Newberry, F. and Burnham, W.M., Post-activation potentiation and the kindling phenomenon, *Electroencephalogr. clin. Neurophysiol.*, 39 (1975) 261–271.
15. Racine, R.J., Paxinos, G., Mosher, J.M. and Kairiss, E.W., The effects of various lesions and knife-cuts on septal and amygdala kindling in the rat, *Brain Res.*, 454 (1988) 264–274.
16. Rashid, K., Van der Zee, C.E.E., Ross, G.M., Chapman, C.A., Sanisz, J., Riopelle, R.J., Racine, R.J. and Fahnestock, M., A nerve growth factor peptide retards seizure development and inhibits neuronal sprouting in a rat model of epilepsy, *Pro.Natl. Acad. Sci. USA*, 92 (1995) 9495–9499.
17. Represa, A. And Ben-Ari, Y., Kindling is associated with the formation of novel mossy fibre synapses in the CA3 region, *Exp. Brain Res.*, 92 (1992) 69–78.
18. Represa, A., Jorquera, I., Le Gal La Salle, G. and Ben-Ari, Y., Epilepsy induced collateral sprouting of hippocampal mossy fibers: does it induced the development of ectopic synapses with granule cell dendrites?, *Hippocampus*, 3 (1993) 257–268.
19. Ribak, C.E. and Peterson, G.M., Intragranular mossy fibers in rats and gerbils form synapses with the somata and proximal dendrites of basket cells in the dentate gyrus, *Hippocampus*, 1 (1991) 355–365.
20. Sloviter, R., Possible functional consequences of synaptic reorganization in the dentate gyrus of kainate-treated rats, *Neurosci. Lett.*, 137 (1992) 91–96.
21. Sutula, T., Reactive changes in epilepsy: cell death and axon sprouting induced by kindling, *Epilepsy Res.*, 10 (1991) 62–70.
22. Sutula, T., He, X.X., Cavazos, J. And Scott, G., Synaptic reorganization in the hippocampus induced by abnormal functional activity, *Science*, 239 (1988) 1147–1150.
23. Van der Zee, C.E.E., Rashid, K., Le, K., Moore, K.A., Sanisz, J., Diamond, J., Racine, R.J. and Fahnestock, M., Intraventricular administration of antibodies to nerve growth factor retards kindling and blocks mossy fiber sprouting in adult rats, *J. Neurosci.*, 17 (1995) 5316–5323.
24. Wanscher, B., Kragh, J., Barry, D.I., Bolwig, T. and Zimmer, J., Increased somatostatin and enkephalin-like immunoreactivity in the rat hippocampus following hippocampal kindling, *Neurosci. Lett.*, 118 (1990) 33–36.

DISCUSSION OF MICHAEL CORCORAN'S PAPER

M. Burnham: Is it correct that in the transected rats you got sprouting and you got a threshold drop? I think that's highly significant. The major problem in epilepsy is not developing motor seizures gradually, but it's threshold. So I think your results are extremely interesting and important. Do you think it was the sprouting that caused the threshold drop?

M. Corcoran: I have no idea. Undoubtedly fimbria-fornix transections have a lot of different physiological effects, as you would expect. Therefore threshold drop could be related to the sprouting, or it could have nothing to do with it.

S. Moshe: As far as I remember, it has been shown in the Tryon bright rats and the Tryon dull rats that the AD threshold does not correlate with the kindling rate.

M. Corcoran: They were inversely related, if I remember correctly.

S. Moshe: Over the years, my impression was that AD thresholds did not predict how fully the epileptogenesis would work. Sometimes it was correlated, sometimes it was not correlated at all. So I do not know what is the meaning of a change in AD threshold.

M. Burnham: The problem in human epilepsy is the onset of spontaneous seizures, which by definition means that there is a low threshold.

S. Moshe: But again, I do not know what is the meaning of the change in the AD threshold. For example, rat pups have very high thresholds and they kindle very fast. We've found the 35 day old animals have the lowest threshold and they require more stimulation to kindle than any others. So we were never able to correlate one change to the other.

J. McNamara: I think it's pretty clear from Michael Corcoran's data and from what Nico Moshé said earlier, that mossy fiber sprouting is neither necessary nor sufficient for kindling, if we define kindling by a class 5 seizure response from an initially subconvulsive stimulation. The way I look at that is I think this is fairly revolutionary. There are obviously multiple mechanisms by which we can enhance synaptic efficacy in communication in networks of neural populations. A P15 rat's brain is entirely different from a mature rat's brain. I think that mossy fiber sprouting in the mature brain is sort of like a model of the synaptic organization that you can measure, that you can see. My suspicion is that these are the sorts of things that probably happen at multiple sites in the brain and we can't see it because we don't have the convenience of the Timm stain with a low background of what we have there. If we had a marker of presynaptic terminals in subsets of neurons, we could get the same sort of information we get from a Timm stain and open our eyes to a whole new world.

M. Corcoran: I couldn't agree more—I think that's the direction we have to go in. We've been obsessed with the dentate gyrus, the mossy fibers, because we have a label, the Timm stain. But if this is reflecting a process that is important for kindling, it wouldn't be just going on in the dentate. It has to be occurring elsewhere, and we need to look at other markers.

J. McNamara: My question is what was the total afterdischarge duration in the fimbria-fornix transected animals? Did you measure that?

M. Corcoran: Yes, but I don't have that number here.

J. McNamara: If indeed that is an activity driven synaptic reorganization and you got a lot more activity, in the form of afterdischarge, then you would expect to see more sprouting.

GENERAL DISCUSSION 4

C. Applegate: You have this tissue. Have you looked at other places, or are there other places that you could look where holes are filled in with the Timm stain? For example, have you looked at the piriform or perirhinal or other areas?

M. Corcoran: The obvious place to look would be CA3. Ron Racine has been looking at that and finding kindling-related increases in Timm stain, but we haven't done that yet. There's a limit to how much you can do, given how often the computer scanner is available, for one thing.

G. Ronduin: Just a comment about this, I think also that you could use immunoreactivity to measure sprouting in the perforant path, in the hippocampus, in the amygdala, where there is overlapping of Timm stain and other markers.

F. Lopes da Silva: Actually I was going to suggest GAP-43 and also SNAP25, which is a good marker that can very well be used in other preparations in other areas of the brain, not just the dentate gyrus and the mossy fibres.

About the apparent cell loss, I think that we have to be very careful on that. Some years ago we looked at reactive staining of GABA cells and the changes intrinsic to the cell. Apparently there is decrease of GABA immunoreactivity especially at long-term kindling. But when you look carefully at this we found two things; first there was not all GABA cells that had this increase. The other most important thing is that when we challenge the cells by using an agent to block GABA transminase so that in that way we increase the proportion of GABA that is used and then we found that there was no change. So it means that the cells were just producing less GABA because not enough was detectable with our levels of optical microscopy using GABA staining. One would have said that there was cell loss, but there was no cell loss, it was a functional apparent cell loss. I suppose that if you could perform a similar analysis, you would find a similar thing.

R. Racine: Maybe I should have made it even clearer in my talk. I do not believe that kindling produces cell loss in the hilus that's measurable with any of the techniques that we're currently using. I agree with everything you've said.

K. Gale: When people do this Timm staining of slides, do you just look at the hippocampus and don't look at any other parts of the brain that happen to be attached? After all, there other cell layers and piriform cortex.

In instances of quantification, certainly, I can understand that you are looking for things that are completely ectopic in the hippocampus and the perirhinal cortex. If you are starting to look at quantification, you certainly can see some changes in density in the hippocampus.

R. Racine: We have looked at a number of other structures, starting in the piriform cortex, because there are Timm bands there. There's a patchy staining in the cortex that I've found kind of intriguing, because of the inherent patchiness of neocortical staining for cytochrome oxydase and NMDA and a number of things. We looked at that, but we didn't look at it very thoroughly; it is basically exploratory. But we haven't found yet any very clear-cut changes, anything quite like in the CA3 or the inner molecular layer for example.

I. Mody: I just want to make a general comment about measuring inhibition that relates to what Ron Racine talked about earlier. I think it's not trivial that one has to be very careful measuring inhibition. Certainly one way of doing it is how Ron has done it with paired-pulse extracellular recordings, that assessed certain things about inhibition and also assesses the excitatory drive of inhibitory cells and then their output onto the dentate granule cells. Another way to completely get rid of excitatory drive of inhibitory cells is to look at spontaneous inhibition and to look at what is described as monosynaptic inhibition. I would caution against calling this necessarily an inhibitory event because now we know that in fact inhibition actually might synchronize cells as opposed to fully inhibit them. It is very clear from several studies done in CA1 that inhibition manages to synchronize the pyramidal cells. It is very very effective, and so enhancement or prolongation of inhibition can actually pace the excitatory output of excitatory cells as opposed to inhibit. I think that has to be considered once we talk about the role of inhibition, as such, in structures like the dentate or the hippocampus.

P. Shinnick-Gallagher: I'd also like to comment about that. I think that there is something that has been rendered as enhanced inhibition that may not be related to GABA. It might be related to a release point of a calcium current that has changed or induced this change. So my point is because you measure paired-pulse inhibition it doesn't necessarily mean that it is actually GABA or inhibition that is being measured. It could be something else, it could be a function of calcium inactivation of calcium ions.

R. Racine: I'd just like to respond to that. Pete Engel did mention this. We had, years ago, done a number of GABA manipulations on those paired-pulse tests, and all of the predicted results were found—the GABA blockers blocked the paired-pulse depression effects, the agonist had reverse effects and enhanced those paired-pulse effects, and so on. Everything that we've done, and that other people have done including intercellular studies going back as far as Lomo, are consistent with those paired-pulse measures tapping into inhibition, during that first few tens of milliseconds.

S. Leung: I think I tend to be a bit more careful about your interpretation because in the dentate there's not paired-pulse facilitation, but maybe in other structures there is paired-pulse facilitation, presynaptic facilitation, and then the story may be more complicated in terms of paired-pulse depression.

Y. Geinisman: Ron Racine stated that there is no cell loss in the hilus. Am I correct?

R. Racine: I said using the measures that we used and the animals that we used and the procedures we used, we found no cell loss.

Y. Geinisman: The unbiased stereological technique has been established which allow us to estimate the total number of neurons or synapses in a brain region. If such techniques are not used, for example was done in many aging studies, the error was plus or minus 40%; so the conclusions were based on the use of other approaches and weren't completely valid.

I. Mody: Have you kindled and have you looked at any changes in cell counts?

Y. Geinisman: No. I haven't done it.

J. Stripling: I think that there's a caveat that one might consider when doing paired-pulse testing and that is that there are activity dependent changes in the threshold for excitation of axons. Thus you might get a different number or population of axons activated by the stimulation, and it is hard to do conventional electrophysiology and measure the presynaptic volley at the recording site.

R. Racine: I want to respond to what Yuri said. I sort of feel that some people are pushing me into a stronger position than I've taken (*laughter from the audience*). I absolutely agree with you that there are probably all kinds of things going on in terms of synaptogenesis, possibly degenerative effects even at the synaptic level, that we're not detecting with any of these measures. I'm responding simply to the phenomena that have been established and reported in the literature and the claims that have been made about those phenomena. The fact of the matter is that we have replicated those phenomena in certain situations. But we can, using the same measures, find completely normal looking cell numbers, compared to control tissue.

R. Adamec: Paired-pulse inhibition is measuring recurrent inhibition. Did you measure feed-forward inhibition?

R. Racine: My own feeling from what I've read is that the paired-pulse measures, at least in the dentate gyrus, are probably tapping into both recurrent and feed-forward inhibition.

R. Adamec: You can't separate them?

R. Racine: No. Bob Sloviter would claim that using his 2 Hz technique that he's tapping in more strongly to feed-forward inhibition. But we find that both of those increased with kindling. That is, there is a resistance to failure as well in kindled animals.

17

REGIONAL SPECIFIC CHANGES IN GLUTAMATE AND GABA$_A$ RECEPTORS, PKC ISOZYMES, AND IONIC CHANNELS IN KINDLING EPILEPTOGENESIS OF THE HIPPOCAMPUS OF THE RAT

Fernando H. Lopes da Silva,[1,2] Guido C. Faas,[1] Willem Kamphuis,[1] Miriam Titulaer,[1] Martin Vreugdenhil,[1] and Wytse J. Wadman[1]

[1]Graduate School Neurosciences Amsterdam
Institute of Neurobiology
University of Amsterdam
Kruislaan 320, 1098 SM Amsterdam, The Netherlands
[2]Institute of Epilepsy "Meer en Bosch"
Achterweg 5, Heemstede, The Netherlands

1. INTRODUCTION

The stimulation of certain pathways of the brain with short series of electrical pulses, repeated at regular intervals, causes progressive changes in the underlying neuronal networks. These changes become manifest as afterdischarges of progressively longer duration. At a given stage, these afterdischarges propagate to related brain areas and eventually lead to the occurrence of seizures of focal onset that can become generalized. Goddard who discovered this phenomenon,[9] named it kindling, a designation that describes in a striking manner the progressive character of the development of this type of epileptogenic focus. We chose to investigate the basic mechanisms responsible for kindling epileptogenesis in the CA1 area of the hippocampus of the rat inducing kindling by stimulating the Schaffer collaterals of the axons of the CA3 pyramidal cells.

In this review of work carried out in our group we concentrate, first, on the effects of kindling on the two main receptors that play a central role as control parameters of the stability of local neuronal networks: the GABA-A and the Glutamate receptors. Second, we consider some of the factors that appear to be important in the regulation of the activity of these receptors and of neuronal excitability in general.

Male Wistar rats (250–400 g), under anesthesia, were implanted with stainless steel electrodes (80 μm diameter) for stimulation and recording using stereotaxic coordinates in

Kindling 5, edited by Corcoran and Moshé.
Plenum Press, New York, 1998.

addition to reference and ground electrodes (screws implanted in the skull). Recordings were made from the stratum radiatum of the CA1 area (coordinates: 3.0 mm posterior to the bregma and 2.4 mm lateral to the midline). Stimulating electrodes were placed in the Schaffer collateral fibre layer (coordinates: 3.2 mm posterior to the bregma and 2.5 mm lateral). In some experiments, we used additional sets of electrodes to measure changes in the fascia dentata (FD): stimulation electrodes were placed in the angular bundle (AB) (coordinates: 7.8 mm posterior to bregma, 4.4 mm lateral), and recording electrodes were positioned in the hilar region of FD (coordinates: 3.0 mm posterior to the bregma and 2.4 mm lateral). The kindling procedure consisted of applying twice daily trains of 1 s duration (50 Hz, 200–300 μA, 0.1 ms duration) to the Schaffer collaterals. These procedures have been described in detail elsewhere.[10,14]

Here we present the experimental data that have been collected during the development of the kindled epileptogenic focus, i.e., during the phase where the behavioral signs and the corresponding electrophysiological phenomena elicited by the kindling procedure become increasingly evident (acquisition phase). This developmental phase lasts, in general, 20–25 sessions. At the end of this phase, a steady-state is reached and most animals present regularly generalized tonic-clonic seizures. A salient feature of the plastic changes, elicited as kindling epileptogenesis develops in the hippocampus, is the finding that an important part of these changes is regionally specific, i.e., is different in the CA fields and in the dentate gyrus (consolidation phase). The following aspects are considered:

1.1. Evolution of Paired-Pulse Evoked Potentials

Changes in excitability of neuronal networks can be assessed easily by recording local field potentials (EPs) in the course of the development of kindling. These EPs are the extracellular reflection of post-synaptic potentials and of compound action potentials (population spikes). To evaluate excitability, it is convenient to use a paired-pulse paradigm. In order to quantify the interaction between the responses to a pair of stimuli given at short intervals, the peak amplitude of the response to the second pulse of the pair is divided by the response to the first. We call this parameter the *paired-pulse index* (PPI). The value of the PPI depends on the intensity of the pulses and on the interval between them. Typically, at low stimulation intensities and at intervals around 20 ms, the PPI presents a value larger than one, indicating the existence of paired-pulse facilitation (PPF). However, at larger intensities the PPI becomes smaller than one, and thus paired-pulse depression (PPD) can be said to be present. This occurs when the second stimulus is given during an IPSP evoked by the first stimulus.

Kindling of the Schaffer collaterals/commissural fibers (SCH) is accompanied by a reduction of PPD of the CA1 responses[10] as illustrated in Fig. 1. This was confirmed by.[48,49]

Taking into consideration that this result was at odds with indications that an enhanced PPD due to kindling was found in the fascia dentata (FD) after stimulation of the angular bundle (AB)/perforant path,[7,26,29,31,43,44] we investigated, in the same animals, whether these differences in PPI could be due to regionally specific plastic changes within the hippocampus. EPs were elicited by stimulation, respectively, of the SCH and of the AB fibers to analyse the two systems in parallel: SCH → CA1, and AB → FD. Fig. 1 shows that at the intensity given, the AB → FD responses presented PPD, and the depression was further accentuated in the course of the development of kindling.[14] Whether PPD was enhanced or not in the FD depended on the stimulus intensity as presented in more detail in Kamphuis et al.[14] This experiment shows that changes in opposite directions of PPI can occur within the same hippocampus depending on sub-area. It implies that the local neuro-

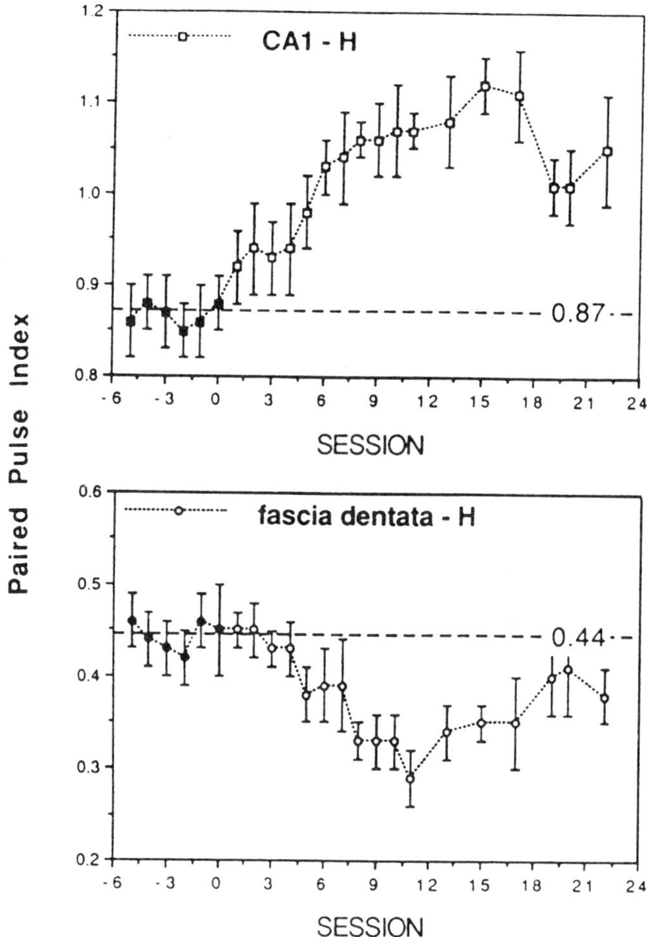

Figure 1. The development of the paired-pulse index (PPI) in response to, above (a) a high (H) stimulus intensity applied to the CA1 SCH-SRr, and below (b) a high (H) stimulus intensity applied to the fascia dentata in the course of kindling. The first 6 closed symbols represent the measurements in the pre-kindling period and the open symbols indicate the recordings during the kindling period. The horizontal dotted line indicates the mean pre-kindling value of PPI. Values represent means ± S.E.M. (n=8) (Adapted from Kamphuis et al. 1992).

nal circuits and elements of the CA1 area and the FD react differently to kindling stimulations. In order to understand the basic processes underlying this phenomenon, we carried out a number of studies in both hippocampal areas in relation to the development of kindling, namely studies of receptor binding, functional studies of the GABA receptor in synaptoneurosomes prepared from both areas, in situ hybrizations of glutamate and GABA receptor subunits and also of different isoforms of Protein Kinase C (PKC).

1.2. Modifications of GABA$_A$ Receptor Binding and of the Expression of mRNAs for GABA$_A$ Receptor Subunits

A quantitative autoradiographic study of the binding of the GABA agonist [^{3}H]Muscimol, of [^{3}H]flunitrazepam that binds to the benzodiazepine site of the GABA$_A$ receptor, and of [^{35}S]t-butylbicyclophosphorothionate (TBPS) that binds to the Cl$^-$channel, was carried out in rats at different stages of the kindling process and corresponding controls. Animals were studied 24 h after the last seizure. The detailed methods are described in Titulaer et al.[38] The main results are schematically presented in Fig. 2.

Several concentrations of [^{3}H]Muscimol were used in the range of the high/intermediate-affinity (5–40 nM) and low-affinity (60–100 nM) binding sites. One of the most salient findings was that the two hippocampal sub-areas reacted differently regarding the

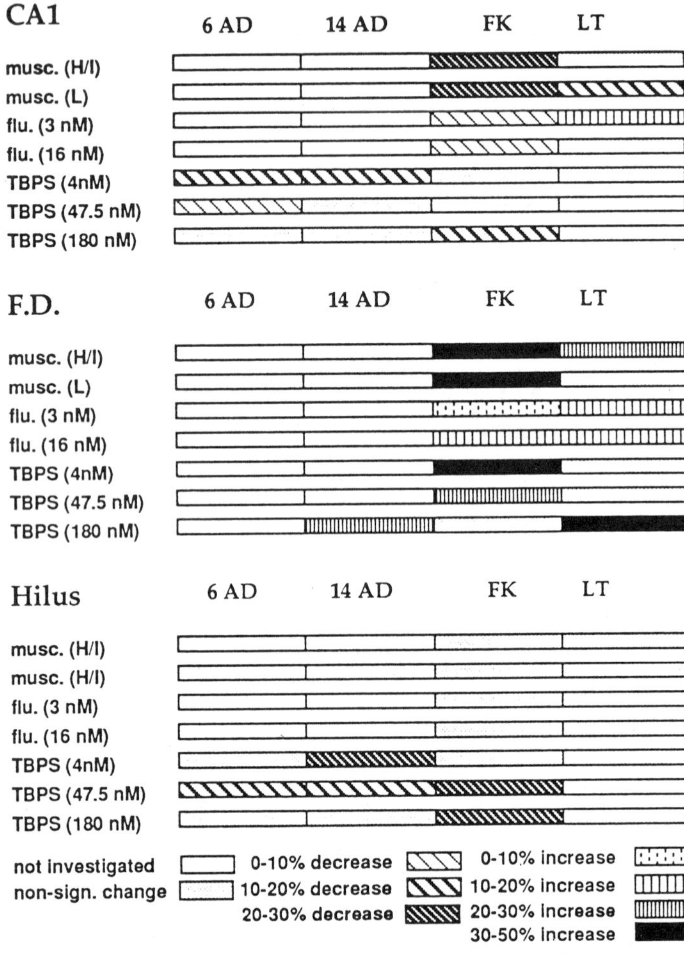

Musc. (H/I) = high/intermediate-affinity (5-40 nM) [^{3}H]muscimol binding;
Musc. (L) = low-affinity (60-100 nM) [^{3}H]muscimol binding;
Flu. (3) = 3 nM (K_D value) [^{3}H]flunitrazepam binding;
Flu. (16) = 16 nM (B_{max} value) [^{3}H]flunitrazepam binding;
TBPS (4) = 4 nM [^{35}S]TBPS binding;
TBPS (47.5) = 47.5 (K_D value) [^{35}S]TBPS binding;
TBPS (180) = 180 nM (B_{max} value) [^{35}S]TBPS binding;

Figure 2. Summary of the relative changes in $GABA_A$ receptor ligand binding during kindling. Note that in CA_1 most changes indicate enhancement of mRNA expression, whereas the opposite is seen in FD (Adapted from Titulaer, 1994).

binding of this $GABA_A$ receptor agonist. In fully kindled rats, the binding of [^{3}H]Muscimol was significantly increased by more than 30% in the FD, while it was decreased in CA1 by 20–30%. It is noteworthy that these changes in [^{3}H]Muscimol binding parallelled the electrophysiological changes both for the CA1 area and the FD. While in the former a *decrease* in PPD occurred in parallel with a *decrease* in [^{3}H]Muscimol binding, the opposite was the case for the FD: i.e., an *increase* in PPD corresponded to an *increase* in [^{3}H]Muscimol binding. Changes in the same opposite directions for the CA1 area and the FD were found for the binding of [^{3}H]Flunitrazepam (at the concentrations of 3 and 16 nM) and for TBPS (4, 47.5 and 180 nM).

Both the electrophysiological observations, using PPI as parameter, and the autoradiographical $GABA_A$ receptor binding studies are indicative that the development of kindling is accompanied in the *CA1 area* by a *decrease* in $GABA_A$ergic inhibition. With regard to the changes in the FD, there is also agreement between the increases in PPD, indicating an increase in $GABA_A$ergic inhibition and the increase in binding of the $GABA_A$ receptor sites found in the autoradiographical studies. The latter changes may be attributed to a reorganization of the mossy fibers, induced by kindling, leading to the formation of new synapses in the supragranular region.[1,4] This process of sprouting may involve also GABAergic interneurons.[6] If this would be so, we may expect that new $GABA_A$ receptors are formed. Therefore we investigated whether these changes of receptor binding could be accounted for by parallel changes at the level of mRNA expression.

A comprehensive investigation using in situ hybridization of mRNAs for the $GABA_A$ receptor subunits revealed indeed an increase in the expression of a number of subunits in the FD at the fully kindled stage as schematically illustrated in Fig. 3.[17] Namely the α_1, α_2, α_4, β_1, β_2, β_3 and the γ_2 subunits showed significant increases (> 20%) in mRNA expression, but in CA1 area a different picture was obtained: there were relatively smaller increases of α_2 and γ_2 accompanied by a small decrease of β_2 in CA3. Most of these changes were more pronounced at the earlier stages of the kindling process. At the long-term, i.e., after a period of at least 4 weeks without stimulations, the only changes of significance were in the subunits α_3 and γ_2. The former, however has a very low abundance and thus this finding does not appear to be relevant. The change in γ_2 mRNA is particularly interesting, since the increase in this subunit is accompanied by a significant decrease in the long variant γ_{2L}. This means that the percentage of γ_{2L} in γ_2 decreases in favour of the short variant γ_{2S}. In contrast to the changes presented above, this change in γ_{2L}/γ_2 occurs in all hippocampal subareas: this ratio decreases from 39±1 to 32±5 in CA1 ($p<0.05$), from 36±1 to 29±3 ($p<0.025$) in CA3, and from 28±1 to 18±3 ($p<0.003$) in FD. This means that at long-term in the steady phase of the kindling process, there is a persistent shift of mRNA splicing preferences in favour of the short variant γ_{2S}. Taking into consideration the fact that the short variant lacks the PKC/calmodulin-dependent protein kinase II phosphorylation sites that are present in the γ_{2L} variant, this change encountered at long-term kindling may have consequences for the capacity of the $GABA_A$ receptor being phosphorylated, and this will likely affect the effectiveness of the $GABA_A$ receptors.

1.3. Changes of Ionotropic Glutamate Receptors (AMPA, NMDA and Kainate)

In addition to the changes in $GABA_A$ receptors, we found that kindling also induces changes in the expression of the AMPA type of glutamate (Glu) receptors, namely of the mRNAs encoding for the Flip and Flop variants of the receptor subunits A, B, and C. In the FD, there was a conspicuous increase of the Flip variant of GluR-A, -B and -C, with-

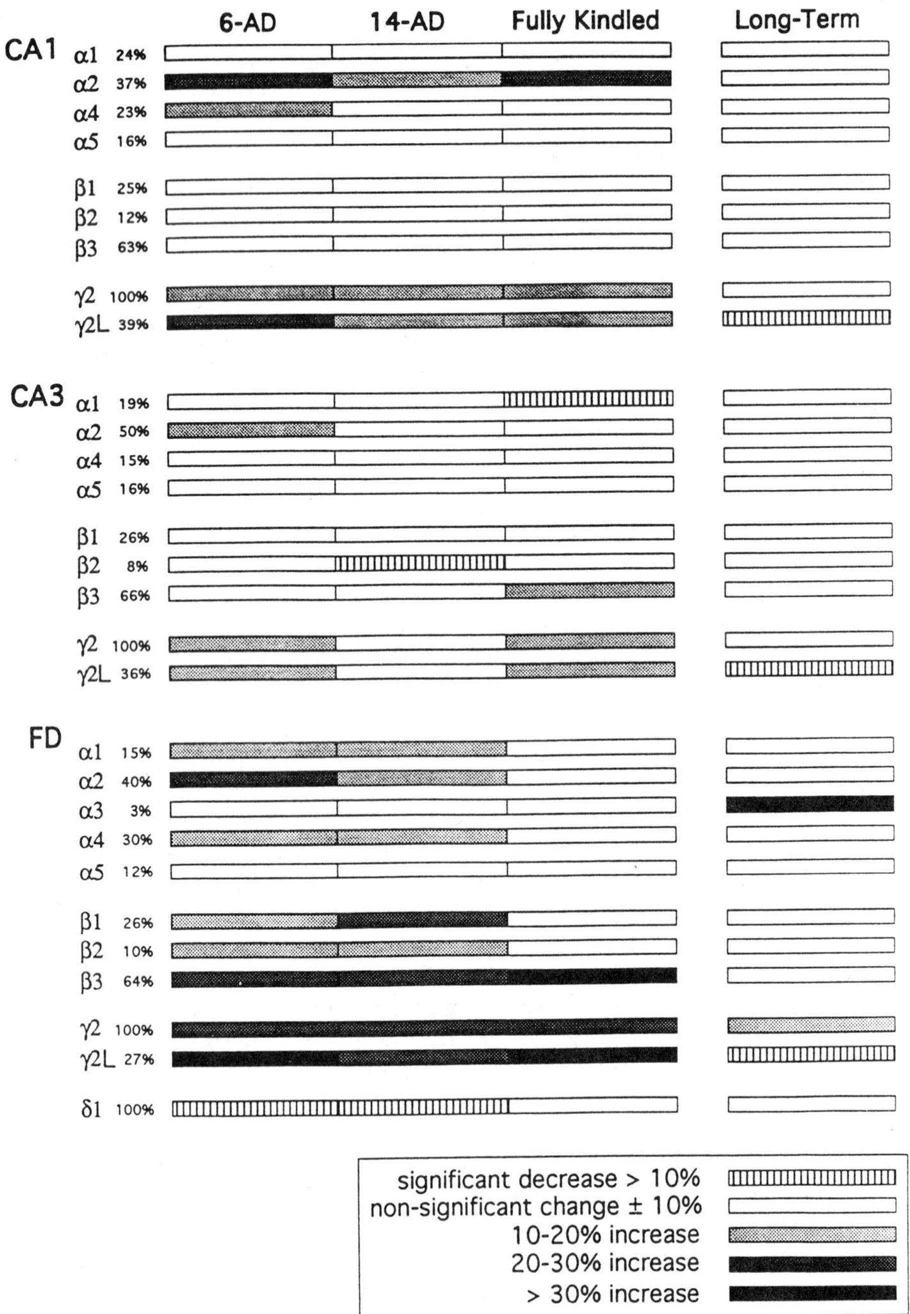

Figure 3. Schematic representation of the results of mRNA in situ hybridization. Note the differences between CA1, CA3 and fascia dentata. Changes in the fascia dentata involve more subunits and increases are of larger magnitude in comparison to CA1 and CA3. Also note the tendency of changes to be more pronounced in the early stages. The percentages at the left represent the contribution of that subunit to the total mRNA population of the class it belongs to. (Adapted from Kamphuis et al 1995a).

out change of the Flop variant, as presented before,[15] that for the Glu R-A persisted at the long-term stage. On the contrary, in the CA1 there was a significant decrease of both Flip and Flop variants of GluR-A, but only at the stage of 14 afterdischarges. Furthermore, we investigated whether there was a change in the editing status of mRNA at the Q/R site of the GluR-A, -B, -5 and -6, since this site is important for the ion selectivity of the corresponding ion channels, but this was not changed.[16] Also the expression levels of the NMDA (NR-1, NR2A and NR2B) and Kainate receptor subunits (-1, -2, GluR-5, -6 and -7) were investigated at the mRNA level. NR1 mRNA levels were slightly decreased in CA1 area of fully kindled animals, whereas in the FD, a minor increase of NR2A and NR2B transcripts was found at all stages of the kindling process. However, none of these changes persisted at long-term.[18]

1.4. Changes in the Expression of Protein Kinase C (PKC) Isozyme ($\alpha - \zeta$) Genes

The fact that kindling of the Schaffer collaterals leads to a substantial increase in excitability of the local CA1 neuronal network, manifested by a reduction of paired pulse inhibition (increase of PPI), and by a diminished sensitivity of the pyramidal neurons to the iontophoretic application of GABA[12] (see below section 1.5), led us to expect that a down-regulation of the GABA$_A$ receptor takes place in the CA1 hippocampal area. Indeed we found a reduction in the binding of GABA$_A$ receptor ligands as described above, but this was not accompanied by a reduction in the expression of genes that encode for the subunits of the GABA$_A$ receptor, with the exception of the decrease in the ratio γ_{2L}/γ_2. Although the latter change indicates a possible alteration of the capacity for phosphorylation of the GABA$_A$ receptor, this change was found only at long-term, while the decrease in paired-pulse inhibition was present already at the induction stages of kindling. GABA$_A$ receptors contain several consensus sequences for phosphorylation by PKC, and the phosphorylation of recombinant GABA$_A$ receptors by PKC results in the reduction of GABA$_A$-activated currents.[21,25] This led us to consider the possibility that the diminished GABA$_A$ receptor function, that becomes manifest in the course of the kindling process, may be the consequence of modifications in phosphorylation conditions. Therefore, we investigated whether the expression of PKC isozyme ($\alpha - \zeta$) genes was changed during kindling.

We found regional specific changes for the different isozymes.[19] In the early stages of kindling (at 6 and 14 afterdischarges), but not at long-term, there were changes in the expression levels of PKC-β, -ε, and -ζ but not of PKC-α, -γ and -δ. PKC-β was decreased in CA1, while PKC-ε and -ζ were increased in CA1, CA3 and FD, as shown in Fig. 4. These results indicate an involvement of PKC-isoform gene expression in the induction stages of kindling but not in the maintenance state. It is interesting to note that calcium-activated forms of PKC were either unchanged or decreased (-α, -β, -ζ), while the calcium-independent forms were enhanced (-ε and -ζ).

A precise translation of these changes at the mRNA levels into functional processes is still an open question. Nevertheless, we may already advance some partial, and tentative, interpretations. The location of PKC-ε in nerve terminals[34] suggests a role for this isoform in the control of presynaptic neurotransmitter release. Indeed an increase in GABA exocytotic release from early stages of kindling was found in our experimental model.[13] The change in PKC-ζ may be related to the finding that a constitutively active kinase generated by the proteolytic cleavage of the regulatory and catalytic domain of PKC-ζ is persistently enhanced in long-term potentiation (LTP).[33]

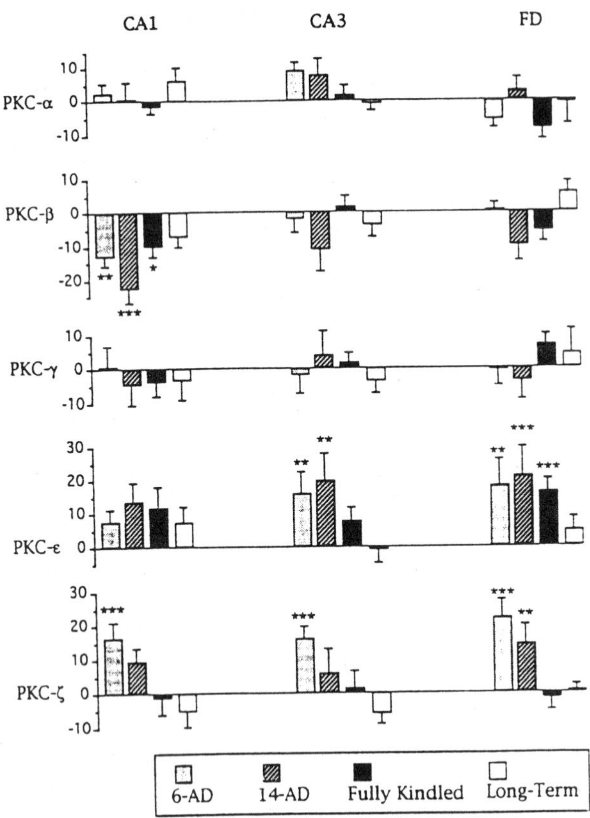

Figure 4. Relative changes in mean extinction values of the in situ hybridization autoradiograms of PKC isozymes in the different kindled groups (% ± S.E.M.). The mean extinction value obtained in the control group was used as reference and set at 100%. Statistical comparisons with respect to controls were carried out directly on the assessed extinction values using a one-way ANOVA, followed by a Student's *t*-test of the different kindled groups vs. the controls. *P<0.05; **P<0.025, *** P<0.010. (Adapted from Kamphuis et al. 1995c).

1.5. Functional Studies of the GABA Receptor in Vivo, in Synaptoneurosomes and in CA1 Pyramidal Neurons Using the Patch-Clamp Technique

A first functional study of GABAergic neurotransmission was carried out in vivo using extracellular recordings of single unit activity recorded from the pyramidal layer of CA1 area.[12] The firing of these neurons was elicited by the iontophoretic application of glutamate; subsequently, GABA was ejected and the ensuing decrease in firing rate was determined. We found a decrease in the sensitivity of these neurons to applied GABA. This finding is in line with the changes encountered in GABA binding sites using autoradiography. However, similar studies were not performed in the FD, so that we are not able to conclude that in this respect the two hippocampal areas behave in opposite directions as occurs with respect to other features.

In order to investigate this question more directly, we applied another technique, namely we isolated synaptoneurosomes, which contain the presynaptic terminal and the attached postsynaptic membrane, from CA1 area and FD and determined the $GABA_A$ mediated $^{36}Cl^-$ fluxes, both for controls and fully kindled animals.[40] In these animals, the muscimol-stimulated $^{36}Cl^-$ uptake was significantly reduced by 21% in the CA area whereas a significant increase of 29% was found in the FD. Thus these findings are in close agreement with the autoradiographic binding data and the results of the paired-pulse electrophysiological observations.

For the CA1 pyramidal neurons, it was possible to perform a more precise analysis of the GABA$_A$ mediated Cl^- currents, in acutely isolated neurons from fully kindled rats and the corresponding controls.[45] Using the whole-cell voltage-clamp technique, no change was found of the maximal Cl^- current amplitude, nor of time-constant of desensitisation. In addition, it was found that Ca^{2+} influx due to activation of voltage-dependent calcium currents appreciably decreased the muscimol-evoked Cl^- current. In this respect it is interesting to note that kindling induces an enhancement of voltage-dependent calcium currents investigated in pyramidal CA1 cells, both in dissociated neurons[46,47] and in slices, in vitro, studied using the in situ patch-clamp technique.[8] In the former, an increased Ca^{2+} influx through high-voltage activated (HVA) Ca^{2+} current was found. It should be added that in this respect, the CA1 area and the FD behave differently, since Mody et al.[28] found a decreased influx in the HVA current in granule cells of the FD, which was attributed to a loss of Ca^{2+}-binding proteins.

The investigation of Faas et al[8] broadened our insight in the behaviour of Ca^{2+} currents in kindling, because they were able to study a low-voltage activated (LVA) current in the in-situ patch-clamp preparation, which is absent in dissociated cells where only HVA currents can be elicited. This LVA current corresponds most probably to the T-type of Ca^{2+} channels. Faas et al.[8] found that in fully kindled animals, both the *transient HVA* and the *LVA currents* were significantly *enlarged*; furthermore these currents inactivated faster.

An important aspect of these changes in Ca^{2+} currents is that they persist at long-term, at least up to 6 weeks after cessation of kindling stimulations in animals that had reached the fully kindled state.

In addition, the enhanced Ca^{2+} currents may contribute to an amplification of neuronal excitability and an increase in the bursting probability of CA1 neurons. It is likely that the increased Ca^{2+} currents may cause a number of changes in the modulation of Ca^{2+} dependent second messenger systems, including a down-modulation of GABA mediated Cl^- currents. Thus, in an indirect way, it may cause a decrease in inhibitory transmission. Indeed it is known that the GABA$_A$-receptor is modulated by calcium-dependent phosphorylation processes.[5,24,36] However, to determine more precisely the effects of an increase in Ca^{2+} influx, one needs to know more about the intracellular Ca^{2+} buffering capacity of these cells.

2. DISCUSSION AND CONCLUSIONS

Kindling of the hippocampus is a model of epileptogenesis that permits the study of how the development of an epileptogenic focus takes place in the course of time. The gradual enhancement of the duration of afterdischarges develops in parallel with the unfolding of successively more severe behavioural seizures. This means that these two phenomena are related. Since the hippocampus is not an output motor structure but projects to a number of target areas related to the motor systems of the forebrain, it is likely that a relatively long hippocampal afterdischarge is necessary for the activation of these structures in order that behavioural seizures may occur.

The evolution of these phenomena in the course of kindling is typically accompanied by gradual changes in electrophysiological parameters, that are characteristic for the excitability of the local neuronal networks. The main feature in this respect is the gradual *decrease* of the paired-pulse depression (PPD) in CA1 area. Surprising is the fact that along with this change in CA1, there is an *opposite* change in FD. We may assume that PPD is a measure of the balance between excitatory (E) and inhibitory (I) processes, i.e., of the *E/I index* that may be considered to be a main control parameter of the stability of the local network. The changes in PPD indicate that a relative increase of the E/I index occurs in CA1 while in the FD there is a decrease in this index. Thus within the hippocampus, the process of epileptogenesis is associated with different, even opposite, changes in PPD. This finding merits further discussion. In this respect, a number of points should be made.

First, a large amount of experimental data and theoretical studies[42] leads to the hypothesis that epileptogenesis is, in general, induced by an increase in E/I index. Thus the change in CA1 found in our kindling model is compatible with such a hypothesis. However this does not apply to the change in FD. We should note that from the functional point of view, these two hippocampal areas occupy quite different positions within the hippocampal circuits; while the FD occupies the position of input interface, the CA1 area is an important source of output signals of the hippocampus. Thus an increase in excitability in the latter will have more direct consequences to target structures, so that the propagation of seizure activity over several brain areas may take place. The change in the FD will have an opposite effect, since an enhancement of inhibition within the local network will lead to a stronger inhibitory input filter action on this network. This may work as a shield to protect the hippocampus from possible disturbing inputs arriving from the entorhinal cortex and adjacent temporal lobe structures.

Second, the finding that the PPD measured in the CA1 and in the FD clearly changes in opposite directions leads directly to the question whether this difference is related to cellular processes that also change in opposite directions within the same hippocampus. Although a complete set of cellular and molecular phenomena, studied using the same kindling protocol in both structures, is not yet available, a number of findings can be considered in this respect, namely (a) the $GABA_A$ receptor binding, (b) the GABA mediated Cl^- fluxes in synaptoneurosomes and the corresponding currents recorded in whole-cell patches, (c) the calcium-buffering capacity of neurons, and (d) the expression of mRNAs for glutamate and $GABA_A$ receptor subunits:

a. The density of the three ligands of the $GABA_A$ receptor studied, i.e., of muscimol binding sites of the high/intermediate affinity class, of benzodiazepine binding sites (flunitrazepam binding) and of TBPS (Cl^- channel) sites, changes in opposite directions, decreasing in CA1 and increasing in FD.[37,39,41]
b. The muscimol-activated Cl^- fluxes in synaptoneurosomes change also in opposite directions, decreasing in CA1 and increasing in FD.[40] The direct measurements of ionic currents present a more complex picture. Vreugdenhil[45] found no change in muscimol activated Cl^- currents in acutely dissociated CA1 pyramidal neurons, but Mody et al[28] reported an increase in GABA mediated inhibitory currents (IPScs) of granule cells in FD after local kindling. Thus in the FD, there is agreement between the results of synaptoneurosomes and the whole-cell patch studies, but this does not appear to be the case for the CA1.

However, measurements in dissociated pyramidal cells are limited to the soma and, at most, the initial part of the dendrites. This fact may be interpreted as indicating that the synaptic structures that contribute to the results of the synaptoneurosome studies correspond mainly to those synapses located at the apical dendrites, which are not included in the measurements carried out in dissociated neurons. This way of reasoning leads to the *hypothesis* that the decrease in GABAergic inhibition, revealed by the synaptoneurosome investigation, should be attributed to changes at the inhibitory synapses situated on the distal dendrites of pyramidal neurons. Nevertheless, the fact that the dissociated pyramidal cells present an increase in Ca^{2+} currents, along with the finding that an intracellular increase in Ca^{2+} depresses $GABA_A$ mediated Cl^- currents, may indicate that GABAergic actions may be depressed in these cells depending on their activity state in dendrites.

c. We observed that in the course of kindling, the immunoreactivity of GABA containing cells was affected, but exclusively of those cells where GABA did not co-localize with the calcium-binding protein parvalbumin,[11] indicating that the GABA containing cells affected by kindling were those that were not protected from an increase in intracellular Ca^{2+} by parvalbumin. It was shown that the GABAergic interneurons that make synaptic contacts with the perisomatic surface of CA pyramidal neurons contain parvalbumin, whereas this calcium-binding protein is absent in those interneurons innervating apical dendrites, which may contain other proteins.[20]

d. Semi-quantitative in situ hybridization techniques to determine levels of mRNAs encoding for specific subunits of glutamate and $GABA_A$ receptors in the kindled hippocampus also revealed clear differences between CA area and FD. The expression level of the mRNAs encoding for the Flip version of the AMPA-receptor subunits A-, B-, and C- was appreciably increased already after 6 afterdischarges, i.e., before overt seizures were detected, and also in fully kindled rats, in the granule cells of FD, whereas in CA1 only some very small decreases were found at initial stages. Furthermore, a number of GABA-A-receptor subunits were appreciably increased in FD but the changes in CA area were slight; only in the case of one subunit β_2 a change in opposite direction, i.e., an increase in FD and a decrease in CA3 area, was encountered but this effect was discrete.[15,17]

What are the possible implications of these changes in relation to kindling? First we consider the changes in glutamate receptors. In the granule cells of the FD, we observed a shift in the ratio of Flip- to Flop-carrying subunits, what may lead to an enhanced sensitivity of the corresponding receptors for L-glutamate and a less desensitizing excitatory response, according to the studies of Sommer et al[32] and Burnashev.[3] This is compatible with the observation that a long-lasting potentiation of the excitatory synaptic responses takes place in the FD in the course of kindling, while this is not the case in CA1.[26,35]

Second, the changes in $GABA_A$ receptor mRNAs indicate an up-regulation of the number of these receptors, since the subunits that presented the largest changes correspond to those that are most abundant under normal conditions. Of course these changes in mRNA expression correlate closely with the enhanced [^{3}H]muscimol, [^{3}H]flunitrazepam and [^{35}S]TBPSbinding, the increased $GABA_A$-mediated Cl^- uptake by synaptosomes prepared from the FD and the gradual strengthening of the PPD in this area. The changes in mRNA levels in CA areas, although contrasting sharply with those found in FD since they are much slighter, are apparently not in line with the changes in receptor binding and in most physiological parameters. This was unexpected. At present, we can only speculate about the processes underlying this finding. This observation, as such, may be interpreted as the result of an aberrant post-translational processing or of a decreased efficiency of the translation of the mRNA into functional $GABA_A$ receptors. The fact that in the course of kindling the $GABA_A$-receptor function is down-regulated in the CA area, due to the increased Ca^{2+} currents and subsequent changes in phosphorylation and in sensitivity of the $GABA_A$-receptor, may lead to a compensatory enhancement of mRNA expression, in order to maintain the balance between excitation and inhibition (E/I index) as close as possible to the normal range.

As a conclusion, we may make an attempt to combine the anatomical data with the physiological findings indicated above, in order to speculate about the significance of the changes encountered for the phenomenon of kindling epileptogenesis. Kindling may affect synaptic processes in dissimilar ways: even within the CA1 area the GABAergic synapses at the level of apical dendrites appear to be affected while those at the perisomatic level are apparently spared. Whether the interneurons would be functionally impaired, namely in their capacity of producing GABA, would depend, among other factors, on their calcium buffering properties.

We may put forward the *hypothesis* that those interneurons that are so efficient in buffering their excessive intracellular Ca^{2+} would become less able to produce GABA, and the corresponding synapses would undergo a decrease in $GABA_A$ receptors. Considering that the corresponding interneurons are those mainly responsible for feedforward inhibition,[2,22,23] the consequent decrease in GABAergic inhibition would lead to a critical decrease in E/I index, within the CA area, that would promote epileptogenesis. The increases in the FD of several parameters, as indicated above, could be related to reactive synaptogenesis, i.e., to sprouting of new synaptic contacts, which is most evident in the territory of the mossy fibers from dentate granule cells in the supragranular layer of the FD and in the infrapyramidal layer of the CA3 region.[30] This would work as a compensatory mechanism to counteract the excessive excitability of the neighbouring CA neuronal networks.

REFERENCES

1. Ben Ari, Y. and Represa, A., Brief seizure episodes induce long-term potentiation and mossy fibre sprouting in the hippocampus, *TINS*, 13 (1990) 312–318.
2. Bulh, E.H., Halsy, K. and Somogyi, P., Diverse sources of hippocampal unitary inhibitory postsynaptic potentials and the number of synaptic release sites, *Nature*, 368 (1994) 823–828.
3. Burnashev, N., Recombinant ionotropic glutamate receptors: Functional distinction imparted by different subunits, *Cell Physiol. Biochem.* 1 (1993) 318–331.
4. Cavazos, J.E., Golarai, G. and Sutula, T. P., Septotemporal variation of the supragranular projection of the mossy fiber pathway in the dentate gyrus of neuronal and kindled rats, *Hippocampus*, 2 (1992) 363–372.
5. Chen, Q.X., Stelzer, A. S., Kay, A. R. and Wong, R. K. S., $GABA_A$ receptor function is regulated by phosphorylation in acutely dissociated guinea-pig hippocampal neurons, *Journal of Physiology*, 420 (1990) 207–221.
6. Davenport, C.J., Brown, W. J. and Babb, T. L., Sprouting of GABAergic and mossy fiber axons in dentate gyrus following intrahippocampal kainate in the rat, *Exp. Neurol.*, 109 (1990) 180–190.
7. de Jonge, M. and Racine, R. J., The development and decay of kindling-induced increase in paired-pulse depression in the dentate gyrus, *Brain Res.*, 412 (1987) 318–328.
8. Faas, G.C., Vreugdenhil, M. and Wadman, W. J., Calcuim currents in pyramidal CA1 neurons in vitro after kindling epileptogenesis in the hippocampus of the rat, *Neuroscience*, (1996) (In Press).
9. Goddard, G.V., McIntyre, D. C. and Leech, C. K., A permanent change in brain function resulting from daily electrical stimulation, *Expl. Neurol.*, 25 (1969) 295–330.
10. Kamphuis, W., Lopes da Silva, F. H. and Wadman, W. J., Changes in local evoked potentials in the rat hippocampus (CA1) during kindling epileptogenesis, *Brain Res.*, 440 (1988) 205–215.
11. Kamphuis, W., Huisman, E., Wadman, W. J., Heizmann, C. W., and Lopes da Silva, F. H., Kindling induced changes in parvalbumin immunoreactivity in rat hippocampus and its relation to long-term decrease in GABA-immunoreactivity, *Brain Res.*, 479 (1989) 23–34.
12. Kamphuis, W., Gorter, J. A. and Lopes da Silva, F. H., A long-lasting decrease in the inhibitory effect of GABA on glutamate responses of hippocampal pyramidal neurons induced by kindling epileptogenesis, *Neuroscience*, 41 (1991a) 425–431.
13. Kamphuis, W., Huisman, E. Veerman, M. J., and Lopes da Silva, F. H., Development of changes in endogenous GABA release during kindling epileptogenesis in rat hippocampus, *Brain Res.*, 545 (1991b) 33–40.
14. Kamphuis, W., Gorter, J. A., Wadman, W. J. and Lopes da Silva, F. H., Hippocampal kindling leads to different changes in paired-pulse depression of local evoked field potentials in area CA1 and in the fascia dentata, *Neuroscience Letters*, 141 (1992) 101–105.
15. Kamphuis, W., De Rijk, T. C., Talamini, L. M. and Lopes da Silva, F. H., Rat hippocampal kindling induces changes in the glutamate receptor mRNA expression patterns in dentate granule neurons, *Eur. J. Neuroscience*, 6 (1994) 1119–1127.

16. Kamphuis, W. and Lopes da Silva, F. H., Editing status at the Q/R site of glutamate receptor -A, -B, -5 and -6 subunit mRNA in the hippocampal kindling model of epilepsy, *Mol. Brain Res.*, 29 (1995) 35–42.
17. Kamphuis, W., De Rijk, T. C. and Lopes da Silva, F. H., Expression of $GABA_A$ receptor subunit mRNAs in hippocampal pyramidal and granular neurons in the kindling model of epileptogenesis: An *in situ* hybridization study, *Mol. Brain Res.*, 31 (1995a) 33–47.
18. Kamphuis, W., Hendriksen, H., Diegenbach, P.C. and Lopes da Silva, N-methyl-D-Aspartate- and kainate receptor gene expression in hippocampal pyramidal and granular neurons in the kindling model of epileptogenesis, *Neuroscience*, 67 (1995b) 551–559.
19. Kamphus, W., Hendriksen, E. and Lopes da Silva, F. H., Isozyme specific changes in the expression of protein kinase C isozyme (α-ξ) genes in the hippocampus of rats induced by kindling epileptogenesis, *Brain Res.*, 702 (1995c) 94–100.
20. Katsumaru, H., Kosaka, T., Heizman, C.W. and Hama, K., Immunocytochemical study of GABAergic neurons containing the calcium-binding protein parvabumin in the rat hippocampus, *Exp. Brain Res.*, 72 (1988) 347–362.
21. Krishek, B.J., Xie, X., Blackstone, C., Huganir, R.L., Moss, S. J. and Smart, T. G., Regulation of $GABA_A$ receptor function by protein kinase C phophorylation, *Neuron*, 12 (1994) 1081–1095.
22. Lacaille, J.C.and Swartzkroin, P.A., Stratum lacunosum-moleculare interneurons of hippocampal CA1 region. II Intracellular response characteristics, synaptic responses, and morphology, *J. Neuroscience*, 8 (1988a) 1400–1410.
23. Lacaille, J.C. and Swartzkroin, P.A., Stratum lacunosum-moleculare interneurons of hippocampal CA1 region. II. Intrasomatic and intradendritic recordings of local circuit synaptic interactions, *J. Neuroscience*, 8 (1988b) 1411–1424.
24. Leidenheimer, N.J., McQuilkin, S. J., Hahner, L.D., Whiting, P. and Harris, R. A., Activation of protein kinase C selectively inhibits the g-aminobutyric acid $_A$ receptor: Role of desensitization, *Mol. Pharmacol.*, 41 (1992) 1116–1123.
25. Macdonald, R.L. and Olsen, R. W., $GABA_A$ receptor channels, *Ann. Rev. Neuroscience*, 17 (1994) 569–602.
26. Maru, E. and Goddard, G. V., Alteration in dentate neuronal activities associated with perforant path kindling. III. Enhancement of synaptic inhibition, *Exp. Neurol.*, 96 (1987) 46–60.
27. Mody, I., Reynolds, J. N., Salter, M. W., Carlen, P. L. and MacDonald, J. F., Kindling-induced epilepsy alter calcium currents in granule cells of rat hippocampal slices, *Brain Res.*, 531 (1990) 88–94.
28. Mody, I., Lasting potentiation of inhibition is associated with an increased number of gamma-ammi-nobutyric acid type $_A$ receptors activated during miniature inhibitory postsynaptic currents, *Proc. Nat. Acad. Sci. USA*, 91 (1994) 7698–7702.
29. Oliver, M.W. and Miller, J. J., Alterations of inhibitory processes in the dentate gyrus following kindling-induced epilepsy, *Exp. Brain Res.*, 57 (1985) 443–447.
30. Represa, A. and Ben-Ari, Y., Kindling is associated with the formation of novel mossy fiber synapses in the CA3 region, *Exp. Brain Res.*, 92 (1992) 69–78.
31. Robinson, G.B., Schabassi, R. J. and Berger, T. W., Kindling-induced potentiation of excitatory and inhibitory inputs to hippocampal dentate granule cells. I. Effects on linear and non-linear response characteristics, *Brain Res.*, 562 (1991) 17–25.
32. Sommer, B., Keinänen, K., Verdoorn, T.A., Wisden, W., Burnashev, N., Herb, A., Kühler, M., Takagi, T., Sakmann, B. and Seeburg, P. H., Flip and Flop: A cell-specific functional switch in glutamate-operated channels of the CNS, *Science*, 249 (1990) 1580–1585.
33. Sacktor, T.C., Osten, P., Valsamis, H., Jiang, X., Naik, M. U. and Sublette, E., Persistent activation of the ξ-isoform of protein kinase C in the maintenance of long-term potentiation, *Proc. Natl. Acad. Sci. USA*, 90 (1993) 8342–8346.
34. Saito, N., Itouji, A., Totani, Y., Osawa, I., Koide, H., Fujisawa, N., Ogita, K. and Tanaka, C., Cellular and intracellular localization of ε-subspecies of protein kinase C in the ratbrain; presynaptic localization of the ε-subspecies, *Brain Res.*, 607 (1993) 2541–2548.
35. Sutula, T. and Steward, O., Facilitation of kindling by prior induction of long-term potentiation in the perforant path, *Brain Res.*, 420 (1987) 109–117.
36. Taleb, O., Feltz, P., Bossu, J. L., Feltz, A. and Pumain, R., Sensitivity of chloride channels to changes in intracellular calcium—investigations on spontaneous and GABA-evoked activity, *Epilepsy Res.*, 8 (1992) 47–56.
37. Titulaer, M.N.G., $GABA_A$ receptor binding and function in the hippocampal model of kindling epileptogenesis in the rat, unpublished doctoral dissertation, University of Amsterdam, (1994) pp. 185.
38. Titulaer, M.N.G., Kamphuis, W., Pool, C. W., Van Heerihuize, J. J. and Lopes da Silva, F. H., Kindling induces time-dependent and regional specific changes in the [3H] muscimol binding in the rat hippocampus: A quantitative autoradiographic study, *Neuroscience*, 59 (1994) 817–826.

39. Titulaer, M.N.G., Kamphuis, W. and Lopes da Silva, F. H., Autoradiographical analysis of [^{35}S] t-butylbicyclophosphorothionate binding in kindled rat hippocampus shows different changes in CA1 area and fascia dentata, *Neuroscience*, 66 (1995a) 547–554.
40. Titulaer, M., Ghijsen, W. E. J. M., Kamphuis, W., De Rijk, T. C. and Lopes da Silva, F. H., Opposite changes in $GABA_A$-receptor function in the CA1–3 area and fascia dentata of kindled rat hippocampus, *J. Neurochem.*, 64 (1995b) 2615–2621.
41. Titulaer, M.N.G., Kamphuis, W., and Lopes da Silva, F. H., Long-term regional specific changes in [^{3}H] flunitrazepam binding in the kindled rat hippocampus, *Neurosci.*, 68(2) (1995c) 399–406.
42. Traub, R.D.and Miles, R., *Neuronal networks of the hippocampus*. Cambridge University Press, New York, 1991.
43. Tuff, L.P., Racine, R. J. and Adamec, R., The effects on GABA-mediated inhibition in the dentate gyrus of the rat. I. Paired pulse depression, *Brain Res.*, 277 (1983) 79–90.
44. Voskuyl, R.A. and Albus, H., Enhancement of recurrent inhibition by angular bundle kindling is retained in hippocampal slices, *Int. J. Neurosci.*, 36 (1987) 153.
45. Vreugdenhil, M., Intrinsic membrane properties of hippocampal pyramidal neurons after kindling epileptogenesis, unpublished doctoral dissertation, University of Amsterdam, (1994) pp.128.
46. Vreugdenhil, M. and Wadman, W. J., Kindling induced long-lasting enhancement of calcium current in hippocampal area CA1 of the rat: Relation to calcium-dependent inactivation, *Neurosci.*, 59 (1994) 105–114.
47. Vreugdenhil, M. and Wadman, W. J., Enhancement of calcium currents in rat hippocampal CA1 neurons induced by kindling epileptogenesis, *Neurosci.*, 49 (1992) 373–381.
48. Zhao, D. and Leung, L. S., Hippocampal kindling induced paired-pulse depression in the dentate gyrus and paired-pulse facilitation in CA3, *Brain Res.*, 582 (1992) 163–167.
49. Zhao, D. and Leung, L. S., Effects of hippocampal kindling on paired-pulse response in CA1 *in vitro*, *Brain Res.*, 564 (1991) 220–229.

DISCUSION OF FERNANDO LOPES DA SILVA'S PAPER

J. McNamara: Since carbamazapine does promote or enhance spike frequency adaptation and there is a reduced responsiveness of the CA1 pyramidal cells to carbamazapine, is there any difference in spike frequency adaptation, or accommodation, in the absence of carbamazapine in the control versus kindled neurons?

F. Lopes da Silva: All this work was done with the voltage-clamp technique; so I think that it is very important to get this relation into a current clamp situation and look at spike adaptation, difference in rise times, decay times and so on. This points to a lot of things that we still have to do.

I. Mody: Do you see any change in the steady state inactivation of the T-channels, and do you have an explanation for the change in kinetics?

F. Lopes da Silva: What I showed you today was just the amplitude of the current. We have also looked at the kinetics, and the kinetics show a change as well, but the change in amplitude and the change in kinetics are going in opposite directions. So we have an increase in amplitude but we also have an increase in the decay, leading to a shorter window for the influx of calcium. We have calculated the total calcium influx, however, and there is still a very significant increase in calcium influx. There were no differences the inactivation of the currents.

B. Adamec: Lovely presentation, very interesting data. You were talking about two types of calcium currents that change; you mentioned the T current, but I don't think that you mentioned what the other type was.

F. Lopez da Silva: What we found was a change in the high voltage activated current, which has two components, a transient component and a sustained component. This current probably corresponds to the L and the N types—we didn't do the pharmacology to characterize these currents farther because in this preparation it is very hard, in that you cannot keep the cell in the patch for such a long time that you can measure the whole tissue currents and activation-activation and then still do the pharmacology. The T types are the low-voltage activated currents—and these are a transient type current—they have no sustained component.

B. Adamec: As you know, some researchers are zeroing in on the protein component of the inactivation gate of the sodium channel, and I was wondering if you had any speculations as to what is going on.

F. Lopez da Silva: No. Not yet.

A. Fernandez-Guardiola: You describe different measures in fully kindled and partially kindled seizures. Did you test electroshock, for example, and compare with fully kindled seizures?

F. Lopez da Silva: No.

KINDLING: A PATHOLOGIC ACTIVITY-DRIVEN STRUCTURAL AND FUNCTIONAL PLASTICITY IN MATURE BRAIN

Devin K. Binder[1] and James O. McNamara[1,2,3]

[1]Department of Neurobiology
[2]Department of Pharmacology
[3]Department of Medicine (Neurology)
Epilepsy Research Laboratory, 401 Bryan Research Building
Duke University Medical Center
Durham, North Carolina 27710

1. KINDLING: ACTIVITY-DRIVEN PLASTICITY IN MATURE BRAIN

Neuroscientists and clinicians are familiar with the idea that physiologic activity is required for stabilization of neuronal connections during development of the mammalian nervous system. Probably the best example is the requirement for physiologic activity in the normal development of the visual system. Hubel and Wiesel[1] demonstrated that suturing an eyelid early in life dramatically modified ocular dominance column formation: neurons in the visual cortex that would normally have been driven by both eyes now were driven only by the eye that remained open. These and related findings led to recognition of the cause of diminished vision in children with strabismus and to treatments which encouraged use of both eyes.

The emerging picture of the cellular and molecular mechanisms by which physiologic activity leads to normal connectivity in the developing nervous system provides a useful framework for thinking about mechanisms underlying the development of kindling in the mature brain. We view kindling as a process analogous to activity-dependent synapse formation during development. In both cases, activity drives formation of novel neuronal connections: physiologic activity drives normal synapse formation during development, whereas pathologic activity in the form of repeated afterdischarges drives abnormal synapse formation in the mature nervous system. The basis for this concept and supporting evidence will be presented below. The power of the concept is that it suggests that the two situations may have overlapping cellular and molecular mechanisms.

Kindling 5, edited by Corcoran and Moshé.
Plenum Press, New York, 1998.

2. HYPEREXCITABILITY OF KINDLED BRAIN: SYNAPTIC PLASTICITY?

In view of the central role of chemical synapses in mediating communication among neurons in the mammalian nervous system, modification of synapses is a logical starting point for investigating mechanisms of hyperexcitability of the kindled brain. One type of synaptic modification could be altered efficacy of preexisting synapses. Indeed, evidence has emerged implicating enhanced function of glutamatergic synapses in the kindled brain (see ref. 2 for an overview).

An alternative (and not mutually exclusive) type of synaptic modification could be formation of novel synapses (i.e. connections in type or number that do not exist in normal brain). Sutula *et al.*[3] discovered that kindling is accompanied by sprouting of the mossy fiber axons of the dentate granule cells of the hippocampus. A similar form of axonal sprouting was found after status epilepticus and neuronal injury by Nadler *et al.*[4] Importantly, the functional consequences of the abnormal synapses formed as a result of the sprouting depend on the target of the anomalous axons. Evidence that this pathologic projection forms a recurrent excitatory synapse emerged from the work of Tauck and Nadler[5]; their electrophysiologic findings were consistent with the idea that the glutamatergic dentate granule cells formed excitatory synapses upon themselves or their neighbors. Recently, Wuarin and Dudek[6] demonstrated spontaneous and evoked bursting and an increase in EPSP frequency using glutamate microstimulation in slices isolated from kainate-treated animals, providing further support for this hypothesis. It is easy to imagine how such an autoexcitatory synaptic loop might contribute to the lasting hyperexcitability of kindling. Moreover, it is unlikely that such pathologic sprouting is restricted to the dentate mossy fiber axons and instead sprouting may well exist in multiple sites in a kindled brain. Given these intriguing observations of a structural reorganization in the kindled brain, how might such a reorganization develop?

3. KINDLING DEVELOPMENT: REQUIREMENT FOR PATHOLOGIC ACTIVITY

The pathologic activity required for development of kindling consists of focal electrical seizures ("afterdischarges" (AD)). Racine[7] demonstrated that evoking an AD is an absolute prerequisite to kindling induction, in that repeated applications of electrical stimulations that fail to evoke an AD are not sufficient to induce kindling. Electrical stimulations are the most convenient method for afterdischarge induction, but repeated induction of focal ADs by microinjection of chemicals such as the cholinergic agonist carbachol[8,9] is also sufficient to induce kindling. The precise cellular events underlying an AD are incompletely understood. These include synaptic events and almost certainly non-synaptic (e.g. ephaptic) events in addition to the synchronous firing of action potentials by large populations of neurons.[10–12] Included in the synaptic events undoubtedly occurring during an AD is the activation of glutamate receptors, because antagonists of glutamate receptors can block focal seizures *in vitro*.[13]

What receptors are activated during an AD that are necessary for kindling development? The receptor most strongly implicated in kindling development is the N-methyl-D-aspartate (NMDA) subtype of glutamate receptor. First, many studies show that eliciting repeated ADs in the presence of diverse structurally distinct NMDA receptor antagonists profoundly retards the development of kindling.[14–23] Pretreatment with either competitive or uncompetitive antagonists of the NMDA receptor results in striking limitation of lengthening of the AD and progression of behavioral seizure intensity. Second, repeated focal microinjection of NMDA itself causes kindling, and this NMDA-induced kindling transfers to electrical kindling.[24] By contrast, a competitive antagonist of the AMPA receptor (NBQX) does not inhibit kindling development at a dose demonstrated to partially inhibit kindled seizures.[25] Third, a recent microdialysis study demonstrated increased glutamate content in the amygdala during a kindled motor seizure.[26] The contribution of activation of other glutamate receptor subtypes (such as kainate receptors or metabotropic receptors) and other receptors and ion channels is still uncertain.

4. KINDLING DEVELOPMENT: A CONSEQUENCE OF GLUTAMATE RECEPTOR-TRIGGERED IMMEDIATE-EARLY GENE EXPRESSION?

Given the pivotal role of ADs and NMDA receptor activation in kindling development, how might hundreds of seconds of NMDA receptor activation in the context of ADs lead to a lifelong structural and functional reorganization exemplified in kindling? How do brief experiences of any sort lead to a lasting modification of brain structure and function? Morgan and Curran[27] and Goelet *et al.*[28] provide an attractive model in which immediate-early genes such as *c-fos* transduce brief episodes of neuronal activity into lasting changes in neuronal structure and function via regulation of gene expression. IEGs such as *c-fos* encode transcription factors which themselves bind to the regulatory elements of target genes to regulate their expression.

What evidence implicates IEGs in kindling development? Results from multiple laboratories have convincingly demonstrated that seizures can induce the transcriptional activation of IEGs. Morgan *et al.*[29] discovered that chemoconvulsant-evoked seizures trigger a marked but transient increase in expression of *c-fos*. Dragunow and Robertson[30] further demonstrated that the necessary event for kindling development, an AD, is sufficient to induce a striking increase in expression of Fos protein in the dentate granule cells of the hippocampus. Simonato *et al.*[31] demonstrated that a brief AD is sufficient to induce increases in expression of multiple IEGs including *c-fos*, *c-jun*, and *NGFI-A* but not *c-myc*. Further analyses of AD-evoked IEG expression in the kindling model revealed other consistent patterns: 1. AD-evoked increases of IEG expression are confined to neurons; no evidence for glial expression has been detected. 2. Generalized limbic and clonic motor (Class 5) kindled seizures induce the expression of IEGs in a small subset of limbic structures with perfect symmetry between the two hemispheres.[32] 3. The anatomic extent of seizure-evoked expression of *c-fos* mRNA expands progressively following focal limbic and clonic motor (Classes 1–3) seizures during the development of kindling.[33] 4. Distinct IEGs exhibit different sensitivities of AD-induced expression with a rank order of thresholds (most sensitive to least sensitive) of: *NGFI-A* > *c-fos* > *c-jun* > *NGFI-B*. Despite these different sensitivities, each IEG is expressed in a subset of the constellation of structures in which the most sensitive IEG (*NGFI-A*) is induced.

The above findings suggest the following conclusions. The progression in anatomic extent of seizure-evoked expression during evolution of kindling fits with the idea that IEG expression may contribute to kindling development. IEG expression occurs in a small subset of limbic structures despite the fact that the seizures themselves are widespread and undoubtedly involve many populations of neurons in which IEG expression is not induced. The distribution of seizure-evoked IEG expression provides an anatomic framework for study of the phenotypic consequences of IEG expression. The similarity in structures expressing different IEGs implies some commonality in mechanism of expression, yet the difference in induction sensitivity also implies some divergence in mechanism.

How do kindled seizures trigger the transcriptional activation of IEGs? Since *c-fos* had been advanced as a marker of neuronal activity, neuronal activity *per se* emerged as an attractive explanation of seizure-induced IEG expression. The hallmark of the neuronal activity of a seizure is epileptiform burst firing. To our surprise, epileptiform burst firing was not sufficient for seizure-induced IEG expression. Unit recording of pars reticulata and pars compacta neurons of substantia nigra during a class 5 kindled seizure demonstrated burst firing,[34,35] yet no evidence for seizure-evoked IEG expression was detected in the substantia nigra.[32] We next considered the possibility that NMDA receptor activation during the seizure was crucial to the IEG induction. Similarity in the anatomic distribution of seizure-evoked expression of IEGs and NMDA receptors was consistent with this idea. Indeed, we demonstrated[36] that two structurally distinct antagonists acting at distinct sites of the NMDA receptor markedly reduced kindled seizure-induced *c-fos* expression in the dentate granule cells of the hippocampus. This inhibition occurred despite an increase in the number of granule cell population action potentials during the seizure.

Taken together, these results provided circumstantial evidence consistent with the idea that glutamate receptor-triggered IEG expression may contribute to kindling development. The necessary event for induction of kindling, an AD, is sufficient to induce IEG expression. The anatomic extent of seizure-induced IEG expression parallels the behavioral and electrophysiologic features of kindling development. Activation of NMDA receptors during ADs is pivotally involved in both kindling development and transcriptional activation of IEGs.

To move from correlation to causation, we aimed to directly determine whether IEG expression is necessary for kindling development. The development of mice carrying a null mutation of *c-fos*[37] (*c-fos* knockout or "fosless" mice) provided a powerful preparation with which to address this question. To this end, we assayed the effect of *c-fos* deletion on kindling development and kindling-induced mossy fiber sprouting.[38] We found that indeed the development of kindling was partially impaired in "fosless" mice. With the knockout of this one IEG, we did not observe a complete abrogation of kindling, but fosless mice were significantly impaired in both afterdischarge lengthening and behavioral seizure development during early kindling stimulations. Second, kindling-induced granule cell axon sprouting into the supragranular region of the dentate gyrus as measured by Timm staining was markedly attenuated in c-*fos* null mutants. We believe that these findings do support the hypothesis that expression of IEGs such as c-*fos* link brief episodes of neuronal activity to lasting modifications of structure and function in the mammalian nervous system.

5. THE FOSLESS PHENOTYPE: IMPAIRED ACTIVATION OF PRO-GROWTH GENE PROGRAMS?

If *c-fos* is necessary for the normal development of kindling and kindling-induced mossy fiber sprouting, what are the target genes of *c-fos* which underlie the "fosless" phenotype? In addition to *c-fos* and other IEGs, seizure activity in the mature brain triggers the transcriptional activation of genes encoding neurotrophic factors (e.g. NGF, BDNF, bFGF), neurotrophic factor receptors (e.g. trkB, FGFR-1), and axonal growth-associated proteins (e.g. GAP-43) in the dentate granule cells.[39–46] Such 'pro-growth' genes are excellent candidates to contribute to seizure induction of mossy fiber sprouting and kindling development in the mature brain. The ability of BDNF or bFGF to selectively enhance the branching of axons but not dendrites of dentate gyrus neurons *in vitro* suggests that neurotrophic factors may contribute to mossy fiber sprouting *in vivo*.[47,48] NGF antibodies have been shown to interfere with kindling development,[49,50] and kindling development is markedly retarded in BDNF +/– mice.[51] Furthermore, transgenic mice overexpressing GAP-43 display spontaneous mossy fiber sprouting (and spontaneous seizures!).[52] The presence of AP-1 sites in the regulatory elements of the bFGF[53] and GAP-43[54] promoter regions strengthens the candidacy of these particular genes in the "fosless phenotype." Although all other possibilities cannot be excluded, we believe that the absence of c-*fos* may limit the transcriptional activation of such growth-related genes. The potential for compensatory or adaptive effects of other members of the FOS family such as *fra*-1, *fra*-2, or *fos*B may explain why inhibition of this structural and functional plasticity is partial instead of complete.[55]

6. IS CELL DEATH NECESSARY FOR KINDLING?

The marked reinduction of such growth-related genes following pathologic activity in the mature nervous system lends support to our concept that seizure activity recapitulates a plastic state in which axonal and synaptic rearrangements occur, now leading to the pathologic outcome termed kindling. However, one possibility that could limit the conceivability of this hypothesis is that other pathologic changes, such as cell death, may accompany pathologic levels of activity. These other changes, not the reactivation of growth-related genes, could in principle be responsible for kindling. Thus, a key question is whether some population of cells must die for kindling to occur.

Initially, reductions in hilar neuronal density were discovered following kindling, which were interpreted to be due to death of hilar neurons.[56,57] Cavazos and Sutula described reductions in hilar neuronal density in rats approximating 15% and 40% after three and thirty Class 5 kindled seizures, respectively. In our recent study, we confirm these findings by demonstrating a reduction in hilar neuronal density of approximately 30% following ten to fifteen Class 5 kindled seizures in *c-fos* +/+ mice.[38] Importantly, however, kindling did not result in any significant change in the total number of hilar neurons in *c-fos* +/+, +/–, or –/– mice. Instead, there were significant increases in hilar volume in all genotypes. Thus, the reductions in hilar neuronal density were due to increases in hilar volume, not to loss of hilar neurons. Although no cell loss was detectable, we cannot exclude the possibility that loss of a small population of hilar neurons escaped detection in these experiments. In similar studies, Lothman and colleagues[58,59] have reported kindling-induced reductions in hilar neuronal density which were due to increases in hilar volume, not to loss of neurons.

Thus, kindling and kindling-induced mossy fiber sprouting do not appear to require death of hilar neurons. In contrast, the kindling-induced increases in hilar volume are reminiscent of the preferential increases in volume identified in those regions of rat neocortex undergoing greater use during development.[60] Accordingly, we favor the idea that the increased hilar volume reflects neuropil elaboration during kindling. (Of course, other possibilities could account for the increase in hilar volume, such as glial proliferation or fluid accumulation in the extracellular or intracellular space, and these warrant careful study.)

7. KINDLING OVERACTIVITY LEADS TO OVERGROWTH OF ADULT NERVOUS SYSTEM

To return to our original conceptualization: in contrast to the effects of physiologic activity on the developing brain, kindling development is the consequence of pathologic activity in mature brain. Just as "pathologic" underactivity leads to "pathologic" undergrowth in the developing visual system, "pathologic" overactivity in kindling leads to "pathologic" overgrowth (mossy fiber sprouting and neosynaptogenesis) in the adult limbic system. In each case, we term the abnormal level of activity "pathologic" because it leads to pathologic outcomes: impaired vision in the former case, epileptogenesis in the latter.

A fascinating possibility is that other pathologic behavioral plasticities in the mature nervous system may share similar mechanisms to kindling. For example, drug sensitization and dependence parallels kindling in that a repeated stimulus (drug administration) leads to long-term pathologic behavioral changes likely due at least in part to abnormal activation of distinct neuronal populations. Mechanistic similarities emerge as well. First, drug sensitization and dependence appears like kindling to be NMDA receptor-dependent in that NMDA receptor antagonists inhibit drug sensitization and dependence in various studies.[61,62] Second, drug administration alters immediate-early gene programs presumably leading to the activation of downstream genes potentially responsible in part for the phenotypes of sensitization and dependence.[63] Third, like kindling, drug sensitization and dependence are robust and long-lasting behavioral changes. While more detailed investigation is crucial, it is intriguing to speculate that abnormal activity-driven plasticity may underlie these and other pathologic states in the adult nervous system, such as post-traumatic stress disorder and central pain sensitization.[64] It is clear that the kindling model has much to offer of heuristic value to the cellular and molecular investigation of these conditions.

Thus, in kindling intermittent seizures activate NMDA receptors, immediate-early genes, and pro-growth gene programs and may lead to elaboration of neuropil and formation of novel functional (predominantly excitatory) synapses. Kindling-induced neuropil elaboration and neosynaptogenesis would superimpose novel dysfunctional circuitry upon existing circuitry, which could then underlie the development and permanence of the hyperexcitable ('kindled') state. The identity and functional importance of the gene programs activated by kindling stimulation in addition to the functional properties of the associated histological and ultrastructural changes continue to provide fascinating and fundamental questions for future study.

ACKNOWLEDGMENTS

This work was supported by NIH grant NS32334. We would like to acknowledge the following colleagues for their contributions to our studies: D.W. Bonhaus, L. Butler, Z. Cao, N. Garcia-Cairasco, D.A. Hosford, R.S. Johnson, D.M. Labiner, L.S. Lerea, H.H. Mansbach, J.V. Nadler, V.E. Papaioannou, M.N. Patel, L. Rigsbee, R.D. Russell, C. Shin, J.M. Silver, M. Simonato, B.M. Spiegelman, J.R. Walters, Y. Watanabe, and G.C. Yeh.

REFERENCES

1. Wiesel, T.N. and Hubel, D.H., Single cell responses in striate cortex of kittens deprived of vision in one eye, *J. Neurophysiol.*, 26 (1963) 1003–1017.
2. McNamara, J.O., Cellular and molecular basis of epilepsy, *J. Neurosci.*, 14 (1994) 3413–3425.
3. Sutula, T., He, X.X., Cavazos, J. and Scott, G., Synaptic reorganization in the hippocampus induced by abnormal functional activity, *Science*, 239 (1988) 1147–1150.
4. Nadler, J.V., Perry, B.W. and Cotman, C.W., Selective reinnervation of hippocampal area CA1 and the fascia dentata after destruction of CA3-CA4 afferents with kainic acid, *Brain Res.*, 182 (1980) 1–9.
5. Tauck, D.L. and Nadler, J.V., Evidence of functional mossy fiber sprouting in hippocampal formation of kainic acid-treated rats, *J. Neurosci.*, 5 (1985) 1016–1022.

6. Wuarin, J.-P. and Dudek, F.E., Electrographic seizures and new recurrent excitatory circuits in the dentate gyrus of hippocampal slices from kainate-treated epileptic rats, *J. Neurosci.*, 16 (1996) 4438–4448.
7. Racine, R.J., Modification of seizure activity by electrical stimulation. II. Motor seizure, *Electroenceph. clin. Neurophysiol.*, 32 (1972) 281–294.
8. Vosu, H. and Wise, R.A., Cholinergic seizure kindling in the rat: comparison of caudate, amygdala, and hippocampus, *Behav. Biol.*, 13 (1975) 491–496.
9. Wasterlain, C.G. and Jonec,V., Chemical kindling by muscarinic amygdaloid stimulation in the rat, *Brain Res.*, 271 (1983) 311–316.
10. Somjen, G.G., Aitken, P.C., Giacchino, J.L. and McNamara, J.O., Sustained potential shifts and paroxysmal discharges in hippocampal formation, *J. Neurophysiol.*, 53 (1985) 1079–1097.
11. Schweitzer, J.S., Patrylo, P.R. and Dudek, F.E., Prolonged field bursts in the dentate gyrus: dependence on low calcium, high potassium, and nonsynaptic mechanisms, *J. Neurophysiol.*, 68 (1992) 2016–2025.
12. Stringer, J.L. and Lothman, E.W., Bilateral maximal dentate activation is critical for the appearance of an afterdischarge in the dentate gyrus, *Neuroscience*, 46 (1992) 309–314.
13. Traynelis, S.F. and Dingledine, R., Potassium-induced spontaneous electrographic seizures in the rat hippocampal slice, *J. Neurophysiol.*, 59 (1988) 259–276.
14. McNamara, J.O., Russell, R.D., Rigsbee, L. and Bonhaus, D.W., Anticonvulsant and antiepileptogenic actions of MK-801 in the kindling and electroshock models, *Neuropharmacology*, 27 (1988) 563–568.
15. McNamara, J.O., Bonhaus, D.W., Nadler, J.V. and Yeh, G.C., N-methyl-D-aspartate (NMDA) receptors and the kindling model, in Wada, J.A. (Ed.), *Kindling 4*, Plenum Press, New York, 1990, pp. 197–208.
16. Callaghan, D.A. and Schwark, W.S., Pharmacological modification of amygdaloid-kindled seizures, *Neuropharmacology*, 19 (1980) 1131–1136.
17. Bowyer, J.F. and Winters, E.D., The effects of various anesthetics on amygdaloid kindled seizures, *Neuropharmacology*, 20 (1981) 199–204.
18. Bowyer, J.F., Phencyclidine inhibition of the rate of kindling development, *Exp. Neurol.*, 75 (1982) 173–178.
19. Bowyer, J.F., Albertson, T.E., Winters, W.D. and Baselt, R.C., Ketamine-induced changes in kindled amygdaloid seizures, *Neuropharmacology*, 22 (1983) 887–892.
20. Holmes, K.H. and Goddard, G.V., A role for the N-methyl-D-aspartate receptor in kindling, *Proc. Univ. Otago Med. Sch.*, 64 (1986) 37–42.
21. Holmes, K.H., Bilkey, D.K., Laverty, R. and Goddard, G.V., The N-methyl-D-aspartate antagonists aminophosphonovalerate and carboxypiperazinephosphonate retard the development and expression of kindled seizures, *Brain Res.*, 506 (1990) 227–235.
22. Cain, D.P., Desborough, K.A. and McKitrick, D.J., Retardation of amygdaloid kindling by antagonism of NMD-aspartate and muscarinic cholinergic receptors: evidence for the summation of excitatory mechanisms in kindling, *Exp. Neurol.*, 100 (1988) 203–208.
23. Vezzani, A., Wu, H.Q., Moneta, E. and Samanin, R., Role of the N-methyl-D-aspartate-type receptors in the development and maintenance of hippocampal kindling in rats, *Neurosci. Lett.*, 87 (1988) 63–68.
24. Croucher, M.J., Cotterell, K.L., and Bradford, H.F., Amygdaloid kindling by repeated focal N-methyl-D-aspartate administration: comparison with electrical kindling, *Eur. J. Pharmacol.*, 286 (1995) 265–271.
25. Durmuller, N., Craggs, M. and Meldrum, B.S., The effect of the non-NMDA receptor antagonists GYKI 52466 and NBQX and the competitive NMDA receptor antagonist D-CPPene on the development of amygdala kindling and on amygdala-kindled seizures, *Epilepsy Res.*, 17 (1994) 167–174.
26. Kaura, S., Bradford, H.F., Young, A.M.J., Croucher, M.J. and Hughes, P.D., Effect of amygaloid kindling on the content and release of amino acids from the amygdaloid complex: in vivo and in vitro studies, *J. Neurochem.* 65 (1995) 1240–1249.
27. Morgan, J.I. and Curran, T., Role of ion flux in the control of *c-fos* expression, *Nature*, 322 (1986) 552–555.
28. Goelet, P., Castellucci, V.F., Schacher, S. and Kandel, E.R., The long and short of long-term memory—a molecular framework, *Nature*, 322 (1986) 419–422.
29. Morgan, J.I., Cohen, D.R., Hempstead, J.L. and Curran, T., Mapping patterns of *c-fos* expression in the central nervous system after seizure, *Science*, 237 (1987) 192–197.
30. Dragunow, M. and Robertson, H.A., Kindling stimulation induces *c-fos* protein(s) in granule cells of the rat dentate gyrus, *Nature*, 329 (1987) 441–442.
31. Simonato, M., Hosford, D.A., Labiner, D.M., Shin, C., Mansbach, H.H. and McNamara, J.O., Differential expression of immediate early genes in the hippocampus in the kindling model of epilepsy, *Mol. Brain Res.*, 11 (1991) 115–124.
32. Hosford, D.A., Simonato, M., Cao, Z., Garcia-Cairasco, N., Silver, J.M., Butler, L., Shin, C. and McNamara, J.O., Differences in the anatomic distribution of immediate-early gene expression in amygdala and angular bundle kindling, *J. Neurosci.*, 15 (1995) 2513–2523.

33. Clark, M., Post, R.M., Weiss, S.R.B., Cain, C.J. and Nakajima, T., Regional expression of *c-fos* mRNA in rat brain during the evolution of amygdala kindled seizures, *Mol. Brain Res.*, 11 (1991) 55–64.
34. Bonhaus, D.W., Walters, J.R. and McNamara, J.O., Activation of substantia nigra neurons: role in the propagation of seizures in kindled rats, *J. Neurosci.*, 6 (1986) 3024–3030.
35. Bonhaus, D.W., Russell, R.D. and McNamara, J.O., Activation of substantia nigra pars reticulata neurons: role in the initiation and behavioral expression of kindled seizures, *Brain Res.*, 545 (1991) 41–48.
36. Labiner, D.M., Butler, L.S., Cao, Z., Hosford, D.A., Shin, C. and McNamara, J.O., Induction of *c-fos* mRNA by kindled seizures: complex relationship with neuronal burst firing, *J. Neurosci.*, 13 (1993) 744–751.
37. Johnson, R.S., Spiegelman, B.M. and Papaioannou, V., Pleiotropic effects of a null mutation in the *c-fos* proto-oncogene, *Cell*, 71 (1992) 577–586.
38. Watanabe, Y., Johnson, R.S., Butler, L.S., Binder, D.K., Spiegelman, B.M., Papaioannou, V.E. and McNamara, J.O., Null mutation of *c-fos* impairs structural and functional plasticities in the kindling model of epilepsy, *J. Neurosci.*, 16 (1996) 3827–3836.
39. Gall, C.M. and Isackson, P.J., Limbic seizures increase neuronal production of messenger RNA for nerve growth factor, *Science*, 245 (1989) 758–761.
40. Ernfors, P., Bengzon, J., Kokaia, Z., Persson, H. and Lindvall, O., Increased levels of messenger RNAs for neurotrophic factors in the brain during kindling epileptogenesis, *Neuron*, 7 (1991) 165–176.
41. Gall, C.M., Seizure-induced changes in neurotrophin expression: implications for epilepsy, *Exp. Neurol.*, 124 (1993) 150–166.
42. Bengzon, J., Kokaia, Z., Ernfors, P., Kokaia, M., Leanza, G., Nilsson, O.G., Persson, H. and Lindvall, O., Regulation of neurotrophin and trkA and trkC tyrosine kinase receptor messenger RNA expression in kindling, *Neuroscience*, 53 (1993) 433–436.
43. Bugra, K., Pollard, H., Charton, G., Moreau, J., Ben-Ari, Y., Khrestchatisky, M., aFGF, bFGF and flg mRNAs show distinct patterns of induction in the hippocampus following kainate-induced seizures, *Eur. J. Neurosci.*, 6 (1994) 58–66.
44. Gall, C.M., Berschauer, R. and Isackson, P.J., Seizures increase basic fibroblast growth factor mRNA in adult rat forebrain neurons and glia, *Mol. Brain Res.*, 21 (1994) 190–205.
45. Bendotti, C., Vezzani, A., Tarizzo, G. and Samanin, R., Increased expression of GAP-43, somatostatin and neuropeptide Y mRNA in the hippocampus during development of hippocampal kindling in rats, *Eur. J. Neurosci.*, 5 (1993) 1312–1320.
46. Meberg, P.J., Gall, C.M. and Routtenberg, A., Induction of F1/GAP-43 gene: expression in hippocampal granule cells after seizures, *Mol. Brain Res.*, 17 (1993) 295–297.
47. Patel, M.N., and McNamara, J.O., Selective enhancement of axonal branching of cultured dentate gyrus neurons by neurotrophic factors, *Neuroscience*, 69 (1995) 763–770.
48. Lowenstein, D.H. and Arsenault, L., The effects of growth factors on the survival and differentiation of cultured dentate gyrus neurons, *J. Neurosci.*, 16 (1996) 1759–1769.
49. Funabashi, T., Sasaki, H. and Kimura, F., Intraventricular injection of antiserum to nerve growth factor delays the development of amygdaloid kindling, *Brain Res.*, 458 (1988) 132–136.
50. Van der Zee, C.E.E.M., Rashid, K., Le, K., Moore, K.A., Stanisz, J., Diamond, J., Racine, R.J. and Fahnestock, M., Intraventricular administration of antibodies to nerve growth factor retards kindling and blocks mossy fiber sprouting in adult rats, *J. Neurosci.*, 15 (1995) 5316–5323.
51. Kokaia, M., Ernfors, P., Kokaia, Z., Elmer, E., Jaenisch, R. and Lindvall, O., Suppressed epileptogenesis in BDNF mutant mice, *Exp. Neurol.*, 133 (1995) 215–224.
52. Aigner, L., Arber, S., Kapfhammer, J.P., Laux, T., Schneider, C., Botteri, F., Brenner, H.-R. and Caroni, P., Overexpression of the neural growth-associated protein GAP-43 induces nerve sprouting in the adult nervous system of transgenic mice, *Cell*, 83 (1995) 269–278.
53. Shibata, F., Baird, A. and Florkiewicz, R.Z., Functional characterization of the human basic fibroblast growth factor gene promoter, *Growth Factors*, 4 (1991) 277–287.
54. Nedivi, E., Basi, G.S., Akey, I.V. and Skene, J.H., A neural-specific GAP-43 core promoter located between unusual DNA elements that interact to regulate its activity, *J. Neurosci.*, 12 (1992) 691–704.
55. Pennypacker, K.R., Hong, J.-S. and McMillian, M.K., Implications of prolonged expression of Fos-related antigens, *Trends Pharmacol. Sci.*, 16 (1995) 317–321.
56. Cavazos, J.E. and Sutula, T.P., Progressive neuronal loss induced by kindling: a possible mechanism for mossy fiber synaptic reorganization and hippocampal sclerosis, *Brain Res.*, 527 (1990) 1–6.
57. Cavazos, J.E., Das, I. and Sutula, T.P., Neuronal loss induced in limbic pathways by kindling: evidence for induction of hippocampal sclerosis by repeated brief seizures, *J. Neurosci.*, 14 (1994) 3106–3121.
58. Bertram, E.H., Lothman, E.W. and Lenn, N.J., The hippocampus in experimental chronic epilepsy: a morphometric analysis, *Ann. Neurol.*, 27 (1990) 43–48.

59. Bertram, E.H. and Lothman, E.W., Morphometric effects of intermittent kindled seizures and limbic status epilepticus in the dentate gyrus of the rat, *Brain Res.*, 603 (1993) 25–31.
60. Purves, D., *Neural activity and the growth of the brain*, Cambridge University Press, Cambridge, UK, 1994.
61. Trujillo, K.A. and Akil, H., Inhibition of morphine tolerance and dependence by the NMDA receptor antagonist MK-801, *Science*, 251 (1991) 85–87.
62. Ohmori, T., Abekawa, T., Muraki, A. and Koyama, T., Competitive and noncompetitive NMDA antagonists block sensitization to methamphetamine, *Pharmacol. Biochem. Behav.*, 48 (1994) 587–591.
63. Nestler, E.J., Hope, B.T., and Widnell, K.L., Drug addiction: a model for the molecular basis of neural plasticity, *Neuron*, 11 (1993) 995–1006.
64. Woolf, C.J. and Thompson, S.W.N., The induction and maintenance of central sensitization is dependent on N-methyl-D-aspartic acid receptor activation: implications for the treatment of post-injury pain hypersensitivity states, *Pain*, 44 (1991) 293–299.

DISCUSSION OF JAMES MCNAMARA'S PAPER

S. Moshe: You reported that the difference in kindling in the mouse without c-*fos* compared to the regular mouse was in the early stages of kindling. Did you do an experiment to examine fiber reorganization after the first few stages, where the real difference is, rather than much later in kindling where the stages were equivalent.

J. McNamara: The answer is no we didn't, and the reason we did the experiment this way was that this was biasing against detecting a difference between the two. What we think is that it is the activity that drives the synaptic reorganization, so that if we killed the mice after 10 stimulations we would find a little bit of sprouting in the wild-type and none in the knockout mice because they haven't had any activity.

S. Moshe: Right then, how do you reach the conclusion in your last slide that you have that the knockout of c-fos impairs kindling and mossy fiber sprouting, when you're really testing mossy fiber sprouting much later when kindling is not impaired.

J. McNamara: Wait a minute, I am not saying that the defect in the mossy fiber sprouting is causing the reduction in kindling. I think that that is a very important possibility, but I am the last one that's going to stand on that one.

S. Moshe: What do you think is the physiological basis of the increase in volume in the hilus.

J. McNamara: I can imagine a number of possibilities. One is that it could be proliferation of glial cells, another one could be that it is an expansion of fluid in the extracellular space or an expansion of fluid in the intracellular space; but what I think is that it is none of those. I think it is an elaboration of neuropil. Why do I think that? If you look, the very first slide I showed is very important conceptually in terms of looking at kindling because all the data on activity-determined plasticity and development provide a road map, a context for understanding kindling. If you look at the development of the nervous system, if you look at barrel cortex in the rat brain as compared to the cortex that is not used very much, what Purves has done is to demonstrate a correlation between heavily used cortex in the expansion of what appears to be neuropil in the barrel cortex whereas unused cortex has a much smaller expansion. I think that this is the same sort of thing with kindling; that's my hypothesis.

I. Mody: Jim, what do you think is so special about calcium entry through NMDA channels that triggers the c-*fos*, as opposed to calcium entering through voltage-gated channels? Also just a comment on the last question, do you think that sprouting itself could expand the hilus?

J. McNamara: I don't know whether it is the mossy fibers themselves that are expanding the hilus, but my suspicion is that this could be one of many contributions. My suspicion is that the mossy fibers provide a little mini window on the neuropil expansion at multiple sites in that nervous system—you can measure it in the mossy fibers. With respect to the calcium and what's so special about the calcium entering through the NMDA channel: This is something that we have spent a lot of time and energy working on, and we've got dentate gyrus neurons in primary culture. What you can demonstrate is that you can turn on *fos* in those cells through calcium entry, either voltage-sensitive calcium channels that are triggered through AMPA receptor activation or directly by calcium going directly through the NMDA receptors. What I think is so special, and this is a hypothesis, is that when calcium goes in through different sites in the cell, it is spatially compartmentalized. There are other proteins and enzymes that are also spatially compartmentalized, and we have demonstrated for example that activation of phospholipase II and oxygenase is required for the NMDA receptor activation of the *fos*, in a calcium-dependent manner, that those enzymes have nothing to do with the AMPA receptor activation of *fos* when it goes through a calcium channel. So I think that the calcium that is going through the NMDA channel is compartmentalized, hooked up to the PSD, and it's locking these things up in its spines. That compartmentalizes the actions of calcium to different enzymes and molecular cascades.

F. Lopez da Silva: My question has to do with the genes. You see the increase in the expression of c-*fos* quite quickly or very early, but one also sees very quickly the expression of *jun* and *zif* and other immediate genes, and these of course are not involved in your model. So there are other pathways that can cause cascades of change that could be important to account for the fact that your mice can still be kindled—they are not impaired in kindling, they are retarded in kindling.

J. McNamara: In fact, we did test *zif*, which is synonymous with NGFIA, and it appears to be relatively unimportant in this. I'm not trying to tell you that *fos* alone is the be-all and end-all of kindling. Obviously kindling was retarded but the animals did kindle and they developed some mossy fiber sprouting. We are using this as a model to dissect out how this might occur. My suspicion is that there are multiple immediate early genes and a whole complex of transcription factors that are activated that must bind to the regulatory elements of a host of different target chains. So it's far more complex than just *fos*, but my suspicion is that not all of the immediate early genes are equally important. For example, perhaps NGFIA is turned on through activation of voltage-sensitive calcium channels, and I'm not convinced that that is causally related to kindling. Who knows what function, if any, this has with respect to kindling.

R. Racine: About the expansion of the hilus, just a couple things. We have, as I reported yesterday, seen astrocyte hypertrophy in the area; so that is no doubt contributing. If you look at the Timm's stain it is certainly very very dark in that whole area, and it is a possibility that there is some expansion. The staining is so heavy anyway that those fibers could spread out and still be black; so it's a little hard to know whether there is any actual sprouting there or not.

ACTIVITIES OF PROTEIN KINASE C IN THE KINDLING MODEL OF EPILEPSY

Kazufumi Akiyama

Department of Neuropsychiatry
Okayama University Medical School
2-5-1 Shikata-cho, Okayama 700, Japan

1. INTRODUCTION

Kindling is the process whereby repeated application of an initially subconvulsive electrical stimulation in a limbic brain structure leads to emergence of progressive epileptiform discharge, and eventually to generalized tonic-clonic motor seizures [4]. Once established, the kindling effect lasts throughout the life time of the animal. Kindling is an excellent model for studying the cellular mechanisms involved in the long-lasting neuronal excitability changes that underlie epilepsy, but the basic mechanism underlying this phenomenon still remains to be studied.

Protein kinase C (PKC) was initially characterized as a serine/threonine protein kinase which is activated by the presence of Ca^{2+} and diacylglycerol, and is now considered to comprise a family of closely related subspecies [20, 21, 31]. It is distributed widely in vertebrate tissues, but particularly high levels are found in the brain. Increase in the intracellular concentrations of calcium triggers moving of PKC molecule from the cytosolic compartment to the membrane, a phenomenon termed translocation, and diacylglycerol enhances the enzyme activity at membrane sites [21]. Putative functions of PKC may, therefore, involve events occurring at membrane sites, such as enhancement of neurotransmitter release [17], ion channel regulations [16, 27, 32], control of growth and differentiation [29] and neuronal plasticity modification [11]. The author and co-workers have investigated activities of PKC in the kindling model of epilepsy [1, 3, 13, 22]. This paper summarizes our findings of long-lasting increase in membrane-associated PKC activities in kindling [1, 3, 13, 22].

2. MATERIALS AND METHODS

2.1. Preparation of Hippocampal- and Amygdala-Kindled Rats

Male Sprague-Dawley rats (Charles River) weighing 250–300 g at the time of surgery were used. A twisted tripolar nichrome electrode was implanted stereotaxically into

Kindling 5, edited by Corcoran and Moshé.
Plenum Press, New York, 1998.

the left dorsal hippocampus (coordinates, AP: –2.6, L:2.3, D:3.2, according to the atlas of Pellegrino et al. [23]). A screw electrode was placed onto the right frontal skull as a reference. After a recovery period of 10 days, the rats received a kindling stimulus of a 1-s train of 60 Hz sine wave pulses at a current intensity of 200–300 μA twice daily. The development of kindled seizure was assessed according to Racine's classification [24]. After the animals had developed stage 5 seizures, the kindling stimulus was administered every other day until at least 5 consecutive stage 5 seizures were elicited. In the amygdala kindling, the electrode was implanted into the left amygdala (coordinates, AP:0, L:5.0, D:8.0, according to the atlas of Pellegrino et al. [23]), and the animals received a kindling stimulus of a 1-s train of 60 Hz sine wave pulses at a current intensity of 200 μA once daily until at least 5 consecutive stage 5 seizures were elicited. Animals that received an electrode implantation in either the left dorsal hippocampus or left amygdala, but no subsequent kindling stimulus, were used as age-matched controls.

2.2. Preparation of PKC-Containing Extracts Using Column Chromatographies

The brain was removed rapidly by decapitation, kept on ice without freezing, and subject to dissection. Fresh rat brain homogenates were centrifuged at 100,000 *g*. The resulting crude extracts of supernatant and pellet which was subsequently dissolved using 1% Triton X-100 were applied to a DEAE-cellulose column (DE-52, Whatman Co.), and the column eluates were taken as cytosolic and membrane-associated PKC-containing crude extracts as described previously [3, 13]. In the Experiment 3, the DE-52 column eluate was applied to a FPLC system (Pharmacia)-coupled hydroxylapatite column (Koken Co.), which had been preequilibrated with potassium phosphate buffer. The a, b and g subspecies were resolved in preprogramed potassium phosphate buffer gradient elution, whereby the concentration of potassium phosphate increased linearly from 20 mM to 215 mM as described previously [7, 12, 22].

2.3. Assay of Protein Kinase C

The PKC assay was performed as described previously [1, 3, 13, 22]. The enzyme preparation in a reaction mixture was either 10 to 30 ml of DE-52 column eluates of each crude extract or 80 μl of hydroxylapatite column eluates. The reaction mixture comprised 5 mmol Tris-HCl, pH 7.5, 1.25 μmol Mg-acetate, 2.5 nmol [γ-^{32}P]ATP, 50 μg H1 histone, 125 nmol $CaCl_2$, 2 μg phosphatidylserine (PS, Serdary Res. Lab.), 0.2 μg 1,2-diolein (DO, Serdary Res. Lab.) and the enzyme preparation. The reaction mixture (final volume of 0.25 ml) was incubated for 3–5 min at 30°C. In parallel with this incubation condition, an equal amount of the enzyme preparation was incubated in the absence of Ca^{2+}, PS and DO, but in the presence of 125 nmol EGTA. The radioactivity trapped on the nitrocellulose filter (pore size 0.45 μm, Toyo-Roshi Inc.), which was thoroughly washed with trichloroacetic acid, was measured using a liquid scintillation spectrometer. Basal activity, which was defined as the radioactivity in the absence of Ca^{2+}, PS and DO, but in the presence of 125 nmol EGTA, was less than 8% of total activity determined in the presence of 125 nmol Ca^{2+}, 2 μg PS and 0.2 μg DO. The radioactivity obtained by subtracting the basal activity from the total activity was transformed into [γ-^{32}P]ATP incorporated into H1 histone/min per mg protein, and the resulting data were shown as PKC activities in the Results.

2.4. In Situ Hybridization

The kindled and matched control rats were sacrificed by decapitation. The frozen brain tissues were sectioned 10-mm thick in a cryostat and thaw-mounted onto glass microscope slides, which were air-dried and stored at −80°C until required for use. Deoxyoligonucleotide antisense probes for PKC α, β, γ, ε and ζ subspecies were synthesized as described elsewhere [9, 19], and 3′-end-labeled with [^{35}S]dATP using terminal deoxyribonucleotidyl transferase. The in situ hybridization was conducted as described previously [5]. For quantification, the experimental slides and standards made of brain paste containing various concentrations of [^{35}S]dATP were exposed to the same tritium-sensitive film.

2.5. Outline of the Study

The present study consists of the four experiments. PKC activities were measured in the membrane and cytosolic fractions 4 and 16 weeks after the last seizure in the hippocampal- (Experiment 1) and amygdala (Experiment 2)-kindling. The activity of each conventional PKC subspecies (α, β, γ) was determined in the bilateral hippocampus 4 weeks after the last hippocampal kindled seizure (Experiment 3). Messenger RNA (mRNA) levels of the conventional subspecies (α, β, γ), and novel and atypical PKC subspecies (ε, ζ) were determined by the in situ hybridization technique 24 hours and 1 week after the last amygdala kindled seizure (Experiment 4).

2.6. Data Analysis

The statistical significance of differences in PKC activities between the right and left brain regions (hippocampus or amygdala/pyriform cortex) of the control was evaluated using Student's t test (unpaired, two-tailed). When there was no significant difference in PKC activities between the right and left brain regions of the control, the statistical significance of differences in PKC activities between the control and kindled group at the same side was evaluated using either Student's t test or one-factor ANOVA followed by a post-hoc test (Bonferroni/Dunn's procedure). P values of less than 0.05 were considered to be significant.

3. RESULTS

3.1. Experiment 1

There was no significant difference in cytosolic PKC activity between the control and the kindled group 4 weeks or 16 weeks after the last hippocampal kindled seizure. At 4 weeks after the last hippocampal seizure, membrane-associated PKC activities increased significantly in the right hippocampus (by 37%, $p<0.01$) and left hippocampus (by 24%, $p<0.05$) and the amygdala/pyriform cortex (by 14%, $p<0.02$) (Fig. 1). At 16 weeks after the last hippocampal seizure, the membrane-associated PKC activities in the kindled group increased significantly in the left hippocampus (by 33%, $p<0.03$) and the amygdala/pyriform cortex (by 62%, $p<0.02$) compared with the control group (Fig. 2).

3.2. Experiment 2

There was no significant difference in membrane-associated or cytosolic PKC activities between the control right and control left hippocampus at any seizure-free interval. 4 weeks after the last kindled seizure, the membrane-associated PKC activity in-

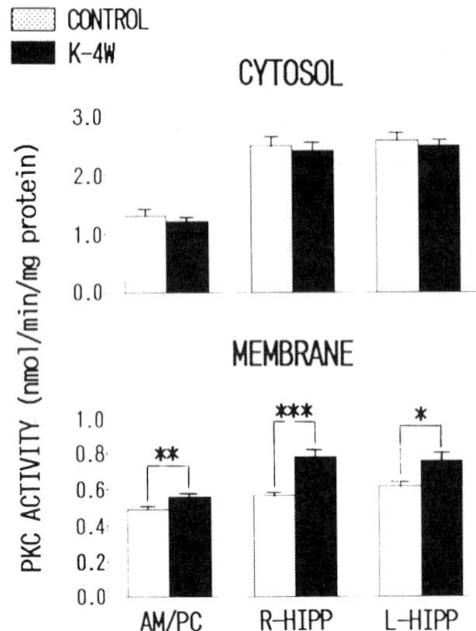

Figure 1. Cytosolic and membrane-associated PKC activity 4 weeks after the last hippocampal kindled seizure. Hippocampal-kindled rats and matched control rats were decapitated 4 weeks after the last kindled seizure. Values of nmol/min per mg protein are expressed as the mean ± S.E.M. of ten determinations. * p<0.05, ** p<0.02, *** p<0.001 as compared to the control (Student's *t* test).

creased significantly in the left hippocampus, which is ipsilateral to the stimulated amygdala (by 35% as compared to the right side control, P<0.03, and by 34% as compared to the left side control, P<0.03, Fig. 3). Sixteen weeks after the last kindled seizure, the membrane-associated PKC activity increased significantly in the left hippocampus (by 24% as compared to the left side control, P<0.05, Fig. 4). Significant difference in the membrane-associated PKC activities was noted between the left hippocampus of the kindled group and right hippocampus of the kindled group at 16 weeks after the

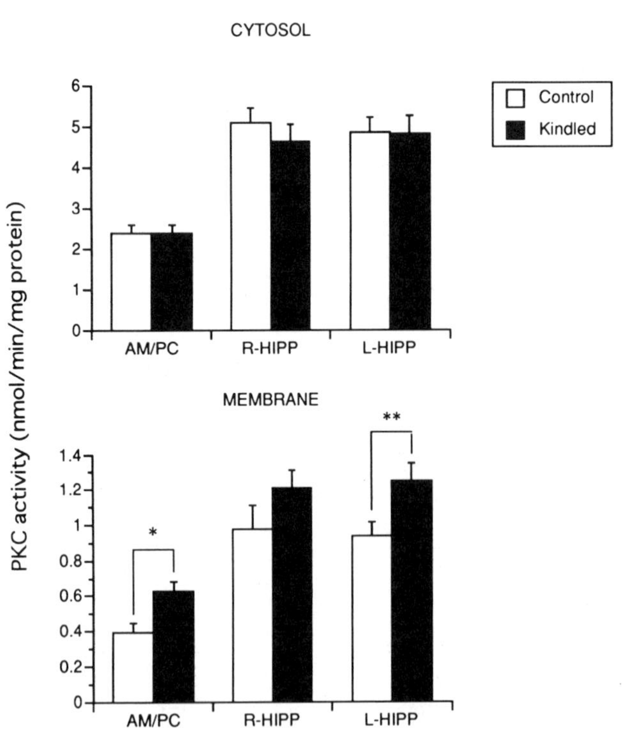

Figure 2. Cytosolic and membrane-associated PKC activity 16 weeks after the last hippocampal kindled seizure. Hippocampal-kindled rats and matched control rats were decapitated 16 weeks after the last kindled seizure. Values of nmol/min per mg protein are expressed as the mean ± S.E.M. of eight determinations. * p<0.02, ** p<0.03 as compared to the control (Student's *t* test).

4 Weeks after the Last Seizure

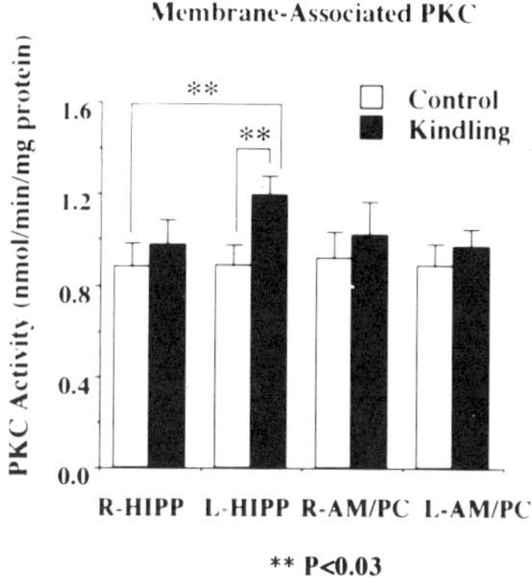

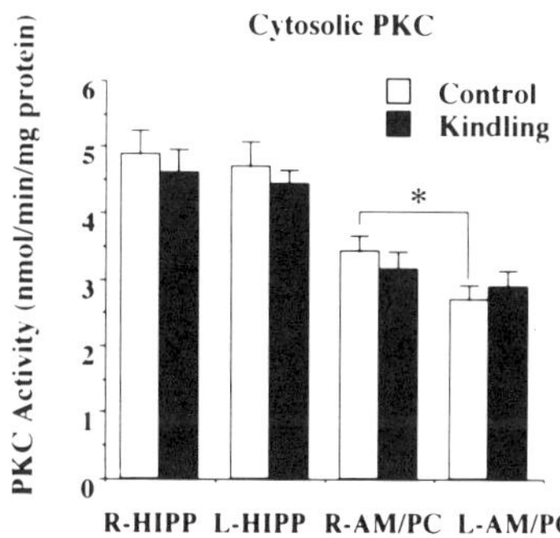

Figure 3. Cytosolic and membrane-associated PKC activity 4 weeks after the last amygdala kindled seizure. Amygdala-kindled rats and matched control rats were decapitated 4 weeks after the last kindled seizure. Values of nmol/min per mg protein are expressed as mean ± S.E.M. of eleven determinations. Bonferroni/Dunn's procedure revealed that the membrane-associated PKC activity increased significantly in the left hippocampus (by 35% as compared to the right side control, P<0.03, and by 34% as compared to the left side control, P<0.03). There was significant (P<0.05, Student's *t* test) difference in cytosolic, and not membrane-associated, PKC activities between the control right and control left amygdala/pyriform cortex.

16 Weeks after the Last Seizure

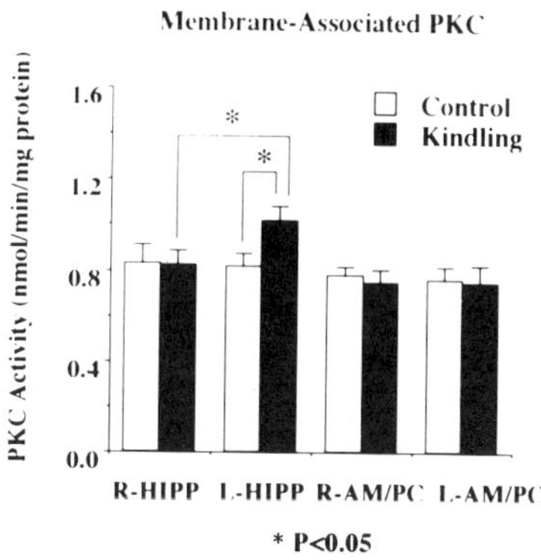

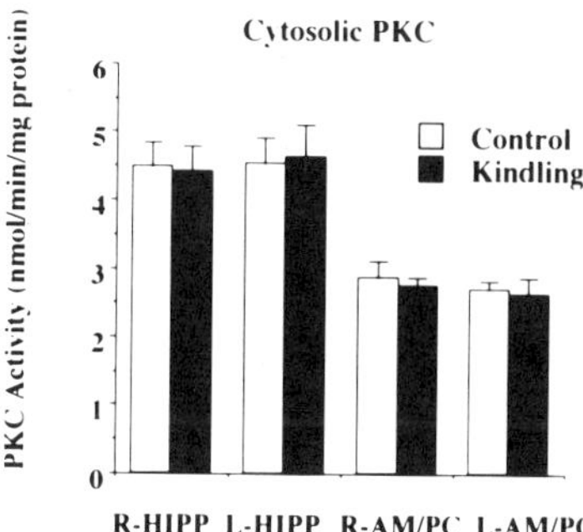

Figure 4. Cytosolic and membrane-associated PKC activity 16 weeks after the last amygdala kindled seizure. Amygdala-kindled rats and matched control rats were decapitated 16 weeks after the last generalized seizure. Values of nmol/min per mg protein are expressed as mean ± S.E.M. of nine determinations. Bonferroni/Dunn's procedure revealed that the membrane-associated PKC activity increased significantly in the left hippocampus (by 24% as compared to the left side control, P<0.05). The membrane-associated PKC activity in the left hippocampus of the kindled group was significantly higher than in the right hippocampus of the kindled group (P<0.05).

last kindled seizure (P<0.05, Fig. 4). The cytosolic PKC activity did not differ between the control and kindled groups in any brain region examined (Fig. 3 and Fig. 4).

3.3. Experiment 3

Fig. 5 shows a representative PKC elution profile from a hydroxylapatite column. The enzymes from both the cytosolic and membrane-associated components separated into three distinct peaks, which were designated types I (fraction no. 13–19), II (fraction no. 20–26)

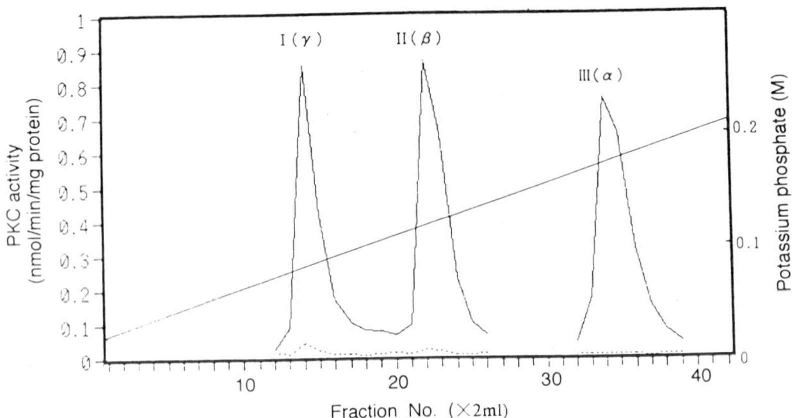

Figure 5. Resolution of PKC activity into three distinct fractions by hydroxylapatite chromatography. The PKC from rat hippocampal tissue homogenates was partially purified using DE-52 anion-exchange chromatoraphy, then subjected to hydroxylapatite chromatography, and PKC activity was assayed. — total PKC activity in the presence of Ca^{2+}, PS and DO, --- basal PKC activity in the presence of EGTA and absence of Ca^{2+}, PS and DO.

and III (fraction no. 32–39), as described by Huang et al. [3]. PKC activities of individual fractions which form each of types I, II and III were summed for the analysis. Western blot analysis showed that the subspecies-selective monoclonal antibodies (anti-γ, β and α) reacted with the type I, II and III-containing fractions from the three peaks eluted from the hydroxylapatite column, respectively, thus confirming their identities (Fig. 6). 4 weeks after the last hippocampal seizure, the membrane-associated activity of the α-subspecies was unchanged, but those of the β- and γ-subspecies in the hippocampal kindled group increased significantly compared with the controls (19%, $p<0.02$ for the β-subspecies, and 19%, $p<0.05$ for the γ-subspecies, Fig. 7). There were no significant differences in cytosolic PKC activity between the control and kindled groups for any subspecies examined.

3.4. Experiment 4

mRNA levels were compared among the three groups (control and two kindled groups fixed either 24 hours or 1 week after the last amygdala seizure). There was no significant difference in mRNA of the α subspecies among the three groups. mRNA levels of the β subspecies in the CA1 increased significantly in the kindled group fixed 1 week after the last seizure as compared to the control and kindled group fixed 24 hours after the last seizure (unpublished data). mRNA levels of the γ subspecies in the dentate gyrus increased significantly in the kindled group fixed 24 hours after the last seizure as compared to the control and kindled group fixed 1 week after the last seizure (unpublished data). mRNA levels of the ε subspecies in the CA1 and dentate gyrus increased significantly in the kindled group fixed 24 hours after the last seizure as compared to the control and kindled group fixed 1 week after the last seizure (unpublished data). There was no significant difference in mRNA of the ζ subspecies among the three groups.

4. DISCUSSION

PKC is now considered to exist as a family of multiple subspecies with closely related structures, but exhibits different biochemical characteristics, distinct tissue distribution and

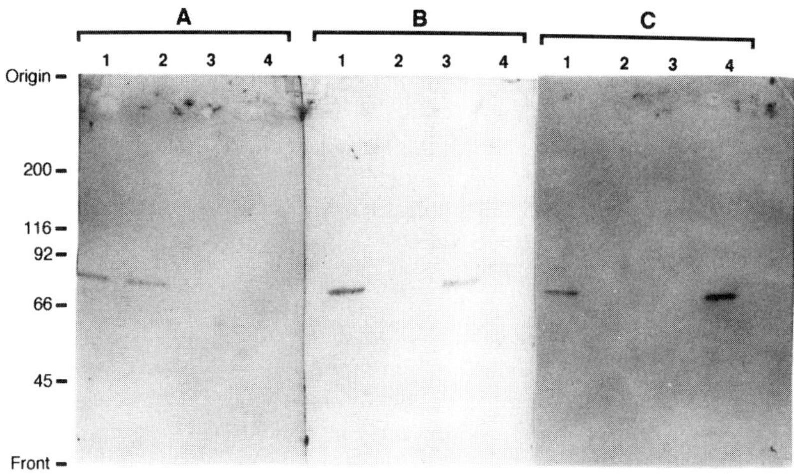

Figure 6. Western blot analysis of PKC subspecies from rat hippocampus. The rat hippocampal PKC subspecies were resolved by hydroxylapatite chromatography, concentrated and subjected to Western blot analysis with subspecies-selective monoclonal antibodies. The DE-52 column eluates (partially purified crude extracts containing α, β, and γ-subspecies) also were subjected to Western blot analysis. The first antibodies, mouse monoclonal antibodies raised against rabbit PKC subspecies, were diluted 1:50 and the second, horseradish peroxidase-conjugated goat anti-mouse immunoglobulin antibodies were diluted 1:2000. The PKC subspecies were detected with antibodies against α- (panel A), β-(panel B) and γ-subspecies (panel C). In each panel, lane 1 represents the DE-52 column eluate; lanes 2, 3, and 4 represent rat hippocampal peaks III, II and I respectively. The position of the origin, gel front and molecular mass standards are shown.

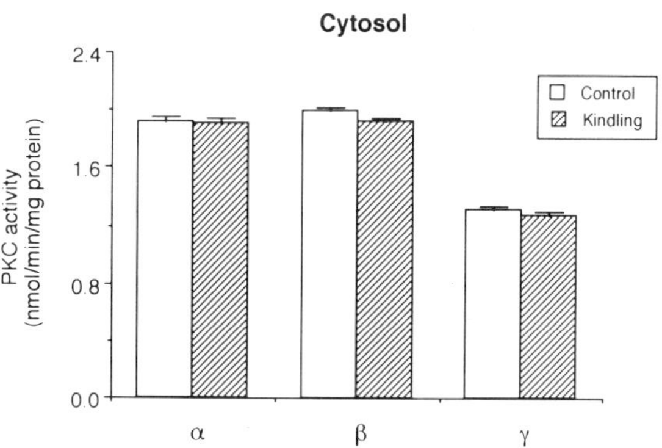

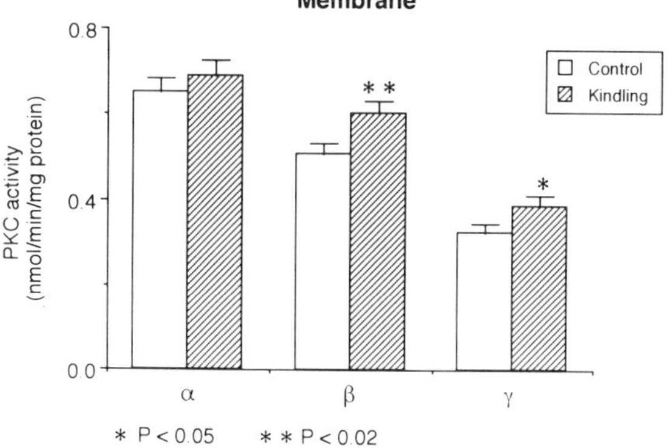

Figure 7. The activity of cytosolic and membrane-associated PKC subspecies in the hippocampus prepared from control and hippocampal-kindled rats. The hippocampal and matched control rats were decapitated 4 weeks after the last seizure of the kindled rats. The data are expressed as the mean ± S.E.M. of 8 experiments; * $p<0.05$, ** $p<0.02$, compared with the control group (Student's t test for unpaired samples).

intracellular localization patterns [20, 31]. The α-, β I-, β II- and γ-subspecies, whose primary structures of their Ca^{2+}-binding domains are highly conserved, appear to form a subgroup, termed conventional PKC. Each of them consists of the regulatory domain and kinase domain [20]. As the β I- and β II-subspecies are derived from a single gene transcript by alternative splicing, but the β II subspecies are predominant in the brain, the two β subspecies were not differentiated in the present study. Other groups of cDNA clones encode novel PKC subspecies (δ, ε, η, θ) and atypical PKC subspecies (ζ, λ), both of which lack the Ca^{2+}-binding domain, and can be activated in Ca^{2+}-independent manner [21, 31].

The main finding of the present study is that both hippocampal-kindling and amygdala-kindling led to increases in the membrane-associated PKC activities in the hippocampus at long-term, that the membrane-associated activities of PKC the β- and γ-subspecies increased in the hippocampus at long-term of the hippocampal-kindling, that mRNA of the γ and ε subspecies were transiently up-regulated, and that mRNA of the β subspecies increased one week after the last amygdala seizure.

Several possible mechanisms may underlie the enduring increase in the membrane-associated PKC activity that results from kindling. The first is translocation of PKC, which is triggered by increased intracellular concentrations of Ca^{2+}. Second, recent studies [6, 21] have suggested that the existence of several other pathways to provide diacylglycerol than receptor-mediated hydrolysis of polyphosphoinositide. Thus, diacylglycerol production resulting from hydrolysis of polyphosphoinositide and phosphatidylcholine is considered to cause further diacylglycerol production from phosphatidylcholine, a process that leads to persistent PKC activation in the absence of elevated intracellular Ca^{2+} concentrations [6, 21]. Third, such delayed elevation of diacylglycerol may induce perturbation of membrane lipid bilayer structure and promote penetration of the PKC molecule into membrane phospholipids, which is termed as a putative form of membrane-inserted constitutive PKC as a complex of protein-lipid structures [2]. The long-lasting increase in PKC activity induced by kindling may be present in the membrane-inserted constitutive PKC form.

The long-lasting increase in the activity of PKC β and γ subspecies in the hippocampus may be involved in regulation of ligand-gated ion channel type of excitatory and inhibitory amino acid receptors. Several lines of evidence have suggested functional modulation by PKC of N-methyl-D-aspartate (NMDA) receptors whose stimulation is essential for induction of kindling [26]. Thus, treatment of *xenopus* oocyte expressing rat brain total mRNA with a phorbol ester, was found to potentiate the NMDA-induced current [33], and PKC was reported to phosphorylate directly the NR1 subunit of NMDA receptor [32]. On the contrary, it was reported that PKC transiently activates heteromeric NMDA receptor channels independent of the phosphorylatable domain [28]. The other type of ligand-gated ion channel which may undergo PKC phosphorylation is $GABA_A$ receptor [16, 30]. Functionally, it was shown that PKC phosphorylation of the β and γ2 subunits of $GABA_A$ receptors caused reduced amplitudes of GABA-activated current [16]. Both NMDA receptors and $GABA_A$ receptors are multimeric proteins composed of homologous subunits. Presently, it is not known whether particular assemblies of these subunits in a certain brain area can undergo PKC phosphorylatoin leading to physiological changes relevant to kindling such as enhanced Ca^{2+} permeability through NMDA receptors [18] or loss of inhibition [10].

Kamphuis et al. [9] reported that mRNA of the PKC ε and ζ subspecies increased during the early stages of kindling, and that increase of mRNA of the ε subspecies was still observed 24 hours, but not one month, after the last full kindled seizure. The present study is consistent with the finding of Kamphuis et al. [9] in that mRNA of the ε subspecies increased in the dentate gyrus 24 hours after the last full kindled seizure. Increase in mRNA of the ε subspecies may be involved in enhanced glutamate release reported in kindling [8] due to the following reasons. First, whereas the β and γ subspecies exist postsynaptically [15], the ε subspecies are immunocytochemically localized on nerve terminals [25, 31]. Second, arachidonic acid, which is considered to be a retrograde neurotransmitter, is able to activate the ε subspecies [14]. It remains to be explored whether presynaptic PKC ε subspecies are involved in enhanced neurotransmitter release in kindling. The increase in mRNA of the PKC ζ subspecies which was reported during the early stage of kindling in the previous report [9] did not occur 24 hours after the last full kindled seizure in the present study. Although it is not well known how the transcripts of each PKC genes are regulated, it may result from the acquisition of epileptogenesis during the early stage of kindling and/or may be the direct effect of kindled seizures per se.

5. SUMMARY

The present study investigated the long-lasting effect of kindling on protein kinase C (PKC) activities and activities of its subspecies in the rat brain. (Experiment 1) The membrane-associated PKC activities in the amygdala/pyriform cortex and both the left and right hippocampus of rats which were kindled from the left hippocampus increased significantly 4 weeks after the occurrence of the last seizure. 16 weeks after the occurrence of the last seizure, the membrane-associated PKC activities increased significantly in the amygdala/pyriform cortex and left hippocampus of the kindled group compared with control rats, whereas the cytosolic PKC activities did not change in any brain region examined. (Experiment 2) In rats kindled from the left amygdala, the membrane-associated PKC activities increased significantly in the hippocampus at 4 weeks and 16 weeks after the last seizure, whereas the cytosolic PKC activities did not change in any brain region examined. (Experiment 3) The membrane-associated activities of the PKC β- and γ-subspecies in the bilateral hippocampus of the hippocampal kindled group increased significantly, compared with the control, 4 weeks after the last seizure, whereas the membrane-associated activities of the a-subspecies were unchanged. As a summary of Experiments 1–3, kindling results in the prolonged activation of PKC after a long-term seizure free interval. However, the underlying mechanism, such as putative membrane-inserted constitutive form, is still a matter to be explored. (Experiment 4) mRNA levels of the PKC γ and ε subspecies were transiently elevated, and mRNA levels of the PKC β subspecies increased 1 week after the seizure. Future study on protein levels of the novel and atypical PKC subspecies in kindling will be required.

ACKNOWLEDGMENTS

This study was supported by the Japanese Epilepsy Research Foundation (recipient; K. Akiyama, 1989–1990 and 1992–1993).

REFERENCES

1. Akiyama, K., Ono, M., Kohira, I., Daigen, A., Ishihara, T. and Kuroda, S., Long-lasting increase in protein kinase C activity in the hippocampus of amygdala-kindled rat. *Brain Res.*, 679 (1995) 212–220.
2. Bazzi, M.D. and Nelsestuen, G.L., Properties of membrane-inserted protein kinase C. *Biochemistry*, 27 (1988) 7589–7593.
3. Daigen, A., Akiyama, K. and Otsuki, S., Long-lasting change in the membrane-associated protein kinase C activity in the hippocampal kindled rat. *Brain Res.*, 545 (1991) 131–136.

4. Goddard, G.V., Development of epileptic seizures through brain stimulation at low intensity. *Nature*, 214 (1967) 1020–1021.
5. Hikiji, M., Tomita, H., Ono, M., Fujiwara, Y. and Akiyama, K., Increase of kainate receptor mRNA in the hippocampal CA3 of amygdala-kindled rats detected by *in situ* hybridization. *Life Sci.*, 53 (1993) 857–864.
6. Huang, K.-P., The mechanism of protein kinase C activation. *Trends Neurosci.*, 12 (1989) 425–432.
7. Huang, K.-P, Nakabayashi, H. and Huang, F.L., Isozymic forms of rat brain Ca^{2+}-activated and phospholipid-dependent protein kinase. *Proc. Natl. Acad. Sci. USA*, 83 (1986) 8535–8539.
8. Jarvie, P.A., Logan, T.C., Geula, C. and Slevin J.T., Entorhinal kindling permanently enhances Ca^{2+}-dependent L-glutamate release in regio inferior of rat hippocampus. *Brain Res.*, 508 (1990) 188–193.
9. Kamphuis, W., Hendriksen, E. and Lopes da Silva, F.H., Isozyme speciifc changes in the expression of protein kinase C isozyme (a-z) in the hippocampus of rats induced by kindling epileptogenesis. *Brain Res.*, 702 (1995) 94–100.
10. Kapur, J., Michelson, H.B., Buterbaugh, G.G. and Lothman, E.W., Evidence for a chronic loss of inhibition in the hippocampus after kindling: electrophysiological studies. *Epilepsy Res.*, 4 (1989) 90–99.
11. Kennedy, M.B., Regulation of synaptic transmission in the central nervous system: long-term potentiation. *Cell*, 59 (1989) 777–787.
12. Kikkawa, U., Ono, Y., Ogita, K., Fujii, T., Asaoka, Y., Sekiguchi, K., Kosaka, Y., Igarashi, K. and Nishizuka, Y., Identification of the structures of multiple subspecies of protein kinase C expressed in rat brain, *FEBS Lett.*, 217 (1987) 227–231.
13. Kohira, I., Akiyama, K., Daigen, A. and Otsuki, S., Enduring increase in membrane-associated protein kinase C activity in the hippocampal-kindled rat. *Brain Res.*, 593 (1992) 82–88.
14. Koide, H., Ogita, K., Kikkawa, U. and Nishizuka, Y. , Isolation and characterization of the e subspecies of protein kinase C from rat brain. *Proc. Natl. Acad. Sci. USA*, 89 (1992) 1149–1153.
15. Kose, A., Ito, A., Saito, N. and Tanaka, C., Electron microscopic localization of g- and bI-subspecies of protein kinase C in rat hippocampus. *Brain Res.*, 518 (1990) 209–217.
16. Krishek, B.J., Xie, X., Blackstone, C., Huganir, R.L., Moss, S.J. and Smart, T.G., Regulation of $GABA_A$ receptor function by protein kinase C phosphorylation. *Neuron*, 12 (1994) 1081–1095.
17. Malenka, R.C., Ayoub, G.S., and Nicoll, R.A., Phorbol esters enhance transmitter release in rat hippocampal slices. *Brain Res.*, 403 (1987) 198–203.
18. Mody, I. and Heinemann, U., NMDA receptors of dentate gyrus granule cells participate in synaptic transmission following kindling. *Nature*, 326 (1987) 701–704.
19. Narang, N. and Crews, F.T., Age does not alter protein kinase C isozymes mRNA expression in rat brain. *Neurochem. Res.*, 20 (1995) 1119–1126.
20. Nishizuka, Y., The molecular heterogeneity of protein kinase C and its implications for cellular regulation. *Nature*, 334 (1988) 661–665.
21. Nishizuka, Y. , Protein kinase C and lipid signaling for sustained cellular responses. *FASEB J* , 9 (1995) 484–496.
22. Ono, M., Akiyama, K., Tsutsui, K. and Kuroda, S., Differential changes in the activities of multiple protein kinase C subspecies in the hippocampal-kindled rat. *Brain Res.*, 660 (1994) 27–33.
23. Pellegrino, L.J., Pellegrino, A.S. and Cushman, A.J., *A Stereotaxic Atlas of the Rat Brain*, Plenum, New York, 1979.
24. Racine, R., Modification of seizure activity by electrical stimulation: II Motor seizure, *Electroencephalogr. Clin. Neurophysiol.*, 32 (1972) 281–294.
25. Saito, N., Itouji, A., Totani, Y., Osawa, I., Koide, H., Fujisawa, N., Ogita, K. and Tanaka, C. , Cellular and intracellular localization of e-subspecies of protein kinase C in the rat brain; presynaptic localization of the e-subspecies. *Brain Res.*, 607 (1993) 241–248.
26. Sato, K., Morimoto, K. and Okamoto, M., Anticonvulsant action of a non-competitive antagonist of NMDA receptors (MK-801) in the kindling model of epilepsy. *Brain Res.*, 463 (1988) 12–20.
27. Shearman, M.S., Sekiguchi, K. and Nishizuka, Y., Modulation of ion channel activity: a key function of the protein kinase C enzyme family. *Pharmacol. Rev.*, 41 (1989) 211–237.
28. Sigel, E., Baur, R. and Malherbe, P. , Protein kinase C transiently activates heteromeric N-methyl-D-aspartate receptor channels independent of the phosphrylatable C-terminal splice domain and of consensus phosphorylation sites. *J. Biol. Cehm.*, 269 (1994) 8204–8208.
29. Spinelli, W. Ishii, D.N., Tumor promoter receptors regulating neurite formations in cultured human neuroblastoma cells, *Cancer Res.*, 43 (1983) 4119–4125.
30. Swope, S.L., Moss, S.J., Blackstone, C.D. and Huganir, R.L., Phosphorylation of ligand-gated ion channels: a possible mode of synaptic plasticity. *FASEB J.*, 6 (1992) 2514–2523.
31. Tanaka, C. and Nishizuka, Y., The protein kinase C family for neuronal signaling. *Annu. Rev. Neurosci.*, 17 (1994) 551–567.

32. Tingley, W.G., Roche, K.W., Thompson, A.K. and Huganir, R.L., Regulation of NMDA receptor phosphorylation by alternative splicing of the c-terminal domain. *Nature*, 364 (1993) 70–73.
33. Urushihara, H., Tohda, M. and Nomura, Y., Selective potentiation of N-methyl-D-aspartate-induced current by protein kinase C in *xenopus* oocytes injected with rat brain RNA. *J. Biol. Chem.*, 267 (1992) 11697–11700.

DISCUSSION OF KAZUFUMI AKIYAMA'S PAPER

F. Lopes da Silva: I would like to congratulate you on this very comprehensive study where you have looked at several aspects of the activity at the mRNA and the protein levels. We have done similar studies, you know, at the mRNA level, and one of the differences with your study is on the PKC subtype ζ. I think that this may probably be due to the fact that you have killed the animals at fully kindled stages and then you have looked at the changes at 24 hours and 1 week afterwards. Now what we found with the ζ subtype is that the mRNA for this PKC subtype is always increased after 6 afterdischarges. This is a very early and transient effect, and disappears at the stage at which you have studied it. What I think is particularly interesting in this case is that a similar change was found in LTP, so this could be a very early change due to kindling that is related to a sort of LTP effect which may appear at the beginning of kindling but is not maintained afterwards.

J. McNamara: It is an interesting dissociation between the protein activity and the message for PKC γ. I just wanted to mention that we have examined the rate of kindling development in mice carrying a null mutation of PKC γ and found no difference in the rate of kindling.

KINDLING INDUCES LONG-TERM CHANGES IN GENE EXPRESSION

Ann C. Rice and Robert J. DeLorenzo

Department of Neurology
Medical College of Virginia
Virginia Commonwealth University
P.O. Box 980599, Richmond, Virginia 23298-0599

1. INTRODUCTION

Kindling is a model of epileptogenesis which involves permanent neuronal changes resulting in a hyperexcitable state in a population of neurons[51,57,96]. The kindled state is achieved by repeated subconvulsive stimulations in a defined pattern which eventually elicit a seizure[25]. The development of the kindled state is progressive. Early in the protocol the stimulations produce focal afterdischarges and later in the paradigm generalized electrographic and behavioral seizures are produced. Once a predefined number of class 5 behavioral seizures[74] is elicited the animal is considered kindled. If a sufficient number of seizures are produced, the animal will exhibit spontaneous seizures[68]. The kindled state is permanent for the life of the animal in that subconvulsive stimulations can produce a seizure months after the last stimulation induced seizure. A variety of kindling protocols exist. The stimulations can be either electrical[25] or chemical[97]. Traditionally electrical stimulations were administered once a day for several weeks; however, Lothman et al.[50] determined that the kindled state could be attained in one day with electrical stimulations administered every 5 min. The stimulations can be applied to different brain regions such as the hippocampus, amygdala, perforant path, septum, entorhinal cortex, piriform cortex or perirhinal cortex to attain the kindled state[17,51,52,96].

Kindling has the advantage over other models of epilepsy in that defined time points after a seizure can be easily characterized. Changes in kindled animals have been described during, immediately following and long-term after the kindling paradigm. The long-term changes are categorized as neuronal plasticity. Several molecular mechanisms that may be involved in the underlying neuronal plasticity include synaptic reorganization[88], long term changes in receptor function[52,60] and long term changes in gene expression[67]. Many of the long-term neuronal changes observed in kindling have also been identified in other models of epilepsy as well as in epileptic foci removed from humans, such as mossy fiber sprouting[1,89] increased activity of NMDA (N-methyl-D-aspartate) receptors[56,60–62] and decreased

Kindling 5, edited by Corcoran and Moshé.
Plenum Press, New York, 1998.

function of $GABA_A$ (γ-amino butyric acid)$_A$ receptors[21,41,79,87]. Long-term or permanent changes are often associated with changes in gene expression[17,67]. Our laboratory is currently studying the role of long-term changes in gene expression as a molecular mechanism for mediating some of the long lasting alterations underlying neuronal excitability. Thus, the role of changes in gene expression in kindling will be the focus of the rest of this chapter.

2. ACUTE CHANGES IN GENE EXPRESSION

The expression of many gene products has been studied during and immediately following completion of the kindling paradigm. The basic trend is similar for most of the genes examined in that there is a transient increase or decrease in expression immediately following a stimulation induced seizure. The immediate early genes (IEGs), which are primarily transcription factors, are the best characterized. In kindled animals c-fos mRNA levels have been shown to be rapidly induced (15 min) and then quickly return to baseline levels (1hr) after the conclusion of the last kindling stimulation using *in situ* hybridization techniques[33] and Northern and slot blot analyses[81,90]. Additionally, c-jun[33,90], jun-B and krox-24 have been demonstrated to be up-regulated in the piriform, perirhinal and entorhinal cortices[33]. NGFI-A (also known as zif)[82], egr-1[11] and tissue-plasminogen activator[73] have been shown to be induced in 30–60 min and then returned to baseline levels by 24 hours after a seizure. Interestingly, c-myc mRNA levels were not elevated in response to the same electrical stimulation[90]. Therefore only specific IEGs are induced in response to kindling. However, the ultimate targets of IEG induction and their role in epilepsy are unknown. This research indicates that specific IEGs are elevated transiently following the kindling stimulation. Since these changes in IEG expression are brief, long-term plasticity changes associated with kindling cannot be explained solely by IEG induction. However, IEGs are transciption factors that regulate the expression of other gene products. Thus, it is possible that these brief changes in IEGs initiate events which elicit a cascade of changes in gene products that ultimately produce long-term changes in gene expression and long-term effects on plasticity.

Neurotrophic factors have been shown to play a role in the development and maintenance of the nervous system[2]. Changes in the expression of neurotrophic gene products have also been observed in kindling. The gene products are up-regulated after the IEGs and remain elevated longer. The neurotrophic factors BDNF, NGF and NT-3 (also known as hippocampal derived neurotrophic factor) have been shown to be transiently increased in response to a kindling stimulation, although the location and duration of the induction is specific for each gene product[19,4]. The neurotrophin tyrosine kinase receptors, trkB (BDNF) and trk C (NT-3), mRNA levels were also elevated, although trk A (NGF) expression did not change[4]. The neurotrophins and their associated receptor genes may play a role in the synaptic reorganization associated with kindling[75]. Increased levels of neurotrophins have been observed in other models of epilepsy concurrent with the presence of mossy fiber sprouting[52,65].

In addition to IEGs and neurotrophic factors several other gene products have been identified as having transiently altered mRNA levels after a stimulation induced seizure. Heat shock protein 73 (HSP 73) mRNA levels are increased in the dentate granule cell layer after seizure activity[52,101]. HSPs 72 and 84 did not show any alteration in expression under the same conditions, further indicating the selectivity of gene regulation in response to seizure discharge. Mineralocorticoid and glucocorticoid receptors also displayed an elevation of mRNA levels in the dentate granule cell layer[14]. Messenger RNA levels were significantly decreased for the calcium binding protein calbindin-D_{28} (CaBP) in the dentate granule cell layer and increased for glutamic acid decarboxylase (GAD) around the

CA1 pyramidal cell layer when grain densities over cells were quantitated by liquid emulsion autoradiography[86]. However, these changes in CaBP and GAD mRNA levels were not observed using Northern or slot blot analysis or by *in situ* hybridization film autoradiography. These results indicate that subtle changes in gene expression may not be detectable by some methods commonly employed and more precise techniques may be required. The role of these transient changes in gene expression in playing a role in the development of the kindled state is unknown.

This research indicates that selective gene products can be transiently regulated by the electrical stimulation paradigm employed in kindling. Some of the functions of these gene products may suggest possible effects in kindled brains by regulating the expression of other genes (IEGs) or initiating synaptic reorganization (neurotrophins). However, none of the changes in expression of these gene products persist beyond a few days. Thus, they cannot ultimately account for the permanent neuronal plasticity associated with kindling. If long lasting changes in gene expression contribute to the maintenance of the kindled state, it should be possible to identify changes in the expression of specific genes. Further research is needed to understand the contribution of the acute transient changes in gene expression to long-term plasticity.

3. LONG-TERM CHANGES IN GENE EXPRESSION

Long-term changes in gene expression represent an ideal mechanism to produce the enduring change in neuronal plasticity associated with kindling. Recent studies have identified gene products that are altered for a long duration after completing the kindling paradigm. Changes in gene expression of ligatin[66,67], calcium calmodulin dependent protein kinase II (CaM kinase II)[7], kainate receptor[30], AMPA (α-amino-3-hydroxy-5-methylisoxazole-4-proprionic acid) receptor[39], NMDA receptor (present study), $GABA_A$ (present study), neuropeptide Y (NPY)[55], prodynorphin[29], and vasopressin[27] (Table 1) provide direct evidence that the kindling process can induce long-term changes in the expression of specific gene products. Small changes in gene expression may be sufficient to upset the finely tuned balance between excitatory and inhibitory processes resulting in a hyperexcitable state. Thus, the permanent neuronal plasticity changes associated with kindling are likely to have underlying long-term changes in gene expression.

3.1. Ligatin

Ligatin is a 10 kDa membrane associated lipoprotein[35], which has been shown to play a role in intercellular adhesion[54]. Ligatin mRNA levels were investigated in kindled animals[67]. These studies used the rapid hippocampal kindling protocol of Lothman et al.[50], in which 50 Hz/10sec trains of 400μA stimulations were administered every 5 min for 6 hr through bipolar twisted electrodes implanted in the ventral hippocampus. A maturation

Table 1. Long-term gene changes in kindling

Neuropeptide Y (1990)[55]	AMPA receptor (1994)[39]
Ligatin (1991,1993)[66,67]	Prodynorphin (1995)[55]
CaM kinase II β (1992)[7]	$GABA_A$ receptor (1996)[present study]
Kainate receptor (1993, 1995)[30,40]	NMDA receptor?[present study]
Vasopressin (1994)[27]	

Listed are genes shown to have altered mRNA levels long-term after kindling followed by the year the report(s) were published.

protocol was also conducted involving 12 stimuli/day every other day beginning on the third day after the initial stimulation and continuing for 5 days. For Northern and slot blot analysis, the brains were rapidly removed and the hippocampi isolated. RNA was extracted and probed as described by Perlin et al.[67]

RNA isolated from hippocampal kindled animals revealed decreased levels of ligatin mRNA at 1wk, 6wks and 4 mos after the last kindling stimuli[66,67]. Fig. 1 depicts a typical

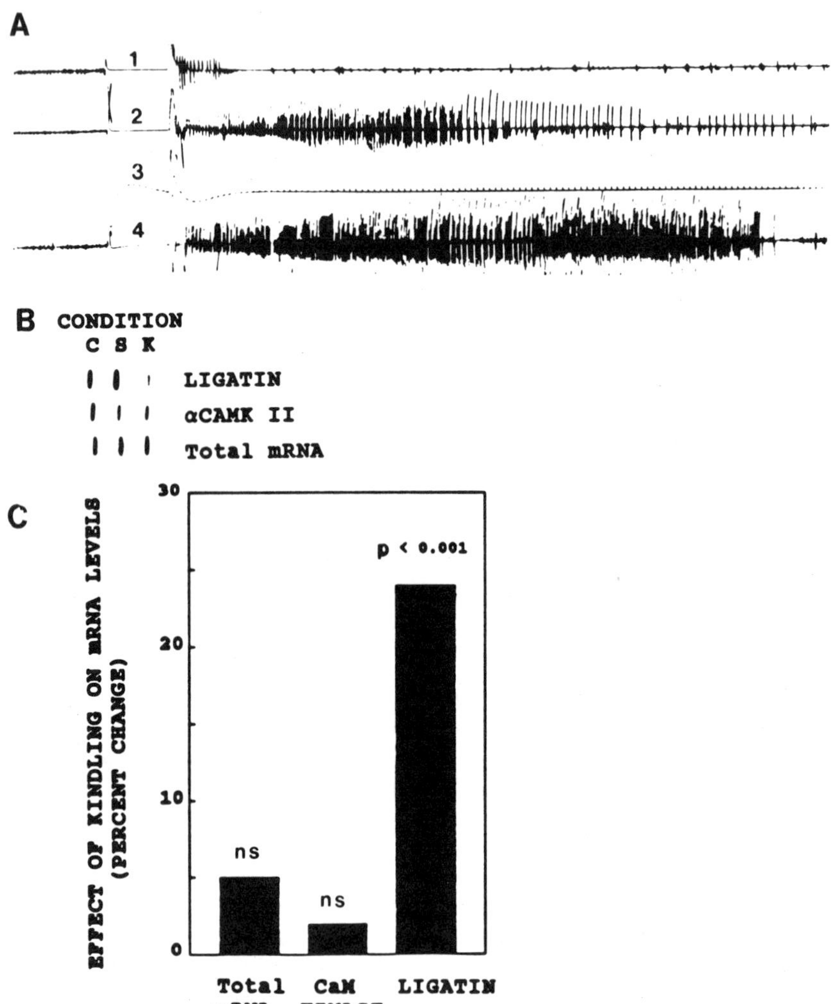

Figure 1. (A) Classical progression of electrographic responses elicited by kindling stimulation to the hippocampus. 1. Early kindling stimulation (identical to a single stimulus response); 2. Late kindling; 3. Time scale (1 second/division); 4. Subsequent expression of a "fully" kindled seizure manifesting Class 4 or 5 behavioral seizures. (B) Cytoslots of hippocampal ligatin, CaM Kinase II, and total mRNA expression in naive control(C), surgical sham control(S), and kindled(K) animals sacrificed 6 weeks after kindling. The data shown are representative of 9 experiments. Autoradiograms were subsequently analyzed by scanning laser densitometry (Ultrascan XL, Pharmacia). The resultant optical densities were used to equilibrate total mRNA per slot for analysis of specific levels. (C) Quantitation of ligatin and CaM Kinase II mRNA expression in surgical sham control, and kindled animals sacrificed over 6 weeks after the last kindling stimuli. Data represent the means of 9 determinations and are expressed as percent change from sham control (normalized to 100%). Standard errors for total mRNA, CaM Kinase II and ligatin expression were 3.8, 5.4 and 6.4 and were omitted for clarity. $p \leq 0.001$ ANOVA; Bonferroni correction. (Reprinted with permission).

afterdischarge elicited (Fig. 1A), slot blot analysis (Fig. 1B) and quantitation (Fig. 1C) of ligatin mRNA isolated from hippocampi 6 wks after the last seizure. Ligatin mRNA levels are significantly decreased by approximately 25% compared to sham operated control animals. *In situ* hybridzation analyses of coronal sections from animals six weeks after the last kindling induced seizure revealed decreased levels of ligatin mRNA throughout the hippocampal formation, with the largest decreases in the CA1–CA3 subfields (Fig. 2A). An undetectable change in mRNA levels of another gene, CaM Kinase II α (Fig. 2B), provides evidence that the decrease in ligatin message is specific to kindling. Immunohisto-

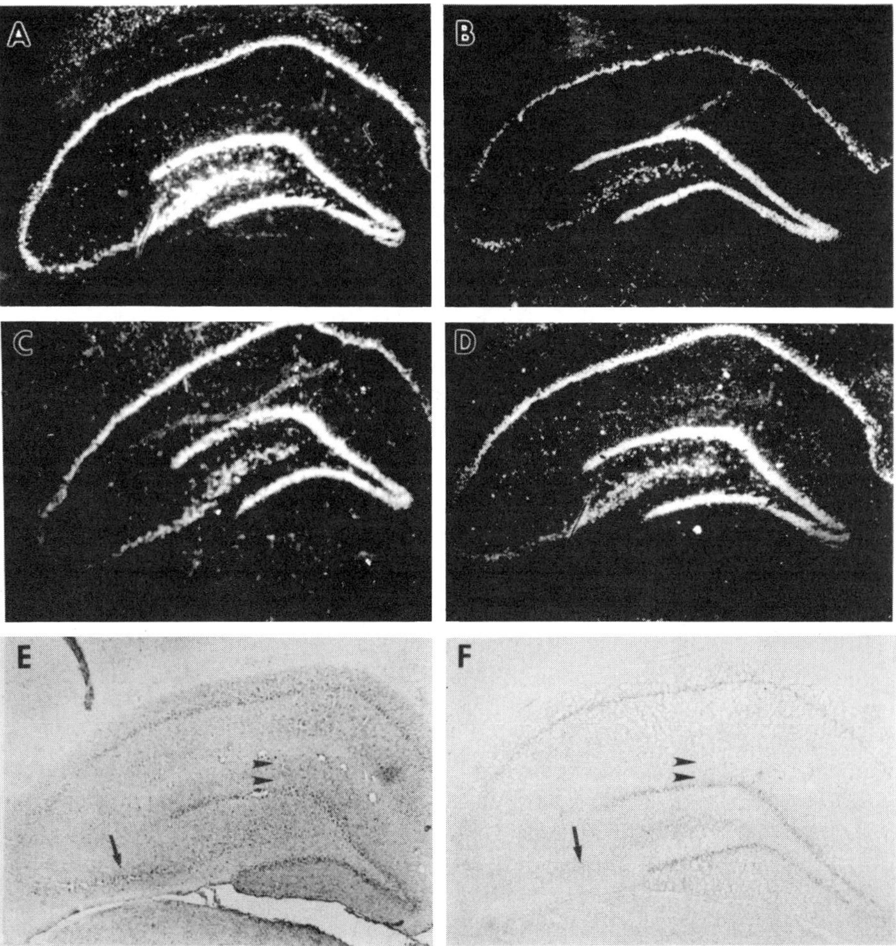

Figure 2. Ligatin gene expression in rat hippocampus 3 mo after kindling using *in situ* hybridization and immunocytochemistry. Dark field photomicrographs [Fig. 3A-D] show *in situ* hybridization of complementary probes to ligatin mRNA. Intense labeling of CA1 to CA3 and the dentate gyrus was observed in control (A) animals. In kindled (B) animals, specific labeling of ligatin mRNA was significantly reduced bilaterally throughout the hippocampus, particularly in the CA3 region. *In situ* hybridization of complementary probes to α CaM Kinase II mRNA in adjacent sections showed no effect of kindling (D) in comparison to control animals (C). Immunocytochemistry using anti-ligatin serum showed labeling of pyramidal cells in the CA 1–3 regions and in the granule cells of the dentate gyrus and significant staining in the synaptic regions of the hippocampus from control animals (E). Kindling (F) produced a reproducible decrease in immunoreactivity in the cell bodies (arrows) and in the synaptic regions (arrowheads). The results are representative of four control, four sham, and four kindled animals. (Reprinted with permission).

chemical studies on adjacent coronal sections using an anti-ligatin antibody indicate that the observed decrease in mRNA levels is reflective of a decrease in the expression of ligatin protein (Fig. 2C). Decreased anti-ligatin antibody staining was observed in the cell body layer as well as in the dendritic areas of the hippocampus. Pretreatment with MK-801retards the development of the kindling state[22–24,58,78,93]. Perlin et al.[67] demonstrated that MK-801 not only blocked the development of kindling, but also blocked the reduction in ligatin mRNA levels. These data represented the first example of the long-term change in expression of a specific gene as a result of electrically stimulated kindling. In addition, MK-801 blocked both the normal development of kindling and the change in expression of this specific gene.

Since both kindling induction and ligatin expression were shown to be NMDA regulated, the effects of glutamate and NMDA receptor activity on the expression of ligatin were studied in the hippocampal neuronal culture (HNC) model of hyperexcitability[64]. Glutamate, the primary excitatory neurotransmitter in the CNS[99], causes neurons in culture to spontaneously depolarize. There is a net decrease in ligatin mRNA levels 1 hr after 6–10 min exposures to glutamate[36,37]. This decrease in mRNA levels persisted for over 24 hrs. Additional experiments in this system demonstrated that the decrease in ligatin mRNA levels was blocked by MK-801 administered before glutamate. Thus, in the HNC model of hyperexcitability, ligatin expression paralleled the changes observed in kindling.

The advantages of the HNC model is that the molecular mechanisms of gene expression can be studied. Using molecular biological techniques, our laboratory has been able to investigate the regulation of glutamate induced changes in ligatin mRNA levels[37,64]. Nuclear run-on experiments revealed that the rate of transcription was not significantly affected. This nuclear run-on data demonstrated that glutamate down regulation of ligatin gene expression in this model is not due to a decrease in the transcription rate of the ligatin gene. In addition mRNA turnover experiments indicated that the half-life of ligatin message was drastically decreased from 10 hr to 1 hr, yeilding a steady state decrease.[36,37] These experiments demonstrated that the NMDA receptor activated decrease in ligatin mRNA levels is at the post-transcriptional level in hippocampal neurons in culture.

In conclusion, these results provide direct evidence that both ligatin mRNA and protein levels remain down regulated indefinitely in parallel to the enduring hyperexcitability observed in the kindled state. In addition, MK-801 blocks the long lasting neuronal plasticity in kindling as well as the down regulation of ligatin, indicating a possible role for ligatin in mediating some of the NMDA-dependent changes in kindling. However, a functional role of ligatin in mediating neuronal hyperexcitability has yet to be determined. Since ligatin has been shown to play a role in the maintenance of synaptic contacts and cell interactions, it is possible that it plays a role in neuronal sprouting. Preliminary results from this laboratory indicate that changes in ligatin protein levels in HNC can alter dendritic architecture and lead to a phenomenon of redirected neuronal outgrowth which appear similar to sprouting. Further studies are needed to determine the role of the changes in ligatin expression in kindled animals, especially the role of ligatin in sprouting or other mechanisms that may contribute to the long-term plasticity changes associated with kindling.

3.2. Calcium-Calmodulin Dependent Protein Kinase II (CaM Kinase II)

CaM kinase II is a calcium activated kinase that is highly concentrated in the brain. It regulates many neuronal processes such as neurotransmitter synthesis and release, cytoskeletal dissociation, ion conductance, neuronal excitabilitiy and induction of long-term potentiation[6,8,13,15,28,43,85]. CaM Kinase II is a multimeric protein complex composed of 10–12 subunits. There are two major subunit forms of CaM Kinase II, α and β. Expression of CaM kinase II β mRNA was assesed in septally kindled rats 2 wks after the last stimulation.[7] There was a significant decrease in CaM Kinase II β mRNA levels throughout the CA1-CA4 regions the fascia dentata and the cerebral cortex. No decrease was observed in the septum, the site of stimulation. This indicated that the changes observed were specific for the regions involved. Our laboratory has examined CaM kinase II α subunit expression[67]. Six weeks after the last stimulation induced seizure, no significant changes were detected in CaM kinase II α mRNA levels (Figs. 1C and 2B). Previous studies have demonstated a decreased CaM kinase II enzymatic activity 1 month after kindling[26,97]. Whether this is a function of the decrease in β subunit mRNA levels or other mechanisms is not known.

CaM kinase II α gene knockout mice exhibit spontaneous seizure activity, increased susceptibility to stimulus evoked afterdischarges and mossy fiber sprouting[10]. This would indicate that changes in CaM kinase II α isoform expression could also have a dramatic effect on hyperexcitability. Studies by Perlin et al.[67] did not observe long-term decrease in the expression of CaM Kinase II α gene expression. However, Bronstein et al.[7] observed a persistent decrease in CaM Kinase II β gene expression. The decrease in CaM Kinase II β expression was determined by counting grain densities over individual cells using liquid emulsion autoradiography[7], whereas the lack of change in CaM Kinase II α mRNA levels was determined by quantitation of *in situ* hybridization using film autoradiography[67]. Therefore it is possible that counting grain densities over individual neurons may reveal more subtle, but significant, changes in CaM kinase II α mRNA levels. This needs further evaluation. Since CaM kinase II regulates many neuronal functions, it is possible that decreased expression of one or both subunits could have profound effects on hyperexcitability and play a key role in kindling.

3.3. Glutamate Receptors

Glutamate is the primary excitatory neurotransmitter in the CNS[99]. Since kindling is a state of hyperexcitability, there is a great deal of interest in the role of the glutamate receptors. There are 3 major classes of ionotropic glutamate receptors identified by discriminatory ligands, kainate, AMPA, and NMDA[3,5,12,18,31,59]. The effects of kindling on the 3 main classes of glutamate receptors has been investigated.

3.3.1. Kainate Receptors. The kainate receptor is primarily a cation channel which has fast synaptic responses. There are 5 known major subunits of this receptor, KA-1, KA-2, GluR-5, GluR-6 and GluR-7, several of which have splice variant isoforms. Changes in some of the kainate receptor subunits were observed in partially and fully hippocampal kindled animals at 24 hr after the last stimulated seizure[40]. KA-2 mRNA expression was increased in the fascia dentata, CA1 and CA3 regions, while KA-1 mRNA expression was not altered. Expression of the GluR-5,-6 and -7 subunits was not altered in the short-term, but GluR-7 was decreased in the fascia dentata at 4 wks after the last stimulated seizure[40]. An increase in KA-2 expression was reported in CA3 at one month after amygdala kindling[30]. Since the KA-2 subunit is expressed throughout the cortex and hippocampal formation, an increase in KA-2 levels could result in increased hyperexcitability. Further studies are needed to investigate the role of long-term changes in the expression of the kainate receptor genes in kindling.

3.3.2. AMPA Receptors. The AMPA receptor is also a cation channel and is responsible for a large part of the fast synaptic responses in the CNS. There are 4 major AMPA receptor subunits referred to as GluR-1(or A), GluR-2 (or B) GluR-3 (or C) and GluR-4 (or D)[5]. Altered expression of AMPA receptor subunits has been examined both acutely (24 hr after last seizure) and chronically (30 days) in the kindling model. Using Northern and slot blot analysis, GluR-1, GluR-2 and GluR-3 expression was shown to be decreased 24 hr after the last seizure in kindled rats in the hippocampus, frontoparietal cortex and amygdala/entorhinal cortex, but not at 30 days[48]. Wong et al. reported that GluR-1 expression was decreased at 24 hr after the last amygdala kindled stimulation[102]. Expression of the GluR-A, -B and -C subunits of the AMPA receptor has been shown to be increased in the DG of hippocampal kindled animals 24 hr after the last seizure[39]. However, only GluR-A expression was still increased 4 wks after the last stimulation induced seizure. It is possible that an increased expression of glutamate receptor subunits after kindling could increase the function of that particular receptor and lead to hyperexcitability of the neuron on which it is expressed.

3.3.3. NMDA Receptors. The third major ionotropic glutamate receptor is the NMDA receptor. It is selective for both Ca^{++} and Na^{+} ions. The NMDA receptor channel also has a Mg^{++} block that is removed by depolarization of the cell, requires glycine as a co-agonist and has much slower kinetics than the other glutamate receptors. Five major subunits have been identified, NR1 (with many splice variants), NR2A, NR2B, NR2C and NR2D[31]. The presence of an NR1 subunit in the receptor is essential for channel function. A number of studies using kindled animals have provided indirect evidence that activation of NMDA receptors is essential for the induction of the long-term plasticity changes associated with kindling. NMDA receptor antagonists have been shown to retard the development of the kindled state[22–24,58,78,93]. Electrophysiological studies indicate that kindled animals[56,60–62] and brain tissue from epileptic humans[34] manifest increased functional activity of NMDA channels compared to control tissue. Binding studies reveal complex results. Some studies demonstrate decreased receptor binding in kindled brains[63]. However under different conditions, increases have been observed[45,103]. These results indicate that long-term changes in NMDA function and expression are complex and require further studies to determine whether alterations of NMDA receptor subunit levels play a role in the kindling phenomenon.

Alterations in NMDA channel function have led several groups to investigate NMDA receptor subunit mRNA levels at various stages during and after kindling. At a partially kindled stage, NR2A and NR2B mRNA levels were significantly decreased in the dentate granule cell layer[70]. In fully kindled animals, there was a decrease in NR1 mRNA levels up to 4 hrs following the last seizure. NR1 mRNA levels returned to baseline by 12 hrs. NR2A exhibited a biphasic pattern of expression. Initially it was decreased at 0 hr and 1 hr, was baseline at 2 hr, increased up to 4 hr and returned to baseline by 12 hrs. NR2B only displayed increased levels at 4 hrs. No changes in NR1, NR2A or NR2B mRNA levels were detected at 24 hrs or 28 days after the last stimulation induced seizure in the kindling paradigm. Slight increases of NR2A and NR2B in the dentate granule cell layer and a small decrease in NR1 in the CA1 subfield were observed at 24 hrs. However, no significant changes were detected at 28 days[40]. In our laboratory, we detect a trend toward increasing expression of NR2A in the CA3 pyramidal cell layer at 6 wks after the last seizure, although larger numbers are needed to determine statistical significance. It is also possible that changes in NR1 splice variants are occurring that have not been detected by the probes used thus far, which could explain the altered electrophysiological and binding data. The role of the NMDA receptor in kindling and other models of epilepsy is an important area for further research.

3.4. Gaba$_A$ Receptor (Gaba$_A$ R)

GABA is the major inhibitory neurotransmitter in the CNS[53]. The GABA$_A$ R is a complex of five subunits which form a Cl^- ion channel[53,94]. There are 6 α, 3 β, 3 γ, 1 δ and 1 ρ subunits identified at this time. Different combinations of these subunits result in different functional activities of the channel. For example, the presence of a γ subunit is required for benzodiazepine (BZ) binding, although the type of α present determines the efficacy of the BZ[71,72].

Alterations in the function of the GABA$_A$ R have been implicated in playing an important role in the induction and maintenance of epilepsy in several experimental models[16,49,51,83,84]. Decreased levels of GABA$_A$ R binding and GABA synthesizing enzymes have been reported in tissue from epileptic patients[49]. Long lasting changes in GABA$_A$ R binding have been described in the kindling model[80,91]. Altered function of the GABA$_A$ R has been described long-term in the kindling and pilocarpine models of epilepsy[9,21]. In conclusion, decreases in function of the GABA$_A$ R have been identified in epileptic tissue from human patients and in several models of epilepsy. It is possible that alterations in the genetic expression of GABA$_A$ R subunits may alter the electrophysiological and pharmacological function of the GABA$_A$ R, leading to the hyperexcitability observed in epilepsy.

3.4.1. Acute Changes in GABA$_A$ Receptor Expression. Expression of the GABA$_A$R subunits has been examined acutely and chronically after the last stimulation induced seizure in kindled animals. Acutely, GABA$_A$ R β1 subunit mRNA expression was increased in the CA1, and GABA$_A$ R β2 mRNA expression was increased in the fascia dentata in hippocampal kindled animals[38]. The GABA$_A$ R β3 was increased throughout the hippocampal formation. A study of GABA$_A$ R α1, β3 and γ2 mRNA levels in the fascia dentata revealed a decrease in expression of all three gene products up to 4 hrs after the last kindled stimulation and then a dramatic increase in expression was observed over a 2 day period. By 5 days the levels of the gene products had returned to baseline[44]. Decreased levels of GABA$_A$ R α1 have been reported 24 hr after kainate induced SE in the CA3 and CA4 regions of the hippocampus[20].

3.4.2. Long-Term Changes in GABA$_A$ Receptor Expression. Research from our laboratory has examined GABA$_A$ R subunit expression 6 wks after the last kindling stimulation. Figure 3 depicts quantitation of GABA$_A$ R mRNA *in situ* hybridization film autoradiography normalized to control animals. Animals were kindled as described previously[66,67]. GABA$_A$ R sequences for oligonucleotide probes are from Seeburg's group[47,69,100] GABA$_A$ R

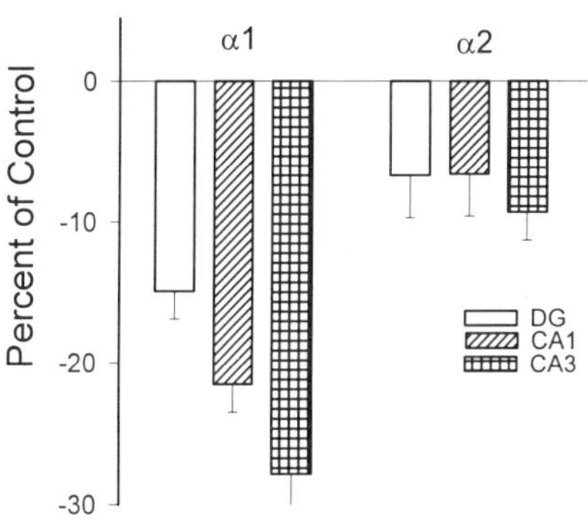

Figure 3. Quantitation of GABA$_A$ receptor subunit mRNA expression. In situ hybridization film autoradiography patterns were quantitated using the Loats quantitative densitometric system for the GABA$_A$ α1 and α2 subunits throughout the hippocampal formation. The data give the values for the kindled animals expressed as a percentage of surgical control animals. The data are expressed as the mean ± SEM.

$\alpha1$ mRNA levels were decreased throughout the hippocampal formation and $GABA_A$ R $\alpha2$ was decreased in CA3. Others have not detected long-term changes in $\alpha1$, $\alpha2$, $\alpha4$ or $\beta1$[48], $\alpha1$, $\beta3$ or $\gamma2$[44], $\beta1$, $\beta2$ or $\beta3$[38] $GABA_A$ R subunit expression. It is possible that slight variations in techniques and different numbers of animals used to determine statistical significance contribute to the discrepancies observed. Further research on $GABA_A$ R subunit expression in kindling is needed to clearly establish the role of long-term changes in $GABA_A$ R expression in the kindling phenomenon.

In the pilocarpine model of epilepsy a decrease $GABA_A$ R $\alpha5$[32,76] and $\alpha2$ mRNA levels in CA1 and an increase in $\alpha5$ in the dentate granule cell layer long-term were detected (Fig. 4)[76]. However, no changes were observed in $\alpha1$, $\beta2$ or $\gamma2$, again indicating specificity. *In situ* hybridization film autoradiography of hippocampal-entorhinal cortical slices incubated in low Mg^{++} revealed a decrease in the $GABA_A$ $\alpha2$ subunit expression[95]. Our preliminary evidence suggests there are $GABA_A$ R subunit gene expression changes occurring in kindled animals as well as evidence indicating changes in expression in other models of epilepsy. It is likely that a shift in expression of specific subunits would result in a shift in the composition of the receptors expressed on the neuronal plasma membrane. The presence of a specific subunit combination likely determines the pharmacology and physiology of the receptor. Thus a shift in $GABA_A$ R isoform expression in CA1 or other areas of the hippocampus may result in altered receptor function and ultimately neuronal physiology.

Messenger RNA turnover experiments were performed in the HNC low Mg^{++} model of epilepsy to assess the mechanism of regulation of the $GABA_A$ R. No alterations in the half-life of the $GABA_A$ receptor subunit mRNA were detected. Therefore the decrease in steady state levels of $GABA_A$ receptor subunits detected in this model could be a result of a decrease in the rate of transcription. These preliminary results indicate that regulation of $GABA_A$ R gene expression is controlled at the transcriptional level.

In conclusion, we have evidence in several models of epilepsy for decreased expression of $GABA_A$ R subunits long-term after the development of the epileptic state. Decreased levels of mRNA of specific $GABA_A$ R subunits may result in shifts in the composition of the receptors expressed on those neurons. Alterations in receptor composition may be sufficient to result in the decreased $GABA_A$ R binding and function observed in the kindling, pilocarpine and low Mg^{++} models of epilepsy. The decreased $GABA_A$ receptor function could result in an upset of the balance between excitatory and inhibitory processes and lead to decreased inhibition or increased excitation, both of which have been observed in human epileptic tissue and in animal models of epilepsy. Thus, we have identified a long-term change in gene expression which could lead to the altered physiology observed in seizure disorders. Further studies need to be done to specifically address the relevance of subtle long-term changes in $GABA_A$ receptor subunit mRNA levels in kindling and other models of epilepsy.

3.5. Peptides

The expression of several neuropeptides has been investigated in the kindling model of epilepsy both short-term and long-term after the last kindling stimulation. Thyrotropin releasing hormone (TRH), neuropeptide Y (NPY), prodynorphin, proenkephalin and vasopressin have been evaluated in kindling. In the dentate granule cell layer THR and NPY were maximally increased 4 hrs post an afterdischarge, but returned to baseline by 24 hrs[77]. However in the pyriform, entorhinal and perirhinal cortices the levels of TRH and NPY were maximally induced at 24 hrs. Another group reports prepro-TRH mRNA induc-

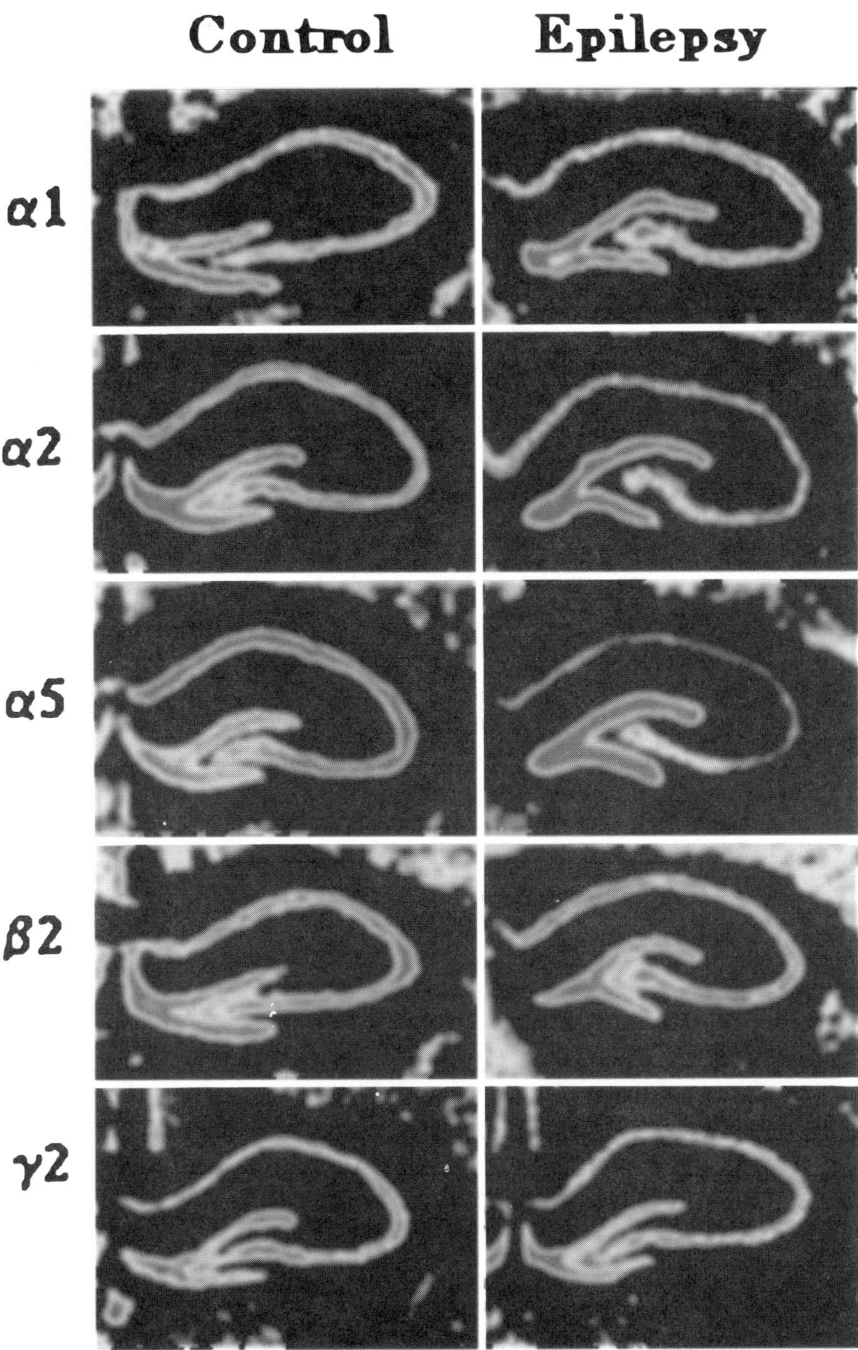

Figure 4. Representative *in situ* hybridization hippocampal patterns for α1, α2, α5, β2 and γ2, $GABA_A$ receptor subunit expression from control and pilocarpine-treated animals. Data are shown as pseudo color images produced on a Loats Quantitative Densitometric System with the intensity scale shown below. Results shown are representative of eight separate experiments. The highest levels of $GABA_A$ receptor subunit mRNA were observed in the neuronal cell body layers of the DG, CA1–2, and CA3 regions of the hippocampus. (Reprinted with permission).

tion peaks 6 and 12 hrs post stimulation in the dentate gyrus, piriform cortex and amygdala[46]. Increased levels of NPY mRNA have been detected in the mossy fibers of pentylenetetrazol kindled and kainic acid treated rats up to 60 days after a seizure[55]. Increased expression of NPY protein long-term was also observed immunohistochemically. These results indicate that both acute and long-term changes in the gene expression of specific neuropeptides occur in the kindling phenomena.

Opioid peptide mRNA expression has been examined in the hippocampal kindling model by *in situ* hybridization[29]. A decrease in prodynorphin mRNA expression at 24 hr after the last stimulus was observed in the dentate gyrus and ventral CA1 and remained decreased at 1 mo in the ventral CA1 region. However, preproenkephalin mRNA expression was increased in the nucleus accumbens and decreased in the entorhinal cortex (EC) at 24 hr, but returned to baseline by one month. Another group reports enkephalin expression was elevated at both 4 and 24 hrs post afterdischarge in pyriform, entorhinal and perirhinal cortices and returned to baseline by 4 days everywhere except the pyriform cortex[77]. Vasopressin mRNA expression was characterized in amygdala kindled rats from 1 day to 4 mos after the last stimulation[27]. An increase in vasopressin expression was detected at 1 wk, 1 mo and 4 mos in the supraoptic nucleus using liquid emulsion autoradiography and counting grain densities, but no increase was observed at 1 day. The role of the long-term decrease in prodynorphin and increase in vasopressin mRNA levels in kindling has yet to be determined.

4. SUMMARY

Evidence has been presented that acute and long-term changes in gene expression occur in the kindling model of epilepsy. These changes in the expression of gene mRNA levels of specific genes could function in several capacities in kindling or other models of hyperexcitability. Gene expression changes could directly lead to some of the hyperexcitability observed. Alterations in the $GABA_A$ receptor α subunits in the CA1-CA3 subfields of the hippocampus and the increase in glutamate receptor KA-2 subunits in the CA3 and GluR A in the dentate gyrus may directly contribute to an alteration in the balance between excitatory and inhibitory systems in the hippocampus. Alternatively some changes in mRNA levels could represent adaptive mechanisms, such as an increase in $GABA_A$ $\alpha5$ in the granule cell layer in the pilocarpine model of epilepsy. Subtle changes in gene expression could be sufficient to upset the finely tuned balance between excitatory and inhibitory influences and lead to the hyperexcitable state. In addition, many of these same changes are seen in other models of epilepsy. Although these observations provide direct evidence for long lasting changes in the expression of both excitatory and inhibitory receptor mRNA levels, further studies are needed to directly determine whether these changes in gene expression contribute to the altered excitability observed in kindling. Some changes in expression could play a role in mossy fiber sprouting, such as the neurotrophins acutely and ligatin long-term. The mechanism for the change in mRNA levels also can vary. They can be regulated at the transcriptional level, which is probably what occurs with the $GABA_A$ R, or post-transcriptionally as with ligatin, where changes in mRNA half-life are occurring.

The induction of the kindled state can alter gene expression acutely and chronically. Selective changes in IEGs, neurotrophins, peptides and neurotransmitter receptors have been observed acutely. Long-term changes in ligatin, CaM kinase II, neurotransmitter receptors and peptides have also been observed. Thus it is clear that selective alteration in gene expression occurs in kindling. The functional role of these gene changes in the long-term plasticity associated with kindling still needs to be determined. However, some evidence suggests that some of these changes could play a role in the altered excitability associated with the kindling phenomenon. Ligatin down regulation could play a role in synaptic reorganization. Increases in excitatory amino acid receptor expression and decreases in inhibitory amino acid receptor expression could result in disruption of the finely tuned balance between excitatory and inhibitory systems and lead to the hyperexcitability observed in kindling. The role of altered gene expression in the kindling phenomenon is an important area for further research.

REFERENCES

1. Babb, T.L., Kupfer, W.R., Pretorius, J.K., Crandall, P.H., and Levesque, M.F., Synaptic reorganization by mossy fibers in human epileptic fascia dentata, *Neuroscience*, 42(1991) 351–363.
2. Barde, Y., Trophic factors and neuronal survival, *Neuron*, 2(1989)1525–1534.
3. Beal, M.F., Role of excitotoxicity in human neurological disorders, *Curr. Op. Neurobiol.*, 2(1992) 657–662.
4. Bengzon, J., Kokaia, Z., Ernfors, P., Kokaia, M., Leanza, G., Nilsson, O. G., Persson, H., and Lindvall, O., Regulation of neurotrophin and trkA, trkB and trkC tyrosine kinase receptor messenger RNA expression in kindling, *Neuroscience*, 53(1993) 433–446.
5. Bettler, B. and Mulle, C., Review: Neurotransmitter receptors II AMPA and kainate receptors, *Neuropharmacology*, 34(1995) 123–139.
6. Braun, A.P. and Schulman, H., The multifunctional calcium/calmodulin-dependent protein kinase: From form to function, *Ann. Rev. Physiol.*, 57(1995) 417–445.
7. Bronstein, J.M., Micevych, P., Popper, P., Huez, G., Farber, D.B., and Wasterlain, C.G., Long-lasting decreases of type II calmodulin kinase expression in kindled rat brains, *Brain Res.*, 584 (1992) 257–260.
8. Browning, M.C., Huganir, R., and Greengard, P. Protein phosphorylation and neuronal function, *J. Neurochem.*, 45 (1985) 11–23.
9. Buhl, E.H., Otis, T.S., and Mody, I., Zinc-induced collapse of augmented inhibition by GABA in a temporal lobe epilepsy model, *Science*, 271(1996) 369–373.
10. Butler, L.S., Alcino, J.S., Abeliovich, A., Watanabe, Y., Tonegawa, S., and McNamara, J.O., Limbic epilepsy in transgenic mice carrying a Ca^{2+}/calmodulin-dependent kinase II a-subunit mutation, *Proc. Natl. Acad. Sci. USA*, 92 (1995) 6852–6855.
11. Chiasson, B.J., Dennison, Z., and Robertson, H.A., Amygdala kindling and immediate-early genes, *Brain Res. Mol. Brain Res.*, 29(1995) 191–199.
12. Choi, D.W., Bench to bedside: the glutamate connection, *Science*, 258 (1992) 241–243.
13. Churn, S.B., Multifunctional calcium and calmodulin-dependent kinase II in neuronal function and disease, *Advances in Neuroimmunology*, (1995) Vol. 5, pp. 241–259.
14. Clark, M., Smith, M.A., Weiss, S.R.B., and Post, R.M., Modulation of hippocampal glucocorticoid and mineralocorticoid receptor mRNA expression by amygdaloid kindling, *Neuroendocrinology* 59 (1994) 451–456.
15. Colbran, R.J. and Soderling, T.R., Calciuim/calmodulin-dependent protein kinase II, *Curr. Top. Cell. Regul.*, 31 (1990) 181–221
16. DeDyne, P., Marescau, B., and MacDonald, R.L., Epilepsy and the GABA hypothesis: A brief review and some examples, *Acta Neurol. Belg.*, 90 (1990) 65–81.
17. DeLorenzo, R.J., The challenging genetics of epilepsy. In: *Genetic strategies in epilepsy research* (Epilepsy Res. Suppl. 4). V.E. Anderson, W.A. Hauser, T.E. Leppik, J.L. Noebels and S.S. Richs (eds). Elsevier Science Publishers, 1991.
18. Dingldine, R., McBain, C.J., and McNamara, J.O., Excitatory amino acid receptors in epilepsy, *Trends Pharmacol. Sci.*, 11 (1990) 334–338.
19. Enfors, P., Bengzon, J., Kokaia, Z., Persson, H., and Lindvall, O., Increased levels of messenger RNAs for neurotrophic factors in the brain during kindling epileptogenesis, *Neuron*, 7 (1991) 165–176.
20. Friedman, L.K., Pellegrini-Giampietro, D.E., Sperber, E.F., Bennett, M.V.L., Moshe, S.L., and Zukin, R.S., Kainate-induced status epilepticus alters glutamate and $GABA_A$ receptor gene expressionin adult rat hippocampus: an in situ hybridization study, *J. Neurosci.* 14(1994) 2697–2707.
21. Gibbs, J.W., Sombati, S., DeLorenzo, R.J., and Coulter, D.A., Epileptogenesis-associated reduction in functional $GABA_A$ receptor density and benzodiazepine modulation in a hippocampal culture model of chronic spontaneous seizures, in press, (1996).

22. Gilbert, M.E., The NMDA-receptor antagonist, MK-801, suppresses limbic kindling and kindled seizures, *Brain Res.* 463 (1988) 90–99.
23. Gilbert, M.E., Potentiation of inhibition with perforant path kindling: an NMDA-receptor dependent process, *Brain Res.* 564 (1991) 109–116.
24. Gilbert, M.E. and Mack, C.M., The NMDA antagonist, MK-801, suppresses long-term potentiation, kindling, and kindling-induced potentiation in the perforant path of the unanesthetized rat, *Brain Res.*, 519 (1990) 89–96.
25. Goddard, G.V., McIntyre, D.C., Leech, C.K., A permanent change in brain function resulting from daily electrical stimulation, *Exp. Neurol.*, 25 (1969) 295–330.
26. Goldenring, J.R., Wasterlain, C.G., Oestreicher, A.B., de Graan, P.N., Farber, D.B., Glaser, G., and DeLorenzo, R.J., Kindling induces a long-lasting change in the activity of a hippocampal membrane calmodulin-dependent protein kinase system, *Brain Res.*, 377 (1986) 47–53
27. Greenwood, R.S., Abdou, A., Meeker, R.B., and Hayward, J.N., Vasopressin mRNA changes during kindling: the effects of kindling site and stage, *Mol. Brain. Res.*, 26(1–2) (1994) 286–292.
28. Hanson, P.I. and Schulman, H., Neuronal Ca2+/calmodulin-dependent protein kinases, *Annu. Rev. Biochem.*, 61 (1992) 559–601.
29. Harrison, M. B., Shumate, M. D., and Lothman, E. W., Opioid peptide expression in models of chronic temporal lobe epilepsy., *Neuroscience,* 65 (1995) 785–795.
30. Hikiji, M., Tomita, H., Ono, M. Fujiwara, Y., and Akiyama, K., Increase of kainate receptor mRNA in the hippocampal CA3 of amygdala-kindled rats detected by *in situ* hybridization, *Life Sci.*, 3 (1993) 857–864
31. Hollmann, M. and Heinemann, S., Cloned glutamate receptors, *Annu. Rev. Neurosci.*, 17 (1994) 31–108.
32. Houser, C.R., Esclapex, M., Fritschy, J.M., and Mohler, H., Decreased expression of the a5 subunit of the $GABA_A$ receptor in a model of temporal lobe epilepsy, *Soc. Neurosci. Absts.* 21 (1995)1475.
33. Hughes, P., Singleton, K., and Dragunow, M., MK-801 does not attenuate immediate-early gene expression following an amygdala afterdischarge, *Exp. Neurol.*, 128 (1994) 276–283
34. Isokawa, M., Levesque, M.F., Babb, T.L., and Engel, J., Jr., Single mossy fiber axonal systems of human dentate granule cells studied in hippocampal slices from patients with temporal lobe epilepsy, *J. Neurosci.*, 13 (1991) 1511–1522.
35. Jakoi, E.R., Kaufman, B., and Vanaman, T.C., Ligatin: A peripheral membrane protein with covalently bound palmitic acid, *J. Biol. Chem.*, 262 (1987) 1300–1304.
36. Jakoi, E.R., Sombati, S., Gerwin, C., and DeLorenzo, R.J., Excitatory amino acid receptor activation produces a selective and long-lasting modulation of gene expression in hippocampal neurons, *Brain Res.*, 582 (1992) 282–290.
37. Jakoi, E.R., Panchision, D.M., Gerwin, C.M., and DeLorenzo, R.J., Post-transcriptional regulation of gene expression in hippocampal neurons by glutamate receptor activation, *Brain Res.*, 693 (1995) 124–132.
38. Kamphuis, W., De Rijk, T. C., and Lopes da Silva, F. H., $GABA_A$ receptor beta 1–3 subunit gene expression in the hippocampus of kindled rats, *Neurosci. Lett.* 174 (1994) 5–8.
39. Kamphuis, W., De Rijk, T. C., Talamini, L.M., and Lopes da Silva, F. H., Rat hippocampal kindling induces changes in the glutamate receptor mRNA expression patterns in dentate granule neurons, *Eur. J. Neurosci.*, 6 (1994) 1119–1127.
40. Kamphuis, W., Hendriksen, H., Diegenbach, P.C., and Lopes da Silva, F.H., N-methyl-D-aspartate and kainate receptor gene expression in hippocampal pyramidal and granular neurons in the kindling model of epileptogenesis, *Neuroscience*, 67 (1995) 551–559.
41. Kapur, J., Stringer, J.L., and Lothman, E.W., Evidence that repetitive seizures in the hippocampus cause a lasting reduction of GABAergic inhibition, *J. Neurophys.*, 61 (1989) 417–434.
42. Kapur, J., Lothman, E.W., and DeLorenzo, R.J., Loss of $GABA_A$ receptors during partial status epilepticus, *Neurology*, 44 (1994) 2407–2408.
43. Kelly, P.T., Calmodulin-dependent protein kinase II. Multifunctional roles in neuronal differentiation and synaptic plasticity, *Mol. Neurobiol.* 5 (1991) 153–177.
44. Kokaia, M., Pratt, G. D., Elmer, E., Bengzon, J., Fritschy, J. M., Kokaia, Z., Lindvall, O., and Mohler, H., Biphasic differential changes of GABAA receptor subunit mRNA levels in dentate gyrus granule cells following recurrent kindling-induced seizures., *Brain Res. Mol. Brain Res.*, 23 (1994) 323–332.
45. Kraus, J.E., Yeh, G.-C., Bonhaus, D.W., Nadler, J.V., and McNamara, J.O., Kindling induces the long-lasting expression of a novel population of NMDA receptors in hippocampal region CA3, *J.Neurosci.*, 14 (1994) 4196–4205.
46. Kubek, M.J., Knoblach, S.M., Sharif, N.A., Burt, D.R., Buterbaugh, G.G., and Fuson, K.S., Thyrotropin-releasing hormone gene expression and receptors are differentially modified in limbic foci by seizures, *Ann. Neurol.*, 33 (1993) 70–76.
47. Laurie, D.J., Seeburg, P.H., and Wisden, W., The distribution of 13 $GABA_A$ receptor subunit mRNAs in the rat brain. II. Olfactory bulb and cerebellum, *J. Neurosci.*, 12 (1992) 1063–1076.

48. Lee S., Miskovsky, J., Williamson, J., Howells, R., Devinsky, O., Lothman, E., and Christakos, S., Changes in glutamate receptor and proenkephalin gene expression after kindled seizures, *Brain Res. Mol. Brain Res.*, 24 (1994) 34–42.
49. Lloyd, K.G., Bossi, L., Morselli, P.L., Murani, C., Rougier, M., and Loiseau, H., Alterations of GABA-mediated synaptic transmission in human epilepsy, *Adv. Neurol.*, 44 (1986) 1033–1044.
50. Lothman, E.W., Hatlellid, J.M., Zorumski, D.F., Conry, J.A., Moon, P.F., and Perlin, J.B., Kindling with rapidly recurring hippocampal seizures, *Brain Res.*, 360 (1985) 83–91.
51. Lothman, E.W., Bertram, E.H. III, and Stringer, J.L., Functional anatomy of hippocampal seizures, *Progress in Neurobiology*, 37 (1991) 1–82.
52. Lowenstein, D.H., Seren, M.S., and Longo, F.M., Prolonged increases in neurotrophic activity associated with kainate-induced hippocampal synaptic reorganization, *Neuroscience*, 56 (1993) 597–604.
53. MacDonald, R.L. and Olsen, R.W., $GABA_A$ receptor channels, *Ann. Rev. Neurosci.*, 17 (1994) 569–602.
54. Marchase, R.B., Harges, P., and Jakoi, R.R., Ligatin from embryonic chick neural retina inhibits retinal cell adhesion, *Developmental Biology*, 86 (1981) 250–255.
55. Marksteiner, J., Ortler, M., Bellmann, R., and Sperk, G., Neuropeptide Y biosynthesis is markedly induced in mossy fibers during temporal lobe epilepsy of the rat., *Neurosci. Lett.*, 112 (1990) 143–148.
56. Martin, D., McNamara, J.O., and Nadler, J.V., Kindling enhances sensitivity of CA3 hippocampal pyramidal cells to NMDA, *J. Neurosci.*, 12 (1992) 1928–1935.
57. McNamara, J.O., Kindling model of epi lepsy, *Adv. Neurol.*, 44 (1986) 303–318.
58. McNamara, J.O., Russell, R.D., Rigsbee, L., and Bonhaus, D.W., Anticonvulsant and antiepileptogenic actions of MK-801 in the kindling and electroshock models, Neuropharmacology (1988) 27: 563–568
59. Meldrum, B. and Garthwaite, J., Excitatory amino acid neurotoxicity and neurodegenerative disease, *Trends Pharmacol Sci.*, 11 (1990) 379–387
60. Mody, I. and Heinemann, U., NMDA receptors of dentate gyrus granule cells participate in synaptic transmission following kindling, *Nature*, 326 (1987) 701–704
61. Mody, I., Stanton, P.K., and Heinemann, U., Activation of N-methyl-D-aspartate receptors parallels changes in cellular and synaptic properties of dentate gyrus granul cells after kindling, *J. Neurophsiol.*, 59(1988) 1033–1054
62. Nadler, J.V., Thompson, M.A., and McNamara, J.O., Kindling reduces sensitivity of CA3 hippocampal pyramidal cells to competitive NMDA receptor antagonists, *Neuropharmacology*, 33 (1994) 147–153.
63. Okazaki, M.M., McNamara, J.O., and Nadler, J.V., N-methyl-D-aspartate receptor autoradiography in rat brain after angular bundle kindling, *Brain Res.*, 482 (1989) 359–364.
64. Panchision, D.M., Gerwin, C.M., DeLorenzo, R.J., and Jakoi, E.R., Glutamate receptor activation regulates mRNA at both transcriptional and posttranscriptional levels, *J. Neurochem.*, 65 (1995) 969–977.
65. Patel, M.N. and McNamara, J.O., Selective enhancement of axonal branching of cultured dentate gyrus neurons by neurotrophic factors, *Neuroscience*, 69 (1995) 763–670.
66. Perlin, J.B. Transient and sustained calcium-dependent biochemical and molecular alterations associated with seizure, epilepsy and status epilepticus. Unpublished doctoral dissertation, Virginia Commonwealth University, 1991
67. Perlin, J.B., Gerwin, C.M., Panchision, D.M., Vick, R.S., Jakoi, E.R., and DeLorenzo, R. J., Kindling produces long-lasting and selective changes in gene expression of hippocampal neurons., *Proc. Natl. Acad. Sci. USA*, 90 (1993) 1741–1745.
68. Pinel, J.P.J. and Rovner, L., Electrode placement and kindling-induced experimental epilepsy, *Exp. Neurol.*, 58 (1978) 335–346.
69. Poulter, M.O., Barker, J.L., O'Carroll, A.-M., Lolait, S.J., and Mahan, L.C., Differential and transient expression of $GABA_A$ receptor α-subunit mRNAs in the developing rat CNS, *J. Neurosci.*, 12 (1992) 2888–2900.
70. Pratt, G.D., Kokaia, M., Bengzon, J., Kokaia, Z., Fritschy, J.-M., Mohler, H., and Lindvall, O., Differential regulation of N-methyl-D-aspartate receptor subunit messenger RNAs in kindling-induced epileptogenesis, *Neuroscience*, 57 (1993) 307–318.
71. Pritchett, D.B., Luddens, H., and Seeburg, P.H., Type I and type II $GABA_A$-benzodiazepine receptors produced in transfected cells, *Science* 245 (1989) 1389–1392.
72. Pritchett, D.B., Sontheimer, H., Shivers, B.D., Ymer, S., Kettenmann, H., Schofield, P.R., and Seeburg, P.H., Importance of a novel $GABA_A$ receptor subunit for benzodiazepine pharmacology, *Nature*, 338 (1989) 582–585.
73. Qian, Z., Gilbert, M.E., Colicos, M.A., Kandel, E.R., and Kuhl, D., Tissue-plasminogen activator is induced as an immediate-early gene during seizure, kindling and long-term potentiation, *Nature*, 361 (1993) 453–457.
74. Racine, R.J., Modification of seizure activity by electrical stimulation: II. Motor seizure, *Electroencephalography and Clinical Neurophysiology*, 32 (1972) 281–294.

75. Rashid, K., Van Der Zee, C.E., Ross, G.M., Chapman, C.A. Stanisz, J., Riopelle, F.J., Racine, R.J., and Fahnestock, M., A nerve growth factor peptide retards seizure development and inhibits neuronal sprouting in a rat model of epilepsy, *Proc. Natl. Acad. Sci. USA*, 92 (1995) 9495–9499.
76. Rice, A., Rafiq, A., Shapiro, S.M., Jakoi, E.R., Coulter, D.A., and DeLorenzo, R.J., Long-lasting reductionof inhibitory function and $GABA_A$ subunit mRNA expression in a model of temporal lobe epilepsy, *Proc. Natl. Acad. Sci. USA*, (in press) (1996).
77. Rosen, J B., Kim, S.Y., and Post, R.M., Differential regional and time course increases in thyrotropin-releasing hormone, neuropeptide Y and enkephalin mRNAs following an amygdala kindled seizure, *Brain Res. Mol. Brain Res.*, 27 (1994) 71–80.
78. Sato, K., Morimoto, K., and Okamoto, M., Anticonvulsant action of a non-competitive antagonist of NMDA receptors (MK-801) in the kindling model of epilepsy, *Brain Res.*, 463 (1988) 12–20.
79. Schwartzkroin, P.A. and Knowles, W.D., Intracellular study of human epileptic cortex: in vitro maintenance of epileptiform activity, *Science*, 233 (1984) 709–712.
80. Shin, C., Pedersen, H.B., and McNamara, J.O., γ-aminobutyric acid and benzodiazepine receptors in the kindling model of epilepsy: A quantitative radiohistochemical study, *J. Neurosci.*, 5 (1985) 2696–2701.
81. Shin, C., McNamara, J.O., Morgan, J.I., Curran, T., and Cohen, D.R., Induction of c-fos mRNA expression by afterdischarge in the hippocampus of naive and kindled rats, *J. Neurochem.*, 55 (1990) 1050–1055.
82. Simonato M. Hosford D A. Labiner D M. Shin C. Mansbach H H. and McNamara J O., Differential expression of immediate early genes in the hippocampus in the kindling model of epilepsy, *Brain Res. Mol. Brain Res.*, 11 (1991) 115–124.
83. Sloviter, R.S., Decreased hippocampal inhibition and a selective loss of interneurons in experimental epilepsy, *Science*, 235 (1987) 73–76.
84. Sloviter, R.S., The functional organization of the hippocampal dentate gyrus and its relevance to the pathogenesis of temporal lobe epilepsy, *Ann. Neurol.*, 35 (1994) 640–654.
85. Soderling, T.R., Calcium/calmodulin-dependent protein kinase II: role in learning and memory, *Mol. Cell Biochem.*, 127–128 (1993) 93–101.
86. Sonnenberg, J.L., Frantz, G.D., Lee, S., Heick, A., Chu, C., Tobin, A.J., and Christakos, S., Calcium binding protein (calbindin-D28k) and glutamate decarboxylase gene expression after kindling induced seizures, *Brain Res. Mol. Brain Res.*, 9 (1991) 179–190.
87. Strowbridge, B.W., Masukawa, L.M., Spencer, D.D., and Shepherd, G.M., Hyperexcitability associated with localizable lesions in epileptic patients, *Brain Res.*, 587 (1992) 158–163.
88. Sutula,T., He, X.X., Cavazos, J., and Scott, G., Synaptic reorganization in the hippocampus induced by abnormal functional activity, *Science*, 239 (1988) 1147–1150.
89. Sutula, T., Cascino, G., Cavazos, J., Parada, I., and Ramirez, L., Mossy fiber synaptic reorganization in the epileptic human temporal lobe, *Ann. Neurol.*, 26 (1989) 321–330.
90. Teskey, G.C., Atkinson, B.G., and Cain, D.P., Expression of the proto-oncogene c-fos following electrical kindling in the rat, *Brain Res. Mol. Brain Res.*, 11 (1991) 1–10.
91. Titulaer, M.N.G., Kamphuis, W., Pool, C.W., van Heerikhuize, J.J., and Lopes da Silva, F.H., Kindling induces time-dependent and regional specific changes in the [^{3}H] muscimol binding in the rat hippocampus: A quantitative autoradiographic study, *Neuroscience*, 59 (1994) 817–826.
92. Titulaer, M.N.G., Ghijsen, W.E.J.M., Kamphuis, W., De Rijk, T.C., and Lopes da Silva, F.H., Opposite changes in $GABA_A$ receptor function in the CA1–3 area and fascia dentata of kindled rat hippocampus, *J. Neurochem.*, 64 (1995) 2615–2621.
93. Tromner, B.L. and Pasternak, J.F., NMDA receptor antagonists inhibit kindling epileptogenesis and seizure expression in developing rats, *Develop. Brain Res.*, 53 (1990) 248–252.
94. Tyndale, R.F., Olsen, R.W., and Tobin, A.J., $GABA_A$ receptors, In: *Handbook of receptors and channels: Ligand- and voltage-gated ion channels*, R.A. North (ed), CRC Press, Cleveland, (1994), pp 261–286
95. Vick, R.S., Rafiq, A., Coulter, D.A., Jakoi, E.R., and DeLorenzo, R.J., $GABA_A$ a2 mRNA levels are decreased following induction of spontaneous epileptiform discharges in hippocampal-entorhinal cortical slices, *Brain Res.*, 721 (1996) 111–119.
96. Wada, J.A. (ed). *Kindling 4*, Plenum Press, New York, (1990).
97. Wasterlain, C.G. and Jonec, V., Muscarinic kindling: Transsynaptic generation of a chronic seizure focus, *Life Sciences*, 26 (1980) 387–391.
98. Wasterlain, C.G. and Farber, D.B., Kindling alters the calcium/calmodulin-dependent phosphorylation of synaptic plasma membrane proteins in rat hippocampus, *Proc. Natl. Acad. Sci. USA*, 81 (1984) 1253–1257.
99. Watkins, J.C. and Evans, R.H., Excitatory amino acid neurotransmitters, *Ann. Rev. Pharmacol. Toxicol.*, 21 (1981)165–204.

100. Wisden, W., Laurie, D.J., Monyer, H., and Seeburg, P.H., The distribution of 13 $GABA_A$ receptor subunit mRNAs in the rat brain. I. Telencephalon, diencephalon, mesencephalon, *J. Neurosci.*, 12 (1992) 1040–1062.
101. Wong, M.L., Weiss, S.R., Gold, P.W., Doi, S.Q., Banerjee, S., Licinio, J., Lad, R., Post, R.M., and Smith, M.A., Induction of constitutive heat shock protein 73 mRNA in the dentate gyrus by seizures., *Mol. Brain Res.*, 13 (1992) 19–25.
102. Wong, M.L., Smith, M.A., Licinio, J., Doi, S.Q., Weiss, S.R., Post, R.M., and Gold, P.W., Differential effects of kindled and electrically induced seizures on a glutamate receptor (GluR1) gene expression, *Epilepsy Res.*, 14 (1993) 221–227.
103. Yeh, G.C., Bonhaus, D.W., Nadler, J.V., and McNamara, J.O., N-methyl-D-aspartate receptor plasticity in kindling: quantitative and qualitative alterations in the N-methyl-D-aspartate receptor-channel complex, *Proc. Natl. Acad. Sci. USA*, 86 (1989) 8157–8160.

DISCUSSION OF ANNE RICE'S PAPER

B. Adamec: I have three sort of related questions with respect to the GABA subunit changes. How long lasting were they after kindling?

A. Rice: These were all 6 weeks after the last stimulation. I think that there are subtle long-term changes that may be affecting the composition of the receptors.

B. Adamec: The second question I had was that you report alpha 1 and alpha 2. But there are many subunit types, and I was wondering if you had also looked at other alphas and gamma subunit types?

A. Rice: In the pilocarpine model we see the alpha 5 go down in CA1 and CA3. In the perirhinal and entorhinal cortex slice with low magnesium model, I think its the alpha 2 that they see going down. So there is not consistency in which isoform we're seeing change and where. In the pilocarpine model and in the slice we do not see the beta 2 change. We've looked at the beta 2 and we've looked at gamma 2 also. We see no changes in gammas.

B. Adamec: My final question was have you looked anywhere else other than the hippocampus?

A. Rice: I have not.

F. Lopez da Silva: About this GABA subunit is very complicated matter, as you know. I was pleased to see that you found this change in alpha 1 because we also found a decrease in alpha 1, but it was very slight and it was only in CA3 area that we could detect it in a significant way. This goes in the same direction but it gives a little bit more emphasis on this, and I wonder if we have to compare some of the technical details to understand this better. I was just wondering about the gamma 2. The gamma 2 subunit was the one in which we found changes at longer periods of kindling in a more persistent way. Gamma 2 appears to exist in multiple subforms, for example gamma 2 short and long, which have different sites for phosphorylation. So which subform is affected could be very important for the function of the GABA receptor. Have you found any changes in gamma 2 at all?

A. Rice: I have not but we have only looked at it in the pilocarpine model, we haven't looked at it in the kindling; so this may be different mechanisms of epilepsy that we are looking at.

M. Burnam: Dr. Richard Olsen was just up in Toronto talking and he has been looking at what he calls alcohol withdrawal kindling and once again finding changes in expression of the GABA-A site.

21

KINDLING IN GENETICALLY ALTERED MICE

Implications for the Role of LTP in Kindling

Donald P. Cain

Department of Psychology and
Graduate Program in Neuroscience
University of Western Ontario
London, Ontario N6A 5C2, Canada

1. INTRODUCTION

Kindling is a neuroplastic process that appears to involve the lasting alteration of synaptic function. This implies that kindling may require a neural growth process for some aspect of its establishment. The fact that inhibition of protein synthesis blocks kindling without affecting the epileptiform afterdischarge (AD) that normally leads to its development [8] is consistent with that suggestion, as are reports of kindling-induced neural alterations and sprouting at the ultrastructural level [17,18,51].

If a neural growth process is involved in kindling, it seems likely that this would require the transcription of information from genes for the subsequent synthesis of protein. Activity-induced gene expression has been proposed as a potential mechanism for the conversion of short term neural activity, such as epileptiform AD, into long term changes in the nervous system, such as kindled seizure susceptibility [15,43]. One method of evaluating this possibility is by measuring gene expression during and after kindling. This approach has shown that kindling is associated with the expression of immediate-early genes [11,15,52]. Although this method is useful, it relies fundamentally on correlative data, and it is not clear whether any of the genes studied so far are crucial for kindling, and if they are crucial, what their role is in the mechanism of kindling.

In addition to measuring gene expression, it is now possible to engineer a defined mutation into a mouse germ line by gene-targeting, thereby creating mutant mice that can be neurologically evaluated [22]. An advantage of gene-targeting is that the interpretation of the seizure phenotype can be simplified by the prior knowledge of the neural expression pattern and biochemical function of the targeted gene, which may provide insights into the molecular mechanisms of epilepsy.

One form of gene-targeting involves a gene knockout technique that creates a mutated version of a targeted gene, rendering it inactive. The result is a mouse that fails to

Kindling 5, edited by Corcoran and Moshé.
Plenum Press, New York, 1998.

express the product of the inactivated gene. A second form of gene-targeting involves modification of a gene in order to increase or decrease its activity. Such transgenic mouse strains express the gene product, but at levels higher or lower than normal. Knockout and transgenic strains have the potential to allow a functional analysis of a gene's role in biological processes.

Among the knockout and transgenic mouse strains developed to date, those developed for the study of long term potentiation (LTP) and learning are of particular interest. LTP is a lasting increase in neural transmission at specific synapses that results from the application of brief high-frequency trains of electrical pulses through electrodes. NMDA-mediated LTP has been studied as a laboratory model of the kind of plastic change that could underlie learning and memory [3], and NMDA/LTP mechanisms have been hypothesized to underlie kindling [2,12,14,30,31,33,34,48,53]. Therefore, it would be of interest to examine kindling in the same strains of mouse that harbor genetic alterations known to affect the induction of LTP. The strains examined in the experiments discussed here harbor genetic alterations in the Fyn tyrosine kinase gene [21], the CaMKII serine-threonine protein kinase gene[32], and the GluR2 subunit of the AMPA receptor gene [27]. Each of these strains has been shown to exhibit both altered LTP and altered behavior. We chose to study electrical kindling in the amygdala, a structure that readily kindles in the mouse [8].

2. GENERAL METHODS

Surgery for the bilateral implantation of indwelling amygdaloid electrodes was accomplished under pentobarbital anesthesia (60–80 mg/kg) after preadministration of 10 mg xylazine. Electrodes were constructed of twisted teflon-insulated Nichrome wire 127 μm in diameter soldered to gold-plated connector pins. Implantation was into the basolateral amygdala at the following coordinates, using standard stereotaxic techniques determined using pilot animals: Anterior-posterior + 2.5 mm relative to interaural zero; medial-lateral 3.3 mm; 5.3 mm ventral to skull surface. A miniature connector and leads attached the pins to brain stimulation and recording equipment. Histological examination confirmed the accuracy of the electrode placements.

After 10 days recovery, trains of biphasic square wave pulses (1.0 msec each, 60 pulse-pairs per sec, for 1.0 sec) were applied through the electrode at increasing intensity to determine AD threshold. Once-daily stimulation at 110% AD threshold was applied beginning 24 hr later until 3 generalized convulsions occurred. Stimulation was applied between 10:00 am and 2:00 pm at the same time for all groups. Electrographic records were obtained from the electrodes before and after each stimulation using a Grass polygraph. AD occurred in response to each suprathreshold stimulation. Kindling sessions of some mice were videotaped, and the tapes were replayed for scoring of the convulsions using Racine's categories [37], with stage 1 indicating brief behavioral immobility with ear flattening or twitching of the facial musculature and stage 5 indicating generalized convulsions. In cases in which videotapes were not made, convulsive behavior was scored by observation of the mice during kindling. After expression of 3 stage 5 convulsions or 30 kindling sessions with AD, mice were allowed 3 to 4 weeks without stimulation and then rekindled with the same electrical stimulation as a measure of retention of kindling.

Spontaneous behavioral activity was measured in some mice using an automated behavior monitoring device (Digiscan, Omnitech) that consisted of 6 monitors (40 × 40 × 30 cm), each of which contained 2 tiers of infrared sensors to measure horizontal (locomotion) and vertical (rearing) movements. A total of 12 behavioral activity variables was then obtained from the pattern of beam interruptions [25]. Mice were observed during a 60-min period.

3. *fyn* KNOCKOUT

The Fyn tyrosine kinase knockout strain was developed for the study of biochemical mechanisms that might underlie both LTP and behavioral learning [21]. The induction of LTP requires a series of signaling steps in both pre- and post-synaptic neurons [3]. The activation of post-synaptic glutamate receptors results in Ca^{2+} influx and signalling that requires the activity of protein tyrosine and serine-theonine kinases [20,29,35]. Fyn is a specific non-receptor tyrosine kinase that is required for the induction of LTP. This was determined by examining mice carrying mutations in a number of different non-receptor tyrosine kinases. Only *fyn* mutants showed a deficit in LTP, in the form of an increase in the threshold for the induction of LTP by tetanic stimulaton [21]. *fyn* mutants also demonstrated spatial learning deficits in the water maze, and structural changes in the hippocampus [21]. Thus, mice carrying a mutation of the *fyn* gene showed impaired synaptic plasticity in the hippocampus and impairments in learning. Thus, if LTP is necessary for kindling, we might expect that *fyn* mutants would also exhibit impaired kindling.

The *fyn* mutation was engineered by homologous recombination into mouse embryonic stem cells and resulted in no detectable expression of Fyn in the brain [21,49]. Since kindling is influenced by genetic background [7] we examined both wild-type (control) and *fyn* mutant mice in the inbred C129Sv strain. All *fyn* mutant mice were confirmed to be homozygous by genomic southern blotting.

The *fyn* mutants exhibited a severe retardation in the development of kindled convulsions (Fig. 1). All mice developed stage 5 generalized convulsions, but the *fyn* mutant group required nearly three times as many evoked ADs as the controls to reach stage 5 (*fyn* mutants, 23.5 ± 4.0, mean ± sem; controls, 9.0 ± 0.4). The ranges of these data do not overlap, and repeated measures analysis of variance yielded a highly significant group difference ($F_{(1,15)}=27.8$, $p<.0001$). The behavioral convulsions of both control and mutant mice were alike, and similar to those described previously for mice [8] and rats [37] kindled in the amygdala. The facts that the kindled convulsions in the mutants were normal and that all mutants reached stage 5 are important findings because they suggest that the retarded kindled seizure development is a specific physiological change, and that it did not result from untoward events that rendered the mutant brain incapable of generating the seizure activity and behaviors required in a generalized stage 5 convulsion.

fyn mutants and control mice were alike in various other respects. These included: (i) similar AD threshold (*fyn*: 40.8μ A; control 40.5 μ A), indicating similar initial sensitivity to the kindling current; (ii) similar electrophysiological patterns of seizure; (iii) similar convulsive behavior (both overall pattern and vigor); (iv) similar propagation of the AD to the contralateral amygdala (Fig. 1C); (v) the expected [4] sudden increase in duration of the AD when stage 5 was attained (session prior to first stage 5, *fyn*: 25.5 ± 0.6 sec, control: 24.7 ± 3.2 sec; first stage 5, *fyn*: 39.5 ± 5.3 sec, control: 37.8 ± 4.2 sec); and (vi) the expected [16] postictal behavioral depression after the first stage 5 convulsion (*fyn*: 177.5 ± 25.9 sec; control: 187.8 ± 17.6 sec). Analysis of variance carried out on the data in i, v, and vi failed to reveal a significant group difference on any measure ($p>.05$). These results are consistent with the earlier suggestion that the retardation of kindling in the mutants was a specific physiological change, and did not result from gross defects in brain mechanisms required for the expression of generalized convulsions.

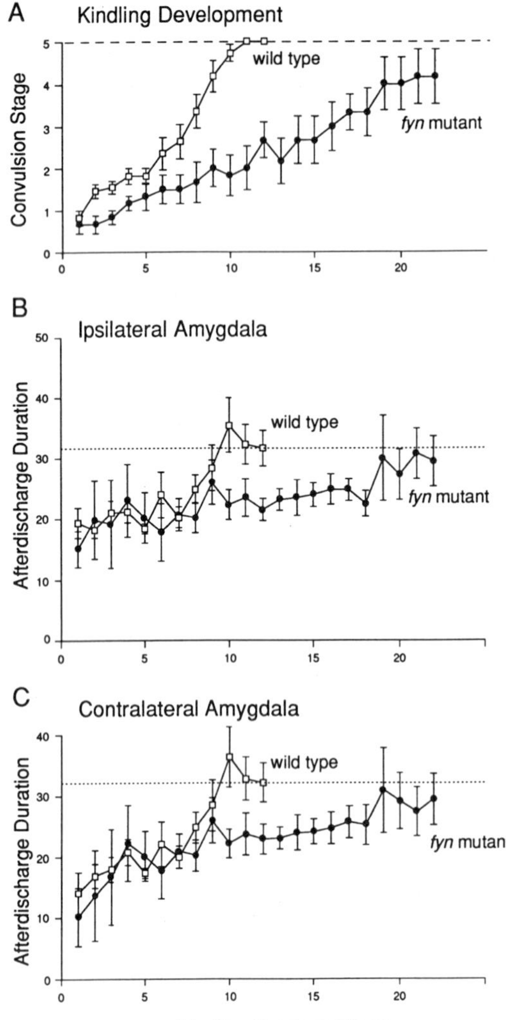

Figure 1. (A) Amygdala kindling is severely retarded in fyn mutant mice. Convulsion stages are from Racine [37]; stage 1 indicates ear flattening or twitching of the facial musculature and stage 5 indicates a generalized behavioral convulsion. The first 22 sessions are shown for the fyn mutants. (B) Afterdischarge duration in the ipsilateral amygdala does not differ between fyn mutant and control mice during the first 9 days. By day 10 most (9/11) control mice had reached stage 5, which is associated with a marked increment in afterdischarge duration [4]. Here and in Fig. 1C the dotted line indicates the stage 5 afterdischarge duration of control mice. Each point represents the mean ± sem. (C) Afterdischarge duration in the contralateral amygdala does not differ between fyn mutant and control mice during the first 9 days.

The persistence of kindling, as evaluated by rekindling 3–4 weeks after the third generalized convulsion, was similar in both groups in terms of both the convulsive and electrographic responses (AD duration on last session before rest period, *fyn*: 34.6 ± 3.5 sec, control: 37 ± 4.7 sec; duration of AD on the first stimulation after the rest period, *fyn*: 50.0 ± 5.8 sec, control: 38.2 ± 2.1 sec; $p>.05$).

There were no group differences among 11 of the 12 behavioral activity variables [25] ($p>.05$). The only variable that differed between groups was mean speed of movement ($F_{(1,24)}=6.0$, $p<.05$), which was 22 percent less in the *fyn* mutants than in the controls. Spontaneous activity distinguishes rats with amygdala damage from those without [47], but the reduction in spontaneous activity that we observed in the mutants in 1 of 12 activity variables was contrary to the expected hyperactivity that results from amygdala damage.

Examination of Nissl stained sections from *fyn* mutant and control mice revealed no systematic group differences in the overall size or position of the nuclei of the amygdala or in surrounding structures. Examination of anterior and posterior hippocampus revealed the expected [21] undulations in the granule cell layer of the anterior dentate gyrus and the pyramidal cell layer of the posterior hippocampal CA3 region.

4. CaMKII SERINE-THREONINE PROTEIN KINASE TRANSGENE

CaMKII is a Ca^{2+}/calmodulin-dependent serine-threonine protein kinase that is required for LTP [24]. Mayford and colleagues [32] found that expression of a Ca^{2+}-independent form of CaMKII was elevated by a transgenic mutation that involved replacement of threonine by aspartate at codon 286. This gave normal LTP when 100 HZ tetany was used to induce LTP, but long term depression (LTD) instead of weak LTP when frequencies of tetany below 10 HZ were used. Thus there was a shift toward LTD instead of LTP when low frequencies of stimulation were applied. Behaviorally, this alteration resulted in a deficit in spatial learning on the Barnes circular maze [1].

The CaMKII transgenic mutation might allow evaluation of the possible roles of LTP and LTD in kindling. Given that the predominant frequencies of amygdala AD spiking during kindling are in the range of stimulation pulse frequencies that produce LTD rather than LTP in these mutants, one would predict that if kindling is dependent on LTP effects produced by AD spiking, and if the spiking produced less excitatory drive as a result of the LTD that occurred, the mutants might kindle slower than controls.

The results of amygdala kindling failed to confirm the expectation, as the mutants and controls kindled at the same rate (Fig. 2). The mean number of ADs required to reach stage 5 did not differ between the groups (mutants, 12.0; controls, 10.9). If anything, the mutants had a greater response to the stimulation as reflected by the longer AD durations throughout the kindling procedure, relative to controls (ipsilateral, $F(1,11)=20.2$, $p<.001$; contralateral, $F(1,11)=12.0$, $p<.005$; Fig. 2). There was no groups X sessions interaction, indicating that although the duration was longer in the mutants, the rate of increase was the same in the 2 groups. AD threshold did not differ between the groups (mutants, 75.4 μA; controls, 111.7 μA). Both groups rekindled to stage 5 rapidly, and did not differ. The predominant frequency of spiking during AD was approximately 3 to 7 Hz.

Behaviorally, the mutants experienced more severe convulsions at the endpoint of kindling. Nearly all of the mutants exhibited running fits that involved very rapid running in circles around the confines of the Faraday cage in which they were kindled. None of the controls exhibited running fits, and none of the other mutants discussed in this report exhibited this form of severe convulsion. The strong tendency of the mutants to exhibit running fits is consistent with their longer AD, but perhaps inconsistent with their failure to develop kindled convulsions faster than controls and with the shift to LTD at tetany frequencies in the range of evoked AD.

5. GluR2 KNOCKOUT

Although N-methyl-D-aspartate (NMDA) receptors are crucial for hippocampal LTP, at least one other glutamate receptor subtype also plays a role in LTP. The α-amino-3-hydroxy-5-methyl-4-isoxazolepropionate (AMPA) receptor mediates fast excitatory synaptic transmission, and may be important for LTP [3]. The GluR2 subunit of the AMPA receptor regulates Ca^{2+} influx, and has been the subject of gene-targeting [27]. Deletion of the GluR2 gene resulted in greatly increased Ca^{2+} influx via AMPA receptors, and a 2-fold increase in the magnitude of LTP induced in the hippocampal CA1 region [27]. Given this finding, one might predict that amygdala kindling would be facilitated in this mutant.

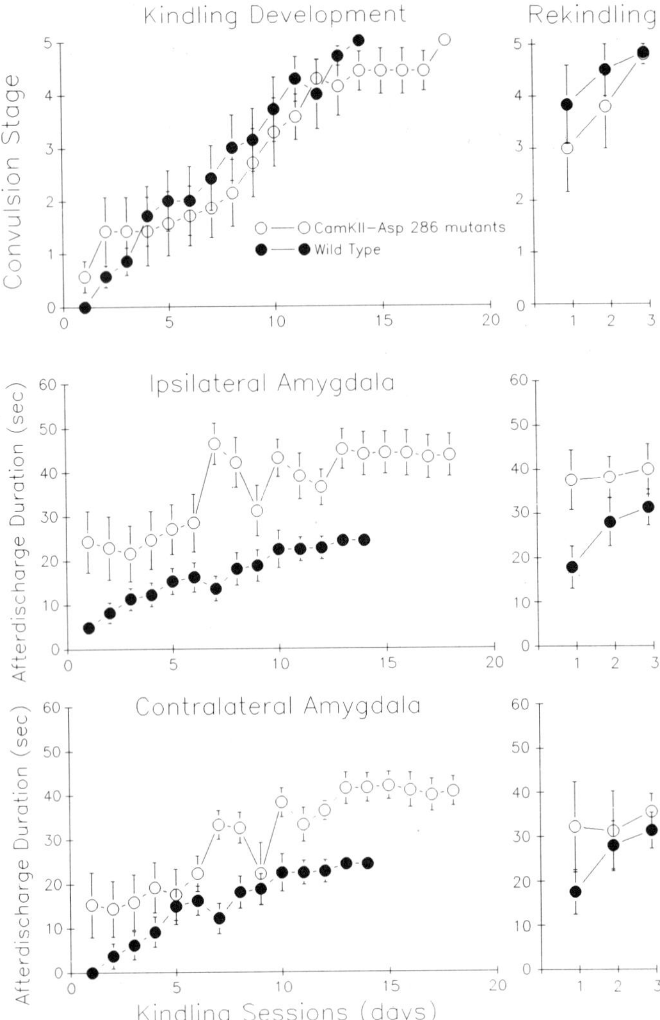

Figure 2. (top) Amygdala kindling does not differ between the groups. (middle) Afterdischarge duration in the ipsilateral amygdala is longer in the mutants than in controls. (bottom) Afterdischarge duration in the contralateral amygdala is longer in the mutants than in controls. (right) Rekindling does not differ between the groups.

This prediction was not upheld. Rather than facilitation, preliminary data from amygdala kindling in this mutant strain revealed truncated kindling, together with a profound attenuation of AD duration and propagation compared to controls and other strains of normal and mutant mouse. In an initial group of mutants (n=5) only 1 mouse reached stage 5. Another mouse reached stage 4, and the other 3 mice reached only stage 3 through session 30, at which point kindling was stopped. Having reached stage 3 or 4 after a mean of 12.5 sessions, the latter 4 mice did not progress further. Background strain controls all reached stage 5 after a mean of 18 sessions. AD duration remained virtually static at approximately 10 sec in the simulated amygdala of the mutants, and only one mutant—the mouse that reached stage 5—displayed any propagation of AD to the the contralateral amygdala. This paucity of AD development and propagation is highly unusual, and is indicative of a striking weakness of AD generation despite robust hippocampal LTP.

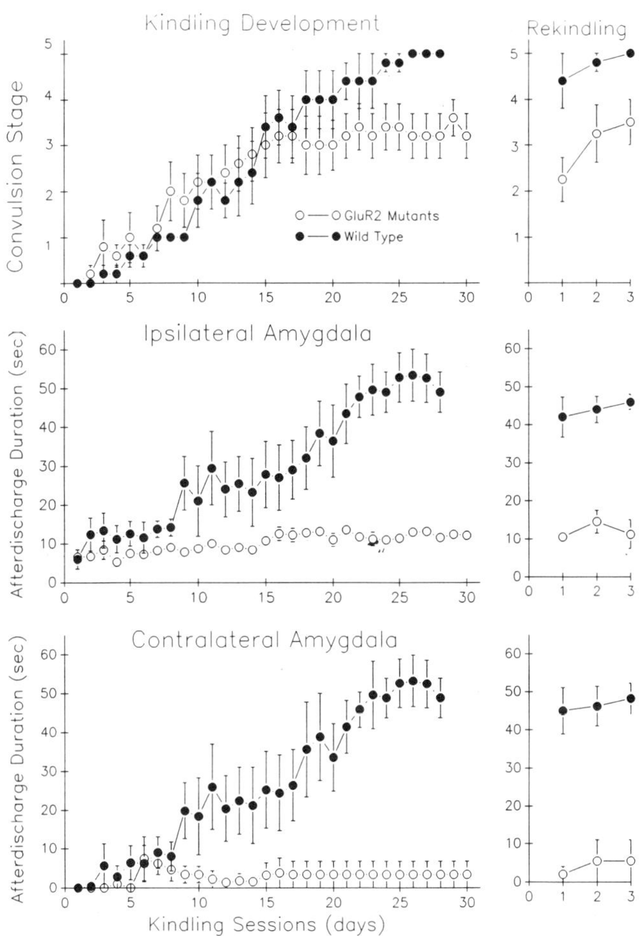

Figure 3. (top) Amydala kindling was truncated in GluR2 mutants, with only one of 5 mutants reaching stage 5. (middle) Afterdischarge duration in the ipsilateral amygdala was severly truncated in the GluR2 mutants, with afterdischarge duration remaining static at about 10 sec throughout the kindling period. (bottom) Propagation of afterdischarge to the contralateral amygdala was strikingly poor in the GluR2 mutants. (right) Convulsive behavior and afterdischarge duration rapidly reached previously kindled levels after a period without stimulation, but never reached the values of the control group.

6. DISCUSSION

There are a number of reasons to be cautious in interpreting the data reported here. First, the genetic engineering techniques that were used are still new and have important limitations. One limitation is that the gene knockout or transgene techniques produce animals that harbor the mutation throughout development, as well as in adulthood. This can lead to developmental defects that are difficult to identify and that can complicate the interpretation of data obtained from adult mutants. For example, the absence of a gene can affect the expression of other genes during development; the mutant animal 'reacts' to the absence of the targeted gene, and the reactions are mostly undocumented [44]. One form that this reaction can take is a compensatory one, in which related proteins take over the function of the one no longer produced [44].

An example of a reaction to the absence of a gene appears to be the proliferation during development, to approximately 125% of normal, of hippocampal CA3 pyramidal cells and dentate granule cells in *fyn* mutants [21]. This results in an undulating appearance in the respective cell layers [10,21], but apart from the blunting of LTP, no abnormality in the normal electrophysiological function of hippocampal circuits has been detected [21]. No other neuroanatomical abnormalities were noted in the brain regions that were examined with the light microscope, including the amygdala [10,21]. However, ultrastructural abnormalities, or abnormalities in brain regions not examined, cannot be excluded.

A second reason to be cautions is that complete details of the biological mechanisms involved with the proteins coded by the genes targeted in these experiments are lacking. Until more is known about the role of the proteins in mechanisms relevant to LTP and kindling, we will be limited in what can be concluded from the experiments.

In the case of the *fyn* mutants, the only kindling measure that differed between the groups was the rate of kindling to stage 5. All of the other kindling measures were similar between the groups, suggesting that the *fyn* mutants were fully capable of producing epileptiform activity and the other phenomena of normal kindling, but that Fyn tyrosine kinase was required for kindling at a normal rate. In the absence of Fyn, kindling can proceed, but at a substantially slower rate. The explanation for this is not known. It does not seem likely that the neuroanatomical abnormality found in the hippocampus of the mutants is responsible. First, apart from the blunting of LTP, hippocampal electrophysiology was normal in *fyn* mutants [21]. Second, the hippocampus is not required for normal amygdala kindling in rats [23,28,41,50].

Alternatively, Fyn may be involved in a biochemical process that is required for normal amygdala kindling. Nonreceptor tyrosine kinases such as Fyn are often activated by transmembrane signaling molecules [49], and may mediate the postsynaptic response of the cell. A role of this kind for Fyn is supported by the fact that tyrosine kinase inhibitors blunt LTP in hippocampal slices from normal mice in a manner similar to the blunting of LTP that is seen in *fyn* mutants [36]. This finding suggests that the blunting of LTP in the *fyn* mutants is the result of the specific lack of Fyn tyrosine kinase, and not an undocumented developmental defect. However, tyrosine kinase inhibitors have not been tested with kindling. The similarity of effects of the *fyn* knockout on LTP and on amydaloid kindling supports the hypothesized functional link between LTP and kindling that was discussed in the Introduction.

The fact that Fyn is necessary to phosphorylate a number of brain proteins including Focal Adhesion Kinase (FAK) [19], another nonreceptor tyrosine kinase, may be relevant to its role in both LTP and kindling. Fyn and FAK may phosphorylate substrates that have been implicated in kindling, including neurotransmitter receptors [9,13,35] and ion channels [26,42,54].

At low pulse frequencies (1–10 HZ) CaMKII-Asp286 mutants produce LTD in the CA1 region of hippocampal slices, rather than weak LTP [32]. This frequency range is also the predominant frequency of spiking during amygdaloid AD. An interpretation of the effects of the CaMKII-Asp286 transgene on kindling in terms of a shift toward the production of LTD at low pulse frequencies depends on the assumption that epileptiform spiking in the range of 1–10 HZ in intact animals mimics in physiologically relevant ways the 1–10 HZ square wave pulses that were applied to hippocampal slices during LTP experiments [32]. Based on the prima facie similarity between LTP and kindling-induced potentiation (KIP) [40], this might be a valid assumption. However, there is experimental evidence that the mechanisms of LTP and KIP are not identical and may differ substantially [5,6,38,39].

In any case, the data show that the CaMKII-Asp286 mutants kindled just as rapidly as controls, had longer AD, and had more severe convulsions despite a shift to LTD in place of LTP at low stimulation frequencies [32]. To the extent that the assumption discussed in the previous paragraph is valid, these findings do not support the hypothesized functional link between LTP and kindling.

The GluR2 mutants provided perhaps the most surprising data of all. Amygdala kindling was highly truncated, and AD duration and propagation were severely attenuated compared to other strains and species, to the point that 80% of the mutants exhibited no AD whatsoever in the amygdala contralateral to the stimulated amygdala, a very unusual finding in the kindling literature. These same mutants also failed to reach stage 5, which is consistent with the general view that widespread propagation of AD is necessary for normal kindling [45]. These deficiencies in kindling occurred in mutants that are known to display LTP that is twice as strong as normal in the CA1 region in the hippocampal slice [27]. This finding does not support the hypothesized functional link between LTP and kindling.

The mixed nature of the outcomes from these experiments does not allow an unambiguous conclusion about the role of LTP in kindling. Only the results from the *fyn* mutants were consistent with a facilitatory role for LTP in kindling. The results from the other 2 mutant strains were contrary to what might have been predicted from the LTP/kindling hypothesis. Although LTP and kindling appear to share many similarities of induction methods and appearance, to date the experimental evidence suggests that these neuroplastic phenomena may have different underlying mechanisms [5,38,39]. Further, pretreatment by systemic administration of a highly selective and competitive NMDA antagonist at a dose known to completely block LTP in the dentate gyrus did not block amygdaloid or hippocampal kindling with either electrical stimulation or carbachol, a cholinergic agonist [46]. Seizure development was slowed during the early kindling stages, but robust seizures and convulsions developed in spite of the pretreatment. Taken together, the data suggest that NMDA/LTP mechanisms are not required for amygdala or hippocampal kindling, although they might normally contribute to it. Despite the apparent similarity between LTP, KIP, and kindling, more research is needed to understand the exact relation between these phenomena [39].

ACKNOWLEDGMENTS

S.G.N. Grant, M. Mayford, E.R. Kandel, D. Saucier, E. Hargreaves, and J. Roder and his colleagues collaborated on some of the experiments discussed here. We thank P. Soriano for providing *fyn* mutant mice, and F. Boon for technical assistance. Supported by a grant to D.P.C. from NSERC, Canada. S.G was supported by the New York State Psychiatric Institute and a grant from the Alzheimers Disease Research Center (AG08702). E.R.K. is a Senior Investigator of the Howard Hughes Medical Institute.

REFERENCES

1. Bach, M.E., Hawkins, R.D., Osman, M., Kandel, E.R. and Mayford, M., Impairment of spatial but not contextual memory in CaMKII mutant mice with a selective loss of hippocampal LTP in the range of the theta frequency, *Cell*, 81 (1995) 905–915.

2. Baudry, M., Long-term potentiation and kindling: Similar biochemical mechanisms? In A. Delgado-Esceuta, A. Ward Jr., D. Woodbury, and R. Porter (Eds.), *Advances in Neurology, Vol. 44*, Raven, New York, 1986, pp. 401–410.
3. Bliss, T.V.P. and Collingridge, G. L., A synaptic model of memory: Long-term potentiation in the hippocampus, *Nature*, 361 (1993) 31–39.
4. Burnham, W.M., Primary and "transfer" seizure development in the kindled rat. In: J.A. Wada (Ed.), *Kindling*, Raven, New York, 1976, pp. 61–83.
5. Cain, D.P., Long-term potentiation and Kindling: How similar are the mechanisms? *Trends. Neurosci.*, 12 (1989) 6–10.
6. Cain, D.P., Boon, F. and Hargreaves, E.L., Evidence for different neurochemical contributions to long-term potentiation and to kindling and kindling-induced potentiation: Role of NMDA and urethane-sensitive mechansisms, *Exp. Neurol.*, 116 (1992) 330–338.
7. Cain, D.P. and Corcoran, M.E., Kindling in the seizure-prone and seizure-resistant Mongolian gerbil, *Electroenceph. Clin. Neurophysiol.*, 49 (1980) 360–365.
8. Cain, D.P., Corcoran, M.E. and Staines, W.A., Effects of protein synthesis inhibition on kindling in the mouse, *Exp. Neurol.*, 68 (1980) 409–419.
9. Cain, D.P., Desborough, K.A. and McKitrick, D.J., Retardation of amygdala kindling by antagonism of NMD-aspartate and muscarinic cholinergic receptors: Evidence for the summation of excitatory mechanisms in kindling, *Exp. Neurol.*, 100 (1988) 179–187.
10. Cain, D.P., Grant, S.G.N., Saucier, D., Hargreaves, E.L. and Kandel, E.R., Fyn tyrosine kinase is required for normal amygdala kindling, *Epilepsy Res.*, 22 (1995) 107–114.
11. Chiasson, B.J., Dennison, Z. and Robertson, H.A., Amygdala kindling and immediate-early genes, *Mol. Brain Res.*, 29 (1995) 191–199.
12. Collingridge, G. and Bliss, T.V.P. NMDA receptors—their role in long-term potentiation, *Trends Neurosci.*, 10 (1987) 288–293.
13. Dennison, Z. and Cain, D.P., Retardation of amygdaloid kindling in the rat by the excitatory amino acid antagonist kynurenic acid, *Synapse*, 4 (1989) 171–173.
14. Dingledine, R., McBain, C.J. and McNamara, J.O., Excitatory amino acid receptors and epilepsy, *Trends. Pharmacol. Sci. Spec. Rep.*, (1990) 49–53.
15. Dragunow, M. and Robertson, H. A., Kindling stimulation induces c-*fos* protein(s) in granule cells of the rat dentate gyrus, *Nature*, 329 (1987) 441–442.
16. Frenk, H., Engel, J. Jr., Ackermann, R.F., Shavit, Y. and Liebskind, J.C., Endogenous opioids may mediate post-ictal behavioral depression in amygdaloid-kindled rats, *Brain Res.*, 167 (1979) 435–440.
17. Geinisman, Y., Morrell, F., deToledo-Morrell, L., Remodeling of synaptic architecture during hippocampal "kindling," *Proc. Natl. Acad. Sci. 85* (1988) 3260–3264.
18. Geinisman, Y., Morrell, F., deToledo-Morrell, L., Alterations of synaptic ultrastructure induced by hippocampal kindling. In J.A. Wada (Ed.), *Kindling 4*, Plenum, New York, 1990, pp. 75–88.
19. Grant, S.G.N., Karl, K.A., Kiebler, M.A. and Kandel, E.R., Focal adhesion kinase in the brain: Novel subcellular localization and specific regulation by Fyn tyrosine kinase in mutant mice, *Genes Dev.*, 9 (1995) 1909–1921.
20. Grant, S.G.N. and O'Dell, T.J., Targeting tyrosine kinase genes and long-term potentiation, *Semin. Neurosci.*, 6 (1994) 45–52.
21. Grant, S.G.N., O'Dell, T.J., Karl, K.A., Stein, P.L., Soriano, P. and Kandel, E.R., Impaired long-term potentiation, spatial learning, and hippocampal development in fyn mutant mice, *Science*, 258 (1992) 1903–1910.
22. Grant, S.G.N. and Silva, A.J., Targeting learning. *Trends Neurosci.*, 17 (1994) 71–75.
23. Grimes, L., McGinty, J., McLain, P., Mitchell, C., Tilson, H. and Hong, J., Dentate granule cells are essential for kainic acid-induced wet dog shakes but not for seizures, *J. Neurosci.*, 8 (1988) 256–264.
24. Hanson, P.I. and Schulman, H., Neuronal Ca^{2+}/calmodulin-dependent protein kinases, *Ann. Rev. Biochem.*, 61 (1992) 559–601.
25. Hargreaves, E.L. and Cain, D.P., Hyperactivity, hyper-reactivity, and sensorimotor deficits induced by low doses of the N-methyl-D-aspartate non-competitive channel blocker MK801, *Behav. Brain Res.*, 47 (1992) 23–33.
26. Huang, X.-Y., Morielli, A.D. and Peralta, E.G., Tyrosine kinase-dependent suppression of a potassium channel by the G protein-coupled m1 muscarinic acetylcholine receptor, *Cell*, 75 (1993) 1145–1156.
27. Jia, Z., Agopyan, N., Miu, P., Xiong, Z., Gerlai, R., Henderson, J., Taverna, F., MacDonald, J., Carlen, P., Abramow-Newerly, W. and Roder, J., Enhanced LTP in the absence of GluR2, manuscript under review.
28. Lee, P.H.K. and Hong, J., Ventral hippocampal dentate granule cell lesions enhance motor seizures but reduce wet dog shakes induced by mu-opioid receptor antagonist, *Neuroscience*, 35 (1990) 71–77.
29. Malenka, R.C. and Nicoll, R.A., Intracellular signals and LTP, *Semin. Neurosci.*, 2 (1990) 335–344.

30. Martin, D., McNamara, J.O. and Nadler, J.V., Kindling enhances sensitivity of CA3 hippocampal calles to NMDA, *J. Neurosci.*, 12 (1992) 1928–1935.
31. Maru, E. and Goddard, G., Alteration in dentate neuronal activities associated with perforant path kindling. I. Long-term potentiation of excitatory synaptic transmission, *Exp. Neurol.*, 96 (1987) 19–32.
32. Mayford, M., Wang, J., Kandel, E.R. and O'Dell, T.J., CaMKII regulates the frequency response function of hippocampal synapses for the production of both LTD and LTP, *Cell*, 81 (1995) 891–904 .
33. McNamara, J.O., Kindling model of epilepsy. In A.Delgado-Esceuta, A. Ward Jr., D. Woodbury and R. Porter (Eds.), *Advances in Neurology, Vol. 44*, Raven, New York, 1986, pp. 303–318.
34. McNamara, J.O., Morrisett, R. and Nadler, J.V., Recent advances in understanding mechanisms of the kindling model. In P. Chavel and A.V. Delgado-Escueta (Eds.), *Advances in Neurology, Vol. 57*, Raven, New York, 1992, pp. 555–560.
35. Moss, S.J., Blackstone, C.D., and Huganir, R.L., Phosphorylation of recombinant non-NMDA glutamate receptors on serine and theonine residues, *Neurochem. Res.*, 18 (1993) 105–110.
36. O'Dell, T.J., Kandel, E.R. and Grant, S.G.N., Long-term potentiation in the hippocampus is blocked by tyrosine kinase inhibitors, *Nature*, 353 (1991) 558–560.
37. Racine, R.J., Modification of seizure activity by electrical stimulation. II. Motor seizure, *Electroenceph. Clin. Neurophysiol.*, 32 (1972) 281–294.
38. Racine, R.J., Burnham, W.M., Gilbert, M and Kairiss, E.W., Kindling mechanisms: I. Electrophysiological studies. In J.A. Wada (Ed.), *Kindling 3*, Raven, New York, 1986, pp. 263–282.
39. Racine, R.J. and Cain, D.P., Kindling-induced potentiation. In F. Morrell (Ed.), *Kindling and Synaptic Plasticity*, Birkhauser, Boston, 1991, pp. 38–53.
40. Racine, R.J., Gartner, J. and Burnham, W.M., Epileptiform activity and neural plasticity in limbic structures, *Brain Res.*, 47 (1972) 262–268.
41. Racine, R.J., Paxinos, G., Mosher, J.M. and Kairiss, E.W., The effects of lesions and knife-cuts on septal and amygdala kindling in the rat, *Brain Res.*, 454 (1988) 264–274.
42. Repp, H., Draheim, H., Rulkand, J., Seidel, G., Neise, J., Preseck, P. and Dreyer, F., Profound differences in potassium current properties of normal and Rous sarcoma virus-transformed chicken embryo fibroblasts, *Proc. Natl. Acad. Sci. USA*, 90 (1990) 3403–3407.
43. Robertson, H.A., Immediate-early genes, neuronal plasticity, and memory, *Biochem. Cell Biol.*, 70 (1992) 729–737.
44. Routtenberg, A., Knockout mouse fault lines, *Nature*, 374 (1995) 314–315.
45. Sato, M., Racine, R.J. and McIntyre, D.C., Kindling: Basic mechanisms and clinical validity, *Electroenceph. Clin. Neurophysiol.* , 76 (1990) 459–472.
46. Saucier, D. and Cain, D.P., Competitive NMDA receptor antagonists do not block cholinergic kindling with carbachol, *Epilepsy Res.*, 1966, in press.
47. Schwartzbaum, J.S. and Gay, P.E., Interacting behavioral effects of septal and amygdaloid lesions in the rat, *J. Comp. Physiol. Psychol.*, 61 (1966) 59–65.
48. Slater, N., Stelzer, A. and Galvan, M., Kindling-like stimulus patterns induce epileptiform discharges in the guinea pig in vitro hippocamopus, *Neurosci. Lett.*, 60 (1985) 25–31.
49. Stein, P.L., Lee, H.-M., Rich, S. and Soriano, P., pp59fyn mutant mice display differential signalling in thymocytes and peripheral T cells, *Cell*, 70 (1992) 741–750.
50. Sutula, T., Harrison, C. and Steward, O., Chronic epileptogenesis induced by kindling of the entorhinal cortex: The role of the dentate gyrus, *Brain Res.*, 385 (1986) 291–299.
51. Sutula, T., Xiao-Xian, H., Cavazos, J. and Scott, G., Synaptic reorganization in the hippocampus induced by abnormal functional activity, *Science*, 239 (1988) 1147–1150.
52. Teskey, G. C., Atkinson, B.G. and Cain, D.P., Expression of the proto-oncogene c-*fos* following electrical kindling in the rat, *Mol. Brain Res.*, 11 (1991) 1–10.
53. Trommer, B.L. and Pasternak, J.F., NMDA receptor antagonists inhibit kindling epileptogenesis and seizure expression in developing rats, *Dev. Brain Res.*, 53 (1990) 248–252.
54. Wilson, G. and Kaczmarek, L., Mode-switching of a voltage-gated cation chanel is mediated by a protein kinase A-regulated tyrosine-phosphatase, *Nature*, 366 (1993), 433–438.

DISCUSSION OF PETER CAIN'S PAPER

B. Adamec: Very interesting. I would like to caution against making general statements about the role of LTP and kindling when you look in one area like the hippocampus. Ron

Racine demonstrated many years ago that there is LTP in many efferent pathways from amygdala foci, for example, that is quite long-lasting. If you don't find a connection in one restricted brain area, it is really hard to make a general statement like that since we don't know where the critical sites of kindling are.

P. Cain: Absolutely, I agree; that was another of the caveats that I alluded to earlier. What I was doing was simple-mindedly making a prediction from what was know about the mutants to what you might expect.

B. Adamec: Hippocampal LTP might in some way be a model for LTP in all relevant pathways in the hippocampus—possibly.

P. Cain: Your comment was why I metioned Deb Saucier's study. If you believe, and I think there are reasons published in the literature to believe, that the treatment that we gave did block NMDA-mediated LTP in widespread areas—not just the ones we discussed in the mutants—then that would be a study perhaps that would get at your question. We found kindling in those animals.

I. Mody: Do you think that the shorter after-discharges in the GluR2 knock-outs are perhaps due to the faster desensitization of the AMPA receptors that don't have GluR2? The second question is, do you have an explanation why these mice are not epileptic when a 30% change in the adding of GluR2 reportedly leads to epilepsy and the mice die within 3 weeks.

P. Cain: No. John Roder wanted to see what would happen with these mice, and predicted that they would be epileptic. We were very surprised to see the opposite, very surprised. I have no explanation for that and I just can't really add to it—the data are the data. As for your first question, I can't say much about that either. I think that one of the problems that I have is that the LTP data and the other slice work with the GluR2 knock-outs are still rather preliminary and in fact unpublished at this point, so I really can't add very much to it.

J. McNamara: Very interesting. I was wondering whether LTP in CA1 is inhibited by APV?

P. Cain: In which knockout?

J. McNamara: You said that there was a two-fold increase in CA1 LTP in slices from the GluR2-less animals. The question is, are they APV sensitive.

P. Cain: They did not do that experiment. They found that NMDA-mediated transmission in the slice was not altered by APV but they did not do the LTP experiment that you asked about.

J. McNamara: The question is whether calcium is going through the NMDA channel to an AMPA channel.

P. Cain: Their interpretation is that it is going through the AMPA channel.

J. McNamara: Hence, APV insensitive LTP.

R. Racine: Just one other caveat to throw in the bucket. You're looking at or referring to LTP, but probably the more relevant potentiation would be kindling-induced potentiation. Did you look at that in these mice at all?

P. Cain: We did not look at KIP in any of these animals. One of the problems is that you have enough trouble with the mutants. A mutant that weighs 20 grams, just getting it to survive your procedures and so on without throwing a bunch of extra electrodes in is difficult, and we just haven't had enough mutants to work with to develop that and to do it. I agree it would be interesting to look at that—this is the first step.

A. Depaulis: Two short questions: Do you have any sprouting data on these guys? And have you tested these mice for sensitivity to other types of seizure?

P. Cain: No to the first question. Regarding the second, we watch the mice carefully for spontaneous seizures and what you might call reflex or noise induced seizures as well as handling induced seizures. We did not see those in any of these mice. However, we did not test systematically for audiogenic seizures or anything else.

P. Engel: You used to kindle with low-frequency stimulation. Did you try that on the transgenic cam-kinase mice, because that's where the difference was in the LTP?

P. Cain: No. Michael Corcoran discovered the effect and he and I then kindled with low-frequency pulses in the range that we were discussing earlier, 1 Hz, and in fact even less than 1 Hz in some cases, and up to 10 Hz. But we did not try that in the mice—again, its a problem of getting enough mutants to work with and getting them to survive. That's something that we could easily do if we could get the mutants and probably will.

C. Applegate: I have a question and a comment. The question first of all is that these GluR2 mice get stuck at stage 3 and are very analogous to guinea pigs, and I wonder if you could comment on AMPA receptor conformation in guinea pig versus these mice.

The comment is that these knock-out mice are an incredibly valuable resource for exploring mechanism, I think, with the caveats that have been brought up by M. Burnam and R. Racine, but one of the issues with these mice is that you have to understand the networks that are responsible for conferring seizure expression and propagation through the brain in order to plug these molecules into a meaningful system. I think that's something to keep in mind when we're looking at these animals as a potential source of defining mechanism.

P. Cain: I completely agree with that. I think that one of the important things in work like this is to know more than we do about any of these knockouts. We need to know more about the anatomy, and I alluded to the difference in the *fin* knock-outs and controls that has just been reported in a paper in press by Glen Proskey at the University of Lethbridge in Alberta. He noted in using these animals that the cerebellar anatomy was different in the knockouts. They have trouble moving, and they have a paucity of neurons in certain parts of the cerebellum, which was not known while Kandel and we were doing our work. Interestingly, just on that note, something that I've become interested in is the question of whether learning is affected in these animals, because that's why of course these strains were developed in the first place, to study LTP and learning. The initial report was that learning in the *fin* mutants was deficient in the water maze. What Proskey has shown is that despite the cerebellar and hippocampal abnormalities and despite their movement disorder, if the animals have a tendency to float in the water maze pool, which many of them do, and you stimulate them by prodding their hind feet briefly with a thin wooden rod it will induce them to begin to swim. Then you take the rod away and they keep swimming and they perform normally in the learning task. It is a very important finding, I think, showing that these animals, despite the impaired LTP, can learn quite well. We need to explore the mutants a lot more.

22

NEUROTROPHINS AND KINDLING EPILEPTOGENESIS

Olle Lindvall,* Zaal Kokaia, Eskil Elmér, Istvan Ferencz, Johan Bengzon, and Merab Kokaia

Section of Restorative Neurology
Wallenberg Neuroscience Center
University Hospital
S-221 85 Lund, Sweden

1. INTRODUCTION

Molecular and cellular mechanisms underlying the development of abnormal excitability in kindling and human epilepsy are poorly understood[39]. One major working hypothesis is that maintenance of the epileptic syndrome is caused by structural rearrangements occurring during epileptogenesis, e. g., sprouting of mossy fibres in the supragranular layer of the dentate gyrus and the infrapyramidal layer of CA3. Such plastic responses could be triggered by trophic factors, the synthesis of which may be influenced by seizure activity. During recent years much interest in this regard has been focussed on the neurotrophin family of trophic molecules, nerve growth factor (NGF), brain-derived neurotrophic factor (BDNF) and neurotrophin-3 (NT-3), and their high-affinity receptors trkA, trkB and trkC[35].

Gall and Isackson (1989)[16] were the first to demonstrate, using a seizure model created by a dentate gyrus hilar lesion, that seizure activity induces elevated NGF mRNA expression in cortical and hippocampal neurons. We subsequently showed that brief, kindling-evoked seizures give rise to increases of both NGF and BDNF gene expression[12], and similar changes were detected in several other models of epilepsy (for references, see[37]). These findings suggested that increased levels of NGF and BDNF protein could trigger the plastic responses observed in epileptic animals and humans and be involved in epileptogenesis. However, besides epileptic seizures, other insults to the brain, not associated with seizure activity, can also cause marked changes of gene expression for the neurotrophins (for references, see[37]). These insults include cerebral ischemia, hypoglycemic coma,

* Correspondence to: Olle Lindvall, M.D., Ph.D., Section of Restorative Neurology, Wallenberg Neuroscience Center, University Hospital, S-221 85 Lund, Sweden. Phone: +46-46-222 05 42; Fax: +46-46-222 05 60.

Kindling 5, edited by Corcoran and Moshé.
Plenum Press, New York, 1998.

cortical spreading depression and traumatic injury. It has therefore been proposed that the neurotrophin response to brain insults might also be a local protective mechanism intended to maintain neuronal function and counteract cell death[37]. The objective of this chapter is to summarise current knowledge of the regulation and function of neurotrophins in kindling. Results from other epilepsy models and insults will not be discussed here.

2. NEUROTROPHIN AND trk LEVELS IN KINDLING

2.1. Changes of mRNA Expression

In our own studies, neurotrophin mechanisms have been analyzed in animals subjected to either a traditional or rapid kindling protocol. In traditional kindling, electrical stimulations have been given once daily with current set just above threshold (usually about 20–100 μA, 100 Hz, 1 ms square wave pulses for 1 s) for inducing afterdischarge. Rapid kindling stimulations have been given with suprathreshold intensity (400 μA, 10 Hz, 1 ms square wave pulses for 10 s) and 5-min intervals.

One brief, focal seizure evoked by hippocampal kindling stimulation induces marked increases of NGF and BDNF mRNA levels in dentate granule cells[3,12]. Interestingly, at least in these cells, the activation of the BDNF gene seems to be an "all-or-none" type of response and dependent on the duration of seizure activity. At 2 h postseizure, BDNF mRNA expression is increased about 8-fold when the afterdischarge duration exceeds 70 s[3].

Forty rapid kindling stimulations in the hippocampus, performed during 3.25 h, induce elevated NGF mRNA levels in dentate granule cells (maximum at 0.5–2 h after the last seizure) and piriform cortex and neocortex (maximum at 4 h)[12]. BDNF mRNA levels are maximally increased at 0.5–2 h after the last seizure in dentate granule cells, CA1 and CA3 pyramidal neurons (Fig. 1), dentate gyrus hilus, amygdala, piriform cortex and neocortex. The levels of both mRNA species have returned to baseline at 24 h and no long-term changes are detected (Fig. 1).

Both the regional and temporal pattern of induction of BDNF mRNA in response to seizure activity is different from that of NGF mRNA[12,18,31]. Elevated BDNF but not NGF mRNA expression is induced in CA1 and CA3 pyramidal neurons. Furthermore, seizure-evoked increases of BDNF mRNA levels develop several hours more rapidly than those of NGF mRNA in brain regions outside the hippocampus.

Kindling-induced seizures lasting more than 70 s also lead to reduced NT-3 mRNA level and increased expression of mRNAs for the functional trkB and trkC receptors in

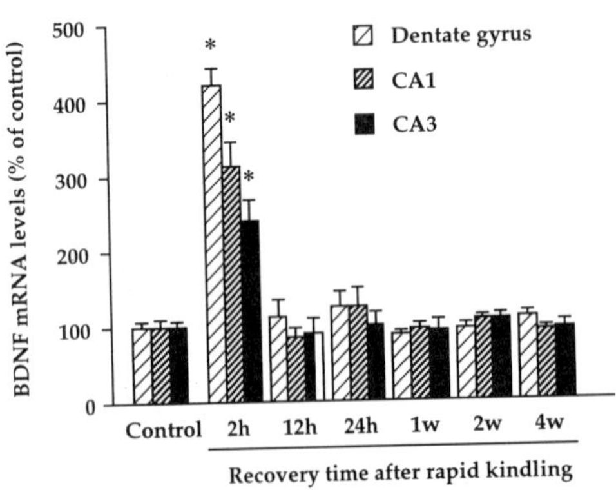

Figure 1. Levels of BDNF mRNA in the dentate granule cell layer and in the CA1 and CA3 pyramidal layers in non-stimulated animals (control) and in rats at various time points after 40 rapid kindling stimulations as quantified by image analysis of *in situ* hybridization autoradiograms. * $p<0.05$ compared to control, one-way ANOVA with post-hoc Bonferroni-Dunn test. Data from Elmér *et al.*[11]

dentate granule cells[3]. The time course of changes of trkB mRNA is the same as for BDNF mRNA, although the increase of BDNF mRNA is more pronounced[3,40]. In fact, both mRNA species increase within the same granule cell[23]. The increase of trkB mRNA is transient, as observed after 40 rapid kindling stimulations, with maximum expression at 0.5 to 2 h after the last seizure, returning to control level at 24 h. Kindled seizures also induce elevated levels of trkB mRNAs encoding truncated receptors, lacking the tyrosine kinase domain, in the dentate hilar region, CA1 and CA3, piriform cortex, and neocortex[3]. There are no changes of trkA mRNA expression after seizures.

2.2. Changes of Protein Levels

Following 40 rapid kindling stimulations, NGF protein levels, determined using an enzyme immunoassay, increase in the dentate gyrus at 4 h after the last seizure and then return to control levels at 12 h[4]. A later, pronounced increase of NGF protein reaches maximum values at 7 days. Marked transient increases are also found in the parietal and piriform cortices, with maximum levels at 24 and 12 h, respectively, after the last seizure. Thus, elevated levels of NGF protein are confined to those brain regions which show increased NGF mRNA levels.

Immunohistochemical evidence has been presented for changes of trkB protein levels after kindling. TrkB immunoreactivity is markedly increased in dentate granule cells and hippocampal pyramidal layer at 2 and 4 h following 40 kindled seizures, but has returned to control level after 24 h[40]. The antibody used by Merlio *et al.*[40] was raised against the extracellular region of the trkB receptor and it is therefore not known if the levels of full-length or truncated trkB receptors or both are elevated after seizures.

Also the regional, kindling-induced BDNF protein levels, as measured using a novel enzyme immunoassay[42], are largely in agreement with the mRNA changes. One focal seizure evoked by hippocampal rapid kindling stimulation gives rise to a significant increase of BDNF protein in the dentate gyrus at 6 h[11]. After 40 stimulations, BDNF protein is elevated in the dentate gyrus, CA1 and CA3 regions and piriform cortex (Fig. 2). Also in the parietal cortex, BDNF protein is slightly increased (not statistically significant). In the hippocampal formation, maximum levels occur at 6 to 24 h whereas the highest BDNF content in the piriform cortex was reached already at 2 h after the last seizure (Fig. 2). The elevated BDNF protein level persists up to 96 h in the dentate gyrus but only up to 6–24 h in the other regions.

3. REGULATION OF NEUROTROPHIN AND trk GENE EXPRESSION

The bulk of the evidence from both *in vitro* and *in vivo* studies indicates that the changes of neurotrophin and trk mRNA levels after kindled seizures and other brain insults are triggered by release of glutamate acting on both NMDA and non-NMDA receptors, depolarization and calcium influx[8,12,17,23,24,36,38,41,49,50]. In addition, gene expression is modulated by several other factors such as glucocorticoids[1,2,30] and GABAergic and cholinergic neural activity[28,34,48]. Of special interest in relation to kindling epileptogenesis are recent studies using selective lesions of the basal forebrain cholinergic system induced by intraventricular injection of 192 IgG-saporin (saporin coupled to a monoclonal antibody against the low affinity NGF receptor). Intraventricular 192 IgG-saporin causes a complete loss of cholinergic afferents to the hippocampus and cerebral cortex, which leads

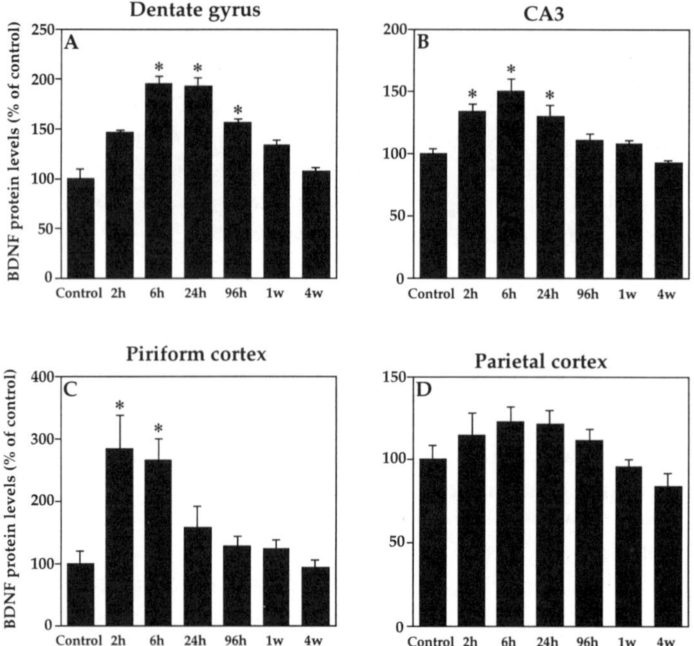

Figure 2. Levels of BDNF protein in dentate gyrus (A), CA3 region (B) and piriform (C) and parietal (D) cortices at various time points after 40 rapid kindling stimulations as measured by ELISA. *$p<0.05$ compared to control, one-way ANOVA with post-hoc Bonferroni-Dunn test. Data from Elmér *et al.*[11]

to about 50 % reduction of basal BDNF mRNA levels in hippocampal subregions and piriform cortex. The lesion markedly attenuates the BDNF mRNA increase in the hippocampal formation and frontal cortex following one generalized seizure evoked by traditional kindling stimulation[22]. In addition, the lesion abolishes the seizure-evoked increase of NGF and trkC mRNA levels and decrease of NT-3 mRNA expression in dentate granule cells. After 40 rapidly recurring kindled seizures, there is no major difference in neurotrophin and trk mRNA expression between denervated and non-denervated rats[13]. These findings suggest that the cholinergic lesion increases the threshold for, but does not prevent the induction of the alteration of neurotrophin and trk gene expression in response to seizures. Interestingly, the 192 IgG-saporin lesion leads to increased responsiveness to stimuli during both rapid and traditional kindling[13,22] which indicates that the cholinergic system has a dampening action on kindling epileptogenesis. Since the neurotrophins are believed to be epileptogenic (see 4.1), it seems unlikely that the seizure-suppressant effect of the cholinergic system is mediated via changes of neurotrophic function.

The BDNF gene comprises four different promoters[46], and alternative usage of these promoters results in transcription of eight different BDNF mRNAs[46]. One kindling-induced hippocampal seizure induces significant increases of exon I, II and III mRNAs in dentate granule cells, whereas exon IV mRNA is unchanged[26]. Maximum levels are detected after 2 h; exon III mRNA increases more rapidly than exon II and, in particular, exon I mRNA. At the end of a series of 40 rapid kindling-evoked seizures, maximum levels of BDNF transcripts have already been reached in the hippocampal formation[26]. The pattern of increases of the various exon mRNAs is region-specific. In dentate granule cells, there are elevated levels of exon I, II and III mRNAs, whereas in the CA3 region significant increases are observed for exon I and III mRNAs and in CA1 only for exon III mRNA. In amygdala, piriform cortex and neocortex marked elevations are detected for exon I and III mRNAs. Various transcripts could give rise to different amounts of BDNF protein and the differential use of multiple BDNF promoters may, therefore, provide additional flexibility and possibilities for fine tuning in the regulation of BDNF synthesis. Such sophisticated regulatory circuits might be necessary to control synaptic plasticity and development of hyperexcitability during kindling epileptogenesis.

4. FUNCTIONAL EFFECTS OF NEUROTROPHINS IN KINDLING

Several lines of evidence indicate that neurotrophins are involved in kindling epileptogenesis. At all stages during the development of kindling and in the fully kindled brain, a seizure episode induces a cascade of gene changes in dentate granule cells including markedly increased expression of BDNF, NGF, trkB and trkC mRNAs and reduced level of NT-3 mRNA. Generalized seizures lead to elevated levels of BDNF mRNA also in other hippocampal subregions, amygdala and piriform and neocortex[3]. The first data suggesting a facilitatory action of NGF in kindling were presented by Funabashi *et al.*[15], who reported that intraventricular administration of an antibody to NGF retards the development of amygdala kindling. Recently, this observation was confirmed by Van der Zee *et al.*[47], who also found that NGF antibody infusion inhibits mossy fibre sprouting. These data indicate that NGF promotes kindling epileptogenesis, and the authors suggest that this effect may be exerted through the stimulaton of mossy fibre sprouting.

To explore the physiological role of BDNF during epileptogenesis, we studied kindling development and maintenance as well as mossy fibre sprouting in mice carrying a deletion in the BDNF gene[21]. Because homozygous BDNF mutant mice (BDNF–/–) die within the first postnatal weeks, only heterozygotes (BDNF+/–) were used. We found that the basal expression of BDNF mRNA is 19–32% lower in cortical and hippocampal neurons in mutants compared to wild-type mice (Fig. 3). Both groups show increased expression of BDNF mRNA after generalized seizures, but the seizure-induced levels of BDNF mRNA are 25 to 51% lower in the BDNF (+/–) mice. The development of amygdala kindling is markedly retarded in the BDNF (+/–) mice (Fig. 4). These mice reach the fully kindled state (third grade 5 seizure) after 37±7 days as compared to 17±3 days in the BDNF (+/+) mice. The deficit in the BDNF mutants mainly reflects dampening of the progression from focal to generalized seizures (Fig. 4). There is no significant difference between the groups in the number of stimulations required to evoke focal seizures (first grade 1 or 2). In contrast, the BDNF mutants spend considerably longer time (17±5 days) than wild-type mice (4±1 days) in focal (grade 2) seizures before they exhibit generalized (grade 4 or 5) seizures. Other seizure characteristics do not differ between the groups.

In order to explore whether the mutation of the BDNF gene influences the maintenance of kindling, BDNF (+/+) and (+/–) mice were stimulated until they had exhibited 10 grade 5 seizures. When a new stimulus was given 9–10 weeks thereafter, there was no difference between wild-type and BDNF mutants in seizure grade, threshold or duration[21]. Thus, the persistence of kindling is unaffected in the BDNF (+/–) mice. Observations in the BDNF +/– mice also provided evidence against the idea that mossy fibre sprouting is an important mechanism underlying the development of hyperexcitability in kindling. In fact, mossy fibre sprouting, as assessed in Timm's stained sections, was clearly more pronounced in the BDNF mutants compared to wild-type animals[21]. The Timm's staining score in the supragranular layer of the dentate gyrus was significantly correlated to the number of kindling

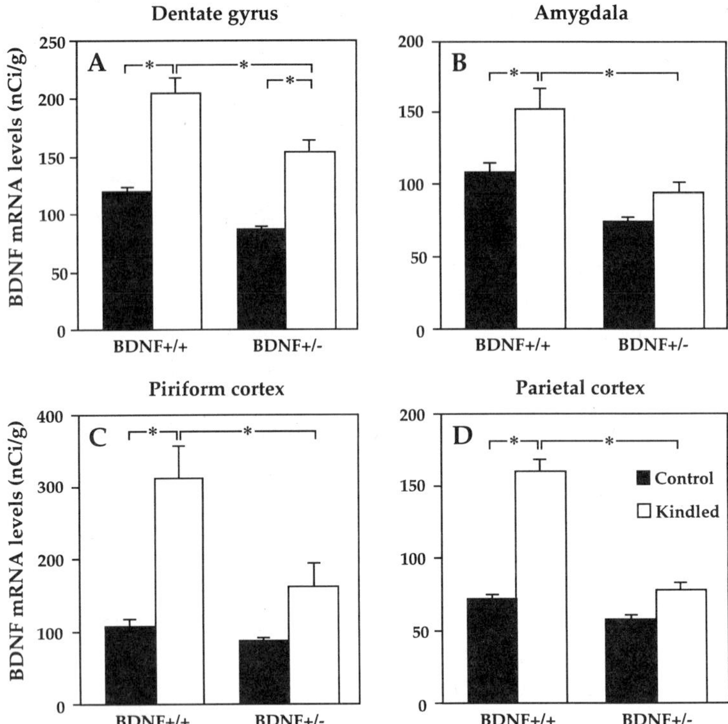

Figure 3. Levels of BDNF mRNA under basal conditions (control) and 2 h after the third grade 5 seizure (kindled) in BDNF +/– and BDNF +/+ mice quantified on *in situ* hybridization autoradiograms in dentate gyrus (A), amygdala (B), piriform cortex (C) and parietal cortex (D). * $p<0.05$ compared to +/+ mice; one-way ANOVA with post-hoc Scheffe's test. Data from Kokaia *et al.*[21]

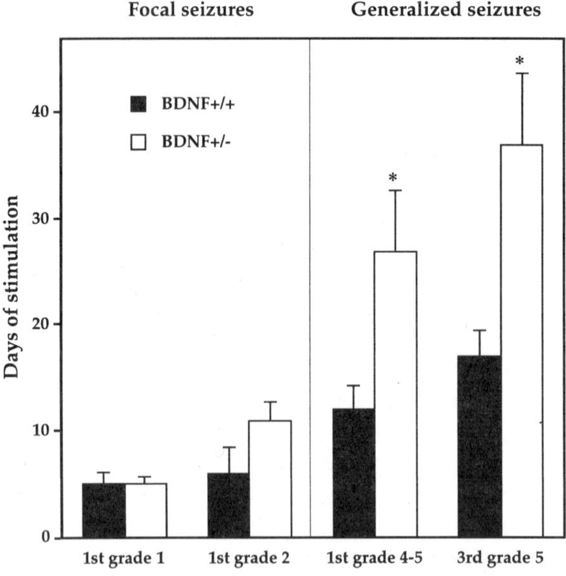

Figure 4. Number of daily amygdala stimulations to reach different seizure grades in BDNF +/+ and BDNF +/– mice. *$p<0.05$ compared to +/+ mice, Student's unpaired t-test. Data from Kokaia *et al.*[21]

stimulations in the different animals. No other morphological differences were observed between the two groups. It therefore seems less likely that BDNF promotes kindling epileptogenesis by triggering mossy fibre sprouting. However, the elevated levels of BDNF following kindling-evoked seizures may induce other changes at the synaptic or cellular level facilitating the development of epilepsy. Presently, the most likely action of BDNF during epileptogenesis seems to be to increase synaptic efficacy. This phenomenon is characteristic of long-term potentiation (LTP) and probably contributes to kindling development[45]. Supporting this idea, kindled seizures and stimulations leading to LTP give rise to similar changes of neurotrophin gene expression in dentate granule cells[3,6,9,12] and hippocampal CA1 neurons[44]. Furthermore, homo- and heterozygous BDNF knockout mice show significant impairment of hippocampal LTP[27,43]. This deficit can be completely reversed by the addition of BDNF[43]. Exogeneous BDNF promotes the induction of LTP in developing hippocampus and a trkB-IgG fusion protein, which scavenges endogeneous BDNF, reduces the magnitude of LTP in the adult hippocampus[14]. Also arguing for an acute role of BDNF in synaptic function are observations in cultured hippocampal neurons of enhanced glutamatergic transmission[32] and increased responsiveness of the postsynaptic neuron to the excitatory input[33] after application of BDNF. Likewise, Kang and Schuman[19] have described a dramatic and sustained (2 to 3 h) enhancement of transmission at the Schaffer collateral—CA1 synapses in hippocampal slices after application of BDNF, probably through a presynaptic mode of action. Directly in favour of an epileptogenic action of BDNF, injection of this factor into the hippocampus can produce epileptiform activity[5].

In contrast to the studies above, the observations of Larmet *et al.*[29] have suggested an inhibitory role of BDNF in kindling epileptogenesis. Chronic infusion of BDNF close to the stimulating electrode during the first week of hippocampal kindling significantly retarded seizure development. The reason for the discrepancy between the the results of Kokaia *et al.*[21] and Larmet *et al.*[29] is yet unclear. However, infusion of BDNF has been shown to rapidly down-regulate the trkB receptor (L. Frank personal communication). It seems possible that such downregulation could attenuate the response to BDNF synthesized and released after kindled seizures.

Recent studies indicate that also NT-3 might have direct effects on synaptic mechanisms. It has been reported that NT-3 can enhance glutamatergic transmission[19] and give rise to epileptiform activity after injection into the hippocampus[5]. Furthermore, NT-3 enhances impulse activity of cortical neurons in culture and induces synchronization of excitatory synaptic currents[20], probably through reduction of GABA-ergic synaptic transmission. We therefore speculated that the levels of NT-3 might be of importance for the rate of kindling epileptogenesis. In order to test this hypothesis, we studied kindling development in heterozygous (+/–) NT-3 mutant mice[10]. These mice exhibit about 30% lower basal and seizure-evoked NT-3 mRNA levels in dentate granule cells as compared to wild type animals (Fig. 5). The development of amygdala kindling is significantly retarded in the NT-3 mutant mice (Fig. 6). These mice do not reach the fully kindled state (third grade 5 seizures) until after 28±4 days as compared to 17±2 days in NT-3 (+/+) mice. Similar to BDNF mutants, the deficit in the NT-3 (+/–) mice mainly reflects dampening of the progression from focal to generalized seizures. The NT-3 mutants spend considerably longer time (13±3 days) than wild-type mice (2±1 days) in grade 2 seizures. When test stimulated 4–12 weeks after having experienced 10 grade 5 seizures, both groups respond with generalized seizures and, thus, the kindled state is maintained. No evidence for any morphological abnormalities have been found in the NT-3 (+/–) mice.

Also in accordance with an involvement of neurotrophins in epileptogenesis are recent data on neurotrophin and trk gene expression in two strains of rats, characterized by

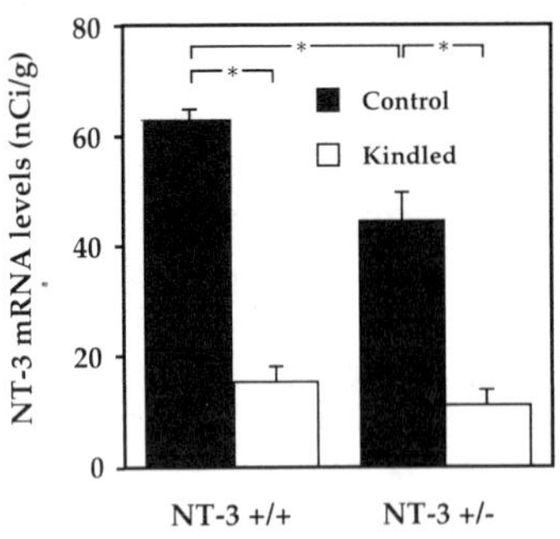

Figure 5. Levels of NT-3 mRNA under basal conditions (control) and 2 h after the last generalized seizure (kindled) in NT-3 +/+ and +/– mice quantified on in situ hybridization autoradiograms in dentate granule cell layer. *p<0.05, one-way ANOVA followed by Bonferroni's post-hoc test. Data from Elmér *et al.*[10]

their different rate of kindling development[25]. In the slow strain, partial seizure development is protracted and secondary generalization is delayed. In contrast, the fast strain rapidly progresses from partial to generalized seizures. At 2 h after the third generalized grade 5 seizure, induced by amygdala kindling, increased expression of BDNF mRNA is detected in the dentate granule cell layer, amygdala, frontoparietal and piriform cortices of the fast kindlers (Fig. 7). Similar seizure-evoked increases of BDNF mRNA levels are also observed in the amygdala and piriform cortex of slow kindlers (Fig. 7). However, in these animals BDNF mRNA expression is not significantly altered by the seizures in the dentate granule cell layer and fronto-parietal cortex. The increased BDNF mRNA expression is thus more widespread after seizures in the fast kindlers than in the slow kindlers. Furthermore, the seizure-induced increase of NGF, trkB and trkC mRNAs and decrease of NT-3 mRNA levels in dentate granule cell layer is only observed in fast, but not in slow kindlers. The observed differences in seizure-evoked neurotrophin and trk synthesis could contribute to the slow and fast kindling rate in these rats.

Studies both *in vitro* and *in vivo* have suggeste that neurotrophins could be neuroprotective after various insults (reviewed in Lindvall *et al.* 1994). These findings raise the possibility that neurotrophins might also counteract cell death caused by kindling. Sei-

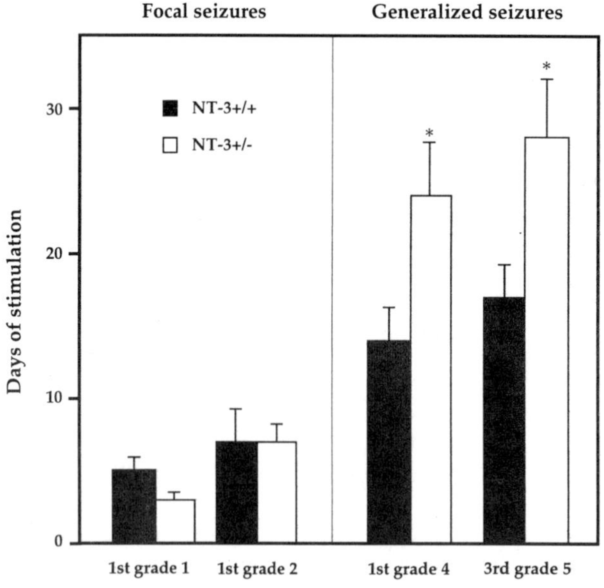

Figure 6. Number of daily amygdala stimulations to reach different seizure grades in NT-3 +/+ and +/– mice. *p<0.05, compared to +/+ mice. Students unpaired t-test. Data from Elmér *et al.*[10]

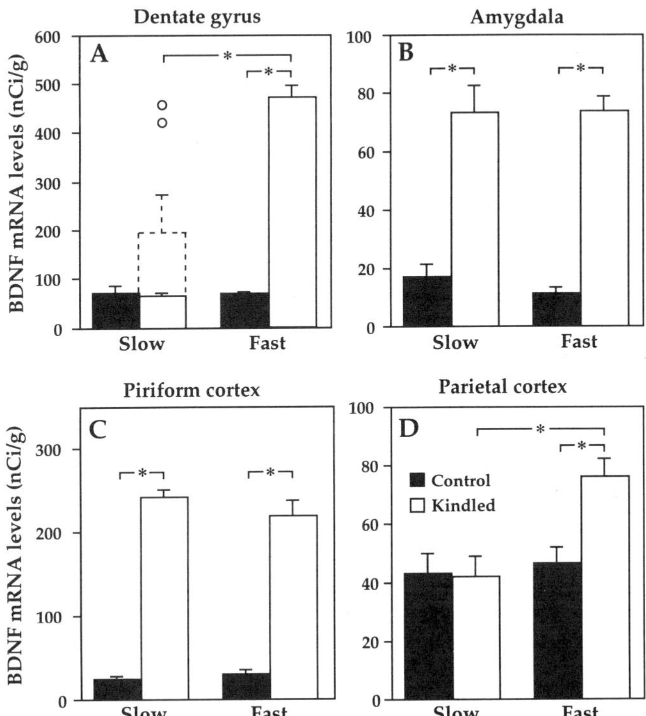

Figure 7. Levels of BDNF mRNA in dentate granule cell layer (A), amygdala (B), piriform cortex (C) and fronto-parietal cortex (D), in non-stimulated animals (control) and at 2 h after the third grade 5 seizure (kindled) in rats of both slow and fast kindling strain as quantified on *in situ* hybridization autoradiograms. Open circles in A denote values for 2 individual animals in the slow kindling group with increased expression of BDNF mRNA and dashed bar represents the mean value for all animals in this group. * $p<0.0001$, one-way ANOVA with Bonferroni-Dunn post-hoc test. Data from Kokaia *et al.*[25]

zure-induced neuronal loss in the hilus of the dentate gyrus has been proposed to play a role for mossy fiber sprouting during kindling epileptogenesis[7]. If BDNF has a neuroprotective action, the lower levels of BDNF in the BDNF +/– mice might make hilar neurons more vulnerable to epileptic insults. Kokaia *et al.*[21] hypothesized that the augmented mossy fiber sprouting in BDNF +/– mice could be due to more marked cell death in these animals. However, there was no difference between mutants and wild-type mice in the number of hilar neurons.

5. CONCLUSIONS

Brief periods of seizure activity, produced by electrical kindling stimulations, rapidly induce marked, transient changes of the levels of both neurotrophins and their receptors in hippocampal and cortical neurons. This neurotrophin response is not unique for epileptic seizures but is also observed after several other brain insults, and may constitute an intrinsic neuroprotective mechanism. However, available data indicate that NGF,[15,47] BDNF,[21] and NT-3[10] promote kindling epileptogenesis. For NGF, this effect may be exerted through the induction of mossy fibre sprouting, whereas it seems more likely that NT-3 and BDNF accelerate kindling by a direct effect on synaptic transmission. These findings suggest that attenuation of the neurotrophin increase after seizures and other brain insults might have antiepileptogenic effects and be prophylactic against epilepsy in humans.

ACKNOWLEDGMENTS

The work of the authors was supported by the Swedish MRC, the Swedish Society for Medical Research, the Kock Foundation, the Wiberg Foundation, the Zoéga Foundation, the Segerfalk Foundation and the Medical Faculty, University of Lund. We thank Marie Lundin for secretarial help.

REFERENCES

1. Barbany, G. and Persson H., Adrenalectomy attenuates kainic acid-elicited increases of messenger RNAs for neurotrophins and their receptors in the rat brain, *Neurosci.*, 54 (1993) 909–922.
2. Barbany, G. and Persson H., Regulation of neurotrophin mRNA expression in the rat brain by glucocorticoids, *Eur. J. Neurosci.*, 4 (1992) 396–403.
3. Bengzon, J., Kokaia Z., Ernfors P., Kokaia M., Leanza G., Nilsson O., Persson H. and Lindvall O., Regulation of neurotrophin and *trkA, trkB* and *trkC* tyrosine kinase receptor mRNA expression in kindling., *Neurosci.*, 53 (1993) 433–446.
4. Bengzon, J., Söderström S., Kokaia Z., Kokaia M., Ernfors P., Persson H., Ebendal T. and Lindvall O., Widespread increase of nerve growth factor protein in the rat forebrain after kindling-induced seizures, *Brain Res.*, 587 (1992) 338–342.
5. Berzaghi, M. P., Gutiérrez R., Heinemann U., Lindholm D. and Thoenen H., Neurotrophins induce acute transmitter-mediated changes in brain electrical activity, *Soc. Neurosci. Abstr.*, (1995) 545.
6. Castrén, E., Pitkanen M., Sirvio J., Parsadanian A., Lindholm D., Thoenen H. and Riekkinen P. J., The induction of LTP increases BDNF and NGF mRNA but decreases NT-3 mRNA in the dentate gyrus, *NeuroReport*, 4 (1993) 895–898.
7. Cavazos, J. E. and Sutula T. P., Progressive neuronal loss induced by kindling: a possible mechanism for mossy fiber synaptic reorganization and hippocampal sclerosis, *Brain Res.*, 527 (1990) 1–6.
8. Comelli, M. C., Guidolin D., Seren M. S., Zanoni R., Canella R., Rubini R. and Manev H., Time course, localization and pharmacological modulation of immediate early inducible genes, brain-derived neurotrophic factor and trkB messenger RNAs in the rat brain following photochemical stroke, *Neurosci.*, 55 (1993) 473–490.
9. Dragunow, M., Beilharz E., Mason B., Lawlor P., Abraham W. and Gluckman P., Brain-derived neurotrophic factor expression after long-term potentiation, *Neurosci. Lett.*, 160 (1993) 232–236.
10. Elmér, E., Kokaia M., Ernfors P., Ferencz I., Kokaia Z. and Lindvall O., Suppressed kindling epileptogenesis and perturbed BDNF and TrkB gene regulation in NT-3 mutant mice, *J. Neurosci.* (1996) submitted.
11. Elmér, E., Kokaia Z., Kokaia M., Carnahan J., Nawa H. and Lindvall O., Widespread increase of brain-derived neurotrophic factor protein in the rat forebrain after kindling-induced seizures, manuscript (1996).
12. Ernfors, P., Bengzon J., Kokaia Z., Persson H. and Lindvall O., Increased levels of messenger RNAs for neurotrophic factors in the brain during kindling epileptogenesis, *Neuron*, 7 (1991) 165–176.
13. Ferencz, I., Kokaia M., Keep M., Elmér E., Metsis M., Kokaia Z. and Lindvall O., Effects of cholinergic denervation on seizure development and neurotrophin mRNA regulation in rapid hippocampal kindling, *Neurosci.* (1996) submitted.
14. Figurov, A., Pozzo-Miller L. D., Olafsson P., Wang T. and Lu B., Regulation of synaptic responses to high-frequency stimulation and LTP by neurotrophins in the hippocampus, *Nature*, 381 (1996) 706–709.
15. Funabashi, T., Sasaki H. and Kimura F., Intraventricular injection of antiserum to nerve growth factor delays the development of amygdaloid kindling, *Brain Res.*, 458 (1988) 132–136.
16. Gall, C. and Isackson P. J., Limbic seizures increase neuronal production of messenger RNA for nerve growth factor, *Science*, 24 (1989) 758–761.
17. Ghosh, A., Carnahan J. and Greenberg M. E., Requirement for BDNF in activity-dependent survival of cortical neurons, *Science*, 263 (1994) 1618–1623.

18. Isackson, P. J., Huntsman M. M., Murray K. D. and Gall C. M., BDNF mRNA expression is increased in adult rat forebrain after limbic seizures: temporal patterns of induction distinct from NGF, *Neuron*, 6 (1991) 937–48.
19. Kang, H. and Schuman E. M., Long-lasting neurotrophin-induced enhancement of synaptic transmission in the adult hippocampus, *Science*, 267 (1995) 1658–1662.
20. Kim, H. G., Wang T., Olafsson P. and Lu B., Neurotrophin 3 potentiates neuronal activity and inhibits γ-aminobutyratergic synaptic transmission in cortical neurons, *Proc. Natl. Acad. Sci. USA*, 91 (1994) 12341–12345.
21. Kokaia, M., Ernfors P., Kokaia Z., Elmér E., Jaenisch R. and Lindvall O., Suppressed epileptogenesis in BDNF mutant mice, *Exp. Neurol.*, 133 (1995) 215–224.
22. Kokaia, M., Ferencz I., Leanza G., Elmér E., Metsis M., Kokaia Z., Wiley R. G. and Lindvall O., Immunolesioning of basal forebrain cholinergic neurons facilitates hippocampal kindling and perturbs neurotrophin messenger RNA regulation, *Neurosci.*, 70 (1995) 313–327.
23. Kokaia, Z., Bengzon J., Metsis M., Kokaia M., Persson H. and Lindvall O., Coexpression of neurotrophins and their receptors in neurons of the central nervous system, *Proc. Natl. Acad. Sci. USA*, 90 (1993) 6711–6715.
24. Kokaia, Z., Gidö G., Ringstedt T., Bengzon J., Kokaia M., Siesjö B. K., Persson H. and Lindvall O., Rapid increase of BDNF mRNA levels spreading depression: regulation by glutamatergic mechanisms independent of seizure activity, *Mol. Brain Res.*, 19 (1993) 277–286.
25. Kokaia, Z., Kelly M. E., Elmér E., Kokaia M., McIntyre D. C. and Lindvall O., Seizure-induced differential expression of mRNAs for neurotrophins and their receptors in genetically fast and slow kindling rats, *Neurosci.*, (1996) in press.
26. Kokaia, Z., Metsis M., Kokaia M., Bengzon J., Elmér E., Smith M.-L., Siesjö B. K., Timmusk T., Persson H. and Lindvall O., Brain insults in rats induce increased expression of the BDNF gene through differential usage of multiple promoters, *Eur. J. Neurosci.*, 6 (1994) 587–596.
27. Korte, M., Carroll P., Wolf E., Brem G., Thoenen H. and Bonhoeffer T., Hippocampal long-term potentiation is impaired in mice lacking brain-derived neurotrophic factor, *Proc. Natl. Acad. Sci. USA*, 92 (1995) 8856–8860.
28. Lapchak, P. A., Araujo D. M. and Hefti F., Cholinergic regulation of hippocampal brain-derived neurotrophic factor mRNA expression: evidence from lesion and chronic cholinergic drug treatment studies, *Neurosci.*, 52 (1993) 575–585.
29. Larmet, Y., Reibel S., Carnahan J., Nawa H., Marescaux C. and Depaulis A., Protective effects of brain-derived neurotrophic factor on the development of hippocampal kindling in the rat, *NeuroReport*, 6 (1995) 1937–1941.
30. Lauterborn, J. C., Berschauer R. and Gall C., Cell-specific modulation of basal and seizure-induced neurotrophin expression by adrenalectomy, *Neurosci.*, 68 (1995) 363–378.
31. Lauterborn, J. C., Isackson P. J. and Gall C. M., Seizure-induced increases in NGF mRNA exhibit different time courses across forebrain regions and are biphasic in hippocampus, *Exp. Neurol.*, 125 (1994) 22–40.
32. Lessman, V., Gottmann K. and Heumann R., BDNF and NT-4/5 enhance glutamatergic synaptic transmission in cultured hippocampal neurones, *NeuroReport*, 6 (1994) 21–25.
33. Levine, E. S., Dreyfus C. F., Black I. B. and Plummer M. R., Brain-derived neurotrophic factor rapidly enhances synaptic transmission in hippocampal neurons via postsynaptic tyrosine kinase receptors, *Proc. Natl. Acad. Sci. USA*, 92 (1995) 8074–8077.
34. Lindefors, N., Ernfors P., Falkenberg T. and Persson H., Septal cholinergic afferents regulate expression of brain-derived neurotrophic factor and beta-nerve growth factor mRNA in rat hippocampus, *Exp. Brain Res.*, 88 (1992) 771–779.
35. Lindsay, R. M., Wiegand S. J., Altar C. A. and DiStefano P. S., Neurotrophic factors: from molecule to man, *TINS*, 17 (1994) 182–190.
36. Lindvall, O., Ernfors P., Bengzon J., Kokaia Z., Smith M.-L., Siesjö B. K. and Persson H., Differential regulation of mRNAs for nerve growth factor, brain-derived neurotrophic factor and neurotrophin-3 in the adult rat brain following cerebral ischemia and hypoglycemic coma, *Proc. Natl. Acad. Sci. USA*, 89 (1992) 648–652.
37. Lindvall, O., Kokaia Z., Bengzon J., Elmér E. and Kokaia M., Neurotrophins and brain insults, *TINS*, 17 (1994) 490–496.
38. Lu, B., Yokoyama M., Dreyfus C. F. and Black I., Depolarizing stimuli regulate nerve growth factor gene expression in cultured hippocampal neurons, *Proc. Natl. Acad. Sci. USA*, 88 (1991) 6289–6292.
39. McNamara, J. O., Bonhaus D. W. and Shin C., The kindling model of epilepsy. In P. A. Schwartzkroin (Ed.), *Epilepsy: models, mechanisms, and concepts*, Cambridge University Press, Cambridge, 1993, pp. 27–47.

40. Merlio, J.-P., Ernfors P., Kokaia Z., Middlemas D. S., Bengzon J., Kokaia M., Smith M.-L., Siesjö B. K., Hunter T., Lindvall O. and Persson H., Increased production of the trkB protein tyrosine kinase receptor after brain insults, *Neuron*, 10 (1993) 151–164.
41. Mudo, G., Persson H., Timmusk T., Funakoshi H., Bindoni M. and Belluardo N., Increased expression of trkB and trkC messenger RNAs in the rat forebrain after focal mechanical injury, *Neurosci.*, 57 (1993) 901–912.
42. Nawa, H., Carnahan J. and Gall C., BDNF protein measured by a novel enzyme immunoassay in normal brain and after seizure: partial disagreement with mRNA levels, *Eur. J. Neurosci.*, 7 (1995) 1527–1535.
43. Patterson, S. L., Abel T. and Deuel T. A. S., Recombinant BDNF rescues deficits in basal synaptic transmission and hippocampal LTP in BDNF knockout mice, *Neuron*, 16 (1996) 1137–1145.
44. Patterson, S. L., Grover L. M., Schwartzkroin P. A. and Bothwell M., Neurotrophin expression in rat hippocampal slices: A stimulus paradigm inducing LTP in CA1 evokes increases in BDNF and NT-3 mRNAs, *Neuron*, 9 (1992) 1081–1088.
45. Sutula, T. and Steward O., Facilitation of kindling by prior induction of long-term potentiation in the perforant path, *Brain Res.*, 420 (1987) 109–117.
46. Timmusk, T., Palm K., Metsis M., Reintam T., Paalme V., Saarma M. and Persson H., Multiple promoters direct tissue-specific expression of the rat BDNF gene, *Neuron*, 10 (1993) 475–489.
47. Van der Zee, C. E., Rashid K. R., Le K., Moore K. A., Stanisz J., Diamond J., Racine R. J. and Fahnestock M., Intraventricular administration of antibodies to nerve growth factor retards kindling and blocks mossy fiber sprouting in adult rats, *J. Neurosci.*, 15 (1995) 5316–5323.
48. Zafra, F., Castern E., Thoenen H. and Lindholm D., Interplay between glutamate and gamma-aminobutyric acid transmitter systems in the physiological regulation of brain-derived neurotrophic factor and nerve growth factor synthesis in the hippocampal neurons, *Proc. Natl. Acad. Sci. USA*, 88 (1991) 10037–10041.
49. Zafra, F., Hengerer B., Leibrock J., Thoenen H. and Lindholm D., Activity dependent regulation of BDNF and NGF mRNAs in the rat hippocampus is mediated by non-NMDA glutamate receptors, *EMBO J.*, 9 (1990) 3545–3550.
50. Zafra, F., Lindholm D., Castren E., Hartikka J. and Thoenen H., Regulation of brain-derived neurotrophic factor and nerve growth factor mRNA in primary cultures of hippocampal neurons and astrocytes., *J. Neurosci.*, 12 (1992) 4793–4799.

DISCUSSION OF OLLE LINDVALL'S PAPER

R. Racine: Just to make the story a little more complicated, Depaulis has infused BDNF and retarded kindling, and we have relicated that. We have infused BDNF with osmotic pumps, and it retards kindling. We've also looked at sprouting and, although it just misses statistical significance so far, it appears to enhance sprouting as well. So that is another potential dissociation between the sprouting and kindling.

O. Lindvall: Yes, I've thought that maybe would have this discussion later today. I think that there are of course pros and cons with these strategies. With the knockouts, I think still the knockout technology may be the best technology to understand what the endogenous BDNF production means, but the problem is of course that these animals have had lowered BDNF levels during their development and one cannot exclude that the deficit is a developmental deficit. We as well as Thoenen's group in Germany have not been able to detect any deficit in the heterozygous BDNF knockouts, but one cannot exclude it. It's very difficult to establish that the brain is normal except that they have lower levels of BDNF. The BDNF infusion of course gives data which now have been reproduced by two groups, but one should also be aware that infusion of BDNF can lead to other changes. For example, people from Regeneron had just shown that you can get a down-regulation of the trk-B receptor and that could mean that if you infuse BDNF and get the down-regulation of the receptor and then kindle, you would have a less responsive system that could turn out as actually a retardation of kindling.

R. Racine: We thought about that possibility, but how would you account for it if the addition of more animals leads to significant increases in sprouting after BDNF infusion?

O. Lindvall: I don't think that I would take that as evidence for the role of BDNF during epileptogenesis.

R. Racine: No, we are talking about the down-regulation of receptors.

O. Lindvall: Yes, it could still be so. What the Regeneron people have shown is the down-regulation of the receptor. They have looked at one functional response, pain, and did not see any change of the functional response on that particular parameter. I am not saying that infusion of BDNF does not show the correct functional effect, but I am saying that I think that one should be aware that infusion of BDNF can change the sensitivity of the receptor and can, according to Thoenen's group, induce seizure activity. It can induce long-term changes of peptide expression, for example. So I would say that there are pros and cons with that technique as well. What we would like to have are conditional knockouts where you can switch off the gene, and I hope that we can have that soon.

A. Depaulis: Two questions: Have you tested the mutant mice in terms of seizure sensitivity, for instance, injecting PTZ or doing electroshock?

O. Lindvall: No. I have the same response as Peter Cain had, I think the answer is that in working with mutants you are limited in numbers. We are now breeding mutants, so we can do all these improvements.

A. Depaulis: And a mean question: How do you reconcile neuroprotection and promotion of epileptogenesis?

O. Lindvall: Yes, that is a very good point. I try to keep that in mind when I write reviews about this. I think that it may be an example of increased synaptic efficacy that goes wrong. If one looks upon a brain insult in a system that tried to protect the cells and increased synaptic efficacy, then I think that that is where we should begin. The problem here is that I've also said that there are data indicating actually BDNF can promote cell death. Then one could fit it with something that actually promotes epileptogenesis. I think it illustrates that we have very good knowledge about the regulation of the gene, the protein synthesis, which cells the neurotrophins act on; but since this is not just a phenomenon that we see in kindling, it could very well be something else and that we are just looking at the very small portion of the phenomenon.

F. Lopez da Silva: I have two questions. One is that what you showed in this heterozygous animals was a retardation of kindling. Do you see any change in afterdischarge duration and threshold?

O. Lindvall: We didn't see any significant changes.

F. Lopez da Silva: So it could perhaps then be interpreted that what you are seeing are effects which are mainly related to the propagation of activity in the brain, not to the generation of epileptogenic activity at the site. Do you have any ideas about that?

O. Lindvall: We don't know that and would like to explore it further, as we have discussed. That is the next step.

F. Lopez da Silva: One small question still. Were these animals tested for memory functions in a comprehensive way?

O. Lindvall: Yes, well, yes, I can't comment on that right now.

J. McNamara: My question goes for Ron Racine as well as Olle: You see increased sprouting with the heterzygous mice and Ron sees increased sprouting when using the BDNF infusion, but what I want to ask whether you have measured the amount of afterdischarge in the hippocampus and the total afterdischarge duration. I think that you've got to control for that in order to meaningfully interpret an increase or decrease in sprouting.

O. Lindvall: What I can say is that we correlated the sprouting in these animals with the kindling, the Timm staining score versus the number of stimulations to reach the tenth stage 5 seizure, and there was a significant correlation between the degree of sprouting and the number of stimulations.

J. McNamara: But that's not the question...

O. Lindvall: Yes, I know that because I don't have the answer to the first question.

D. McIntyre: Let me just add to that, in epileptic status experiments when we're measuring metabolic activation with deoxyglucose, electrographic seizures and metabolic activity are often unrelated as well, so even having an electrographic seizure that is the same in two animals doesn't mean that they have the same metabolic activity.

23

SOMATOSTATIN- AND NEUROPEPTIDE Y-MEDIATED NEUROTRANSMISSION IN KINDLING EPILEPTOGENESIS

Annamaria Vezzani,[1] Charles Piwko,[2] Marco Gobbi,[1] Christoph Schwarzer,[3] Gunther Sperk,[3] and Daniel Hoyer[2]

[1]Mario Negri Institute for Pharmacological Research
Milano, Italy
[2]Preclinical Research
Sandoz Pharma Ltd, Basel
[3]Department of Pharmacology
University of Innsbruck, Innsbruck

1. SUMMARY

It has been shown that the release of somatostatin (SRIF) and neuropeptide Y (NPY) were significantly enhanced in the hippocampus during kindling epileptogenesis. To investigate the neuronal populations involved in this effect and the consequences of enhanced extracellular concentrations of neuropeptides on their receptors, we measured SRIF and NPY-immunoreactivity (IR) and their receptor binding sites *during* and at different times *after* electrical kindling of the rat dorsal hippocampus using immunocytochemistry and quantitative receptor autoradiography.

In the hilar region, SRIF and NPY-IR were strongly increased in interneurons of the polymorphic cell layer and in their presumed projections to the outer molecular layer of the dentate gyrus at the preconvulsive stage 2 and after three consecutive tonic-clonic seizures (stage 5). NPY-IR was also markedly increased in type 1 and type 2 basket cells located below the granule cell layer at both stages of kindling. NPY-IR was *transiently* expressed in the granule cells/mossy fibres after stage 2 and two days but not one week after stage 5. Similar effects were observed in the hippocampus ipsi- and contralateral to the electrical stimulation and in its septal and temporal poles. The intensity of these changes was similar two days after stages 2 or 5 of kindling, but the effects were less pronounced one week and one month after complete kindling. After a single afterdischarge (AD), peptide-IR was similar to shams except for a *transient* increase in NPY in the mossy fibres.

Kindling 5, edited by Corcoran and Moshé.
Plenum Press, New York, 1998.

During and after kindling, there was a significant decrease (about 40%) in SRIF receptor binding sites in the molecular layer of the dentate gyrus as determined using $SRIF_1$ receptor-selective and non-selective ligands. No changes were observed in the brain of rats after a single AD. Binding to NPY-Y_1 receptors was not significantly modified by kindling, while NPY-Y_2 receptor binding rose significantly—by 220%—in the terminal field of mossy fibres. This effect was still observed one month after the last stage 5 seizure.

These results are discussed in relation to the functional consequences of changes in neuropeptide-mediated neurotransmission and their possible involvement in the establishment of a chronic epileptic focus.

2. INTRODUCTION

Alterations in peptide-mediated neurotransmission have been hypothesized in recent years to be implicated in seizures. Among the various peptides in the CNS, somatostatin (SRIF) and neuropeptide Y (NPY) are of particular interest for the following reasons: (i) they are co-localized with GABA and glutamate, which are significantly involved in triggering and propagating seizures[25,26]; (ii) electrophysiological evidence has shown that they may affect synaptic transmission in the hippocampus in either an inhibitory or excitatory manner depending on their site of release and the receptor subtypes with which they interact[2,3,22]; (iii) long-lasting modifications have been reported in the levels of expression of their mRNAs, immunoreactivity, release and receptor status after the acute phases of limbic seizures[23]; (iv) pharmacological manipulation of peptide-mediated neurotransmission affects seizures in their acute phase and chronic seizure susceptibility ensuing after status epilepticus or kindling[16,28,30]; (v) the biochemical and morphological modifications in SRIF- and NPY-containing neurons in the hippocampus closely resemble those in patients with temporal lobe epilepsy (TLE)[5,20]. This evidence indicates that seizures induce functional changes in peptide-containing neurons in limbic areas and suggest that peptides are involved in seizure modulation and possibly in the establishment of a chronic epileptic focus.

The changes in peptide expression have been mainly characterized in experimental models of status epilepticus, and information is still scarse in the kindling model of limbic epilepsy. Kindling is a gradual process of epileptogenesis considered to be a model of certain aspects of human epilepsy of focal onset[18]. We have shown by *in situ* hybridization histochemistry that the expression of SRIF and NPY mRNA increased in neurons of the dentate hilus and strata oriens and radiatum CA1/CA3 of the hippocampus during kindling and one week but not one month after generalized stage 5 seizures, suggesting enhanced synthesis of the peptides in the related neurons[1]. In addition, we found that the tissue concentration and release of SRIF and NPY from rat hippocampal slices were significantly enhanced both during kindling and in the longer run after its acquisition[19,29].

To clarify the functional significance of the changes in neuropeptide-containing neurons during kindling epileptogenesis, it is important to assess where the peptides are released in the hippocampus and the status of their receptor subtypes. In this study we report the immunocytochemical pattern of SRIF and NPY in the hippocampus during kindling and at different times after its acquisition. We also studied SRIF and NPY receptor binding sites using quantitative receptor autoradiography.

We have compared these results with those reported in experimental models of status epilepticus, and discuss their implications on the development and establishment of a chronic epileptic focus.

3. MATERIALS AND METHODS

3.1. Experimental Animals

Male-Sprague Dawley rats (250–280 g, Charles River, Italy) were used. The animals were housed at constant temperature (23°C) and relative humidity (60%) with a fixed 12-h light-dark cycle and free access to food and water. Procedures involving animals and their care were conducted in conformity with the institutional guidelines that are in compliance with national (D.L. N.116, G.U., suppl. 40, 18 febbraio 1992) and international laws and policies (EEC Council Directive 86/609, OJ L 358, 1, 12 December 1987; NIH Guide for the Care and Use of Laboratory Animals, NIH Publication No. 85–23, 1985).

3.2. Kindling

The electrodes were implanted in the dorsal hippocampus, under Equithesin anesthesia (1% pentobarbital/4% chloral hydrate; 3.5 ml/kg, i.p.), according to the following coordinates (mm) from bregma: nose bar −2.5 below the interaural line, AP −3.5, L ±2.3, H 2.9 below dura. Electroencephalographic recordings were made using bilateral cortical and hippocampal electrodes in unanesthetized, freely moving animals after a postoperative period of seven days. Constant current stimuli (50 Hz, 2 ms monophasic rectangular wave pulses for 1 s, the current intensity ranging between 60 and 200 μA) were delivered unilaterally to the dorsal hippocampus through a bipolar electrode (recording electrode) twice daily for five days at intervals of at least 6 h. Behavior was observed and the duration of the afterdischarge (AD) after each stimulation was measured in the stimulated hippocampus for every animal.

Before electrical stimulation, the rats were randomly assigned to two groups and received 12±1 and 27±2.5 stimuli (mean±SEM) to reach respectively stage 2 (stereotypies, occasional retraction of a forelimb) and 5 (tonic-clonic seizures with rearing and falling) of kindling according to Racine's classification[18]. Animals were considered fully kindled when they experienced at least three consecutive stage 5 seizures. Controls were implanted with electrodes, but were not electrically stimulated (referred to here as sham stimulation).

Rats kindled at stages 2 and 5 and the corresponding shams were killed respectively two days or one week after the last electrical stimulation. These intervals were chosen on the basis of previous studies showing mRNA and release changes for SRIF and NPY related to kindling-induced plasticity but not to the recent experience of seizure activity[1,19,29]. Six different rats received a single stimulation inducing an AD and were killed two or seven days later.

3.3. Tissue Preparation for Immunocytochemistry

Rats after a single AD (n=6) or kindled at stages 2 (n=7) and 5 (n=8) and their respective shams (n=7) were anesthetized with Equithesin and perfused through the ascending aorta with 50 ml phosphate buffered saline (PBS, 50 mM, pH 7.4) followed by 200 ml chilled 4% paraformaldehyde in PBS. The brains were postfixed in the same fixative for 90 min at 4°C and then transferred to 20 % sucrose in PBS for 24 h at 4°C. The brains were then immersed in −70°C isopentane for 3 min and stored in tightly sealed vials at −70°C.

3.4. Immunocytochemistry

Coronal and horizontal sections (40 μm in thickness) were obtained from the dorsal and ventral hippocampus respectively. The indirect peroxidase-antiperoxidase technique of Sternberger[27] was used as already described in detail[23]. Primary antisera for SRIF and NPY were raised in rabbits against the synthetic peptides which had been covalently bound to egg albumin, and were characterized by radioimmunoassays. No cross-reactivity was found with various other neuropeptides[23]. The antisera were used at the following dilutions: SRIF 1:1500 and NPY 1:1000. For controls the primary antisera was preadsorbed with the respective neuropeptide (5 μM, 24 h, 4°C) and the slices were incubated without the primary antisera.

3.5. Tissue Treatment for Receptor Autoradiography

Rats after one AD (n=3) or kindled to stages 2 and 5 (n=5–8) and their shams (n=5–8) were decapitated and the brains rapidly removed from the skull. The brains were immediately immersed in –70°C isopentane for 3 min and stored in tightly sealed vials at –70°C. Brains were cut in 10 μm thick slices using a microtome-cryostat, thaw-mounted onto microscope slides and stored at –20°C. Receptor autoradiography analysis was carried out in the cerebral cortex, the limbic system and hippocampus.

3.6. Receptor Autoradiography

3.6.1. Somatostatin. Receptor autoradiography for SRIF receptor subtypes ($SRIF_2$ family, including sst_1 and sst_4 receptors and $SRIF_1$ family, including sst_2, sst_3 and sst_5 receptors) was done as follows: 20 min of preincubation in buffer containing 50 mM Tris-HCl pH 7.4, 0.2% bovine serum albumin, 10 μg/ml bacitracin, 2 mM EGTA and 5 mM $MgCl_2$ (for $[^{125}I]Tyr^3$-octreotide, a $SRIF_1$ receptor-selective ligand and $[^{125}I]$CGP 23996, a non-selective receptor ligand) or 120 mM NaCl (favouring $[^{125}I]$CGP 23996 binding to the $SRIF_2$ receptor family) at room temperature. The slides were incubated for 2 h at room temperature in the same medium supplemented with approximately 50 pM $[^{125}I]$ligand. Radioligands were custom synthesized by Anawa (Wangen, Switzerland). Non-specific binding was determined in a set of adjacent slices by incubation in the presence of 1 μM SRIF-14. After the washing steps, the labelled sections were quickly dried under a stream of cold air.

3.6.2. Neuropeptide Y. NPY receptor binding was performed according to Dumont et al.[6] as previously described in detail[21]. The sections were incubated in the assay buffer supplemented with 0.1% bovine serum albumin, 10 μg/ml bacitracin and 15 pM $[^{125}I]$-peptide YY (PYY) (2200 Ci/mmol, New England Nuclear-DuPont, Boston, MA) at room temperature for 2 h. Y_2 specific binding was determined by incubating the sections in the presence of 60 nM of $[Leu^{31}][Pro^{34}]$NPY, a selective Y_1 receptor agonist. Non-specific binding was determined by including 1 μM NPY in the incubation medium. At the end of incubation, sections were washed and rapidly dried under a stream of cold air.

Autoradiograms were generated by apposing the labelled tissues and 10 μm thick autoradiographic $[^{125}I]$micro-scales (Amersham, Buckinghamshire, UK) to ^{3}H-Hyperfilms (Amersham, Buckinghamshire, UK) at 4°C for three to ten days depending on the radioligand. Autoradiography sections were then stained with 0.5% Cresyl Violet and brain regions were localized according to Paxinos and Watson[15].

3.7. Data Analysis

Autoradiograms were densitometrically quantified with a computerized image analysis system. Optical density was measured in several subfields of the hippocampal formation, limbic system and in different regions of the cerebral cortex and non-specific values subtracted to obtain the specific optical density in the area investigated. The values listed in the tables are the mean fmol/mg protein ± S.E.M. To calculate the amount of protein in fmol/mg we used 10 μm thick [^{125}I]micro-scales (Amersham, Buckinghamshire, UK) and followed the manufacturer's instructions.

4. RESULTS

We previously showed that pyramidal and granule neurons were preserved in fully kindled rats in the dorsal hippocampus at the site of electrical stimulation and contralaterally as assessed by light microscopic analysis of Nissl stained sections. However, a 26% decrease on average was found in neurons of the hilus in both hippocampi at stage 5[23].

4.1. Immunocytochemistry

Fig. 1 shows the changes in SRIF and NPY-IR in the dorsal (A) and ventral hippocampus (B) two days after stage 2 and one week after stage 5 of kindling compared to shams. SRIF cell bodies were numerous in strata oriens CA1/CA3 and in stratum radiatum CA3. NPY-IR neurons were similarly distributed as predicted by their extensive co-existence with SRIF[10]. In the dentate gyrus stained cell bodies were numerous in the hilus but absent in the granule cells and molecular layer. NPY-IR neurons similar to type 1 and type 2 basket cells were located respectively within or close to the inner surface of the granule cell layer (Fig. 2). Peptide-positive fibres were found mainly in the outer molecular layer and stratum lacunosum moleculare (Fig. 1a).

SRIF-IR increased in the dorsal and ventral hippocampus in the hilar interneurons and in their presumed projections to the outer molecular layer two days after stages 2 and 5 of kindling; the staining was also increased in the stratum lacunosum moleculare (Fig. 1A and B). The changes in IR were less pronounced one week after stage 5 (Fig. 1) and returned almost to control values after one month (not shown).

NPY-IR in kindling was similar to SRIF. However, staining was also increased in presumed GABAergic pyramidal-shaped basket cells in the subgranular region (Fig. 2).

Expression of NPY was also increased in the terminal field of mossy fibres at stage 2 (Fig. 1e) and one day (not shown) but not one week (Fig. 1f) after stage 5. All the changes induced by kindling occurred bilaterally to a similar extent.

SRIF- and NPY-IR in the hilus were similar to controls two days after a single AD, while NPY-IR increased in mossy fibres two days but not one week after the electrical stimulus, like in stage 2 (not shown).

4.2. Receptor Autoradiography

4.2.1. Somatostatin. Fig. 3 depicts the autoradiograms of the total binding of SRIF receptor ligands in shams (C), kindled rats one week after stage 5 (K), and rats after a single AD. Significant decreases ($p<0.01$) were selectively observed in the molecular

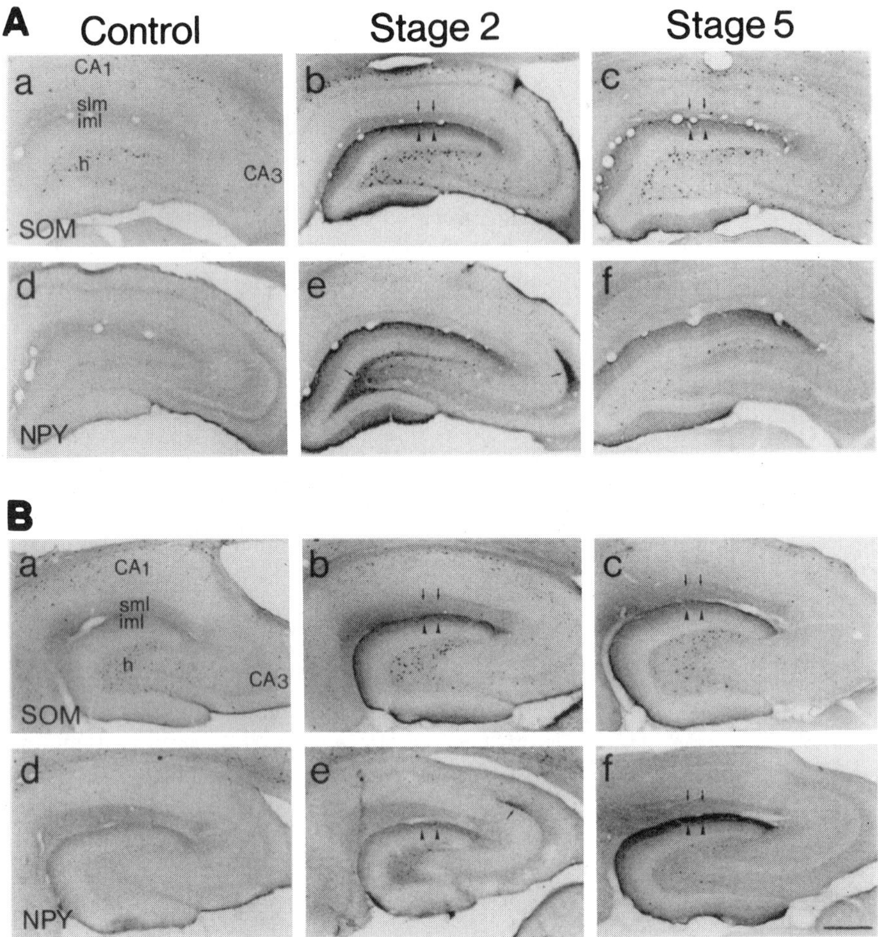

Figure 1. Photomicrographs showing somatostatin- (a-c) and neuropeptide Y-IR (d-f) in the dorsal (A) and ventral (B) hippocampus of shams (a,d), stage 2 (b,e) and stage 5 (c,f) kindled rats. Peptide IR was studied respectively two days and one week after stages 2 and 5 of kindling. IR was markedly increased in interneurons of the hilus and in the outer molecular layer (arrowheads in b and c) and/or stratum lacunosum moleculare (arrows in b and c) at stages 2 and 5. Note the increase of NPY-IR in the terminal field of mossy fibres at stage 2 (arrows in e). Scale bar: 50 μm. (Reprinted from Schwarzer et al., Neuropeptides-immunoreactivity and their mRNA expression in kindling: functional implications for limbic epileptogenesis, Brain Res. Reviews, 22(1996) 27–50, with kind permission from Elsevier Science-NL, Sara Burgerhartstraat 25, 1055 KV Amsterdam, The Netherlands).

layer of the dentate gyrus in the binding of [^{125}I]Tyr^3-octreotide (40% on average) and [^{125}I]CGP 23996 (Mg^{++}-buffer) (36% on average) in the stimulated and contralateral hippocampus (Table 1) at both stages of kindling. No differences were observed in the binding of [^{125}I]CGP 23996 when assessed in Na$^+$-buffer which favours binding to the SRIF$_2$ receptor family (not shown). One month after stage 5 seizures binding to all receptor ligands was decreased by 14% on average (not shown). No changes were observed after a single AD. In all other regions of the brain examined (subiculum, entorhinal cortex, amygdala and frontal cortex) kindling had no effect on binding of the radioligands (not shown).

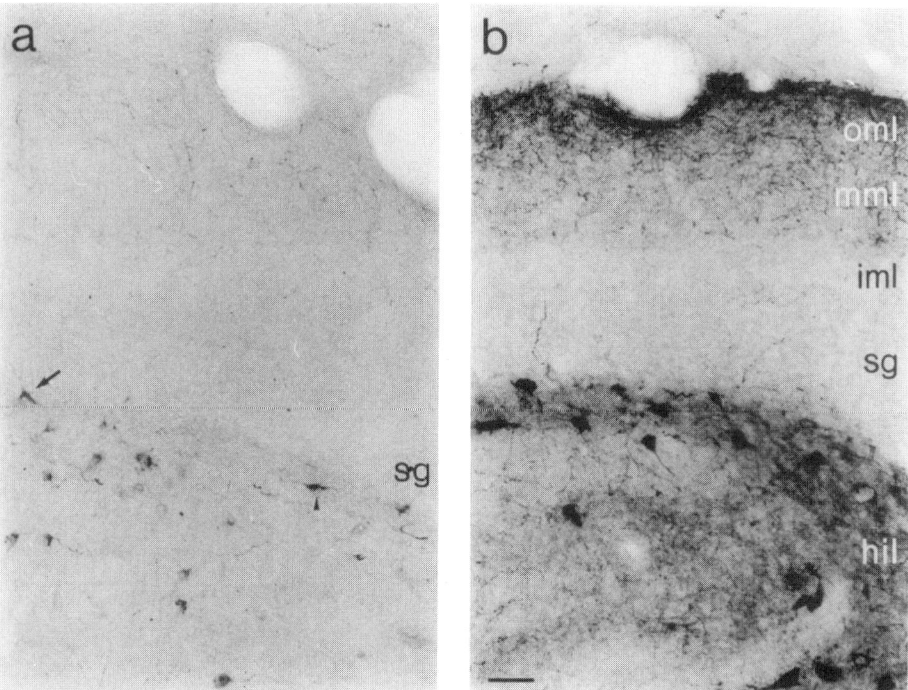

Figure 2. High magnification photomicrographs of neuropeptide Y-IR in the dorsal dentate gyrus of sham (a) and stage 2 (b) kindled rats. Note the increased IR in the hilar interneurons and in the type 1 (arrow in a) and type 2 (arrowhead in a) basket cells below the stratum granulosum (sg). NPY-IR was also enhanced in fibres in the hilus (hil) (b). oml, outer molecular layer; mml, middle molecular layer; iml, inner molecular layer. (Reprinted from Schwarzer et al., Neuropeptides-immunoreactivity and their mRNA expression in kindling: functional implications for limbic epileptogenesis, Brain Res. Reviews, 22(1996) 27–50, with kind permission from Elsevier Science-NL, Sara Burgerhartstraat 25, 1055 KV Amsterdam, The Netherlands).

4.2.2. Neuropeptide Y. Fig. 4 shows the total and Y2 specific binding of [^{125}I]PYY to representative sections of shams (a,c) and one month after stage 5 (b,d). In shams, Y_2 specific binding was mainly present in strata oriens and radiatum CA1/CA3 (80% to 90%), while Y_1 receptor binding (assessed by subtracting Y_2 specific binding from total binding) was predominant in the molecular layer of the dentate gyrus (70%). In the hilar region each receptor subtype amounted to about 50% of the total binding. In kindled rats Y_2 binding selectively increased, by 220% compared to shams, in the hilus of the dentate gyrus along the area of mossy fibre projections ($p<0.01$, Table 2). No significant changes in Y_1 receptor sites were observed in kindled rats except for a 30% decrease in the molecular layer that did not reach statistical significance.

5. DISCUSSION

5.1. Changes in Immunoreactivity

The kindling model of limbic epilepsy enables us to investigate the progression of epileptogenesis at various defined points. Thus, the biochemical changes occurring in the kindled tissue may help in understanding the mechanisms involved in the establishment of an epileptic focus.

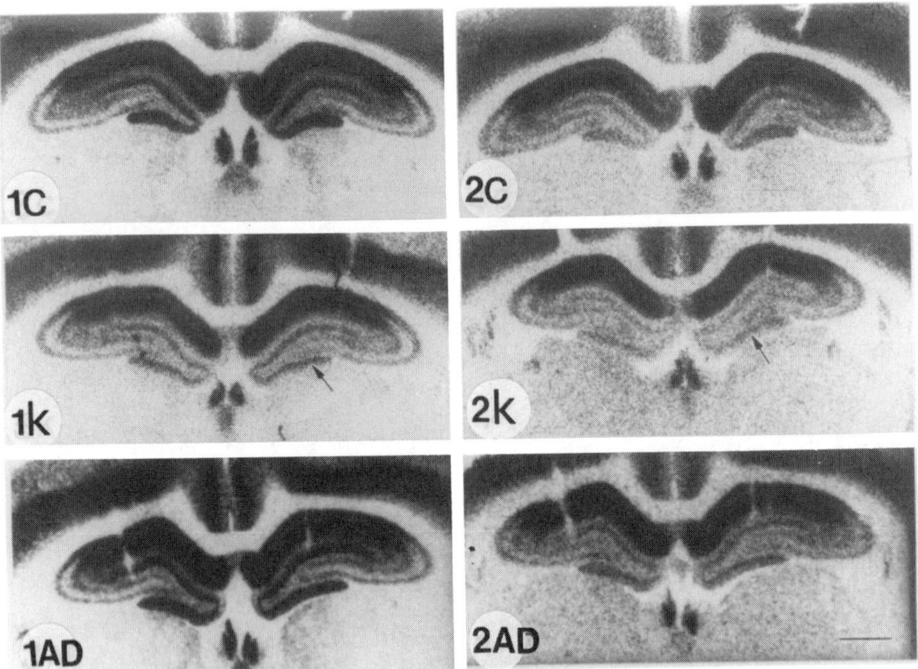

Figure 3. Autoradiographic distribution of SRIF receptor sites in sections showing the hippocampus of shams (C), stage 5 kindled rats (K) and rats after a single AD (AD), using [^{125}I]Tyr^3-octreotide (1) and [^{125}I]CGP 23996 (Mg^{++} buffer) (2). Scale bar: 2 mm.

Table 1. Autoradiographic analysis of somatostatin receptors in control and hippocampal kindled rats after stages 2 and 5

Area	Sham	Stage 2 (fmol/mg protein)	Sham	Stage 5
[^{125}I]Tyr^{3}octreotide				
molecular layer of DG	116 ± 7	68 ± 4*	113 ± 8	69 ± 3*
granular layer of DG	39 ± 5	34 ± 5	35 ± 4	36 ± 3
stratum oriens of CA1	88 ± 4	86 ± 4	87 ± 3	85 ± 2
stratum radiatum of CA1	85 ± 6	89 ± 4	86 ± 5	90 ± 4
stratum oriens of CA2	31 ± 2	31 ± 2	29 ± 3	29 ± 2
stratum radiatum of CA2	33 ± 2	35 ± 2	32 ± 2	33 ± 3
stratum oriens of CA3	23 ± 2	25 ± 2	22 ± 2	23 ± 1
stratum radiatum of CA3	23 ± 3	24 ± 3	24 ± 2	23 ± 2
[^{125}I]CGP 23996 in Mg^{++}-buffer				
molecular layer of DG	26 ± 2	17 ± 3**	29 ± 3	18 ± 2*
granular layer of DG	9 ± 2	8 ± 1	9 ± 1	7 ± 2
stratum oriens of CA1	53 ± 4	55 ± 4	49 ± 5	54 ± 4
stratum radiatum of CA1	72 ± 6	68 ± 6	67 ± 4	65 ± 5
stratum oriens of CA2	22 ± 2	21 ± 3	19 ± 3	22 ± 3
stratum radiatum of CA2	23 ± 2	26 ± 3	27 ± 2	22 ± 2
stratum oriens of CA3	16 ± 1	15 ± 2	18 ± 2	19 ± 1
stratum radiatum of CA3	16 ± 2	18 ± 3	14 ± 2	15 ± 2

Data are fmol/mg protein ± S.E.M. (three rats per experimental group). $^*p < 0.05$; $^{**}p < 0.01$ by two-tailed t-test; DG, dentate gyrus.

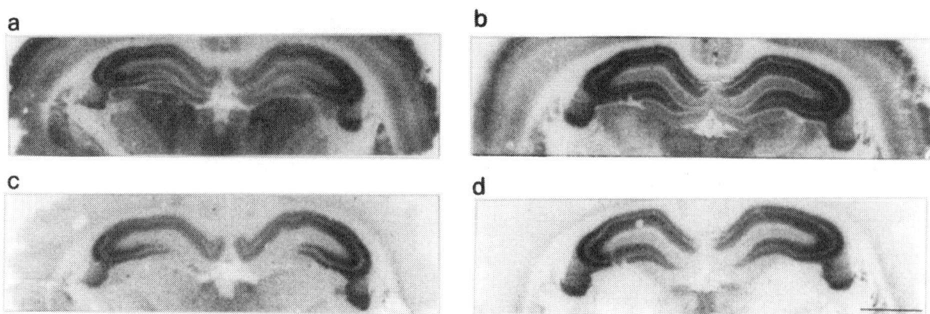

Figure 4. Representative autoradiograms showing total [^{125}I]PYY binding (a,b) and Y_2 specific binding (c,d) in controls (a,c) and stage 5 rats (b,d), killed 30 days after the last seizure. Note the enhanced binding of PYY at Y_2 receptors in the hilus of kindled rats. Binding to Y_2 receptors was measured in the presence of 60 nM [Leu^{31}][Pro^{34}]NPY which selectively displaces [^{125}I]PYY from Y_1 receptors. Scale bar: 500 μm.

Our immunocytochemical evidence shows increased staining in hilar SRIF- and NPY-containing neurons at the early preconvulsive stages of kindling, maintained after kindling acquisition. This very likely indicates an increase in peptide content consequent to its enhanced synthesis, as suggested by the enhanced mRNA expression in the same neuronal populations. Interestingly, immunostatining was also increased in the outer molecular layer of the dentate gyrus, probably reflecting accumulation of peptides in the terminal projections of the hilar interneurons. In this area, peptide-immunoreactive dendrites establish symmetric, thus inhibitory, synaptic contacts with granule cell dendrites[12,14], which in turn receive excitatory afferents from the entorhinal cortex[9]. Thus, peptides released in larger amounts during kindling[19,29] may help to control granule cell excitability, altered during kindling[11]. There is electrophysiological and pharmacological evidence of this for SRIF. Thus, although somatic depolarization of pyramidal neurons has been described, lasting pressure ejection or bath application of SRIF induces dendritic hyperpolarization on hippocampal neurons[22].In addition, application of SRIF analogs in the hippocampus has anticonvulsant effects[16,30] and endogenous SRIF has a tonic inhibitory action on kindling epileptogenesis[13].

The immunoreactive pattern in kindled rats differs from that reported in animal models of status epilepticus induced by kainic acid (KA), sustained electrical stimulation of the ventral hippocampus, or tetanus toxin. After status epilepticus extensive neuronal damage was found in a subpopulation of SRIF- and NPY-containing neurons in the hilus[24,26]. It is

Table 2. Autoradiographic analysis of neuropeptide Y receptors in the hippocampus 30 days after stage 5 of kindling

	Receptor subtypes % of control	
Area	Y_1	Y_2
Stratum oriens CA1/CA3	n.d.	80±10
Stratum radiatum CA1/CA3	n.d.	99±16
Hilus	113±10	223±7**
Molecular layer of DG	69±5	n.d.

Data are mean ± SEM (5-6 rats per experimental group) expressed as a percentage of sham values. *p<0.05; **p<0.01 vs respective control group by two-tailed t-test. Statistics were done on absolute values.
n.d., not detected because the level of receptor binding was too low to be reliably quantified (<20% of total binding).

also interesting to note that NPY was only transiently expressed in granule neurons of kindled rats as well as after a single AD, but there was a persistent increase of the peptide in the terminal field of mossy fibres for at least 30–60 days after status epilepticus only in rats with *sustained* motor convulsions[26]. The lack of motor convulsions at stage 2 or the induction of brief generalized seizures at stage 5 may be associated with milder granule cell activation than in rats after status epilepticus. These findings suggest that NPY synthesis is enhanced in granule neurons as a consequence of their level of excitation.

The functional consequences of an increase of NPY in mossy fibres, which do not contain the peptide constitutively, are still largely unexplored. This aspect requires the discussion of the results concerning the plastic changes induced by seizures in its receptor subtypes.

5.2. Receptor Changes

5.2.1. SRIF Receptor Subtypes. Based on operational and structural considerations, two classes of SRIF receptors can be distinguished: the $SRIF_1$ family (sst_2, sst_3 and sst_5) that shows intermediate to high affinity for short cyclic analogs of SRIF (octreotide, seglitide and somatuline), and the $SRIF_2$ family that displays virtually no affinity for them[8].

SRIF receptor sites were selectively decreased in the molecular layer of the dentate gyrus during and after kindling, with no changes in their mRNA expression[17]. The $SRIF_1$ family of receptors appears to be involved since binding of [^{125}I]Tyr^{3}octreotide (a $SRIF_1$ selective radioligand) was decreased whereas there was there was no change in the binding of CGP 23996 in the presence of Na^+, which favours binding to the $SRIF_2$ family.

The decreased binding in the molecular layer may indicate receptor down-regulation on dendrites of granule neurons in response to enhanced release of the peptide. Since SRIF has a tonic inhibitory action on kindling epileptogenesis[13] and sst2 receptors mediate the anticonvulsant effects of the peptide in the hippocampus[16,30], the decrease in $SRIF_1$ receptor binding may have some role in favouring the hyperexcitability of the kindled tissue by impairing inhibition on granule cell dendrites. This effect, however, is only transient; so it is presumably not involved in maintenance of the kindled state.

The consequences of kindling and status epilepticus on SRIF receptors clearly differ. Thus, one month after KA sst_3 and sst_4 receptor mRNA and SRIF binding decreased in the area of neurodegeneration (CA1 and CA3), while sst_1 and sst_2 receptors mRNAs were unaltered[16]. This is in line with the immunocytochemical evidence of degeneration of hilar SRIF neurons and no increase of immunoreactivity in the outer molecular layer[26].

5.2.2. Neuropeptide Y Receptors. Y_2 receptor sites, presumably located on mossy fibres, were increased after kindling. This increase was long-lasting, since it was detected one month after the last stage 5 seizures. The same effect was observed 30 days after status epilepticus induced by KA[21]. On the other hand, a 30% decrease on average was found in Y_1 receptor sites in kindled rats and after KA[21], although in kindling it did not reach statistical significance.

The immunocytochemical patterns of NPY in these two models of limbic epilepsy differ considerably, indicating that the enhanced release of the peptide[16,19,28,29] largely occurs at different synaptic sites, possibly affecting hippocampal excitability differently in spite of similar changes in the receptors. However, NPY-IR was also enhanced in the hilus of the dentate gyrus in kindling. Thus, we cannot exclude that, in addition to the stratum moleculare, the release is increased at this site too, resulting in enhanced NPY-mediated neurotrasmission through Y_2 receptors.

NPY has inhibitory effects on synaptic transmission in the hippocampus acting on presynaptic Y_2 receptor subtypes on Schaffer's collaterals and on mossy fibres[4]. This is very likely due to the fact that the peptide reduces glutamate release from these terminals[7]. Conversely, it excites granule cells acting on postsynaptic Y_1 receptor subtypes in the molecular layer[2].

We recently found that the infusion of a selective antibody against NPY in KA-treated rats lowered their susceptibility to metrazol-induced convulsions[28]. The same effect was found in rats treated i.c.v. with BIBP 3226, a selective Y_1 receptor antagonist (unpublished), suggesting that NPY released from mossy fibres may have proconvulsant effects through Y_1 receptors. Thus, the effect of NPY on seizure susceptibility depends on the balance between its excitatory and inhibitory actions mediated by the different receptor subtypes.

6. CONCLUSIONS

The changes in peptide IR in kindling probably reflect functional modifications in peptidergic neurotransmission, as indicated by release and receptor binding studies in hippocampal slices from kindled rats[16,19,21,29]. Since these changes take place in the early preconvulsive stages they cannot be a mere consequence of seizures, but are more likely part of the plastic changes of synaptic transmission during epileptogenesis.

Comparing these data with those reported in experimental models of limbic status epilepticus, two main differences must be commented: (i) SRIF and NPY expression were increased in hilar interneurons and their presumed projections to the outer molecular layer in kindling, but these neurons were less intensively stained or degenerated after status epilepticus. We suggest that these neurons exert an inhibitory control on granule cell excitability, so their loss after status epilepticus may facilitate epileptogenesis and contribute to spontaneous seizures; (ii) NPY was persistently expressed in granule cells and their mossy fibres after status epilepticus, but only transiently in kindling. The functional consequences of this change on hippocampal excitability presumably depend on how much Y_1 and Y_2 receptor subtypes contribute to NPY-mediated neurotransmission.

Thus, seizures may lead to dramatic changes in the expression of neuromodulatory peptides[23] and in the phenotype of different neuronal populations in the hippocampus, or to nerve cell degeneration. Further electrophysiological and pharmacological studies are needed to cast light on how these changes affect synaptic physiology and the synaptic plasticity accompanying limbic epilepsy.

ACKNOWLEDGMENTS

We gratefully acknowledge M. Rizzi, M. Gariboldi and D. Cavaleri for their contribution to kindling procedure. This work was supported by a grant to A.V. form Sandoz Pharma Ltd, Basel, Switzerland and by Consiglio Nazionale delle Ricerche, Rome, Contract No 95.01080.CT04.

REFERENCES

1. Bendotti, C., Vezzani, A., Tarizzo, G. and Samanin, R., Increased expression of GAP-43, somatostatin and neuropeptide Y mRNA in the hippocampus during development of hippocampal kindling in rats, *Eur. J. Neurosci.*, 5 (1993) 1312–1320.

2. Brooks, P.A., Kelly, J.S., Allen, J.M., Smith, D.A.S. and Stone, T.W., Direct excitatory effects of neuropeptide Y (NPY) on rat hippocampal neurons in vitro, *Brain Res.*, 408 (1987) 295–298.
3. Colmers, W.F., Modulation of synaptic transmission in hippocampus by neuropeptide Y: presynaptic actions. In J.M. Allen and J.I. Koenig (Eds.) *Central and Peripheral Significance of Neuropeptide Y and its Related Peptides*, Ann.NY Acad.Sci., New York, 1990, pp. 206–218.
4. Colmers, W.F., Klapstein, G.J., Fournier, A., St-Pierre, S.and Treharne, K.A., Presynaptic inhibition by neuropeptide Y in rat hippocampal slice *in vitro* is metiated by a Y2 receptor, *Br. J. Pharmacol.*, 102 (1991) 1–44.
5. DeLanerolle, N.C., Kim, J.H., Robbins, R.J. and Spencer, D.D., Hippocampal interneuron loss and plasticity in human temporal lobe epilepsy, *Brain Res.*, 495 (1989) 387–395.
6. Dumont, Y., Fournier, A., St.-Pierre, S. and Quirion, R., Comparative characterization and autoradiographic distribution of neuropeptide Y receptor subtypes in the rat brain, *J. Neurosci.*, 13 (1993) 73–86.
7. Greber, S., Schwarzer, C. and Sperk, G., Neuropeptide Y inhibits potassium-stimulated glutamate release through Y2 receptors in rat hippocampal slices *in vitro*, *Br. J. Pharmacol.*, 113 (1994) 737–740.
8. Hoyer, D., Bell, G.I., Berelowitz, M., Feniuk, W., Humphrey, P.P.A., O'Carroll, A.M. and Patel, Y.C., Classification and nomenclature of somatostatin receptors,*TiPS*, 16 (1995) 86–88.
9. Jones, R.S.G., Entorhinal-hippocampal connections: a speculative view of their function, *TINS*, 16 (1993) 58–64.
10. Kohler, C., Eriksson, L., Davis, S. and Chan-Palay, V., Co-localization of neuropeptide tyrosine and somatostatin immunoreactivity in neurons of individual subfields of the rat hippocampal region, *Neurosci. Lett.*, 78 (1987) 1–6.
11. McNamara, J.O., Cellular and molecular basis of epilepsy, *J. Neurosci.*, 14 (1994) 3413–3425.
12. Milner, T.A. and Bacon, C.E., Ultrastructural localization of somatostatin-like immunoreactivity in the rat dentate gyrus, *J. comp. Neurol.*, 290 (1989) 544–560.
13. Monno, A., Rizzi, M., Samanin, R. and Vezzani, A., Anti-somatostatin antibody enhances the rate of hippocampal kindling in rats, *Brain Res.*, 602 (1993) 148–152.
14. Nitsch, R. and Leranth, C., Neuropeptide Y (NPYè- immunoreactive neurons in the primate fascia dentata; occasional coexistence with calcium-binding proteins: a light and electron microscopic study, *J. comp. Neurol.*, 309 (1991) 430–444.
15. Paxinos, G. and Watson, C., *The rat stereotaxic atlas*, Academic Press, New York, 1986,
16. Peréz, J., Vezzani, A., Civenni, G., Tutka, P., Rizzi, M., Schupbach, E. and Hoyer, D., Functional effects of D-Phe-c-(Cys-Tyr-D-Trp-Lys-Val-Cys)-Trp-NH_2 and differential changes in somatostatin receptor messenger RNAs, binding sites and somatostatin release in kainic acid-treated rats, *Neuroscience*, 65 (1995) 1087–1097.
17. Piwko, C., Thoss, V.S., Samanin, R., Hoyer, D. and Vezzani, A., Changes in somatostatin receptor messenger RNAs and binding sites in rat brain during kindling epileptogenesis (submitted).
18. Racine, R.J., Modification of seizure activity by electrical stimulation. II. Motor seizure,*Electroenceph. clin. Neurophysiol.*, 32 (1972) 281–294.
19. Rizzi, M., Monno, A., Samanin, R., Sperk, G. and Vezzani, A., Electrical kindling of the hippocampus is associated with functional activation of neuropeptide Y-containing neurons, *Eur. J. Neurosci.*, 5 (1993) 1534–1538.
20. Robbins, R.J., Brines, M.L., Kim, J.H., Adrian, T., deLanerolle, N., Welsh, M.S. and Spencer, D.D., A selective loss of somatostatin in the hippocampus of patients with temporal lobe epilepsy, *Ann. Neurol.*, 29 (1991) 325–332.
21. Roder, C., Schwarzer, C., Vezzani, A., Gobbi, M., Mennini, T. and Sperk, G., Autoradiographic analysis of neuropeptide Y receptor binding sites in the rat hippocampus after kainic acid-induced limbic seizures, *Neuroscience*, 70 (1996) 47–55.
22. Scharfman, H.E., Presynaptic and postsynaptic actions of somatostatin in area CA1 and the dentate gyrus of rat and rabbit hippocampal slices. In T.V. Dunwiddie and D.M. Lovinger (Eds.) *Presynaptic Receptors in the Mammalian Brain*, Birkhauser, Boston, 1993, pp. 42–70.
23. Schwarzer, C., Sperk, G., Samanin, R., Rizzi, M., Gariboldi, M. and Vezzani, A., Neuropeptides—immunoreactivity and their mRNA expression in kindling: functional implications for limbic epileptogenesis, *Brain Res. Rev.*, (1996) (In press)
24. Schwarzer, C., Williamson, J.M., Lothman, E.W., Vezzani, A. and Sperk, G., Somatostatin, neuropeptide Y, neurokinin B and cholecystokinin immunoreactivity in two chronic models of temporal lobe epilepsy, *Neuroscience*, 69 (1995) 831–845.
25. Sloviter, R.S. and Nilaver, G., Immunocytochemical localization of GABA- cholecystokinin-, vasoactive intestinal polypeptide-, and somatostatin-like immunoreactivity in the area dentata and hippocampus of the rat, *J. comp. Neurol.*, 256 (1987) 42–60.

26. Sperk, G., Marksteiner, J., Gruber, B., Bellman, R., Mahata, M. and Ortler, M., Functional changes in neuropeptide Y and somatostatin containing neurons induced by limbic seizures in the rat, *Neuroscience*, 50 (1992) 831–846.
27. Sternberger, L., Immunocytochemistry, Wiley, New York, 1979.
28. Vezzani, A., Civenni, G., Rizzi, M., Galli, A., Barrios, M. and Samanin, R., Enhanced neuropeptide Y release in the hippocampus is associated with chronic seizure susceptibility in kainic acid treated rats, *Brain Res.*, 660 (1994) 138–143.
29. Vezzani, A., Monno, A., Rizzi, M., Galli, A., Barrios M. and Samanin, R., Somatostatin release is enhanced in the hippocampus of partially and fully kindled rats, *Neuroscience*, 51 (1992) 41–46.
30. Vezzani, A., Serafini, R., Stasi, M.A., Vigano', G., Rizzi, M. and Samanin, R., Somatostatin and its octapeptide analog SMS 201–995 modulate seizures induced by quinolinic and kainic acids differently in the rat hippocampus, *Neuropharmacology*, 30 (1991) 345–352.

DISCUSSION OF ANNAMARIA VEZZANI'S PAPER

C. Wasterlain: There is an increase in NPY expression in the mossy fibers—is it related to the increase in GAD, and is it actually something functional?

A. Vezzani: I don't know if it is related to the initial expression of GAD actually. However, as you have suggested, both of them are increased in mossy fibers in a transient fashion, at least in kindled animals. I think that the increase in NPY mossy fibers is functional, because we found an enhanced release from hippocampal slices taken from these animals as compared to sham controls. I haven't looked at NPY in kindling but only in status epilepticus rats, where NPY is stably expressed in mossy fibers. We found that if we infuse an antibody selective against NPY in the hippocampus of kainic acid treated rats one month after status epilepticus, we can protect from increased susceptibility to Metrazol induced seizures, which is a pharmacological method to show that these animals have an innate response to generalized seizures. So this would suggest that the endogenous NPY is proconvulsant. Then we did the pharmacological study using a selective antagonist of NPY1 receptors and found protection from Metrazol induced seizures, tonic-clonic seizures, in these kainic acid treated rats. So it is possible that NPY, released from mossy fibers and acting on NPY1 receptors of the granule cell dendrites, may have proconvulsant actions. I don't know about kindling, because I haven't done the experiments yet.

F. Lopes da Silva: My question is on the status epilepticus model, where you show the increase of NPY and the disappearance of the hilar cells. Were these animals sacrificed after having spontaneous seizures, or was it in the silent period before they have spontaneous seizures, and at what time after the status did you in fact make these observations?

A. Vezzani: We killed the animals one month after the status epilepticus, and we only know that the animals had spontaneous seizures. At that time, I was collaborating with Eric Lothman in this project, and unfortunately we didn't monitor the animals at that time. So we are going to do that now to understand that if what we see is a long-term effect due to the status epilepticus or just a reflection of the disappearance of the seizures, but I don't know now.

24

AMYGDALA KINDLING AND RODENT ANXIETY

Robert Adamec

Department of Psychology
Memorial University of Newfoundland
232 Elizabeth Avenue
St. John's, Newfoundland A1B 3X9, Canada

1. INTRODUCTION

1.1. Epilepsy and Psychopathology

Kindling of the mammalian limbic system has been suggested as a model of epileptogenesis in complex partial seizure disorder[2] (CPS). The most commonly agreed upon problems of an affective nature associated with epilepsy are anxiety and depression[2,42,87]. An extensive literature implicates the amygdala in the production of fearful and anxiety related states in animals and humans. It is of interest, then, that anterior temporal lobectomy in human epileptics resecting the amygdala and the anterior hippocampus reduces a preexisting anxiety disorder[43]. Data like these, and a great deal of other data[1], implicate alteration of amygdala functioning in affective disturbance in epilepsy.

1.2. Modelling Epileptically Induced Changes in Affect—The Feline Partial Kindling Model

Direct evidence in favour of this possibility has been obtained in studies of the behavioral effects of partial kindling in felines. Partial limbic kindling, which repeatedly activates the amygdala, lastingly increases defensive response to several species relevant threats in cats[2–7,11–14]. Most recent data suggest that changes in excitability within the amygdala as well as N-methyl-D-Aspartate (NMDA) dependent long term potentiation (LTP) in efferents from the right basomedial amygdala to the right periacqueductal gray (PAG) are critical mediators of lasting increases in feline anxiety-like behavior[10].

1.3. Modelling Epileptically Induced Changes in Affect—Rodent Kindling Models

Experimentally induced seizure activity produces long lasting LTP in rodent amygdala efferents[65]. Moreover, LTP occurs in rodent amygdala nuclei[19,33,83,84]. One might

Kindling 5, edited by Corcoran and Moshé.
Plenum Press, New York, 1998.

suspect, then, that kindling in rodents should also change anxiety-like behavior. If true then a rodent model of increased anxiety associated with epilepsy would be available. Development of such a model has several advantages. Among the most important are that a rodent model should accelerate progress in our understanding the relationship between pathophysiology of limbic system epilepsy and affective disturbance. A great deal is known about the impact of kindling on brain function in rodents. Therefore, there is a rich knowledge base from which to proceed to decipher which brain changes induced by kindling are responsible for lasting changes in rodent affect.

The history of reports of lasting changes in rodent affect is long, but sparse (reviews[2,13]). Very few studies have directly addressed the question of does amygdala kindling alter anxiety-like behavior in rodents? Moreover, the apparent inconsistency of findings of studies addressing this issue calls into question the suitability of the rodent kindling model as a reliable model of epileptically induced interictally maintained changes in anxiety.

The purpose of this chapter is to review recent studies of the impact of amygdala kindling on anxiety-like behavior in rodents. Findings from my laboratory, in conjunction with findings from other laboratories, point to a number of factors which may account for past inconsistencies. Moreover, this partial meta analysis of the literature suggests an interesting reorientation of thinking about the function of different rodent amygdala nuclei in each hemisphere in lasting changes in affect.

2. EFFECTS OF KINDLING ON RODENT MODELS OF ANXIETY-LIKE BEHAVIOR

Studying rodents has the advantage of access to several pharmacologically validated models of anxiety. Prior to 1994, there have been several studies utilizing such models with apparently contradictory results. Such findings, however, may be better understood when one takes into consideration the location of the kindled focus, as well as possibly the strain of the rat used.

2.1. Histological Representation of Kindled Foci

As pointed out above, the location of the focus may be a critical factor in behavioral effects of kindling on rodent affect. Therefore, the locations of electrodes in the studies cited in this chapter were carefully examined and plotted on sections of the Paxinos and Watson atlas[59].

2.1.1. Calculation of Average Electrode Location. When the location of each electrode was shown in the published report, their coordinates in the lateral and vertical plane for each anterior-posterior plane (AP plane) section were visually determined with the aide of the Brain Browser program[17]. AP plane was determined directly from the paper if the Paxinos and Watson atlas was used, or mapped on the Paxinos and Watson system trigonometrically. Then the average lateral and vertical location in a given AP plane was determined. If the data in the vertical or lateral planes were not normally distributed, the median rather than the mean was used as the measure of central tendency for that plane. The average/median location for each AP plane in the published report was then plotted. When the AP plane calculated from another atlas was not among the plates given in the Paxinos and Watson atlas, the plane closest to it was used in the figure. The figures shown do provide AP plane plots which encompass the 95% confidence intervals of the electrode locations in the AP plane.

In some reports cited, only target coordinates were given without histology. In such cases, the electrode locations were taken as the target coordinates. These less informative locations are plotted as single points rather than ranges of locations. Where appropriate, they will also be clearly noted in the text. Otherwise placements will be plotted without additional comment.

2.1.2. Estimating Area of Tissue Activation during a Stimulus Train. Though electrically triggered seizure discharges spread intrinsically within the amygdala[85], it is of theoretical interest to represent the possible spread of subconvulsant activation. As pointed out previously, LTP of efferents from the amygdala is important in feline behavioral change. If similar processes mediate rodent affective change, then tissue engaged by high frequency trains prior to onset of seizure discharge would be that tissue whose efferents are experiencing LTP during the stimulus train. Those pathways might then have additional reinforcement of the subconvulsant LTP once a seizure is triggered. This process would result in efferents from the stimulated focus being strengthened even more than efferents in other amygdala areas to which the seizure activity spreads.

Watson et al.[85] reported on the spread of activation of neural tissue undergoing high frequency, kindling-like, stimulation in albino (Sprague-Dawley) rats using 2 DG autoradiographic estimates of glucose utilization. The stimulus and electrode parameters used were those commonly employed in kindling studies. Subconvulsant activation was recorded while the animals were anaesthetized with xylazine and ketamine. Subconvulsant activation produced a spherical distribution of uptake which varied in diameter for different nuclei. These distributions were used to estimate diameters of a sphere of activation in the figures in this chapter. Diameter in this paper was taken as the cross section of the glucose uptake plots in Watson et al. where relative isotope concentration had declined to .2 mCi/g (to 25% of maximum). These values varied with amygdala nucleus, as will be apparent in the figures. Watson et al.'s[85] estimates of current spread and activation fit electrophysiological estimates of current spread in dorsal columns of cat and rabbit spinal cord[15]. Bagshaw and Evans[15] also showed a 3.4-fold increase in spatial spread of current for each 10 fold increase in current intensity. This latter correction factor was used to adjust the estimates of diameter of spheres of activation when a given study employed stimulus intensities different from those used by Watson et al.[85]

3. FACTORS IMPORTANT FOR INTERICTAL BEHAVIORAL OUTCOME FOLLOWING KINDLING OF THE RODENT AMYGDALA

A main point of this chapter is that there are a number of factors contributing to the lasting effects of amygdala kindling on rodent anxiety-like behavior. The factors are: strain of rat used, hemisphere of the focus, amygdala nucleus of the focus, location of the focus within a nucleus in the anterior-posterior plane. Baseline level of anxiety prior to kindling is also a factor and will be the topic of another publication.

3.1. Strain of Rat Used

McIntyre[53] found that central amygdala kindling facilitated muricide in Wistar but not hooded rats. Since that time much of the work on kindling effects on affect has been done in albino rats. It remains an open question if strain differences exist when anxiety is being investigated. It is possible that a subtle strain difference exists with respect to susceptibility to change following left amygdala kindling. Kalynchuk et al.[46] report no effects on anxiety after 20 kindling stimulations in the left posterior centrolateral—basolateral amygdala area of hooded rats, though the animals developed stage 5 seizures. More stimulations (60–100), however produced lasting changes. In contrast, Adamec and Morgan[9] reported that after 4 stage 5 seizures (average of 13 stimulations) there was a lasting change in anxiety in Wistar rats.

3.2. Hemisphere of the Focus

Only recently have the effects of unilateral amygdala kindling on rodent anxiety been investigated. With one exception, left amygdala kindling appears to be anxiolytic. In contrast right amygdala kindling is lastingly anxogenic, or anxiolytic, or ineffective depending on the location of the focus. The variety of focus locations investigated is greater in the right than in the left hemisphere, so hard generalizations about the left hemisphere are not warranted at this time.

3.3. Right Hemisphere Kindling—Effects of Right Amygdala Kindling on Vulnerability to Stress and Anxiety

Two of the first studies of effects of right amygdala kindling on anxiety showed an increase in anxiety one week after four stage 5 seizures in Wistar rats[1,8]. Electrode locations appear in Figure 1.

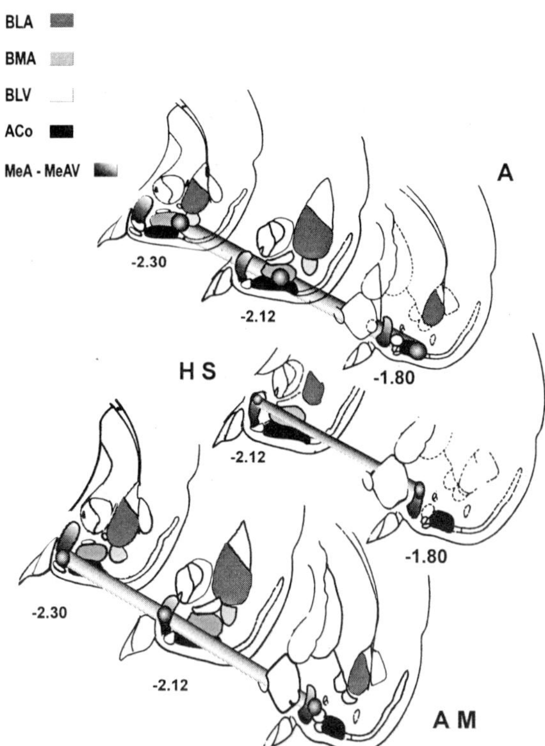

Figure 1. Spheres of activation around mean electrode locations in the Adamec[1] (A) and Adamec and McKay[8] studies (AM). Also plotted are electrode positions of Henke and Sullivan[41] (HS) for comparison.

Table 1. Summary of effects of kindling difference amygdala nuclei on behavior

	Left hemisphere	Right hemisphere
Cortico-medial group of nuclei		
Ant Aco	?	Anxiogenic
Post ACo-PLCo	?	Anxiolytic
MeA	?	Anxiogenic
Me(mid)	?	Neutral
MeP	?	?
Basolateral group of nuclei		
Ant BMA	Anxiolytic	Anxiogenic
Post BMA	Anxiolytic	Neutral
BM		?
BLP-BMP	?	Anxiogenic
BLV	?	Anxiolytic
BLA	Anxiolytic/ Anxiogenic?	Anxiogenic
Central group of nuclei		
Anterior	Anxiolytic?	Anxiolytic
Mid	Anxiolytic?	Neutral
Posterior	Anxiolytic	Anxiogenic

Anatomical abbreviations: nomenclature (adapted from Paxinos and Watson)
ACo: Anterior cortical nucleus
BLP: Posterior basolateral nucleus
BLV: Ventral basolateral nucleus
BMA: Anterior basal (basomedial, accessory basal)
BM: Basal
BMP: Posterior basal nucleus
BLA: Anterior basolateral nucleus
CeL: Lateral central nucleus
CeM: Medial central nucleus
LA: Lateral nucleus (includes DL, VM, VL)
MeA: Anterior medial nucleus
Me: Medial nucleus
MeP: Posterior cortical nucleus (dorsal and ventral parts)
PLCo: Posterior lateral cortical nucleus

All tracings in this and other figures are from the atlas of Paxinos and Watson[59]. AP Plane identification in all figures is in mm from bregma. Anatomical abbreviations follow Paxinos and Watson[59] and are also summarized in Table 1.

Anxiety is assessed in my lab with the commonly used novel elevated plus maze test. Open arm exploration (frequency/duration) expressed as a ratio of total arm exploration is the primary measure of anxiety in this test (Ratio Entry and Ratio Time for frequency and duration respectively). Decreased open arm exploration is taken to indicate an increase in anxiety, provided it cannot be shown to be due to a decrease in exploratory tendencies. For this reason, rats are usually tested in a novel hole board (open field apparatus) prior to plus maze testing. This apparatus assesses activity and exploration independently of the plus maze.

In the A and AM studies in Figure 1, increases in plus maze anxiety were observed 7 days after the fourth stage 5 seizure. Anxiety increase was not due to changes in exploratory tendency or activity in either the holeboard test or in the plus maze test (total arm entries). While there was decreased exploratory behavior in the holeboard in both studies (head dips into the holes), decreased exploration was unrelated to the changes in anxiety. Removing the effects of head dip changes from the open arm entry measure of anxiety did not alter the changes produced by kindling. This is a common but not universal pattern of results in kindling studies using these tests.

Of interest is the close correspondence of the AM and HS foci (Figure 1). This correspondence was intentional. Henke and Sullivan[41] (HS) showed that kindling, partial kindling, or even one afterdischarge increased stress susceptibility (stomach ulceration to cold restraint) one day later in Wistar rats.

3.4. AP Plane Position of the Right Amygdala Kindled Focus Affects the Nature of the Kindling Induced Change in Anxiety

AP plane position of the kindled focus is important for behavioral effects of kindling. Increases, decreases, or no change in rodent anxiety-like behavior are produced depending on focus position in a given nucleus. On the other hand, in some nuclei, AP plane position does not seem to be important.

AP plane is important in the anterior cortical and basomedial nuclei. We have found that kindling of the anterior part of the cortical nucleus is anxiogenic ("A" placements in Figure 2). In contrast kindling of the posterior part of this same nucleus is anxiolytic[1,8] (Figure 2 "AM" placements). There were no changes in exploration or activity in the hole-board or plus maze accompanying the anxiolytic effects of kindling of these nuclei.

Implanted controls with electrodes in the posterior cortical nucleus (AM –2.56 to –2.80 mm Figure 2) were more anxious than anterior cortical nucleus implanted controls or unoperated handled controls, which did not differ[8]. Moreover, anxiety levels in animals kindled in the posterior cortical nucleus equalled anxiety levels in the unoperated controls. It seems that the posterior part of the anterior cortical nucleus may exert a tonic anx-

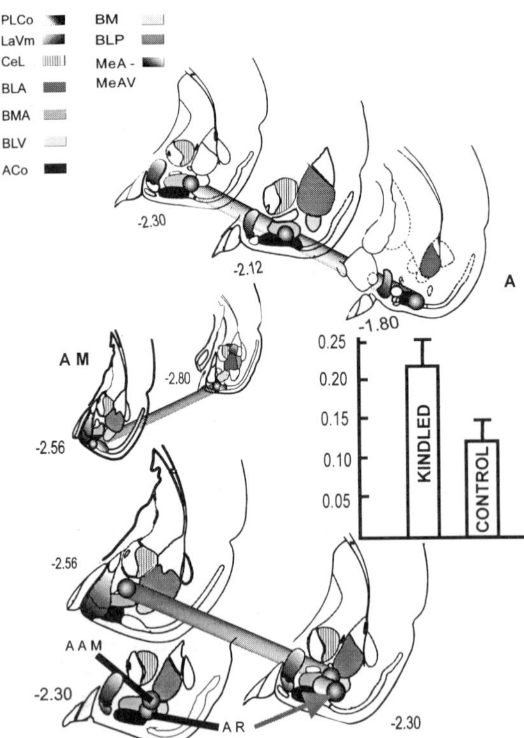

Figure 2. Spheres of activation around mean "anxiogenic" kindled focus electrode locations in the Adamec[1] (A) and the more posterior "anxiolytic" kindled foci in Adamec and McKay[8] (AM). In the "A" plot, note particularly AP plane –1.80 to –2.12 mm from bregma for the anterior part of the anterior cortical nucleus. The lower three plates show a close up of the basomedial electrode locations extending from –2.30 to –2.56 mm in the Adamec and Morgan[9] (AAM) study. Additional placements from a recent unpublished study (AR) are superimposed. In the AR study electrodes were tightly clustered in the vicinity of AP –2.30 mm. The sphere extending to the right of the plane of the plate represents the extent of the activation taking into account the 95% confidence interval of the variation in placements in the AP plane. The actual coordinates range is –2.28 to –2.36 mm from bregma, around a mean of –2.32. The bar graph insert shows the Ratio Time data from the "AR" study.

iolytic-like influence on behavior. Damage by the electrode reduced this action. Kindling, then, may have restored anxiolytic action by increasing local excitability in the undamaged tissue. Similar phenomena are observed in left hemisphere[9].

AP plane is also important in the basomedial (accessory basal) nucleus. Adamec and Morgan[9] found kindling over a range of AP plane positions in this area tended to increase anxiety in the plus maze ($p<.09$) (see Figure 2 for foci). Moreover there was a correlation between AP plane and anxiety levels in kindled rats. More posterior placements were associated with reduced anxiety. The trend toward an anxiogenic effect may have been due to the electrode locations spanning both anxiogenic and anxiolytic or neutral foci, with the summed effect being a nearly signficant behavioral change. This view is supported by recent data in our laboratory (Adamec et al., in preparation, Figure 2, "AR" placement). Kindling of the right basomedial amygdala with tightly clustered foci centered on –2.32 mm from bregma was anxiogenic one week after 4 stage 5 seizures ($F\{1,56\}=6.35$, $p<.015$, Ratio Time measure, see Figure 2). Increased anxiety was not associated with changes in activity or exploration. It is unclear if kindling of the posterior basomedial nucleus would be anxiolytic, though the correlation with AP plane suggests it should be. Studies kindling the posterior basomedial nucleus are needed.

3.4.1. Mechanisms Underlying AP-Plane Differences in the Cortical and Basomedial Nuclei. This discussion is based on a speculative assumption. The assumption is that behavioral changes depend in part on selective LTP of efferents arising from cells activated by stimulation of the focus. Such a selective potentiation of amygdala efferent function occurs following repeated seizures in cats with behavioral consequences[2,10,12,75]. In addition, LTP of rodent amygdala efferent pathways occurs, and is strengthened by kindled seizures[65]. As seizures begin, and spread in the amygdala, LTP in the primary pathway is assumed to be reinforced more than in other efferents whose cells become engaged by the seizure. With more seizures, one might expect some mixed behavioral effects. Fewer seizures ought to induce neural changes with more restricted behavioral effects. It is possible, however, that with sufficient overlap of LTP in efferents with antagonistic behavioral functions, no effects of kindling on behavior would be observed. A possible instance of this was described above for the basomedial nucleus, and other examples are encountered later in this chapter.

Under this assumption, different efferent pathways should be identifiable from anterior and posterior foci, the potentiation of which could explain the graded anxiogenic to anxiolytic effects of stimulation of these foci. One of the primary efferent pathways from amygdaloid nuclei is the stria terminalis. There is an anterior-posterior plane difference in the origin and targeting of the stria terminalis which may be relevant. The rostral medial, basomedial and cortical nuclei project to the core of the ventromedial hypothalamus (VMH) via the ventral component of the stria terminalis, while the posterior portions of these nuclei project to the shell around the VMH via the dorsal stria[18,26,35,49]. The effect of amygdala stimulation on cells in the core of the VMH is excitatory, with an inhibitory component carried via a stria input to inhibitory interneurons in the shell of the VMH[28,54].

Evidence in the cat suggests that excitatory input to the VMH from the amygdala facilitates defensive response to environmental threat[6,13,50,54,75]. Moreover kindling or drug induced NMDA dependent LTP of amygdalo-VMH input is associated with lasting increases in defensiveness in the cat[7]. In addition, activation of the VMH (electrically or glutamatergically) increases rodent defense[55,57,73]. Moreover, defensive excitability of the VMH in rodents may be under tonic GABA mediated inhibitory control[52,58,64,73]. A kindling induced LTP of rostral basomedial-cortical inputs to the VMH core might enhance defensive (anxious) response to threat in rats, as the data suggest it does in the cat. Kindling of more caudal nuclei could induce LTP of stria inputs to the inhibitory shell, potentiating its function. LTP of GABAergic inhibition does occur following limbic kindling in cats and rats[2,12]. Potentiation of VMH shell GABA function might enhance the tonic GABA suppression present, and reduce the excitatory drive of the anterior nuclei on VMH shell neurons, attenuating defensive (anxious) response to threat.

Selective changes in other relevant efferents are possible. These speculations are meant to be illustrative, not exhaustive. The afferent-efferent anatomy of the rodent amygdala is complex and highly organized, and more is being learned each year.

3.5. AP Plane and Right Central Nucleus

In a recent study (in preparation) we targeted the nucleus basalis, anterior central, mid central and posterior central amygdala. The AP plane ranges for the central nucleus division were: –1.80 to –2.29 (anterior), –2.30 to –2.79 (mid), and –2.80 to –3.3 (posterior) (all in mm from Bregma using Paxinos and Watson[59]). Rats were kindled to 4 stage 5 seizures and their behavior tested one week later. The results from the central amygdala placements will be described here. The nucleus basalis results parallel those for the anterior central nucleus. Significant effects on behavior were observed following kindling of anterior (anxiolytic) and posterior (anxiogenic) foci, but not with kindling of mid range foci (Figure 3). The behavior most affected was Risk Assessment[16].

Risk Assessment is taken as frequency of stretch attend postures into the open arms of the plus maze with both hindepaws in the closed arms. Frequency is then expressed as a

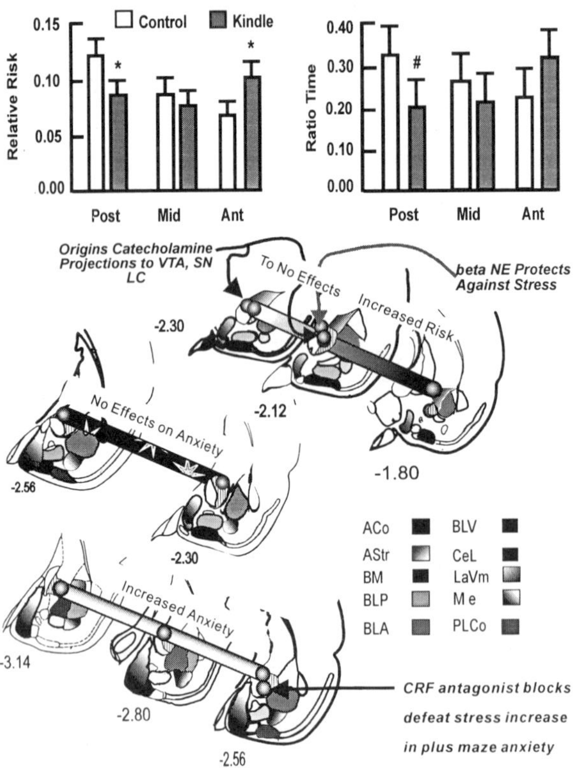

Figure 3. In the upper bar graphs, mean Relative Frequency Risk Assessment and Ratio Time for Kindled and Control groups are plotted for each focus location in the central nucleus. Means marked with an asterisk differ from their respective implanted but unkindled control. The mean marked with a "#" tends to differ from control (p<.08, 1 tailed t test). The three sets of rat atlas plates below the bar graph show electrode locations and spheres of activation for the central nucleus placement generating the data in the bar graphs. The anterior (Ant) placements are in the upper set, the middle placements (Mid) are in the middle set, and the posterior (Post) placements appear in the lower set of rat atlas plates. Superimposed on the anterior and posterior sets are locations from other studies of relevance (e.g. "origins catecholamine . . .") and described in more detail in the text.

ratio of time in the closed arms (see[9]). In our hands, reductions in this measure are usually accompanied by decreased ratio time (an anxiogenic effect). Conversely increases in Risk Assessment are associated with anxiolytic effects (increases in Ratio Time)[9]. There were no effects on Ratio Time, though there was a trend toward a reduction in Ratio Time (anxiogenic) effect with posterior central kindling ($t\{80\}=1.43$, $p=.078$, one tailed test, Figure 3).

These findings are of interest from several perspectives. First, they provide evidence that two commonly used indices of anxiety-like behavior in rodents may be controlled by separate substrates, and therefore may be measuring different aspects of rodent anxiety like behavior. Second, another clear instance of AP plane effects on anxiety is apparent in the central nucleus, though it is reversed with respect to a similar dependence in the basomedial and cortical nuclei. In the central nucleus, the more anterior the placement the less the anxiety, and the more posterior the placement, the greater the anxiety. The lack of effects with more central locations might be due to joint activation of two substrates with opposite behavioral effects. Careful examination of focus location in this study, combined with other studies of central nucleus function support this speculation, and suggest mechanisms of behavioral change.

3.5.1. Mechanisms of AP Plane Effects on Anxiety in the Right Central Nucleus—Anxiolytic Catecholaminergic Mechanisms in the Anterior Nucleus, Anxiogenic CRF Mechanisms in the Posterior Nucleus. The overlap of anxiolytic sites and sites providing protection from stress induced stomach ulceration (beta NE site in Figure 3) are of interest. Ray et al.[67] showed that β noradrenergic agonist infusion into the anterior central nucleus of male Wistar rats protects against cold restraint stress induced ulcers. This might be expected from activation of an area with anxiolytic effects. Moreover, there is a close overlap of anxiolytic kindled foci, adrenergic anti-stress areas, and the origins in the amygdala of catecholaminergic (noradrenergic and dopaminergic) projections to the brain stem (Wallace et al.[82], Figure 3, "Origins Catecholamine . . ."). Kindling in this area might in some way potentiate functioning in these brain stem sources of ascending catecholaminergic influences. Engel et al.[30] reported increase glucose utilization in the substantial nigra at the transition to stage 3 seizures kindled from the amygdala. So there is a potentiation of efferent activity to brain stem, at least during a seizure. If there is some lasting after effect of this growing activation, there might be lasting behavioral consequences.

Figure 3 also shows the locations of mid and posterior nucleus foci in our unpublished study. Of interest is the fact that the posterior anxiogenic foci overlap with locations of the highest concentrations of CRF peptide and mRNA containing cells in hooded rats,[38] and mRNA for CRF[51] (AP plane range −2.56 to −3.14, highest concentration at −2.80). In addition, social stressors (defeat stress) increase CRF content in these areas[52], associated with increased anxiety in the elevated plus maze[40] ("CRF antagonist . . ." site, Figure 3). Moreover defeat stress anxiety is dependent on CRF release in this area, since cannulation of a CRF antagonist into the site shown prevents defeat stress increases in anxiety[40]. Kindling might potentiate the release of CRF in the amygdala to mild stressors. Then the stress of the novel plus maze could engage this potentiated CRF anxiety facilitating mechanism. Exposure to the plus maze is mildly stressful (raises corticosteroid levels)[31]. The work of Stenzel-Poore et al[78] supports this idea as well. They developed a transgenic mouse model of CRF overproduction. In adulthood, overproducing mice were more anxious in the elevated plus maze than controls. Central CRF receptors are involved, since increased anxiety is blocked by icv administration of a CRF antagonist.

The central nucleus is also rich in peptidergic as well as non-peptidergic efferent pathways via the VAF and stria teminalis to the bed nucleus of the stria terminalis and to the PAG, among other targets[69]. CRF is carried in these pathways and targets the PAG[37] as well as the bed nucleus of the stria terminalis[69]. Modulation of PAG excitability is important in plus maze anxiety[36,73,74]. Moreover, cannulation of CRF into the PAG promotes defensive immobility to signalled shock[80]. Potentiation of function in these pathways, perhaps via some form of LTP, might also contribute to increased anxiety.

Mid central foci without behavioral effects are positioned in such a way that they could activate both the anterior anxiolytic sites, and the more posterior foci (Figure 3). Following the LTP hypothesis proposed above, stimulation in this area might potentiate function in both the anterior and posterior central nuclei producing behavioral effects which cancel each other out.

3.6. Importance of Amygdala Nucleus in the Right Hemisphere for Kindling Effects on Behavior

Effects of kindling of several different nuclei in the same AP planes in the right amygdala are summarized in Figure 4. It is clear from this figure that slight shifts in focus location in the same plane produce very different effects of kindling on rodent anxiety. That is, every possible effect is observed from no effect (mid central nucleus) to increased (basolateral and basomedial nuclei) and decreased (basolateral ventral nucleus, BLV).

We (Adamec and Morgan[9]) found that kindling of the BLV is anxiolytic . In addition the electrode lesion in implanted controls appeared to be anxiogenic. There may be some tonic anxiolytic function of the BLV as suggested for the cortical nucleus. In addition, the basolateral foci used by Helfer and colleague[42] are shown ("BLA, BLP, BMP anxiogenic" plates in Figure 4). Helfer et al.[39] kindled male Wistar rats in these sites to 15 stage 5 seizures, or partial kindling to stage 3. One week later, kindled and partially kindled rats were more anxious in the plus maze and social interaction tests. No changes in exploration or activity were produced by kindling. Moreover, the anxiogenic effects of kindling were reduced by a benzodiazepine anxiolytic (chlordiazepoxide HCl). Of further interest is the

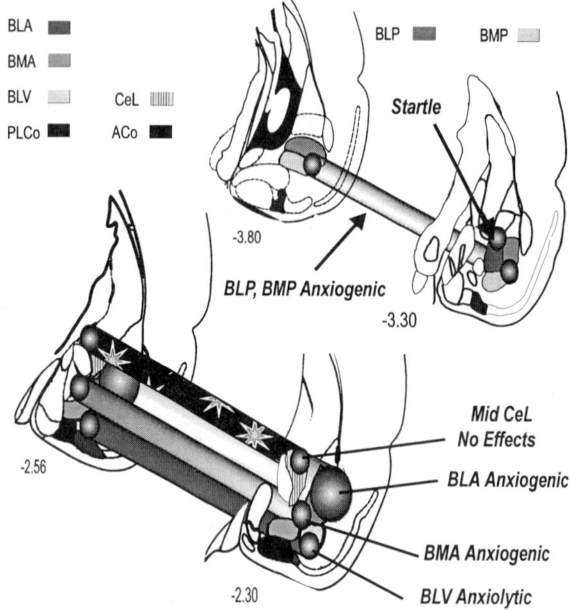

Figure 4. Spheres of activation of foci in the right amygdala producing a variety of effects in plus maze anxiety. Foci are identified by effect. Sources of effects are described in the text. The single focus labelled "Startle" is a site where Rosen et al[68] find partial kindling increases fear potentiated startle.

correspondence in site yielding increased anxiety in Helfer et al. and a recent report by Rosen et al.[68] that acoustic startle is increased 24 hours after partial kindling of the posterior basolateral nucleus. Startle reactions are increased in some anxiety disorders, such as in Post Traumatic Stress Disorder[81]

The Helfer et al.[39] study is the first rodent kindling study to show lasting effects of partial amygdala kindling on rodent anxiety. Moreover, this study examined the effects of kindling on depressive like behaviors (swim stress, sucrose preference), and found no effects. These preliminary findings are consistent with the human clinical literature which implicates left hemisphere dysfunction in depression, and right hemisphere dysfunction in affective disorders associated with epilepsy[32,70].

Of interest is the fact that there is no evidence of AP plane effects on behavioral outcome in Helfer et al.[39], since some electrode placements extended into the posterior basolateral nuclei (Figure 4, BLP, BMP). The absence of an AP plane dependence for behavioral effects in the right BLA is suggestive of mechanisms mediating behavioral change. *Phaseolus* anterograde tracer studies reveal a converging projection of posterior and anterior BLA neurons to a mid planar position with strong efferent projections to the posterior central nucleus (AP –2.80 to –3.80)[72]. This is within the CRF concentrating anxiogenic region discussed above. If the anatomy defines the flow of potentiation during kindling, then a potentiation of output of the BLA onto central nucleus might be one route of the anxiogenic effects produced by kindling nearly anywhere within the BLA. Of course there are other possible efferent routes from the BLA, but these are sparse. The other strong projections from the mid BLA is to the anterior amygdaloid area[72]. This area and its efferents might also be implicated in the anxiogenic effects of BLA kindling.

4. HEMISPHERIC DIFFERENCES IN THE EFFECTS OF KINDLING ON AFFECT IN RODENTS

As stated at the outset, the predominant effect of left amygdala kindling on rodent anxiety to date is to reduce anxiety. Moreover, kindling of comparable areas in the left and right hemisphere yields opposite behavioral effects. Finally there is no evidence of AP plane dependencies in left hemisphere kindling. Part of the reason may be that most foci are in the BLA, which does not show AP plane dependency in the right amygdala either. Nevertheless other foci include the basomedial amygdala and posterior central nucleus. Kindling these nuclei in the left hemisphere decreases plus maze anxiety one day to one week after stage 5 seizures[9,46]. These points are anatomically summarized in Figure 5.

There are no direct data to date on the effects of left anterior central nucleus kindling on anxiety. McIntyre[53] kindled Wistar rats bilaterally in the anterior central nucleus and produced a lasting decrease in latency to attack mice. This effect is consistent with the anxiolytic effect of right anterior central nucleus kindling in similar placements in my laboratory. If both hemispheres contributed to McIntyre's findings, then left anterior central nucleus kindling might also be anxiolytic. In contrast, left posterior central nucleus kindling is anxiolytic[46], whereas right posterior central nucleus kindling is anxiogenic (Figures 3 and 5).

4.1. Effects of Left Hemisphere Kindling on Rodent Anxiety

Witkin et al.[86] reported that kindling enhanced the anxiolytic action on punished responding of subconvulsant high frequency stimulation of the left basolateral amygdala. After kindling of the same site in the left basolateral amygdala, but not frontal cortex, the

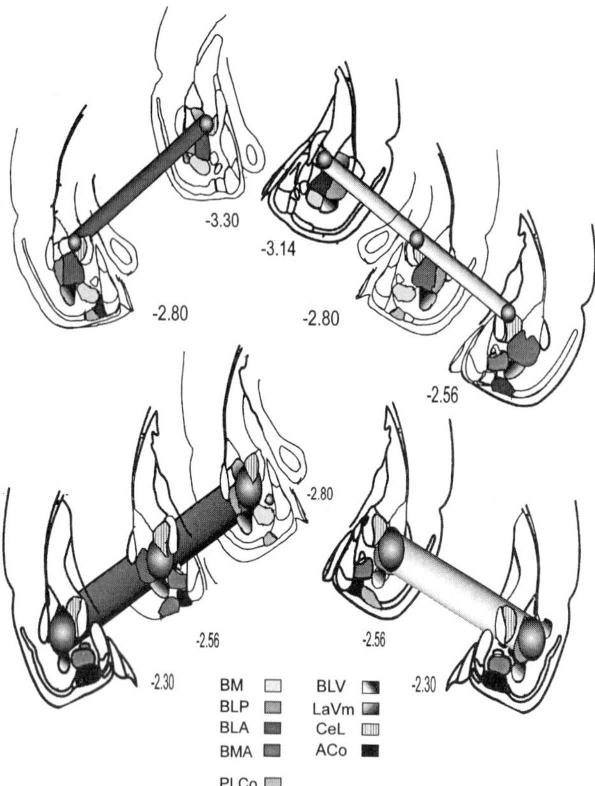

Figure 5. Plots of mean electrode locations and spheres of activation of studies involving kindling of comparable foci in the left[9] and right basolateral[39] (lower set of plates); and posterior central amygdaloid nuclei (upper set of plates). Posterior central placements depicted are from Adamec et al. (in preparation) for right central nucleus, Kalynchuk et al.[46] for the left central nucleus. Right foci are anxiogenic, left foci are anxiolytic.

anxiolytic effects of left amygdala stimulation were increased over prekindling levels at 3 and 60 min after the train. The average location of their electrodes with spheres of kindling stimulation activation appears in Figure 6. Adamec and Morgan[9] also found an anxiolytic effect in the plus maze of left basolateral (as well as basal accessory) nucleus kindling in male Wistar rats (Figure 6). Considering the BLA alone, kindling increased Ratio Time relative to implanted controls ($F\{1,33\}=4.80$, $p<.04$, adapted from Adamec and Morgan[9]). There were no changes in behavior in the holeboard test. However, less anxious kindled rats showed increased total arm entries in the plus maze ($F\{1,33\}=5.65$, $p<.03$). Increased total arm entries could reflect increased exploratory and motor responses to the stress of the novel plus maze, or be a release from inhibition of exploration by reduced anxiety. This issue will be addressed below in the context of possible dopaminergic involvement in left hemisphere anxiolytic effects.

Though the two studies just cited report anxiolytic effects of left basolateral amygdala kindling, Neiminen et al.[56] found left amygdala kindling to be lastingly anxiogenic in the elevated plus maze. Effects were observed in albino rats (Han Wistar males) two weeks after three stage 5 seizures. Kindling reduced open arm exploration, but had no effect on learning in the Morris water maze task.

These contradictory findings are troublesome. The locations from Neiminen et al.[56] clearly overlap with anxiolytic sites from Adamec and Morgan[9] (Figure 6). However, the plotted site is the reported target location, not the average position of electrodes. No histology was given in the paper nor was any reported (or done, personal communication). Therefore electrode location differences may be important in understanding the discrepan-

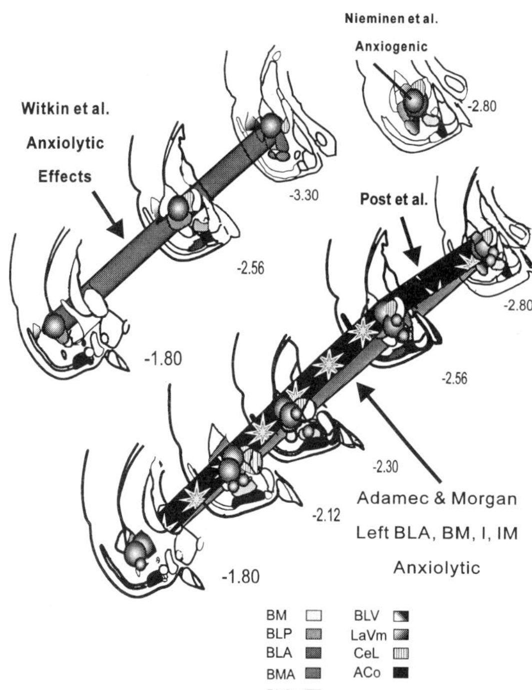

Figure 6. Spheres of activation of all locations of left hemisphere kindled foci of Witkin et al[86]. Also plotted are the foci of activation from Adamec and Morgan[9] in the left amygdala, including the basolateral nucleus, among others. Superimposed on the this plot are the locations of foci in the Post et al.[63] study discussed in detail in section 4.3. Finally the reported unconfirmed target of electrodes in the Nieminen et al. study appears in the uppermost single plate.

cics. As has already become clear in this chapter, behavioral outcome of kindling is very sensitive to location of the focus. Moreover, there are reasons to believe that Nieminen et al. were kindling outside of the left basolateral area. Adamec and Morgan[9] and Post et al.[63] reported kindling rates in nearly identical foci in the left basolateral amygdala which were faster than those observed by Nieminen et al.[56] with comparable train parameters. That is it took 7.9 ± 2.9 and 8.6 ± 1.7 stimulations to stage 5 (means ± 95% confidence intervals for Post and Adamec studies respectively). These values are considerably lower than the average of 17 stimulations to stage 5 described by Nieminen et al.[56]

A third most recent study of left basolateral kindling reports anxiolytic effects in the plus maze. Kalynchuk et al.[46] found that 60 to 100 kindling stimulations with many stage 5 seizures increased open arm exploration in the elevated plus maze one day after seizures ceased. Behavioral effects were long lasting but reversible, lasting as long as 1 month after kindling ceased (Kalynchuk, personal communication). The 60 to 100 stimulation animals were stimulated in sites overlapping with those of Adamec and Morgan[9] and Post et al.[63]

Consistent with Adamec and Morgan[9], there was an increase in total arm entries, in all stimulation conditions. In addition, Kalynchuk's 60 to 100 stimulation animals were more resistant to capture in an open field, but not in their home cages, replicating an earlier finding of Pinel et al.[62] The predominant defensive response was to flee from the experimenter's hand. In addition, 60 to 100 stimulation kindled animals, but not 20 stimulation kindled rats, were less active for the first 30 sec of exposure to a novel open field. All stimulated groups were more thigmotactic, spending more time near the walls of the open field. All of these effects increased the more the animals were stimulated.

The increases in total arm entries is consistent with our findings, as is the lack of effect of 20 stimulations on thigmotactic behavior. In fact, we found a trend toward a decrease in thigmotactic behavior in the novel holeboard in kindled animals made less anxious in the plus maze (adapted from data of Adamec and Morgan[9]; time near wall in holeboard, $F\{1,33\}=2.43$, $p<.13$, 234.9 ± 9.7 vs 213.0 ± 10.25, means ± SEM. control and kindled respectively). In addition we found no changes in vertical (rearing) or general activity in the novel holeboard, consistent with Kalynchuk et al.[46]

An important difference between our findings and those of Kalynchuk et al.[46] is that 20 stimulations did not decrease anxiety, though there was a trend. In contrast we found a decrease in anxiety with half that number of stimulations. The electrode locations overlapped considerably, so focus location is likely not a factor. Other differences are time since the last seizure, with Kalynchuk measuring one day after the last seizure, and Adamec and Morgan measuring one week after the last seizure. Another difference is strain of rat used. Long Evans hooded rats were used by Kalynchuk et al.[46], and Wistars were used in the Adamec and Morgan[9] study. The hooded rats used by Kalynchuk et al.[46] are naturally more anxious in the plus maze than are Wistars (Adamec et al., in preparation). Perhaps a stronger defensive disposition is more difficult to change by kindling.

Kalynchuk et al.[46] suggested that the increased exploration of the open arms might really be an attempt to escape from the maze, driven by a shift to escape rather than an immobility defensive tendency. They defended this view by other behavioral changes which may be defensive, such as resistance to capture and reduced exploration in the open field. Moreover, at one month post kindling with 60–100 stimulations to the left BLA, hooded rats become more anxious, not less anxious, in the elevated plus maze[47]. In further support of their escape hypothesis, they point to the growing tendency to jump off the maze by 60 and 100 stimulation animals. This behavior would be consistent with an escape hypothesis. However, in our studies kindling anxiolysis in the plus maze was associated with fewer instances of falling off the open arms of the maze (number of falls: 14.4 among 18 controls vs 2 among 16 kindled, $F\{1,33\}=9.54$, $p<.004$). This suggests that increased "escape" tendency is not mediating open arm exploration in our kindled animals, at least. This does not rule out the possibility that with 60 or more stimulations, open arm exploration reflects escape attempts, however.

4.2. Effects of Left Amygdala Kindling, Anxiolytic or Anxiogenic?

The findings of these studies suggest several possible interpretations of the effects of left amygdala kindling on rodent anxiety. Perhaps the simplest is that there is a graded effect of left amygdala kindling, ranging from an initially anxiolytic profile with fewer kindled seizures (4–5 stage 5) to a possibly anxiogenic profile with enhanced escape tendencies with 60 stimulations or more. This formulation follows if one accepts Kalynchuk et al.'s[46] interpretation of their data. There are other possibilities. One is that left amygdala kindling is anxiolytic, regardless of the number of stimulations. What changes with the increased number of kindled seizures is a recruitment of change in the substrates of other behavioral systems. What the animal does depends then on the situation in which it is tested. This suggests that a rat might appear more defensive in one test situation, but less anxious in another. This could happen if the substrates mediating the different behavioral responses were parallel in operation and not highly interdependent. This kind of finding is not without precedent. D'Aquila et al.[25] recently reported that chronic exposure to a mild (CMS) unpredictable stress reduced consumption of sucrose, increased defensive behavior in a resident-intruder paradigm, decreased male sexual behavior, but had an anxiolytic profile in the elevated plus maze. In fact, Pinel[61] in this volume reports increased defensive behavior in the resident intruder paradigm with left basolateral kindling which also produces an anxiolytic profile in the plus maze.

It is possible, then, that kindling with fewer seizures is indeed anxiolytic in the elevated plus maze, as our findings suggest. Continuation of kindling to many more seizures might continue this anxiolytic trend, but overlay on it other more defensive behaviors as other substrates are potentiated. This hypothesis is testable. Future tests of the effects of kindling on rodent anxiety should include a variety of tests of affective behavior.

4.3. Effects of Left Hemisphere Kindling on Dopamine Function, Suggestions for Mechanisms of Changes in Rodent Anxiety-like Behavior

Post et al.[63] reported a lasting (14 day) increase in behavioral response to dopamine challenge following left basolateral amygdala kindling in Sprague Dawley rats after 20 kindling stimulations The nearly exact overlap of the placements in the Post et al[63], Adamec and Morgan[9] and to some extent the Kalynchuk et al.[46] studies makes these findings of particular interest (Figure 6). Post et al.[63] observed an increase in vertical and horizontal motor activity in response to apomorphine (4 mg/kg). Accompanying these effects was a decreased response to cocaine, indicating a possible chronic reduction in dopamine (DA) neurotransmission with an upregulation (supersensitivity) of postsynaptic dopamine receptors.

These findings are relevant to both the changes in exploratory locomotion in the plus maze (arm entries) and to changes in anxiety. A variety of data point to increased dopamine (DA) transmission in the nucleus accumbens (NAcc) as a mediator of increased locomotion in stressful novel situations[71]. Kindling induced potentiation in DA transmission might increase locomotion in the novel plus maze, exposure to which is stressful[31]. Changes in hole board activity might not occur, because the accumulated stress of two novel experiences may be required, in Wistar rats at least. Combined effects of stressors on facilitation of DA transmission in the NAcc have been observed[48]. Potentiation of DA transmission might also be anxiolytic. Recently, it has been shown that a DA D_2/D_3 agonist (quinpirole) given systemically acutely or chronically is anxiolytic in the elevated plus maze in long evans hooded rats[29]. This is accompanied by persistent forward locomotion (Einat, personal communication). These data suggest that an increase in DA transmission in the mesolimbic dopamine system might be anxiolytic in the plus maze. On the other hand the increased locomotion might also reflect an increased exploratory drive.

In contrast, other data suggest that potentiation of mesolimbic dopamine functioning has anxiogenic consequences. Potentiation of dopamine input to the nucleus accumbens produces lasting increases in defensiveness. Stevens and Livermore[79] showed that repeated stimulation of the cat ventral tegmental area led to lasting increases in defensive social withdrawal which was dopamine dependent. Of particular interest is the fact that the right, not the left, VTA was stimulated. Perhaps left VTA activation would be anxiolytic. On the other hand, in the rat, bilateral facilitation of DA transmission effects on D_2 receptors by CCK-8 in the posterior nucleus accumbens is anxiogenic in the plus maze[23,24,27]. Unfortunately in these studies unilateral hemisphere effects were not studied.

Some clue regarding what kinds of changes in DA transmission might lead to increased or decreased anxiety come from recent work on rats differing in response to novelty and anxiety (in the plus maze)[24]. Less anxious more exploratory rats show potentiated responses to DA agonists[44,76], decreased DA turnover in the prefrontal cortex (PFC) and increased turnover in the NAcc in either basal conditions or after 120 min in a novel environment[60]. Moreover, there is evidence of increased post synaptic responsiveness to DA in less anxious rats in the accumbens[44]. This suggests that increased DA transmission with elevated postsynaptic responsiveness in the nucleus accumbens, plus diminished PFC DA transmisssion, is associated with increased exploratory response and decreased anxiety.

It is tempting to speculate that left basolateral amygdala kindling establishes such an anxiolytic like pattern in mesolimbic and mesocortical dopamine functioning. This change could be accomplished by upregulation of dopamine receptors in the nucleus accumbens and perhaps no change or reduction in DA transmission in the PFC. There is some evidence that this may be happening[66]. In this study, no histology was given, but the target of kindling was such that tissue activated would likely span from AP –2.56 to –3.72 in the BLA. Rada and Henandez[66] found that immediately after the third stage 5 kindled seizure in Wistar rats, there is a complex pattern of change in DA turnover in NAcc and PFC ipsilateral to the side of stimulation (which varied from side to side). There was an increase in turnover in the PFC and a decrease in NAcc lasting at least 120 minutes. Repeated patterns of activation like this might alter dopamine receptors differentially in the two brain areas, with a downregulation in the PFC and an upregulation in the NAcc.

More recently, upregulation of DA D_2 receptors has been reported following left basolateral amygdala kindling to 5 stage 5 seizures in Sprague Dawley rats[20,21]. No histology was given, but the target was in the vicinity of the sphere of activation in the basolateral amygdala ranging from AP –2.0 to AP –3.14 (Paxinos and Watson[59] coordinates). This certainly would overlap with the basolateral placements used by Post et al.[63] and Adamec and Morgan[9]. Of particular interest is the laterality of the changes. Csernansky et al.[20,21] report a lasting (2 days to 2 weeks) increase in ^{3}H spirperidol binding in the left but not right Nacc following left amygdala or dorsal hippocampal kindling. Binding in left or right amygdala, or caudate, was unchanged. Consistent with these findings are lasting bilateral increases in mRNA for D_2 receptors in the NAcc 30 days following left amygdala kindling the BLA near AP-2.56 mm from Bregma[34]. In light of Csernansky's work, the data could suggest some unilateral disturbance in the transcription process is caused by kindling.

It is possible that anxiolytic effects of such changes will only occur when they appear in the left NAcc and PFC. Studies of individual differences in less anxious exploratory rats do not distinguish between hemispheres, so laterality data are not available. Nor are there enough kindling studies specifying the hemisphere of the focus to address this question by literature review. It must remain as a question for future research.

If left basolateral kindling produces an anxiolytic pattern of dopamine transmission in the PFC and NAcc, one would expect to see increased exploration in a novel environment. This is seen in the novel plus maze but not in the holeboard or open field in kindled rats. If locomotion changes are stress driven, it is possible that the plus maze is more stressful than a novel open field or hole board. Alternatively, the combined stress of the holeboard and plus maze might sum to potentiate DA release in the NAcc in the plus maze, increasing locomotion. Such effects have been reported in unkindled rats in the microdialysis studies of Ladurelle et al.[48]

Furthermore, it is of interest that the decrease in anxiety seen in the Adamec and Morgan[9] study following left amygdala kindling is eliminated when arm entries are removed by analysis of covariance ($F\{1,31\}=2.91$, $p<.10$). This suggests that the increases in arm entries (activity/exploration) in the plus maze and the decreases in anxiety are related. The dependence of anxiolytic effects in the plus maze on arm entries suggests the possibility that the anxiolytic interpretation of increased open arm exploration may be in error. That is changes in dopamine transmission may increase exploratory/activity tendencies in the plus maze, without altering defensiveness, or may mask an increased defensiveness. A marker of this kind of action may be increased total arm entries. In support of this masking hypothesis is the fact that the initially anxiolytic plus maze profile seen by Kalynchuk et al.[46] reverses to an anxiogenic profile at one month after kindling. Perhaps kindling induced increases in exploratory tendencies produced by DA transmission changes wane before the effects of kindling on defensive substrates promoting immobility in the plus maze.

Kindling of the posterior part of the right anterior cortical nucleus is also anxiolytic, but without changes in exploratory behavior in either the hole board or plus maze[8]. These data suggest that mechanisms different from those just suggested for left amygdala kindling are operative when decreases in anxiety are produced by right hemisphere kindling.

Clearly more work is required to unravel an apparently complex pattern of findings.

5. SUMMARY AND CONCLUSIONS

A summary of effects of kindling of different nuclei appears in Table 1. From the table, it is clear that more details are known about the right than the left amygdala. As stated at the outset, kindling effects on rodent affect depend on hemisphere of the focus. Moreover, in the right hemisphere at least, which nucleus is kindled and in which AP plane are also important. Careful consideration of the anatomy of these areas also provides clues as to mechanisms governing these changes in behavior. In most instances, kindling seems to enhance normal functions, as has been suggested in the cat.

Previous attempts to relate kindling in rodent models to affective change in epilepsies have been inconclusive. The data reviewed here suggest why. Previous studies paid insufficient attention to location of kindled foci. Often histology was not reported, nor was hemisphere of the focus. Clearly the amygdala of the rodent has the same degree of functional specificity as that described in the cat many years ago[45,75]. Progress in rodent models will be facilitated if careful attention is paid to the apparently highly organized functional and anatomical differentiation within the rodent amygdala.

5.1. Clinical Implications

Further investigation of the effects of kindling in the left (as well as the right) hemisphere might be guided by several considerations. The first is a recognition of the possibility that kindling induces a variety of behavioral effects, some of which might appear paradoxical. Given that we have shown that LTP of specific amygdala efferent pathways is closely related to lasting changes in defensiveness in cats, it is possible that LTP of many efferent pathways occurs with spread of seizures. Potentiation of different behavior modifying pathways during kindling might also be expected to grow with more and more kindled seizures. A process like this would predict more complex patterns of interictal behavioral change with more extensive kindling.

These considerations suggest that the studies of the behavioral effects of kindling in future should carefully monitor changes in a variety of behaviors in the same rat. Such observations should be combined with careful examination of effects over different time frames following kindling with different numbers of kindled seizures. Results of these studies might have interesting clinical implications. One characteristic of affective change in limbic epilepsy is a deepening of a variety of affective states, and a reported mood lability, in addition to increased anxiety[2,77]. The degree of these reported affect changes varies directly with the reported frequency and intensity of aura experiences thought to reflect limbic system discharges[2]. It has been argued that aura measures such as these might be comparable to the number of limbic seizures experienced. If so, the clinical data suggest the more limbic seizures, the more variable and labile is mood. If increased kindled seizures lead to parallel and complex changes in a variety of affective substrates, then it may offer a way to model complexity of affective change in epileptics.

ACKNOWLEDGMENTS

The work from this laboratory described in this paper was supported by the Medical Research Council of Canada grant to R. Adamec (MT 702). The invaluable aid of Tanya Shallow, John Budgell, and Paul Burton is also gratefully acknowledged.

REFERENCES

1. Adamec, R., Amygdala Kindling and Anxiety in the Rat, *NeuroReport*, 1 (1990) 255–258.
2. Adamec, R., Does kindling model anything clinically relevant?, *Biol. Psychiat.*, 27 (1990) 249–279.
3. Adamec, R., Behavioral and epileptic determinants of predatory attack behaviour in the cat. In: J.A. Wada (Ed.). *Kindling*, Raven Press, New, York, (1976), pp. 135–154.
4. Adamec, R., Normal and abnormal limbic system mechanisms of emotive biasing, In: K.E. Livingston and O. Hornykiewicz (Eds.), Limbic Mechanisms, Plenum Press. New York, (1978), pp. 405–455.
5. Adamec, R., Partial Kindling of the Ventral Hippocampus:Identification of Changes in Limbic Physiology which Accompany Changes in Feline Aggression and Defence, *Physiol. Behav.*, 49 (1991) 443–453.
6. Adamec, R., Individual differences in temporal lobe sensory processing of threatening stimuli in the cat, *Physiol. Behav.*, 49 (1991) 455–464.
7. Adamec, R., Transmitter systems involved in neuroplasticity underlying increased anxiety and defence following traumatic stress, *Neuroscience and Biobehavioral Reviews*, (1996) in press.
8. Adamec, Robert E. and McKay, D., Amygdala kindling, anxiety and corticotrophin releasing factor (CRF), *Physiol. Behav.*, 54 (1993) 423–431.
9. Adamec, R., Morgan, H. (1994) The effect of kindling of different nuclei of the amygdala on anxiety in the rat, *Physiol. Behav.*, 55 (1994) 1–12.
10. Adamec, R. (1994) Modelling anxiety disorders following chemical exposures, *Tox. Indust. Health*, 10 (1994) 391–420.
11. Adamec, R. and Stark-Adamec, C., Partial kindling and emotional bias in the cat: Lasting after-effects of partial kindling of ventral hippocampus. I: Behavioral Changes, *Behav. Neur. Biol*, 38 (1983) 205–222.
12. Adamec, R. and Stark-Adamec, C., Partial kindling and emotional bias in the cat: Lasting after-effects of partial kindling of ventral hippocampus. II: Physiological Changes, *Behav. Neur. Biol*, 38 (1983) 223–239.
13. Adamec, R. and Stark-Adamec, C., Limbic kindling and animal behavior—Implications for human psychopathology associated with complex partial seizures., *Biol. Psychiat.*, 18 (1983) 269–293.
14. Adamec, R.E. and Stark-Adamec, C. (1986). Partial kindling and behavioral change—Some rules governing the behavioral outcome of repeated limbic seizures, In: Juhn Wada (Ed.), *Kindling 3*, Raven Press, New York, (1986), pp. 195–212.
15. Bagshaw, E.V. and Evans, M.H., Measurement of current spread from microelectrodes when stimulating within the central nervous system, *Exp. Brain Res.*, 25 (1976) 391–400.
16. Blanchard, D.C., Blanchard, R.J. and Rodgers, R.J., Pharmacological and neural control of anti-predator defense in the rat, *Aggressive Behavior*, 16 (1990) 165–175.
17. Bloom, F.E. and Young, W.G., *Brain Browser*. Academic Press, New York, (1993).
18. Canteras, N.S., Simerly, R.B. and Swanson, L.W., Connections of the posterior nucleus of the amygdala, *J. Comp. Neurol.*, 324 (1992) 143–179.
19. Chapman, P.F. and Bellavance, L.L., Induction of long-term potentiation in the basolateral amygdala does not depend on NMDA receptor activation, *Synapse*, 11 (1992) 310–318.
20. Csernansky, J.G., Mellentin, J., Beauclair, L., and Lombrozo, L., Mesolimbic dopaminergic supersensitivity following electrical kindling of the amygdala, *Biol. Psychiatry*, 23 (1988) 285–294.
21. Csernansky J.G., Kerr S., Pruthi R., Prosser E.S., Mesolimbic dopamine receptor increases two weeks following hippocampal kindling, *Brain Res.*, 449 (1988) 357–60
22. Dauge, V., Dor, A., Feger, J. and Roques, B.P., The behavioral effects of CCK8 injected into the medial nucleus accumbens are dependent on the motivational state of the rat, *Eur. J. Pharmacol.*, 163 (1989) 25–32.

23. Dauge, V., Steimes, V., Derrien, M., Beau, N., Roques, B.P. an Feger, J., CCK8 effects on motivational and emotional states of rat involve CCK-A receptors of the postero-median part of the nucleus accumbens, *Pharm. Biochem. Behav.*, 34 (1989) 157–163.
24. deCabo, C., DeSousa, N.J., Traubici, M.E. and Vaccarino, F.J., Anxiety-like response I the plus maze is predicted by combined individual differences in sugar feeding and novel exploration, *Soc. Neurosci. Abstr.*, 21 (1995) 448.
25. D'Aquila, P.S., Brain, P. and Wilner, P., Effects of chronic mild stress on performance in behavioural tests relevant to anxiety and depression, *Physiol. Behav.*, 56 (1994) 861–7.
26. De Olmos, J.S., The amygdaloid projection field in the rat as studied with cupric-silver method, In B.E. Eleftheriou (Ed.) *The Neurobiology of the Amygdala*. Plenum Press, New York (1972), pp. 145–204.
27. Derrien, M., Durieux, C., Dauge, V., Roques, B.P., Involvement of D_2 dopamine receptors in the emotional and motivational responses induced by injection of CCK8 in the posterior part of the nucleus accumbens, *Brain Res.*, 617 (1993) 181–188.
28. Dreifuss, J.J., Effects of electrical stimulation of the amygdaloid complex on ventromedial hypothalamus. In. B.E. Eleftheriou (Ed.) *The Neurobiology of the Amygdala, Advances in Behavioral Biology*, Vol. 2, Plenum Press, New York, (1972), pp. 295–318.
29. Einat, H. and Szechtman, H., An anxiolytic-like effect of quinpirole in the plus maze. Abstracts of the Canadian College of Neuropsychopharmacology, 19th Annual Meeting, June 2–5, 1996.
30. Engel, J. Jr., Wolfson, L. and Brown, L., Anatomical correlates of electrical and behavioral events related to amydaloid kindling, *Ann. Neurol.*, 3 (1978) 538–544.
31. File, S.E., Johnston, A.L. and Baldwin, H.A., Anxiolytic and anxiogenic drugs: changes in behavior and endocrine responses, *Stress Med.*, 4 (1988) 221–230.
32. Flor-Henry, P., Epilepsy and psychopathology, In K. Granville-Grossman (Ed.) *Recent Advances in Clinical Psychiatry*. Churchill Livingston, New York (1976), pp. 262–294.
33. Gean, P.-W., Chang, F.-C., Huang, C.-C., Lin, J.-H. and Way, L.-J., Long-term enhancement of EPSP and NMDA receptor-mediated synaptic transmission in the amygdala, *Brain Research Bull.*, 31 (1993) 7–11.
34. Gelbard HA, Applegate CD Persistent increases in dopamine D2 receptor mRNA expression in basal ganglia following kindling, *Epilepsy Res.*, 17 (1994) 23–9
35. Gomez, d. M. and Winans Newman, S., Differential projections of the anterior and posterior regions of the medial amygdaloid nucleus in the syrian hamster, *J. Comp. Neurol.*, 317 (1992) 195 218.
36. Graeff, F.G., Silveira, M.C.L., Nogueira, R.L., Audi, E.A. and Oliveira, R.M.W., Role of the amygdala and periaqueductal gray in anxiety and panic, *Behav. Brain Res.*, 58 (1993) 123–131.
37. Gray, T.S. and Magnuson, D.J., Peptide immunoreactive neurons in the amygdala and the bed nucleus of the stria terminalis project to the midbrain central gray in the rat, *Peptides*, 13 (1992) 451–460.
38. Harrigan, E.A., Magnuson, D.J., Thunstedt, G.M. and Gray, T.S., Corticotropin releasing factor neurons are innervated by calcitonin gene-related peptide terminals in the rat central amygdaloid nucleus, *Brain Res. Bull.*, 33 (1994) 529–534.
39. Helfer, V., Deransart, C., Marescaux, C. and Depaulis, A., Amygdala kindling in the rat: anxiogenic-like consequences, *Neuroscience*, (1996) in press.
40. Heinrichs, S.C., Pich, E.M., Miczek, K.A., Britton, K.T. and Koob, G.F., Corticotropin-releasing factor antagonist reduces emotionality in socially defeated rats via direct neurotropic action, *Brain Res.*, 581 (1992) 190–197.
41. Henke, P.G. and Sullivan, R.M., Kindling in the amygdala and susceptibility to stress ulcers, *Brain Res. Bull.*, 14 (1985) 5–8
42. Hermann, B.P. and Whitman, S., Behavioral and personality correlates of epilepsy: A review, methodological critique, and conceptual model., *Psych. Bull.*, 95 (1984) 451–497.
43. Hermann, B.P., Wyler, A.R., Ackerman, B. and Rosenthal, T., Short-term psychological outcome of anterior temporal lobectomy, *J. Neurosurg. [JD3].*, 71 (1989) 327–334.
44. Hooks, M.S., Jones, G.H., Smith, A.D., Neill, D.B. and Justice, J.B., Response to novelty predicts the locomotor and nucleus accumbens dopamine response to cocaine, *Synapse*, 9 (1991) 121–128.
45. Kaada, B.R., Stimulation and regional ablation of the amygdaloid complex with reference to functional representations, In B.E. Eleftheriou (Ed.) *The Neurobiology of the Amygdala, Advances in Behavioral Biology*, Vol. 2, Plenum Press, New York, (1972), pp. 205–282.
46. Kalynchuk, L.E., Pinel, J.P.J., Treit, D. and Kippin. T.E., Changes in emotional behavior produced by long-term amygdala kindling in rats, *Biol. Psychiat.*, (1996) (in press).
47. Kalynchuk, L.E., Pinel, J.P.J., Barr,K.N., Kippin,T.E. and Treit, D., Amygdala kindling in rats results in increased defensive behavior which is lasting but not permanent, *Neuroscience and Biobehavioral Reviews*, Abstract (1996), in press.

48. Ladurelle, N, Roques, B.P., and Dauge, V., The transfer of rats from a familiar to a novel environment prolongs the increase of extracellular dopamine efflux induced by CCK8 in the posterior nucleus accumbens, *J. Neurosci.*, 15 (1995) 3118–27.
49. Luiten, P.G.M., Ono, T., Hishijo, H. and Fukuda, M., Differential input from the amygdaloid body to the ventromedial hypothalamic nucleus in the rat, *Neurosci. Lett.*, 35 (1983) 253–258.
50. Maeda, H. and Hirata, K., Two-stage amygdaloid lesions and hypothalamic rage: A method useful for detecting functional localization, *Physiol. Behav.*, 21 (1978) 529–530.
51. Makino, S., Gold, P.W., Schulkin, J., Coricosterone effects on corticotropin-releasing hormone mRNA in the central nucleus of the amygdala and the parvocellular region of the paraventricular nucleus of the hypothalamus, *Brain Res.*, 640 (1994) 105–112.
52. Merlo Pich, E., Koob, G.F., Sattler, S.C., Menzaghi, F., Heilig, M., Heinrichs, S.C., Vale, W. and Weiss, F., Stress-induced release of corticotropin releasing factor in the amygdala measured by *in vivo* microdialysis, *Soc. Neurosci. Abstr.*, 18 (1992) 535
53. McIntyre, D., Amygdala kindling and muricide in rats, *Physiol. Behav.*, 21 (1978) 49–56.
54. Murphy, J.T., The role of the amygdala in controlling hypothalamic output, In. In B.E. Eleftheriou (Ed.) *The Neurobiology of the Amygdala, Advances in Behavioral Biology*, Vol. 2, Plenum Press, New York, (1972), pp. 371–96.
55. Narita, K., Yokawa, T., Nishihara, M. and Takahashi, M., Interaction between excitatory and inhibitory amino acids in the ventromedial nucleus of the hypothalamus in inducing hyper-running, *Brain Res.* , 603 (1993) 243–247.
56. Nieminen, s., Sirvio,J., Teittinen, K., Pitkanen, A., Airaksinen, M.M., and Riekkinen, P., Amygdala kindling increased fear-repsonse, but did not impair spatial memory in rats, *Physiol. Behav.*, 51 (1992) 845–849.
57. Oakes, M.E. and Coover, G.D., Aggression and social behavior after four different medial hypothalamic lesions, *Soc. Neurosci. Abstr.*, 19 (1993)
58. Ogawa, S., Kow, L.-M. and Pfaff, D.W., Effects of GABA and related agents on the electrical activity of hypothalamic ventromedial nucleus neurons in vitro, *Experimental Brain Research*, 85 (1991) 85–92.
59. Paxinos, G. and Watson, C., *The Rat Brain in Stereotaxic Coordinates*, Second Edition, Academic Press, London, 1986.
60. Piazza, P.V., Rogue-Pont, F., Deminier, J.M., Kharouby, M., LeMoal, M., Simon, H., Dopaminergic activity is reduced in the prefrontal cortex and increased in the nucleus accumbens of rats predisposed to develop amphetamine self-administration, *Brain Res.*, 567 (1991) 169–174.
61. Pinel, J.P.J., Effects of kindling on rodent defense (this volume).
62. Pinel, J.P.J., Treit, D and Rovner,L.I., Temporal lobe aggression in the rats, *Science,* 197 (1977) 1088–1089.
63. Post, R., Squillace, K.M., Pert, A. and Sass, W., The effect of amygdala kindling on spontaneous and cocaine-induced activity and lidocaine seizures, *Psychopharmacology,* 72 (1981) 189–196.
64. Priestley, T., The effect of baclofen and somatostatin on neuronal activity in the rat ventromedial hypothalamic nucleus *in vitro*, *Neuropharmacology*, 31 (1992) 103–109.
65. Racine,R.J, Milgran,N.W. and Hafner, S., Long-term potentiation phenomena in the rat limbic forebrain, *Brain Res.*, 260 (1983) 217–231.
66. Rada, P. and Hernandez, L., Opposite changes of dopamine turnover in prefrontal cortex and nucleus accumbens after amygdaloid kindling, *Neurosci.Lett.*, 117 (1990) 144–148.
67. Ray, A., Henke, P.G. and Sullivan, R.M., Noradrenergic mechanisms in the central amygdalar nucleus and gastric stress ulcer formation in rats, *Neurosci. Lett.*, 110 (1990) 331–336.
68. Rosen, J.B, Hamerman, E., Sitcoske, M. and Glowa, J.R., Hyperexcitability: Exaggerated fear-potentiated startle produce by partial amygdala kindling, *Beh. Neuroscience,* 110 (1996) 43–50.
69. Roberts, G.W., Neuropeptides: Cellular Morphology, Major Pathways, and Functional Considerations, In John P. Aggleton (Ed.) *The Amygdala, Neurobiological Aspects of Emotion, Memory, and Mental Dysfunction.* Wiley-Liss, New York (1992), pp. 115–142.
70. Sackeim, H.A., Emotion, disorder of Mood, and Hemispheric Functional Specialization. In B.J. Carrol and J.E. Barrett (Eds.) *Psychopathology and the Brain*. Raven Press, New York (1991), pp. 209–242.
71. Salamone, J.D., The behavioral neurochemistry of motivation: Methodological and conceptual issues in studies of the dynamic activity of nucleus accumbens dopamine, *Neurosci. Method.*, 64 (1996) 137–149.
72. Savander, V., Go, C.G., LeDoux, J.E. and Ptikanen, A., Intrinsic connections of the rat amygdaloid complex: Projection originating in the basal nucleus, *J. Comp. Neurol.*, 361 (1995) 345–368.
73. Silveira, M.C.L. and Graeff, F.G., Defense reaction elicited by microinjection of kainic acid into the medial hypothalamus of the rat: Antagonism by a $GABA_A$ receptor agonist, *Behav. Neural Biol.*, 57 (1992) 226–232.

74. Silveira, M.C.L., Sandner, G. and Graeff, F.G., Induction of Fos immunoreactivity in the brain by exposure to the elevated plus-maze, *Behav. Brain Res.*, 56 (1993) 115–118.
75. Siegel, A., Anatomical and functional differentiation within the amygdala—behavioral state modulation, In R. Bandler (Ed.) *Modulation of Sensorimotor Activity During alterations in Behavioral States*. Alan R. Liss, Inc. New York (1984), pp. 299–323.
76. Sills, T. and Vaccarino, F.J., Individual differences in sugar consumption predict individual differences in sensitization to the locomotor activating effect of amphetamine, *Soc. Neurosci. Abstr.*, 19 (1993) 334.10.
77. Stark-Adamec, C. & Adamec, R.E., Psychological methodology vs clinical impressions: Different perspectives on psychopathology and seizures, In B.K. Doane and K.E. Livingston (Eds.) *The Limbic System: Functional Organization and Clinical Disorders*. New York, Raven Press, (1986), pp. 217–227.
78. Stenzel-Poore M.P., Heinrichs S.C., Rivest S., Koob G.F., Vale W.W., Overproduction of corticotropin-releasing factor in transgenic mice: a genetic model of anxiogenic behavior, *J Neurosci*, 14 (1994) 2579–84
79. Stevens, J.R. and Livermore, A.Jr. Kindling of the mesolimbic doapmine system: animal model of psychosis, *Neurology*, Jan. (1978) 37–46.
80. Tershner, S.A. and Helmstetter, F.J., Pretraining injections of corticotropin releasing factor into the ventral periaqueductal gray enhance freezing to an auditory conditional aversive stimulus, *Soc. Neurosci. Abstr.*, 19 (1993)
81. Van der Kolk, B.A., The body keeps score: memory; the evolving psychobiology of posttraumatic stress disorder, *Harvard Rev. Psychiat.*, Jan/Feb (1994) 253–265.
82. Wallace, D.M., Magnuson, D.J. and Gray, T.S., Organization of amygdaloid projections to brainstem dopaminergic, noradrenergic, and adrenergic cell groups in the rat, *Brain Res. Bull.*, 28 (1992) 447–454.
83. Watanabe, Y., Ikegaya,Y., Saito, H. and Abe, K., Roles of $GABA_A$, NMDA and muscarinic receptors in induction of long-term potentiation in the medial and lateral amygdala in vitro, *Neurosci. Res.*, 21 (1995) 317–322.
84. Watanabe, Y., Saito, H. and Abe, K., Nitric oxide is involved in long-term potentiation in the medial but not the lateral amygdala neuron synapses in vitro,. *Brain Res.*, 688 (1995) 233–236.
85. Watson, R.E. Jr., Troiano, R., Poulakos, J., Weiner, S., Block, C.H. and Siege, A., A {[4]2-Deoxyglucose Analysis of the functional neural pathways of the limbic forebrain in the Rat. I. The amygdala, *Brain Res. Rev.*, 5 (1983) 1–44.
86. Witkin, J.M., Lee, M.A. and Woolsack, DD., Anxiolytic properties of amygdaloid kindling unrelated to benzodiazepine receptors, *Psychopharmacology*, 96 (1988) 296–301.
87. Whitman, S. and Hermann, B.P., The architecture of research in the epilepsy/psychopathology field, *Epilepsy. Res. [EMA]*., 3 (1989) 93–99.

DISCUSSION OF ROBERT ADAMEC'S PAPER

Karen Gale: You portrayed the data as averages, and I was wondering if you did it on an animal by animal basis, left versus right. Also, how did you determine the percent?

B. Adamec: The anxiolytic effect is demonstrated statistically; so you have a comparably implanted group, you measure their "anxiety level," and then you compare that statistically to an "anxiety level" of animals that are kindled. Now to do an animal by animal comparison is kind of difficult, because what would you use as your control level? You could use the average of your controls, but then why not just use the average of the kindled animals?

K Gale: Have you ever actually done one side and then transferred to the other side and seen whether it switches?

B. Adamec: Oh, I see. No, it's a good idea, but I have not done it.

K. Gale: These are all across-animal data then.

B. Adamec: Yes, but the histological figures that I showed you are electrode placements averaged within the A-P plane. The A-P plane range I showed you captures the 95% confidence interval, and the center of those spheres was the mean or median position if they weren't normally distributed.

K. Gale: If you then analyzed the data by taking the average as your usual point, what kind of distribution do you get around that? Are 100% of the animals at the beginning anxiogenic here on the left or the right side?

B. Adamec: No, its not 100%. There is going to be some overlap of the two distributions, it is not totally separated, but it is statistically significant.

A. Depaulis: Are the kindling parameters exactly the same between sides? In terms of the evolution of kindling, did you compare between sides whether the number of stimulations reached a certain stage?

B. Adamec: For the most part yes, but not always. It isn't tied to behavior.

P. Engel: Not all rats are right handed. There is literature on lateralization in rats. There are tests to see which front paw they prefer to dig things out of a hole with, and when you hold them by the tail they rotate in different directions consistently. Have you thought about taking that into consideration?

B. Adamec: Absolutely, it is on my agenda. Because I think actually that they may be a dopaminergic component to the apparent anxiolytic effects in the left hemisphere. Bob Post showed a long time ago that kindling in almost exactly the same sites in the basal lateral amygdala in which we find an anxiolytic effect produced an enhancement in apomorphine induced movement. If you look at the literature that has evolved since then, the action is likely in the nucleus accumbens. There are some studies now showing very long lasting increases in D2 receptors following kindling, and also there is a recent study that shows that quinperol, a D2/D3 agonist, in fact has anxiolytic effects in the plus maze. So I think attention to dopamine function in this model may well be an important clarifier, and certainly those hemispheric differences might in fact make a difference. Theoretically, a right sided dominant animal might in fact show an anxiolytic effect.

J. Wada: Are there sex differences?

B. Adamec: These are all done in males so I don't know. I am the usual rat chauvinist pig, and I certainly agree that it should also be done in females.

LONG-TERM AMYGDALA KINDLING AND DEFENSIVE BEHAVIOR IN RATS

John P. J. Pinel,[1] Lisa E. Kalynchuk,[1] and Dallas Treit[2]

[1]Department of Psychology
University of British Columbia
Vancouver, British Columbia, Canada
[2]Department of Psychology
University of Alberta
Edmonton, Alberta, Canada

1. INTRODUCTION

Epilepsy is a chronic disorder that is characterized by spontaneously recurring seizures. There are several different forms of epilepsy. Of these, temporal lobe epilepsy represents the biggest problem: It is the most prevalent form of epilepsy, comprising 55% of all cases in adults; it is the most resistant to treatment; and it is often characterized by severe interictal behavioral disturbances, which can be more problematic than the seizures themselves[16,17]. The interictal behavioral disturbances associated with temporal lobe epilepsy are the focus of this paper

Gaining an understanding of the nature and cause of the interictal behavioral disturbances associated with temporal lobe epilepsy is important for at least two reasons. First, they constitute a serious medical problem: They can disable epileptic patients to the point where they cannot work, sustain normal relationships, or otherwise function normally in society. Second, they provide a means of inferring the role of the temporal lobes in normal human psychological functioning.

1.1. Interictal Emotionality in Temporal Lobe Epileptics

Since the early 1900s, there have been numerous anecdotal and case study reports suggesting a relation between temporal lobe epilepsy and interictal psychopathology[15]. However, it was not until 1977 that the first systematic assessment of the interictal behavioral changes associated with temporal lobe epilepsy was published. In a questionnaire study, Bear and Fedio[7] confirmed that temporal lobe epileptics scored higher than non-epileptic controls on 18 behavioral traits, all of which had been linked to temporal lobe epilepsy in earlier anecdotal and case study reports, and they concluded that all 18 of these

Kindling 5, edited by Corcoran and Moshé.
Plenum Press, New York, 1998.

traits were a consequence of a general increase in emotionality[8]. Since Bear and Fedio's seminal study, the presence of interictal emotional disturbances in temporal lobe epileptics has been well documented[15], but considerable controversy still remains over their nature and cause. Particularly problematic is the widely-held belief that temporal lobe epileptics are prone to aggression, despite the fact that there is little empirical support for this view[19].

It has proven difficult to resolve the controversy over the nature and cause of interictal emotionality in temporal lobe epileptics because of problems inherent in the study of epileptic patients. For example, the interictal emotional disturbances associated with temporal lobe epilepsy per se are often clouded by the side effects of antiepileptic medication[25], by the heterogeneity of the seizures that commonly occur in epileptics, by the experience of suffering from a disorder that is both traumatic and unpredictable[19], and from the emotional impact of the social stigma that is attached to it[17]. Moreover, the diffuseness and variability of the structural and functional brain pathology in temporal lobe epileptics[6,17] makes it difficult to link the emotional changes associated with temporal lobe epilepsy to changes in particular cerebral structures. Consequently, the availability of a useful animal model of the interictal emotional disturbances associated with temporal lobe epilepsy would greatly facilitate their study.

1.2. Kindling Model of the Emotional Behavior Associated with Temporal Lobe Epilepsy

Kindling is the most widely studied animal model of temporal lobe epilepsy. Several lines of evidence support the view that rats and other animals kindled by amygdala stimulation are valid models of human temporal lobe epilepsy. First, drug effects on amygdala-kindled convulsions in rats are predictive of drug effects on complex partial seizures in humans[32,37]. Second, kindled rats display patterns of neuronal damage[10,41,39] and axon sprouting[42,43] similar to those observed in the brains of human temporal lobe epileptics. And third, extensive kindling ultimately results in the recurrence of spontaneous convulsions (i.e., motor seizures), which are the defining feature of clinical epilepsy[34].

Adamec was the first to document the effects of kindling on interictal emotional behavior[1]. He studied the behavioral effects of partial kindling in cats in several noteworthy experiments. He found that partial kindling (i.e., kindling that produces afterdischarges but no convulsions) of the amygdala or ventral hippocampus in cats results in behavioral changes that appear to be independent of convulsions or interictal spiking for their maintenance[2]. After partial kindling, cats displayed increased defensive responses when they were exposed to rats, mice, and conspecific threat vocalizations[1] or when they received electrical stimulations of the ventromedial hypothalamus[40]. These behavioral changes were reversible, lasting from several days to several weeks[2]. Adamec's studies of partial kindling have provided important data regarding the effects of repeated seizures on defensive behavior; the advantage of such studies of partial kindling is that they assess behavioral changes at a stage in kindling before afterdischarges have become generalized.

Pinel, Treit, and Rovner[36] were the first to document amygdala-kindling-induced increases in interictal emotional behavior in rats. In their experiment, rats received 99 stimulations of the amygdala, hippocampus, or caudate and their response to a pencil tap on the back and their resistance to capture were assessed. The amygdala- and hippocampal-kindled rats displayed a significantly greater response to tail tap and greater resistance to capture than both the sham-stimulated control rats and the caudate-kindled rats.

Since the seminal experiments of Adamec and of Pinel and his colleagues, most investigators interested in the interictal emotional disturbances associated with temporal lobe epilepsy have studied the changes in emotional behavior that accompany short-term amygdala kindling[2,14]. Short-term kindling refers to protocols in which animals receive enough stimulations to induce three consecutive generalized convulsions—generally between 15 and 25 stimulations in amygdala-kindled rats. The subjects, typically rats, are tested at least 24 hr after the final kindling stimulation, in order to be sure that any apparent behavioral differences are not due to postictal electrical activity. Using this protocol, amygdala kindling in squirrel monkeys has been shown to cause increases in defensiveness and social withdrawal[31]; and in rats, it has been shown to decrease exploratory behavior[33,22], increase corticotrophin releasing-factor-induced defensive fighting[44] and increase stress-induced stomach ulcers[23]. However, this protocol has produced no increases in tests of depression[22], and no anterograde memory impairments[33,26]. Thus, amygdala-kindling-induced alterations in behavior appear to be specifically related to changes in fear or anxiety.

Although the results of studies of short-term amygdala kindling have consistently demonstrated increases in interictal emotional behavior, they have not totally consistent with respect to the precise nature of the emotional changes produced by kindling. For example, the effects of short-term kindling in rats have been inconsistent with respect to behavior on the elevated plus maze—left basolateral-amygdala kindling has been associated with both anxiolytic[4] and anxiogenic[33] effects.

1.3. Long-Term Amygdala Kindling as a Model of the Emotional Behavior Associated with Temporal Lobe Epilepsy

The experiments described in this paper are studies of the effects of long-term (i.e., 100 stimulations) amygdala kindling on interictal emotional behavior in rats. Why did we choose to study long-term, as opposed to short-term, kindled rats? The reason is that kindling is a progressive disorder that is far from complete once three consecutive generalized convulsions have been elicited: If the program of stimulations is continued in rats, the severity of their motor seizures increases (i.e., multiple fits of rearing and falling, running fits, and tonic motor seizures develop), interictal epileptic spikes begin to punctuate the EEG records, and after about 250 stimulations, motor seizures begin to recur spontaneously[34]. This suggested to us that long-term kindling might produce some changes in interictal emotional behavior that are not apparent after short-term kindling and some changes that are larger and more reliable than those that are apparent after short-term kindling. We selected 100 stimulations as our standard treatment because our experience with long-term kindling suggested that 100 stimulations would be enough to guarantee that all subjects would be well kindled, but not so well kindled that they would be displaying spontaneous convulsions, which would confound the behavioral testing.

2. METHODS

The following is a brief description of the methods that were used in our experiments. A more complete description has been published elsewhere[27].

2.1. Kindling

All rats had a bipolar stimulating electrode (Plastic Products MS-302) implanted in the basolateral amygdala. Following a postsurgical recovery period of at least 7 days, some of the rats received a convulsive stimulation (1 sec, 60 hz, 400 μA) three times per day, 5 days per week and some received sham stimulations. A sham stimulation consisted of attaching the stimulation lead to a rat's electrode but not passing any current through it. There was a minimum of 2 hr between consecutive stimulations.

2.2. Behavioral Testing

One day after the final kindling stimulation, each rat was placed by itself in an unfamiliar open field for 5 min while an experimenter, who had not previously handled the rats and who was unaware of their experimental history, sat quietly in the room out of sight of the rat. The open field was a large, topless, wooden box, 60 × 60 × 60 cm, which was located on the floor. After the 5 min, the rat was forcefully picked up from above by the experimenter, who was wearing a leather glove unfamiliar to the rat. The rat's resistance to being picked up was scored according to the following 7-point scale adapted from Albert and Richmond[5]: 0 = easy to pick up, 1 = vocalizes or shies away from hand, 2 = shies away from hand and vocalizes, 3 = runs away from hand, 4 = runs away and vocalizes, 5 = bites or attempts to bite, 6 = launches a defensive jump attack.

Some of the kindled rats were tested as intruders in a resident-intruder paradigm[9]. Each rat was placed in the cage of an unfamiliar weight- and age-matched resident rat for 10 min, and the interaction of the two rats was videotaped for later analysis.

3. EXPERIMENTAL RESULTS

3.1. Effect of Number of Amygdala Stimulations on the Development of Increased Emotionality

We began by replicating Pinel et al.'s[36] finding that 99 amygdala stimulations greatly increase the resistance to capture of rats compared to sham-stimulated controls. The location of the stimulation electrode within the amygdala (basolateral vs. central nucleus) had no significant effect[27].

Next, we compared the behavior of kindled rats that had received different numbers of stimulations—to our knowledge, the effect of number of stimulations on kindling-induced changes in emotionality had not been previously assessed.

The rats were divided into six groups after surgery: Three stimulation groups received 20 (n=14), 60 (n=13), or 100 (n=14) convulsive stimulations; and three sham-stimulation groups received either 20 (n=6), 60 (n=6), or 100 (n=6) sham stimulations. One day after the final stimulation, each rat's resistance to capture was assessed.

Figure 1 shows that amygdala-kindling produced substantial increases in resistance to capture from the open field, and that the magnitude of these changes was dependent on the number of stimulations that the rats had received. The 100-stimulation rats displayed significantly more resistance to capture than did the 20-stimulation rats or the sham-stimulation rats ($p<.01$), and the 60-stimulation rats displayed significantly more resistance to capture than did the sham-stimulation rats ($p<.01$). Accordingly, these results confirm and extend previous reports of increases in emotionality following short-term amygdala kindling[2,14].

3.2. Role of Novelty in the Expression of Kindling-Induced Hyperemotionality

In our initial experiments, resistance-to-capture testing was done in an environment unfamiliar to the subjects and by an experimenter unfamiliar to the subjects, the hypothe-

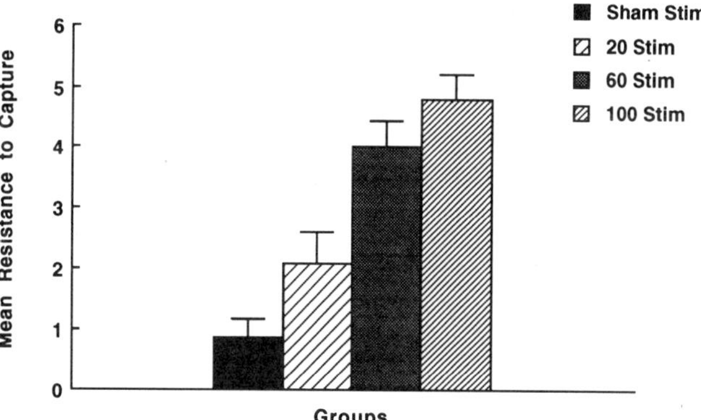

Figure 1. The mean resistance-to-capture score displayed by the rats in each group one day after its last kindling stimulation (error bars indicate standard errors). The 100-stimulation rats were signficantly more resistant to capture than both the 20-stimulation and the sham-stimulation rats; the 60-stimulation rats were significantly more resistant to capture than the sham-stimulation rats.

sis being that the reactions of kindled rats to mild forms of threat, such as being picked up from above, would be greater in a strange situation. We tested this hypothesis in two ways: by comparing the resistance-to-capture scores of kindled rats (n=13) in their home cages as opposed to the unfamiliar open field and by assessing the effects of repeated testing of kindled rats (n=13) in the open field, one trial per day for 5 days.

The results of these two tests confirmed our hypothesis; they are summarized in Figure 2. When tested one day after the last stimulation, the kindled rats were substantially more resistant to capture in the unfamiliar open field than in their home cages ($p<.001$), and resistance to capture scores declined monotonically with repeated daily testing in the initially unfamiliar open field ($p<.01$).

3.3. Increased Emotionality Produced by Long-Term Amygdala Kindling Is Enduring

Whether or not kindling-induced hyperemotionality persists after the kindling stimulations have been discontinued is an important issue because it has implications for understanding the mechanisms that underlie this hyperemotionality. If the hyperemotionality were permanent, it would suggest that the mechanisms underlying it are the same as those underlying the kindled state; alternatively, if the hyperemotionality were to quickly dissipate, it would suggest that the mechanisms underlying it are related to some other, less enduring, consequence of the stimulations. The permanence of interictal increases in emo-

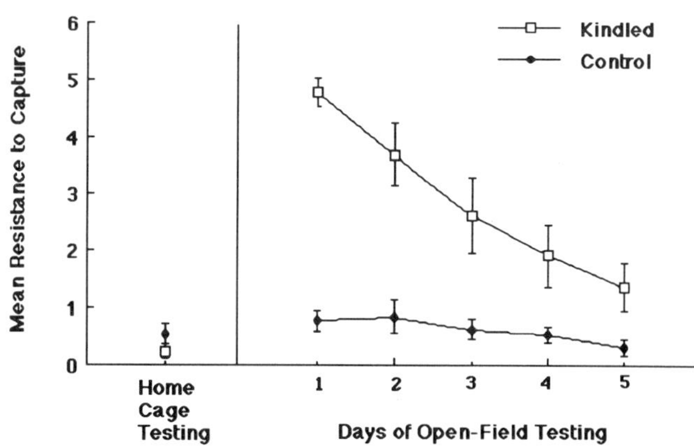

Figure 2. The mean resistance-to-capture score displayed by the rats tested in their home cage and after repeated daily testing in an intially unfamiliar open field (error bars indicate standard errors). The kindled rats displayed significantly more resistance to capture from the open field than from their home cage; the initial high levels of resistance to capture from the open field also declined significantly with repeated exposure to the open field.

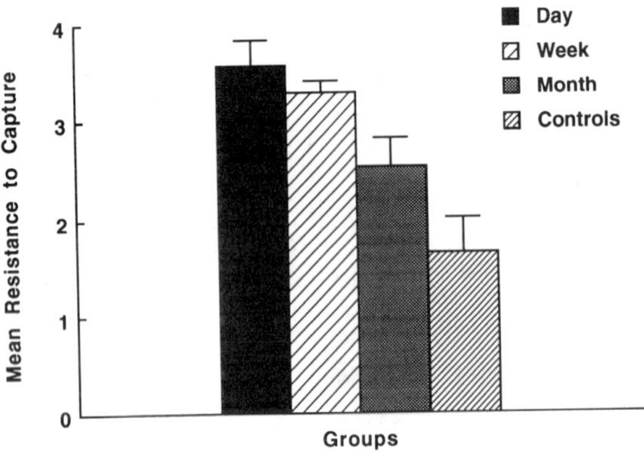

Figure 3. The mean resistance-to-capture score displayed by the rats tested 1 day, 1 week, or 1 month after the last kindling stimulation (error bars indicate standard errors). Compared to the sham-stimulated controls, the rats tested 1 day and 1 week after the last stimulation displayed significant resistance to capture but the rats tested 1 month after the last stimulation did not.

tionality also has important implications for the development of strategies for the treatment of interictal emotional disturbances in human epileptics.

To assess the permanence of the hyperemotionality produced by long-term kindling, we tested the resistance to capture from a novel open field of six groups of rats. The rats in three experimental groups received 99 kindling stimulations and were tested 1 day (n=12), 1 week (n=14), or 1 month after their last stimulation (n=13); and three sham-stimulation control groups were tested after the same three intervals (total n=14).

Figure 3 illustrates the results of this experiment. Both the 1 day and 1 week rats were significantly more resistant to capture from the open field than were the sham-stimulation control rats ($p<.03$). However, there were no significant differences in resistance to capture among the 1 day, 1 week, and 1 month rats ($p>.05$). Thus, amygdala-kindling-induced increases in resistance to capture do not significantly dissipate within 1 month of the cessation of stimulations.

Interestingly, in another experiment, rats received 99 amygdala stimulations and were tested for resistance to capture. They were then kept unstimulated for 60 days, subjected to an additional 0, 1, 10, or 30 stimulations, and finally retested for resistance to capture. The 60-day break from stimulations was sufficient to induce a significant dissipation of the initial high levels of resistance to capture but 30 additional stimulations reinstated asymptotic levels of resistance to capture.

3.4. Fundamental Nature of Kindling-Induced Hyperemotionality: Aggression or Defense?

It is widely believed that temporal lobe epileptics are prone to outbursts of aggression[18], despite the fact that little empirical evidence exists to support this claim. Alternatively, it has been suggested that the emotional outbursts are fundamentally defensive in nature[19]. Which of these two views is correct? We attempted to answer this question by comparing the behavior of kindled (n=13) and sham-stimulated control (n=13) rats as intruders in the resident-intruder paradigm.

In the resident-intruder paradigm, the topographies of aggressive and defensive behavior are readily distinguishable. This can be seen most easily when the interactions of a large resident male (aggressor) and a small male intruder (defender) are assessed[9]. The resident first sniffs the perianal area of the intruder and chases it around the cage. The intruder, unable to escape from the apparatus, eventually turns to face the resident and rears up on its haunches in a "boxing" posture. Then, the resident approaches the intruder side-

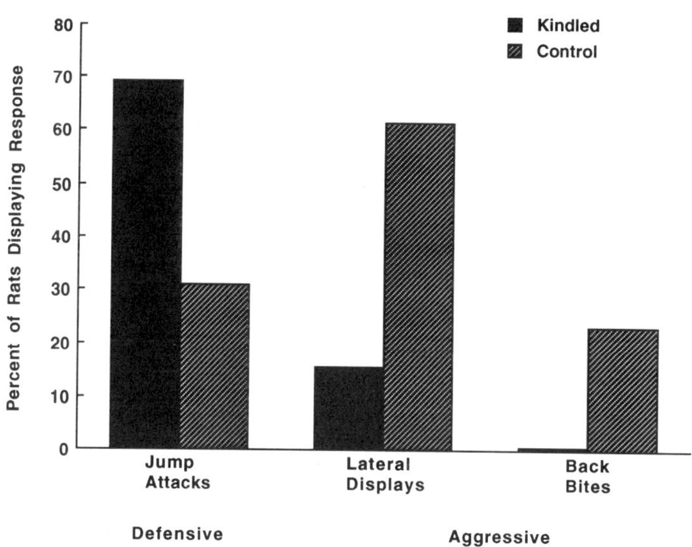

Figure 4. The percent of kindled and control rats that engaged in defensive and aggressive behaviors when tested as intruders in a resident-intruder paradigm. The kindled intruders displayed significantly more defensive attacks and significantly less aggressive lateral displays and bites to the resident's back than the control rats did.

ways (lateral approach) so that it is in a position to make a darting attack around the intruder to deliver a bite to its back, which is the target site of all aggressive social attacks by rats. The intruder defends itself by pivoting on its hindlegs and fending off the resident with its forepaws; however, if sufficiently pressed, it will launch a defensive biting jump attack directly at the face of the intruder. Accordingly, we attempted to resolve the question of whether interictal hyperemotionality is fundamentally aggressive or defensive by determining whether the male rats subjected to 99 amygdala stimulations would display more aggressive lateral attacks and back bites or more defensive jump attacks than controls when tested as intruders in the resident-intruder paradigm.

The results of the resident-intruder tests are summarized in Figure 4. Intruders that had been subjected to long-term kindling were much more likely to launch defensive attacks than were the controls ($p<.05$), and they were also much less likely to display aggressive lateral attacks and back bites ($p<.05$). Accordingly, by these measures, rats that have been subjected to long-term amygdala kindling are more defensive but less aggressive than controls.

4. DISCUSSION

In this chapter, we have reported five findings: (1) that long-term amygdala kindling produces a marked increase in the resistance to capture of rats, (2) that this increase in resistance to capture is significantly greater following long-term kindling than short-term kindling, (3) that it occurs only when the rats are tested in an unfamiliar environment, (4) that it is enduring for at least 1 month following the cessation of stimulations, and (5) that it is fundamentally defensive in nature.

Due to space limitations, we have restricted the description of our results to two tests of kindling-induced hyperemotionality: the resistance-to-capture test and the resident-intruder test. However, we recorded several measures of emotionality in each of our experiments. In addition to the effects already described, we have found that long-term amygdala kindling decreases open-field activity, increases thigmotaxia, and increases escape behavior from an elevated plus maze[27].

The pattern of behavioral changes that we have observed after long-term amygdala kindling—primarily increases in defensive behavior—suggests that long-term amygdala kindling increases the level of fear experienced in threatening situations. Our observation that kindling-induced increases in resistance to capture are potentiated by testing in strange situations is also consistent with this view. Others have reached a similar conclusion: Nieminen and his colleagues[33] concluded that the decreased activity in a novel open field, decreased open-arm activity in an elevated plus maze and impaired performance on an elevated-bridges test observed in their short-term amygdala-kindled rats was indicative of increased levels of fear; and Rosen and his colleagues[38] concluded that the increased potentiated startle seen in their partially amygdala-kindled rats was also indicative of increased levels of fear.

Our hypothesis that long-term amygdala kindling induces an increase in fearfulness is consistent with the extensive research literature linking the amygdala to the expression of fear-motivated behavior[12,29]. For example, electrical stimulation of the amygdala elicits feelings of fear or anxiety in humans[21] and a pattern of behavioral changes that is analogous to that produced by stressful or fearful stimuli in rats[13]. In addition, lesions of the amygdala in rats abolish conditioned fear[11,24], decrease freezing in novel situations[20], and attenuate fear-induced increases in heart rate[28].

The link between the amygdala and fear-motivated behavior led us to test the hypothesis that the effect of kindling-induced hyperemotionality is specific to the amygdala and related structures. We compared the ability of long-term amygdala kindling, hippocampal kindling, and caudate kindling to increase several measures of interictal hyperdefensiveness. Although the exact nature of the results depended on the particular measure of defensiveness, in general, amygdala kindling produced large increases, hippocampal kindling produced intermediate increases, and caudate kindling had little or no effect[35].

The present findings are at odds with the widely held notion that temporal lobe epileptics are highly aggressive[18]. They suggest instead that temporal lobe epileptics tend to become excessively fearful and display heightened levels of defensive behavior when threatened—indeed, amygdala kindled rats displayed lower levels of aggressive behavior in the resident-intruder paradigm. These results provide support for the results of recent retrospective studies of human temporal lobe epileptics: although epileptics tend to respond excessively to threatening situations, few engage in acts of premeditated aggression[19].

4.1. Conclusions

The present experiments had three purposes: to establish the potential of long-term amygdala kindling as a model of the interictal hyperemotionality associated with temporal lobe epilepsy, to identify some of the major variables that influence the expression of interictal hyperemotionality, and to characterize its fundamental nature. These purposes were accomplished. First, the present experiments established the potential of long-term kindling as a model of the interictal hyperemotionality associated with temporal lobe epilepsy by demonstrating large, reliable, and systematic increases in emotional behavior that are similar in major respects to those reported in temporal lobe epileptics and to those reported following short-term amygdala kindling. Second, the present experiments identified the number of seizures, the testing environment, and the time since the last seizure as factors influencing the expression of interictal hyperemotionality—these variables may account for some of the diversity of interictal psychopathology in human temporal lobe epileptics[16]. And third, the present experiments buttress recent conclusions based on the study of temporal lobe epileptics that the fundamental interictal emotional change is an increase in defensiveness rather than an increase in aggression[19].

In comparison to studies of kindled seizures themselves, studies of kindling-related interictal behavioral changes are small in number. This chapter and the preceding one by Adamec[3] suggest that a partial shift in focus is long overdue: Studies of the interictal effects of short- and long-term kindling converge to provide information of substantial clinical, social, and scientific relevance.

ACKNOWLEDGMENTS

This work was supported by the Natural Sciences and Engineering Research Council of Canada. Lisa E. Kalynchuk is a recipient of a Medical Research Council of Canada Postgraduate Scholarship.

REFERENCES

1. Adamec, R.E., Behavioral and epileptic determinants of predatory attack behaviour in the cat, In J.A. Wada (Ed.), *Kindling*, Raven Press, New York, 1976, pp. 135–154.
2. Adamec, R.E., Does kindling model anything clinically relevant? *Biol. Psychiatry*, 27 (1990) 249–279.
3. Adamec, R.E., Amygdala Kindling and Rodent Anxiety, In M. Corcoran and S. Moshe (Eds.), *Kindling V*, Plenum Press, New York, in press.
4. Adamec, R.E. and Morgan, H.D., The effect of kindling of different nuclei in the left and right amygdala on anxiety in the rat, *Physiol. Behav.*, 55 (1994) 1–12.
5. Albert, D.J. and Richmond, S.E., Septal hyperreactivity: A comparison of lesions within and adjacent to the septum, *Physiol. Behav.*, 15 (1975) 339–347.
6. Armstrong, D.D., The neuropathology of temporal lobe epilepsy, *J. Neuropathol. Exp. Neurol.*, 52 (1993) 433–443.
7. Bear, D.M. and Fedio, P., Quantitative analysis of interictal behavior in temporal lobe epilepsy, *Arch. Neurol.*, 34 (1977) 454–467.
8. Bear, D.M., Temporal lobe epilepsy—A syndrome of sensory-limbic hyperconnection, *Cortex*, 15 (1979) 357–384
9. Blanchard, R.J., Brain, P.F., Blanchard, D.C. and Parmigiani, S., *Ethoexperimental approaches to the study of behavior*, Kluwer Academic Publishers, Dordrecht, 1989.
10. Cavazos, J.E., Das, I., and Sutula, T.P., Neuronal loss induced in limbic pathways by kindling: Evidence for induction of hippocampal sclerosis by repeated brief seizures, *J. Neurosci.*, 14, (1994) 3106–3121.
11. Coover, G.D., Murison, R., and Jellestad, F.K., Subtotal lesions of the amygdala: The rostral central nucleus in passive avoidance and ulceration, *Physiol. Behav.*, 51 (1992) 795–803.
12. Davis, M., The role of the amygdala in fear and anxiety, *Ann. Rev. Neurosci.*, 15 (1992) 353–375.
13. Davis, M., Rainnie, D. and Cassell, M., Neurotransmission in the rat amygdala related to fear and anxiety, *TINS*, 17 (1994) 208–214.
14. Depaulis, A., Helfer, V., Deransart, C., and Mareascaux, C., Anxiogenic-like consequences in animal models of complex partial seizures, *Neuroscience and Biobehavioral Reviews*, in press.
15. Devinsky, O., Interictal behavioral changes in epilepsy, In O. Devinsky and W.H. Theodore (Eds.), *Epilepsy and Behaviour*, Wiley-Liss, New York, 1991, pp. 1–21.
16. Dodrill, C.B. and Batzel, L.W., Interictal behavioral features of patients with epilepsy, *Epilepsia*, 27 (suppl 2) (1986) S64-S75.
17. Engel, J. Jr. and Rocha, L.L., Interictal behavioral disturbances: a search for molecular substrates, *Epilepsy Res.*, suppl 9 (1986) 341–350.
18. Fenwick, P., Aggression and epilepsy, In O. Devinsky and W.H. Theodore (Eds.), *Epilepsy and Behaviour*, Wiley-Liss, New York, 1991, pp. 85–96.
19. Gloor, P., Role of the amygdala in temporal lobe epilepsy, In J.P. Aggleton, (Ed.), *The Amygdala: Neurobiological Aspects of Emotion, Memory, and Mental Dysfunction*, Wiley-Liss, New York, 1992, pp. 505–538.

20. Grijalva, C.V., Levin, E.D., Morgan, M., Roland, B. and Martin, F.C., Contrasting effects of centromedial and basolateral amygdala lesions on stress-related responses in the rat, *Physiol. Behav.*, 48 (1990) 495–500.
21. Halgren, E., The amygdala contribution to emotion and memory: current studies in humans, In Y. Ben-Ari (Ed.), *The Amygdaloid Complex* , Elsevier, Amsterdam, 1981, pp. 395–408.
22. Helfer, V., Deransart, C., Marescaux, C. and Depaulis, A., Amygdala kindling in the rat: Anxiogenic-like consequences, *Neuroscience*, (1996).
23. Henke, P.G. and Sullivan, R.M., Kindling in the amygdala and susceptibility to stress ulcers, *Brain Res. Bull.*, 400 (1985) 360–364.
24. Hitchcock, J. and Davis, M., Lesions of the amygdala, but not of the cerebellum or red nucleus, block conditioned fear as measured with the potentiated startle system, *Behav. Neurosci.*, 100 (1986) 11–22.
25. Hirtz, D.G. and Nelson, K.B., Cognitive effects of antiepileptic drugs., In T.A. Pedley and B.S. Meldrum (Eds.), *Recent Advances in Epilepsy, vol 2,* Churchhill Livingstone, London, 1985, pp. 161–182.
26. Holmes, G.L., Chronopoulos, A., Stafstrom, C.E., Mikati, M.A., Thurber, S.J., Hyde, P.A. and Thompson, J.L., Effects of kindling on subsequent learning, memory, behaviour, and seizure susceptibility, *Dev. Brain Res.*, 73 (1993) 71–77.
27. Kalynchuk, L.E., Pinel, J.P.J., Treit, D. and Kippin, T.E., Changes in emotional behaviour produced by long-term amygdala kindling in rats, *Biol. Psychiatry*, in press.
28. Kapp, B.S., Frysinger, R.C., Gallagher, M. and Haselton, J.R., Amygdala central nucleus lesions: Effects on heart rate conditioning in the rabbit, *Physiol. Behav.*, 23 (1979) 1109–1117.
29. LeDoux, J.E., The amygdala: contributions to fear and stress, *Sem Neurosci.*, 6 (1994) 231–237.
30. Letty, S., Lerner-Natoli, M. and Rondouin, G., Differential impairments of spatial memory and social behaviour in two models of limbic epilepsy, *Epilepsia*, 36 (1995) 973–982.
31. Lloyd, R.L., Kling, A.S. and Ricci, O., Amygdaloid kindling in the squirrel monkey: Relation to temporal lobe epilepsy and schizophrenia, *Neurosci. Res. Comm.*, 5 (1989) 53–61.
32. Löscher, W., Jackel, R. and Czuczwar, S.J., Is amygdala kindling in rats a model for drug-resistant partial epilepsy? *Exp. Neurol.*, 93 (1986) 211–226.
33. Nieminen, S.A., Sirvio, J., Teittinen, K., Pitkanen, A., Airaksinen, M.M. and Riekkinen, P., Amygdala kindling increased fear-response, but did not impair spatial memory in rats, *Physiol. Behav.*, 51 (1992) 845–849.
34. Pinel, J.P.J., Spontaneous kindled motor seizures in rats, In J.A. Wada (Ed.), *Kindling 2*, Raven Press, New York, 1981, pp. 179–187.
35. Pinel, J.P.J., Kalynchuk, L.E. and Treit, D., Amygdala kindling produces more "defensive" behavior than hippocampal or caudate kindling in rats, *Soc. for Neurosci. Abstr.*, 21 (1995) 2114.
36. Pinel, J.P.J., Treit, D. and Rovner, L., Temporal lobe aggression in rats, *Science,* 197 (1977) 1088–1089.
37. Racine, R.J. and Burnham, W.M., The kindling model. In P.A. Schwartzkroin and H.V. Wheal (Eds.), *The electrophysiology of epilepsy,* Academic Press, New York, 1984, pp. 153–171.
38. Rosen, J.B., Hamerman, E., Sitcoske, M., Glowa, J.R. and Schulkin, J., Hyperexcitability: Exaggerated fear-potentiated startle produced by partial amygdala kindling, *Behavioral Neuroscience*, 110 (1996) 43–50.
39. Scharfman, H.E. and Schwartzkroin, P.A., Responses of cells of the rat fascia dentata to prolonged stimulation of the perforant path: sensitivity of hilar cells and changes in granule cell citability, *Neuroscience,* 35 (1990) 491–504.
40. Siegel, A., Anatomical and functional differentiation within the amygdala: Behavioral state modulation, In R. Bandler (Ed.), *Modulation of sensorimotor activity during alterations in behavioral states*, Alan R. Liss, New York, 1984, pp. 299–324.
41. Sloviter, R.S., Decreased hippocampal inhibition and a selective loss of interneurons in experimental epilepsy, *Science,* 235 (1987) 73–77.
42. Sutula, T.P., Experimental models of temporal lobe epilepsy: new insights from the study of kindling and synaptic reorganization, *Epilepsia,* 31 (1990) S45-S54.
43. Wasterlain, C.G. and Shirasaka, Y., Seizures, brain damage and brain development, *Brain Dev.*, 16 (1994) 279–295.
44. Weiss, S.R.B., Post, R.M., Gold, P.W., Chrousos, G., Sullivan, T.L., Walker, D. and Pert, A., CRF-induced seizures and behavior: Interaction with amygdala kindling, *Brain Res.*, 372, (1986) 345–351.

DISCUSSION OF JOHN PINEL'S PAPER

D. McIntyre: John, do you make a predetermination as to which rat is going to be kindled? In the real world, of course, animals tend to be either dominant or not, as you indicated.

J. Pinel: No, it's just random.

D. McIntyre: I wondered the ease with which you could take a very aggressive animal and turn it into a defensive one.

J. Pinel: We don't do pretesting on them. The problem with a lot of these tests is that if you test them more than once you start to have complicated things happening because of the repeated testing. We certainly get very clear results just by random assignment. It might be interesting to do so though.

D. McIntyre: Yes, if an animal loses an encounter, very often it is a different animal.

A. Depaulis: Maybe just a suggestion. I don't think that you measured 22–28 kHz ultrasonic vocalizations here?

J. Pinel: No we haven't.

A. Depaulis: I would strongly suggest to you to do so because then there would be a nice confirmation of the defensive nature of the pre-defensiveness that you could measure. What is also interesting is that during the afterdischarge you have production of ultrasonic vocalizations as well, in the same range. So I was wondering if there was some relationship between these two kinds of vocalizations?

J. Wada: I have a quick question for you, John. Which side are the animals kindled on?

J. Pinel: Always on the left.

J. Wada: The left, good. Some time ago, we were interested in defensive behavior in kindled cats. There appears to be an arrest of defensive behaviours in stressful situations. What we have done in cats is kindled in the left amygdala, and before kindling we measured the threshold of the hypothalamic rage. We found a bit of a change. Then we measured after the secondary site was kindled and found a steady decrease after three months of secondary site stimulation. If you identify which side is first kindled and then go to the secondary site, what do you see as the consequences of that?

J. Pinel: I didn't do that. Only one side was kindled.

B. Adamec: If the speculation that I made about the anterior/posterior plane differences in the central nucleus may answer your question, then at least in the rodent I would expect that if you found a site that increased in anxiolytic effects in the left side and then kindled the right side in a comparable anxiogenic area that you might end up with no effect at all. They might cancel each other out. The speculation that I have about the central nucleus is that it may be spreading to engage anterior and posterior systems that mediate opposite behavioural effects.

K. Gale: From what you described, you were looking at kindling of the intruder animal. What happens if you do the kindling of the resident?

J. Pinel: We have done that. We have looked at the tapes, they haven't been scored yet, but mainly it's quite boring. Usually the resident will attack, but when the resident is kindled and you put in the intruder, the resident just kind of stays away from it and not too much happens.

K. Gale: So you actually lose the resident attacks?

J. Pinel: Yes.

W. M. Burnham: Just a comment. First of all, the emotionality that we see after multiple ECS has the same effect as what you are describing. I'm a little confused about one thing, though. Bob Adamec said that the left side is anxiolytic, and you find that it is anxiogenic. You are applying stimulation three times a day or more. Is it possible that you are affecting the system as though you are lesioning it in some way?

J. Pinel: In our experiments where we have looked at some 20 stimulations, we get a small anxiogenic effect with 20, and with subsequent stimulation it just gets bigger and bigger.

26

THE NEUROBEHAVIORAL CONSEQUENCES OF KINDLING

Theresa D. Hernandez, Lisa A. Warner, and Sylvia Montañez

Department of Psychology
Campus Box 345
The University of Colorado
Boulder, Colorado 80304

1. BACKGROUND

Diverse neural alterations are responsible for and a consequence of seizures, epileptogenesis and epilepsy. Many of these changes are transient and tied to the seizures, themselves, while others are more permanent in nature and thought to reflect the long-term epileptogenic state. Seizures are characterized by the sudden and excessive discharge of neuronal activity [42]; epileptogenesis is the process by which distinct seizure events increase the likelihood of recurrence; epilepsy is the resulting disorder of recurrent seizures. The behavioral disturbances that are associated with each of these in certain measures of learning, memory and cognition have been fairly well characterized [9, 10, 22, 49, 52, 54, 55, 60]. The bulk of the data, however, has been collected from non-brain injured subjects with epilepsy (in the case of humans) or experimentally-induced models of epilepsy (in the case of animals). Much scarcer are studies assessing the neurobehavioral consequences of seizures or epileptogenesis following brain damage [3, 19], and their impact on functional recovery [20, 24, 39, 40]. Depending upon the severity, brain injuries carry a degree of risk for post-traumatic seizures (i.e., non-recurrent seizure(s) following brain injury) and post-traumatic epilepsy (i.e., recurrent seizures that cannot be linked to causes other than the brain injury). These issues are significant given the high incidence of brain injury each year, 1.5–2 million [44, 69] and the overall increase in survival rates following brain injury [70]. At the same time, fire-arm associated mortal injuries now surpass those of motor vehicles [70]. This increase in the type of brain injuries (e.g., penetrating missile type) that carry the highest risk for post-traumatic epilepsy translates into more individuals with both brain damage-associated morbidity and a high propensity for post-traumatic epilepsy. Of necessity in this situation is a better understanding of the functional consequences of seizures, epileptogenesis and epilepsy after brain injury, as well as the impact of those treatment strategies aimed at their prevention (e.g., anti-convulsant prophylaxis). This is a particularly important means by which to study epilepsy given that structural abnormalities are so prevalent a cause for this

Kindling 5, edited by Corcoran and Moshé.
Plenum Press, New York, 1998.

disorder [28, 35]. Only with such discovery can post-injury treatment practices be advanced to the point of having no significant functional cost to the organism.

1.1. Developing a Model

To study these issues in humans would be optimal. However, ethical and practical concerns make this difficult, except via retrospective studies. Addressing these issues in animals and developing a truly representative animal model of post-traumatic epilepsy poses quite a challenge. Because of the traumatic nature of most brain injuries, it is not necessarily desirable to exactly mimic this in animals. Moreover, reliably eliciting trauma-induced seizures is not easily accomplished. Willmore and colleagues [75] have proposed a model of post-traumatic epilepsy which utilizes intracortical injections of iron to produce persistent epileptiform discharges and histopathological alterations that bear resemblance to the epileptic foci in humans. It is advantageous in that it allows for the induction of a chronic epileptic focus by methods thought to parallel events that occur after brain injury in humans, yet because the seizures are spontaneous, it is difficult to measure the impact of distinct seizure events on behavioral function. While there may be no exact way in which to model post-traumatic epilepsy, it is still possible to determine the degree to which differing levels of seizure activity and epileptogenesis affect recovery from behavioral deficits and how the seizure-associated changes in recovery are affected by anti-convulsant administration. This has been successfully accomplished in our laboratory by combining two experimentally-induced events, i.e., focal brain damage via cortical lesion and focal epileptogenesis via electrical kindling [40]. Certain criteria have been identified that strengthen the validity of this model. First, the region of the brain that is damaged, the anteromedial cortex, produces behavioral deficits similar to those seen in humans and is measured using analogous techniques to those utilized in humans. Second, electrical kindling is an extremely well characterized model of epileptogenesis. Finally, the combination of these two allows for experimental control over the type, severity and number of seizures that occur after brain damage. Using this model, we have begun to delineate the functional consequences of seizures and epileptogenesis after brain damage and how these patterns are altered by anti-convulsant administrations.

1.1.1. Anteromedial Cortex Lesion. The electrolytic lesion technique, while a very "old" or traditional method [67] of inducing damage, remains advantageous for a variety of reasons. It is more reliable than the suction method in yielding hemorrhage-free cortical lesions of relatively uniform shape and size in both the horizontal and vertical dimensions ([7] and unpublished observation). Such lesions create focal and complete neuronal loss. Thus, in contrast to contusion models that tend to produce more diffuse damage, focal brain lesions offer the capability of answering questions about localized behavioral deficits relating to the area of injury. In addition, when accomplished with a stainless steel electrode, there is a certain amount of iron deposited in the region of damage which mimics the type of damage most prone to post-traumatic epilepsy.

There are many cortical regions from which to choose as a potential lesion site. The region of interest with which we have begun our investigations, the anteromedial cortex [6], has been particularly fruitful (see Figure 1). The region includes the medial precentral, pre-limbic, medial agranular and anterior cingulate cortices [4]. Damage to this region produces deficits that can be readily assessed in rats using tests analogous to those used in patients with frontal or parietal cortex lesions (i.e., the method of 'simultaneous extinction') [68]. Recovery from the lesion-induced somatosensory asymmetries occurs within a

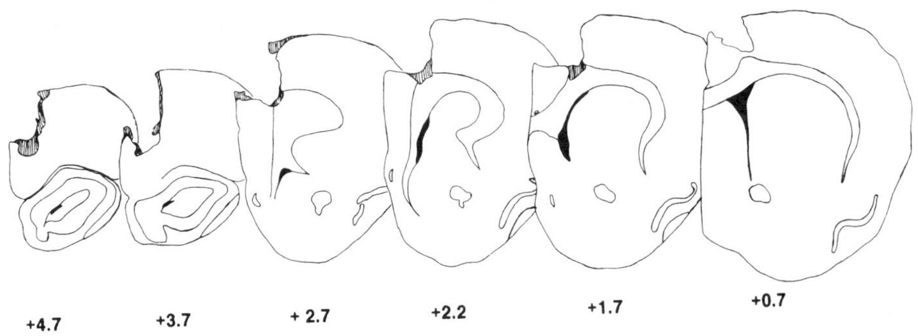

Figure 1. Representative tracing of a unilateral anteromedial cortex lesion at several coordinates relative to bregma (in mm, based on [59]).

reasonably short period of time (3–4 weeks) which makes alterations in the recovery pattern (i.e., facilitation or retardation) detectable. By contrast, lesions of the sensorimotor cortex in rat also produce somatosensory deficits, yet it typically takes the animal at least 60 days to recover from these deficits. Consequently, even though facilitated recovery is easily measured after sensorimotor cortex lesions, this long recovery pattern does not lend itself to studies of delayed recovery. The recovery pattern after anteromedial cortex lesions has already been shown to be very sensitive to pharmacological intervention [36, 64] and a critical period has been identified as being a minimum of 12–96h(4d) and a maximum of 6 days [38].

1.1.2. Assessment of Behavioral Deficits and Recovery: Tactile Extinction. The method of 'simultaneous extinction' when used in humans following stroke has been found to be one of the best predictors of ultimate functional outcome [63]. The bilateral tactile stimulation tests, which are the tactile extinction analog for animals, are unique in that these assess somatosensory asymmetries reliably and rapidly in the home cage [66] and can be used in rats [64], as well as in non-human primates [2]. In using this test with rats, animals are removed from the home cage and equally sized pieces of adhesive-backed paper (1/2 in; 113 mm^2) are placed bilaterally and simultaneously on the radial aspect of each forepaw. Upon return to the home cage, rats will typically contact and remove each adhesive stimulus, one at a time, with their teeth. Rats with unilateral brain damage typically contact and remove the stimulus ipsilateral to the lesion first, before contacting and removing the contralateral stimulus. All rats with an ipsilateral asymmetry (i.e., on greater than 70% of the trials the ipsilateral stimulus was contacted first) are given an additional test in which the magnitude of their asymmetry is measured. In this more sensitive test, the size of the contralateral stimulus is progressively increased and the size of the ipsilateral stimulus is simultaneously decreased by an equal amount (14.1 mm^2). With sufficient increase in the contralateral/ipsilateral ratio, an ipsilateral bias can be reversed, such that the rat will no longer respond preferentially to the stimulus ipsilateral to the lesion, and will instead, preferentially contact the stimulus contralateral to the lesion first. The contralateral/ipsilateral size ratio necessary to reverse a response bias reflects the magnitude of asymmetry. Each incremental change in the contralateral/ipsilateral size ratio corresponds to a number or "level" from 1–7, with stimuli of equal size considered as level 0. For each level, the adhesive stimulus pairs have a predetermined contralateral/ipsilateral size ratio: level 1=1.3/1; level 2=1.7/1; level 3=2.2/1; level 4=3/1; level 5=4.3/1; level 6=7/1; and level 7=15/1. As an example, if a rat has an asymmetry magnitude of 4.0, then the contralateral stimulus needs to be more than three times the size of the ipsilateral stimulus in order to reverse the ipsilateral response bias. This latter test provides a more sensitive measure of somatosensory asymmetry for two reasons. First, the initial post-lesion contralateral/ipsilateral ratio necessary to reverse an ipsilateral bias is proportional to the degree of brain damage, and second, as an animal recovers, the size of the contralateral stimulus necessary to reverse an ipsilateral bias, decreases [5, 65, 66]. An animal is said to be "recovered" when it no longer exhibits an ipsilateral response bias that is different from sham operated controls, which typically fluctuate between a magnitude of 0 and 0.5 (unpublished observation).

1.1.3. Amygdala Kindling. Kindling refers to the brief, repeated electrical stimulation of particular brain regions that initially produces only epileptiform afterdischarge, yet no convulsive behavior; however, over days there is a progressive increase in both the convulsions and seizure activity [31]. Amygdala kindling has been proposed as a suitable animal model of certain types of epilepsy [1, 50, 51, 53]. Electrical kindling of the amygdala is a useful means by which to produce post-lesion epileptogenesis and is preferable over chemical kindling because this latter methodology would add another pharmacological variable that might make interpretation of the studies in which anti-convulsants are utilized difficult. In addition, amygdala kindling has been shown to produce highly reproducible, long-term changes in several aspects of neural function that correlate well with given seizure stages (for review see [14, 61]). Perhaps the greatest advantage is that amygdala kindling allows for the study of individual kindled seizures of distinct types, acquisition of kindled seizure susceptibility (i.e., epileptogenesis) and the "state" of kindled seizure susceptibility (i.e., the resulting, relatively stable state of increased seizure susceptibility) [61]. Consequently, the impact of each of these can be correlated with changes in behavioral recovery.

In our laboratory, kindling occurs in the home cage and consists of a 1-s train of 100 Hz biphasic square waves, each 1 ms in duration. This always follows the bilateral tactile stimulation tests in order to minimize the effects of post-ictal depression on behavioral measures. The stimulus current for kindled rats (100–300μA, base-to-peak) is one that elicits an afterdischarge (i.e., post-stimulation epileptiform neuronal activity). Duration of EEG seizure activity, or afterdischarge, is recorded each day that the rat was stimulated. Assessment of behavioral convulsions are recorded and rated on a scale adapted from Racine's stages of behavioral seizures [62]: Stage 0=immobility; Stage 1=robust chewing or jaw clonus; Stage 2=head nodding; Stage 3=bilateral forelimb clonus; Stage 4=rearing onto hindlimbs with full extension of the spine while maintaining balance and/or righting reflex; and Stage 5=rearing and loss of righting reflex.

2. KINDLED SEIZURES AND FUNCTIONAL RECOVERY

Prior to these studies, only chemically- or electrically-induced seizures had been elicited after brain lesion and functional recovery assessed: recovery from somatosensory and motor deficits was improved [24, 39]. While these studies are suggestive, they may not mimic the type of seizure activity that would occur after brain damage, i.e., endogenous electrically-induced seizures with varying degrees of epileptogenicity. In order to study this, we have elicited distinct seizure stages (Stage 0, 1 or 5) during the post-lesion critical period [40, 73]. Animals (Stage 0 and Stage 1 groups) sustained unilateral electrolytic lesions of the anteromedial cortex in the same surgery in which an electrode was implanted into the ipsilateral amygdala. Amygdala kindling began forty-eight hours later and always took place after behavioral testing. Kindling was initiated at this time because it is within the "critical period" after anteromedial cortex lesions during which the recovery process has been found to be particularly vulnerable to pharmacological intervention [36, 38]. This delay was also chosen because of our desire to begin initiating seizure activity as soon as possible after brain lesion without interfering with ultimate lesion size, which appears to reach a peak at approximately 24 hours after surgery [76]. Furthermore, we have seen no difference in rate of kindling and seizure threshold when kindling began 48 hours after lesion, as compared to beginning 7 days after lesion (unpublished observation). To elicit Stage 1 seizure activity this soon after lesion, animals were stimulated 2–3 times on the first day of kindling, twice on the second day of kindling and once daily thereafter until each responded with a Stage 5 seizure. Animals in the Stage 0 group were stimulated no more than twice on the first day of kindling and once per day thereafter until a Stage 5 seizure was provoked. A slightly different procedure was required to elicit Stage 5 seizures within the first six days after cortex lesion: animals were kindled to a Stage 5 *prior to* anteromedial cortex lesion and then stimulated once per day for a total of 7 days beginning 48h after lesion. As a control for this dual surgery procedure and to determine if kindling to Stage 5 prior to brain lesion affects recovery, a group of animals was pre-kindled to a Stage 5 *prior to* lesion, but then experienced no seizure activity during the critical period [73]. This dual surgery procedure had no effect on functional recovery.

2.1. Electrical Kindling after Brain Lesion

As can be seen in Figure 2, all animals in the Early Stage 1 group responded with at least one reliable Stage 1 seizure on or before post-operative day 6. In contrast, animals in

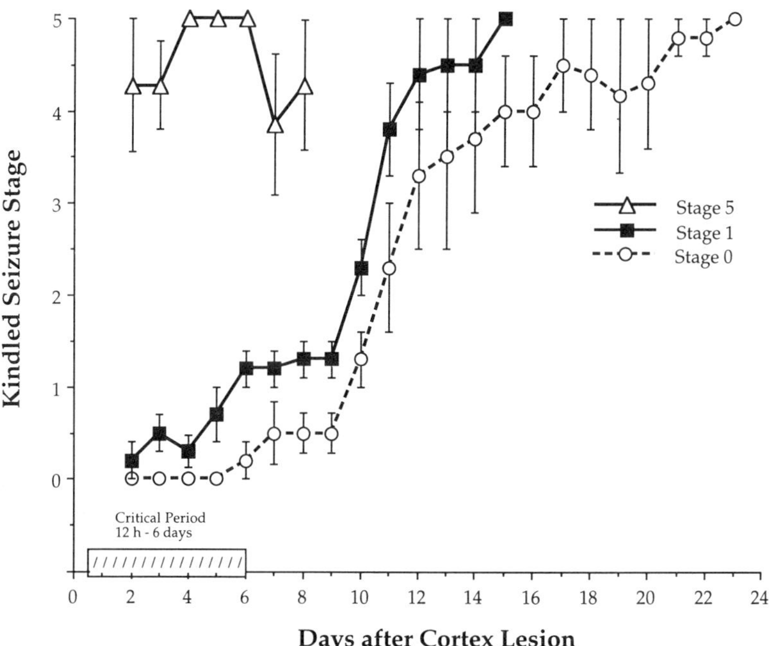

Figure 2. Average (±SEM) kindled seizure stage exhibited on days after surgery in the Stage 0, Stage 1 and Stage 5 groups. Group assignment was based on the seizure stage that occurred during the post-lesion critical period (12 h–6 days after lesion).

the Early Stage 0 group only exhibited reliable Stage 0 seizures during the first 6 days after surgery and did not respond with Stage 1 seizures until after post-operative day 6. All rats in the Daily Stage 5 group responded with a Stage 5 seizure on at least 4 of the 7 days of post-lesion stimulation, and only 2 out of the 7 animals had sub-convulsive seizure activity on at least 1 day of stimulation.

All animals exhibited characteristic AD in response to kindling stimuli and the duration of it invariably increased over days. Within the critical period of 6 days after lesion, the range of cumulative AD in animals in the Stage 0 and Stage 1 groups (combined) was 88–402 seconds. Because of technical difficulties with these particular groups, the differences in AD between groups could not be assessed. In the Stage 5 group, however, there were no such technical difficulties and the cumulative AD duration (mean in seconds ± S.E.M.) during this same critical post-lesion period was 408 ± 40.51 (range = 295–547 seconds).

2.2. Recovery from Somatosensory Deficits after Lesion: Seizure Stage and Outcome

As can be seen in Figure 3, kindled seizures had distinct effects on behavioral recovery depending upon which seizure stage occurred during the post-lesion critical period. Non-kindled animals recovered between 35 and 63 days, and this was not significantly different from the group experiencing daily Stage 5 seizure activity during that same post-lesion period. In contrast, Stage 1 seizure activity during the critical period appeared to prevent functional recovery during 4 months of testing (behavioral data from months 3 and 4 not shown in figure). Finally, Stage 0 seizure activity had no statistically significant

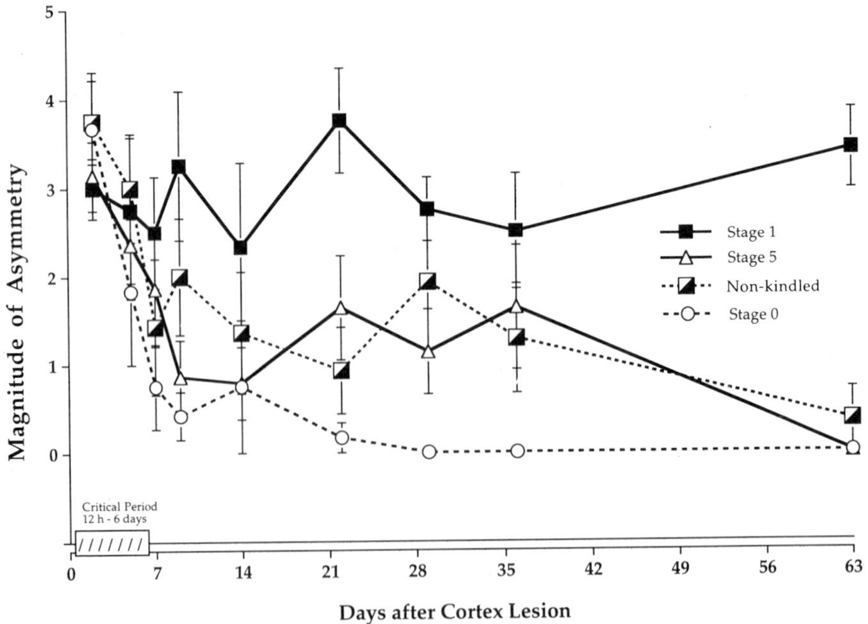

Figure 3. Average (±SEM) magnitude of somatosensory asymmetry is plotted as a function of days after unilateral anteromedial cortex lesions in three groups of kindled rats. Those that experienced Stage 0, Stage 1 or Stage 5 seizure activity during the post-lesion critical period. Post-lesion Day 2 was the first day of kindling and kindling always occurred after behavioral testing.

impact on functional recovery compared to non-kindled controls. Animals in this former group recovered from somatosensory deficits in approximately 3 weeks of testing.

On the first day of testing (Day 2), all groups exhibited an equivalent lesion-induced magnitude of asymmetry (mean ± SEM): 3.7 ± 0.64 = Stage 0; 3.0 ± 0.34 = Stage 1; 3.14 ± 0.39 = Stage 5 and 3.75 ± 0.47 = Nonkindled. With this degree of asymmetry, the contralateral stimulus needed to be at least 3 times as large as the simultaneously applied ipsilateral stimulus in order to reverse an ipsilateral bias in all groups. By Day 7, however, the Stage 0 group showed a marked decrease in asymmetry magnitude (0.75 ±0.48) and by Day 22, this group had recovered (0.17 ± 0.17) to the level of sham operated controls (unpublished observation). This recovery was stable and enduring through 63 days of testing. Animals in the Nonkindled group, however, continued to exhibit a significant degree of asymmetry up to 35 days of testing (1.3 ± 0.61), yet by post-operative Day 56 (data not shown in figure), they too had recovered (0.78 ± 0.57). This is similar to the recovery pattern seen in the Stage 5 group which recovered within 42 days (0.75 ± 0.38). In contrast to these groups, the Stage 1 group continued to display a significant magnitude of asymmetry at Day 63 (3.4 ± 0.45) and through 4 months after lesion (data not shown in figure) this group exhibited a significant degree of asymmetry (2.17 ± 0.78). Therefore, recurrent Stage 0 or Stage 5 seizure activity during the post-lesion critical period had no detrimental impact on behavioral recovery, and yet as few as a single Stage 1 during this same time after lesion completely interfered with recovery during 4 months of testing.

2.3. Discussion

Kindled seizures can have distinct effects on functional recovery depending upon kindled seizure type [40]. Stage 1 kindled seizures occurring within a sensitive period of 6 days following anteromedial cortex lesion prevented recovery from somatosensory deficits. Conversely, Stage 0 kindled seizure activity occurring within this same period had no significant impact on recovery. Based on these results, we hypothesized that Stage 1 kindled seizures were detrimental to recovery due to the plastic epileptogenic process that underlies this type of seizure activity and not to the seizures themselves. In support of this is our finding that kindling to Stage 5 seizure prior to cortex lesion has no significant impact on recovery and daily fully kindled seizures during the post-lesion critical period are not detrimental to recovery from cortex lesion. This seems particularly striking given that as few as a single Stage 1 seizure during the same time period completely disrupted recovery. In fact, Stage 5 seizures were more similar to Stage 0 in that neither was deleterious to recovery. Therefore, it seems that the severity of amygdala-kindled seizures during the critical period is not the key factor in whether recovery can occur unimpeded. Instead, it is the degree to which seizures are potentially epileptogenic in nature that determines whether recovery is affected. That is, recurrent Stage 0 or Stage 5 seizures did not affect recovery because they may be less epileptogenic or the changes they elicit are slower than those brought about by Stage 1 seizures.

3. KINDLED SEIZURES, PHENOBARBITAL, AND FUNCTIONAL RECOVERY

The administration of certain anti-convulsants after brain lesion appears to delay or prevent functional recovery. Diazepam [37, 64] and phenobarbital [36] have each been found to impede recovery from somatosensory deficits in animals following cortex lesion.

Phenytoin [20] administration after brain injury in humans is associated with impaired neurobehavioral function as measured on a battery of neuropsychological tests. In the studies of animals, there was no evidence of seizure activity, suggesting that in the absence of post-lesion seizures, anti-convulsant administration may be a detriment. What is not known from these studies is the impact of these drugs on functional recovery when seizure activity does occur. We have some data addressing these issues. Following electrolytic lesions of the anteromedial cortex, animals experienced Stage 0 seizure activity during the post-lesion critical period of 6 days coupled with a 7-day phenobarbital regimen. As in all of our studies, behavioral testing always occurred prior to any drug treatments or kindling. Phenobarbital or saline was injected twice daily (30 mg/kg a.m. and 15 mg/kg p.m.) beginning either 1 hour prior to or after amygdala kindling. This dose regimen was chosen because it has been found to delay functional recovery and should yield phenobarbital levels at or above the high therapeutic range of 45–85 ng/ml throughout the treatment period, with a relatively steady state (80–85 ng/ml) achieved within the first three days of drug treatment. Thus, the goal of this study was to determine if phenobarbital, at relatively constant anti-convulsant levels, altered the recovery pattern associated with Stage 0 seizure activity after lesion.

3.1. The Effects of Phenobarbital on Electrical Kindling after Brain Lesion

All animals, regardless of drug treatment, experienced Stage 0 seizure activity during the first 6 days after lesion (see Figure 4). As was expected, phenobarbital administration delayed kindled seizure progression to Stage 5 and had its most significant impact

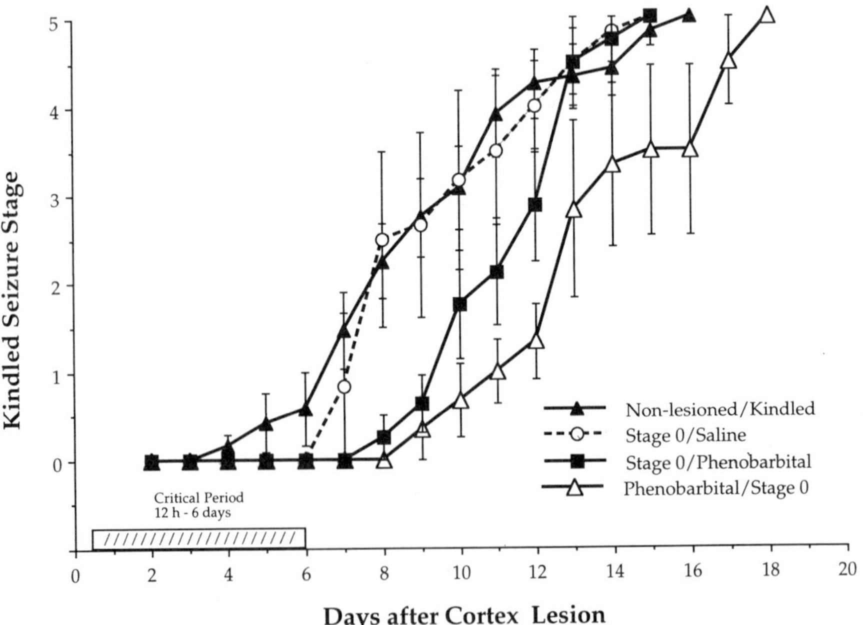

Figure 4. Average (±SEM) kindled seizure stage exhibited on days after surgery in kindled animals experiencing Stage 0 seizure activity coupled with phenobarbital administration 1 hour prior to (phenobarbital/Stage 0) or after (Stage 0/phenobarbital) kindling stimulation. While animals were kindled to Stage 5, the phenobarbital regimen was only 7 days. Also included are two groups of kindled controls: those that did not receive the drug (Stage 0/saline) or were not lesioned (non-lesioned/kindled).

when administered *prior to* kindling stimulation. Nonetheless, all animals eventually responded with a Stage 5 seizure within 17 days after lesion.

There were no differences in the cumulative AD duration (mean in seconds ± S.E.M.) experienced by each group during the first 6 days after lesion: Stage 0/saline = 55.17 ± 4.84; Stage 0/phenobarbital = 52.25 ± 3.53 and Phenobarbital/stage 0 = 44.0 ± 5.30.

3.2. The Effects of Phenobarbital on Seizure-Associated Recovery Patterns

Phenobarbital administration coupled with post-lesion Stage 0 seizure activity interfered with functional recovery (see Figure 5). In agreement with the results outlined above, animals in the Stage 0/saline group recovered from somatosensory deficits within about 3 weeks. By comparison, phenobarbital administration *after* Stage 0 seizure activity delayed functional recovery to approximately 63 days. In contrast, when phenobarbital was injected *before* kindling stimulation, recovery from somatosensory deficits was prevented during the 63 days of testing.

All groups exhibited an equivalent lesion-induced magnitude of asymmetry (mean ± S.E.M.) on the first day of testing (Day 2): phenobarbital/Stage 0 = 3.083 ± 0.327, Stage 0/phenobarbital = 3.438 ± 0.651 and Stage 0/saline = 3.667 ± 0.459. There was a dramatic decrease in this asymmetry magnitude in the Stage 0/saline group such that they had recovered by Day 23 (0.33 ± 0.61). The Stage 0/phenobarbital group did not fully recovery to the level of asymmetry of sham operated controls until Day 63 (0.19 ± 0.19). Finally, phenobarbital administration prior to daily kindling stimulation appeared to prevent func-

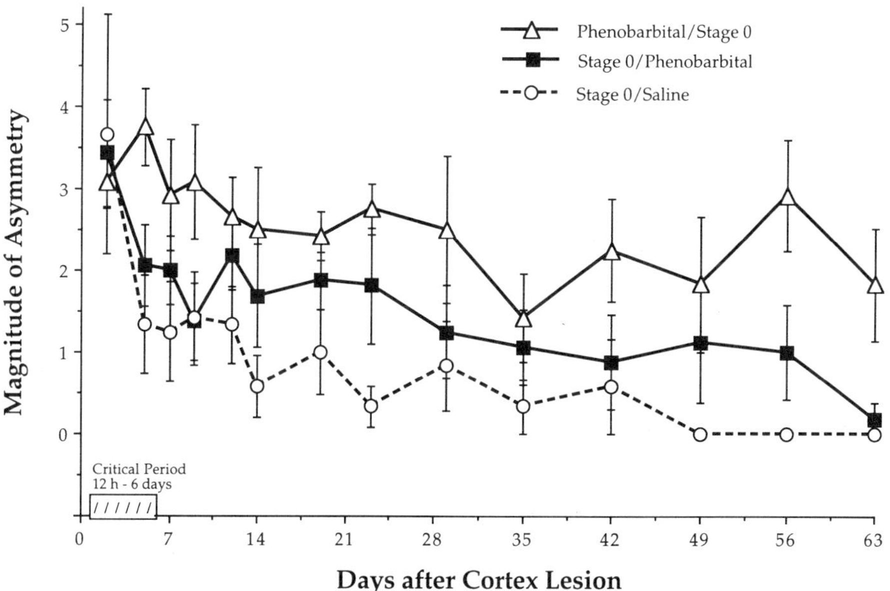

Figure 5. Average (±SEM) magnitude of somatosensory asymmetry is plotted as a function of days after unilateral anteromedial cortex lesions in three groups of kindled rats. Those that experienced Stage 0 seizure activity coupled with phenobarbital administration 1 hour prior to (phenobarbital/Stage 0) or after (Stage 0/phenobarbital) kindling stimulation. Also included is a group of non-drugged, kindled controls (Stage 0/saline). Kindling and/or drug administration always occurred after behavioral testing.

tional recovery in that the phenobarbital/Stage 0 group maintained a significant deficit even 63 days after lesion (1.83 ± 0.69).

3.3. Discussion

The anti-convulsant phenobarbital was capable of reversing the neutral effect of post-lesion Stage 0 seizure activity to the point of blocking recovery. However, this only occurred when phenobarbital was injected before electrical kindling. When phenobarbital was injected after Stage 0 seizure activity, the recovery pattern was delayed, but not prevented. A possible explanation for these differences may be in neurochemical changes brought forth by the kindling process itself coupled with phenobarbital levels present in the brain. Indeed, various neurotransmitters have been implicated in the process of epileptogenesis, but we have focused on the role of GABA. One hypothesis brought forth is that as epileptogenesis is established, GABA mediated inhibition is activated but subsequently collapses while the excitatory system is intensified gradually [46, 57]. Therefore, the balance between excitation and inhibition systems are disrupted as the kindling process is established. In line with the above hypothesis, as a result of kindling, an enhanced release of GABA would compensate for the recurrent depolarization. Enhanced GABA release has been observed in fully [21, 45, 46] and some partially kindled animals [21]. Thus, in the phenobarbital/Stage 0 group, kindled seizure-associated increases in GABA levels would coincide with phenobarbital-induced potentiation of GABA (which peaks 1 hour after injection). This potentiation of GABA would be greater than that of phenobarbital alone, explaining why recovery in the phenobarbital/Stage 0 group was not simply delayed, but prevented. In contrast, when kindling occurs before phenobarbital administration (Stage 0/phenobarbital group), any kindling-associated potentiation of GABA would not coincide with peak phenobarbital levels in the brain. Hence, in this latter group, recovery is only delayed.

4. GENERAL DISCUSSION

It has been found that following brain injury, neural function is vulnerable to manipulation which can alter behavioral recovery patterns. Of particular import in this regard is the state of post-traumatic neural depression [23, 71] that has been characterized metabolically, neurochemically and electrophysiologically after brain damage [11, 13, 16, 27, 41, 47, 56, 58]. This state of neural depression has been correlated with certain behavioral deficits, and recovery from those deficits has been correlated with the re-establishment of normal neuronal activity [17, 29, 30]. Pharmacological manipulations (e.g., diazepam, phenobarbital, phenytoin, haloperidol) that augment this neural depression and in general depress neural function, have been found to delay functional recovery in laboratory [12, 25, 36–38, 64, 74] and clinical [20, 32, 34] studies. One possible mechanism by which functional recovery is impeded comes from studies with diazepam, which has been shown to augment the degree of subcortical degeneration that is seen following cortex lesions [43].

In contrast, those agents or interventions that produce post-injury central nervous system stimulation appear to improve functional recovery in animals [18, 25, 26, 39, 48, 72] and humans [15, 33]. Facilitation of recovery is thought to be linked to the rapid reversal or arrest of post-traumatic neural depression. For example, the chemoconvulsant pentylenetetrazol [39] and electroconvulsive shock [24] have each been shown to facilitate recovery from lesion-induced behavioral deficits. Based on this information, it has been hypothesized that central nervous system stimulation following brain damage may serve to counteract the post-traumatic neural depression that typically accompanies brain injury and that post-traumatic seizure activity may initially serve as an adaptive mechanism by which the brain attempts to counteract post-traumatic neural depression [64]. While this notion is an interesting one, it does not address the consequences of recurrent, epileptogenic seizures after brain injury. Our data suggest that this latter type of seizure activity may be indicative that this "adaptive" mechanism has gone awry and could be a significant detriment to the functional outcome of the organism.

5. UNANSWERED QUESTIONS

The question of the underlying mechanism(s) by which kindled seizures with and without anti-convulsants exert their distinct effects on functional recovery remains important. To this end, we are beginning to look at site specificity of both the kindling focus and lesion. Following damage, different regions of the cortex (anteromedial cortex and sensorimotor cortex) rely on the ipsilateral or contralateral cortices for functional recovery [4, 8]. With this in mind, we will electrically kindle both ipsilateral and contralateral structures, beginning with the amygdala, and measure functional recovery after regionally specific cortical lesions. In addition, we know that subcortical degeneration is enhanced by procedures that interfere with recovery [43]. Consequently, we are measuring such changes after different types of kindled seizures in brain lesioned animals. To better understand the degree to which our results are due to seizures vs. epileptogenesis, functional recovery will be measured in animals pre-kindled to various seizure stages prior to brain lesion. After this, behavioral recovery will be compared between groups that are pre-kindled only to a given stage and those that are kindled beyond that given stage during the post-lesion critical period. Finally, other anti-convulsants, particularly those that may not interfere with functional recovery in the absence of seizure activity, will be combined with amygdala kindling after brain lesion and behavioral recovery will be assessed.

6. CONCLUSIONS

Brain injury occurs frequently and at a significant cost to the individual and society. The morbidity associated with most brain injuries is only exacerbated by the presence of post-traumatic epilepsy and treatment with anti-convulsant drugs. A better understanding of how and why different types of seizures affect functional recovery is essential for improved treatment strategies that do both of the following for survivors of brain injury: minimize the occurrence of post-traumatic epilepsy and maximize functional outcome.

ACKNOWLEDGMENTS

We thank Tess Gasser and Anthony Kline for their able and talented technical assistance. This work was supported by NINDS Grant No. NS-30595 and the Alfred P. Sloan Foundation. TDH is an Alfred P. Sloan Research Fellow.

REFERENCES

1. Albright, P.S. and Burnham, W.M., Development of a new pharmacological seizure model: Effects of anti-convulsants on cortical- and amygdala-kindled seizures in the rat, *Epilepsia*, 21 (1980) 681–689.

2. Annet, L.E., Rogers, D.C., Hernandez, T.D. and Dunnett, S.B., Behavioural analysis of unilateral monoamine depletion in the marmoset, *Brain*, 115 (1992) 825–856.
3. Armstrong, K.K., Sahgal, V., Block, R., Armstrong, K.J. and Heinemann, A., Rehabilitation outcomes in patients with post-traumatic epilepsy, *Arch. Phys. Med. Rehab.*, 71 (1990) 156–160.
4. Barth, T.M., Jones, T.A. and Schallert, T., Functional subdivisions of the rat somatic sensorimotor cortex, *Behav. Brain Res.*, 39 (1990) 73–95.
5. Barth, T.M., Lindner, M.D. and Schallert, T., Sensorimotor asymmetries and tactile extinction in unilateral frontal cortex-damaged and striatal dopamine depleted rats, *Soc. Neurosci. Abstr.*, 9 (1983) 482.
6. Barth, T.M., Parker, S.M. and Sinnamon, H.M., Unilateral lesions of the anteromedial cortex in the rat impairs approach to contralateral visual cues, *Physiol. and Behav.*, 29 (1982) 141–147.
7. Barth, T.M. and Schallert, T., Somatosensorimotor function of the superior colliculus, somatosensory cortex and lateral hypothalamus in the rat, *Exper. Neurol.*, 95 (1987) 661–678.
8. Barth, T.M. and Stanfield, B.B., The recovery of forelimb-placing behavior in rats with neonatal unilateral cortical damage involves the remaining hemisphere, *J. Neurosci.*, 10 (1990) 3449–3459.
9. Becker, A., Grecksch, G., Rüthrich, H.-L., Pohle, W., Marx, B. and Matthies, H., Kindling and its consequences on learning in rats, *Behav. Neural Biol.*, 57 (1992) 37–43.
10. Beldhuis, H.J.A., Everts, G.J., Van der Zee, E.A., Luiten, P.G.M. and Bohus, B., Amygdala kindling-induced seizures selectively impair spatial memory. 1. Behavioral characteristics and effects on hippocampal neuronal protein kinase C isoforms, *Hippocampus*, 2 (1992) 397–410.
11. Boyeson, M.B. and Feeney, D.M., Striatal dopamine after cortical injury, *Exp. Neurol.*, 89 (1985) 479–483.
12. Brailowsky, S., Knight, R.T. and Efron, R., Phenytoin increases the severity of cortical hemiplegia in rats, *Brain Res.*, 376 (1986) 71–77.
13. Cooper, R.M. and Thurlow, G.A., 2-Deoxyglucose uptake in the thalamus of awake rats after neocortical ablations, *Exper. Neurol.*, 86 (1984) 261–267.
14. Corcoran, M.E., Characteristics and mechanisms of kindling. In: P. Kalivas and C. Barnes (Eds.), *Sensitization of the nervous system*, The Telford Press, Caldwell, N.J., 1988, 81–116.
15. Crisostomo, E.A., Duncan, P.W., Propst, M., Dawson, D.V. and Davis, J.N., Evidence that amphetamine with physical therapy promotes recovery of motor function in stroke patients, *Ann. Neurol.*, 23 (1988) 94–97.
16. Dauth, G.W., Gilman, S., Frey, K.A. and Penney, J.B., Basal ganglia glucose utilization after recent precentral ablation in the monkey, *Ann. Neurol.*, 17 (1985) 431–38.
17. Deuel, R.K. and Collins, R.C., The functional anatomy of frontal lobe neglect in the monkey: behavioral and quantitative 2-deoxyglucose studies, *Ann. Neurol.*, 15 (1984) 521–529.
18. Dietz, M.A. and McDowell, F.H., Potentiation of rehabilitation: medication effects on the recovery of function after brain injury and stroke, *J. Stroke Cerebrovasc. Dis.*, 1 (1991) 37–48.
19. Dikmen, S. and Reitan, R.M., Neuropsychological performance in posttraumatic epilepsy, *Epilepsia*, 19 (1978) 177–183.
20. Dikmen, S.S., Temkin, N.R., Miller, B., Machamer, J. and Winn, H.R., Neurobehavioral effects of phenytoin prophylaxis of posttraumatic seizures, *JAMA*, 265 (1991) 1271–1277.
21. During, M.J., Craig, J.S., Hernandez, T.D., Anderson, G.M. and Gallager, D.W., Effect of amygdala kindling on the in vivo release of GABA and 5-HT in the dorsal raphe nucleus of freely moving rats, *Brain Res.*, 584 (1992) 36–44.
22. Feasey-Truger, K.J., Kargl, L. and ten Bruggencate, G., Differential effects of dentate kindling on working and reference spatial memory in the rat, *Neurosci. Lett.*, 151 (1993) 25–28.
23. Feeney, D.M., Pharmacological modulation of recovery after brain injury: a reconsideration of diaschisis, *J. Neuro. Rehab.*, 5 (1991) 113–128.
24. Feeney, D.M., Bailey, B.Y., Boyeson, M.G., Hovda, D.A. and Sutton, R.L., The effects of seizures on recovery of function following cortical contusion in the rat, *Brain Injury*, 1 (1987) 27–32.
25. Feeney, D.M., Gonzalez, A. and Law, W.A., Amphetamine, haloperidol and experience interact to affect rate of recovery after motor cortex lesions, *Science*, 217 (1982) 855–857.
26. Feeney, D.M. and Sutton, R.L., Pharmacotherapy for recovery of function after brain injury, *CRC Crit. Rev. Neurobiol.*, 3 (1987) 135–197.
27. Feeney, D.M., Sutton, R.L., Boyeson, M.G., Hovda, D.A. and Dail, W.G., The locus coeruleus and cerebral metabolism: recovery of function after cortical injury, *Physiol. Psychol.*, 13 (1985) 197–203.
28. Forsgren, L., Bucht, G., Ericksson, S. and Bergmark, L., Incidence and clinical characterization of unprovoked seizures in adults: a prospective population-based study, *Epilepsia*, 37 (1996) 224–229.
29. Gilman, S., Dauth, G.W., Frey, K.A. and Penney Jr., J.B., Experimental hemiplegia in the monkey: basal ganglia glucose activity during recovery, *Ann. Neurol.*, 22 (1987) 370–376.
30. Glassman, R.B. and Malamut, D.L., Recovery from electroencephalographic slowing and reduced evoked potentials after somatosensory cortical damage in cats, *Behav. Biol.*, 17 (1976) 333–354.

31. Goddard, G.V., McIntyre, D.C. and Leech, C.K., A permanent change in brain function resulting from daily electrical stimulation, *Exp. Neurol.*, 25 (1969) 295–330.
32. Goldstein, L.B., Pharmacologic modulation of recovery after stroke: clinical data, *J. Neuro. Rehab.*, 5 (1991) 129–140.
33. Goldstein, L.B., Basic and clinical studies of pharmacological effects on recovery from brain injury, *J. Neur. Transplant. Plast.*, 4 (1993) 175–192.
34. Goldstein, L.B., Prescribing of potentially harmful drugs to patients admitted to hospital after head injury, *J. Neurol. Neurosurg. Psychiatry*, 58 (1995) 753–755.
35. Hauser, W.A., Annegers, J.F. and Kurland, L.T., Incidence of epilepsy and unprovoked seizures in Rochester, Minnesota: 1935–1984, *Epilepsia*, 34 (1993) 453–468.
36. Hernandez, T.D. and Holling, L.C., Disruption of behavioral recovery by the anticonvulsant phenobarbital, *Brain Res.*, 635 (1994) 300–306.
37. Hernandez, T.D., Jones, G.H. and Schallert, T., Co-administration of the benzodiazepine antagonist Ro 15–1788 prevents diazepam-induced retardation of recovery, *Brain Res.*, 487 (1989) 89–95.
38. Hernandez, T.D., Kiefel, J., Barth, T.M., Grant, M.L. and Schallert, T., Disruption and facilitation of recovery of function: implication of the gamma-aminobutyric acid/benzodiazepine receptor complex. In: M. Ginsberg and W.D. Dietrich (Eds.), *Cerebro-Vascular Diseases*, Raven Press, New York, 1989, 327–334.
39. Hernandez, T.D. and Schallert, T., Seizures and recovery from experimental brain damage, *Exper. Neurol.*, 102 (1988) 318–324.
40. Hernandez, T.D. and Warner, L.A., Kindled seizures during a critical post-lesion period exert a lasting impact on behavioral recovery, *Brain Res.*, 673 (1995) 208–216.
41. Hovda, D.A., Sutton, R.L. and Feeney, D.M., Recovery of tactile placing after visual cortex ablation in cat: a behavioral and metabolic study of diaschisis, *Exp. Neurol.*, 97 (1987) 391–402.
42. Jackson, J.H., On convulsive seizures. In: J. Taylor (Eds.), *Selected Writings of John Hughlings Jackson: On Epilepsy and Epileptiform Convulsions*, Basic Books, New York, 1958, 412–457.
43. Jones, T.A. and Schallert, T., Subcortical deterioration after cortical damage: effects of diazepam and relation to recovery of function, *Behav. Brain Res.*, 51 (1992) 1–13.
44. Kalsbeek, W.D., McLaurin, R.L., Harris, B.S.H. and Miller, J.D., Report on the national head and spinal cord injury survey, *J. Neurosurg.*, 53 (1980) 519–531.
45. Kamphuis, W., Huisman, E., Veerman, M.J. and Lopes da Silva, F.H., Development of changes in endogenous GABA release during kindling epileptogenesis in rat hippocampus, *Brain Res.*, 545 (1991) 33–40.
46. Kamphuis, W., Huisman, H., Dreijer, A.M.C., Ghijsen, W.E.J.M., Verhage, M. and Lopes da Silva, F.H., Kindling increases the K+-evoked Ca2+-dependent release of endogenous GABA in area CA1 of rat hippocampus, *Brain Res.*, 511 (1990) 63–70.
47. Kempinsky, W.H., Experimental study of distal effects of acute focal injury, *Arch. Neurol. Psychi.*, 79 (1958) 376–389.
48. Kline, A.E., Chen, M.J., Tso-Olivas, D.Y. and Feeney, D.M., Methylphenidate treatment following ablation-induced hemiplegia in rat: experience during drug action alters effects on recovery of function, *Pharmacol. Biochem. Behav.*, 48 (1994) 773–779.
49. Knowlton, B.J., Shapiro, M.L. and Olton, D.S., Hippocampal seizures disrupt working memory performance but not reference memory acquisitions, *Behav. Neurosci.*, 103 (1989) 1144–1147.
50. Löscher, W., Jäckel, R. and Czuczwar, S.J., Is amygdala kindling in rats a model for drug-resistant partial epilepsy?, *Exp. Neurol.*, 93 (1986) 211–226.
51. Löscher, W. and Schmidt, D., Which animal models should be used in the search for new antiepileptic drugs? A proposal based on experimental and clinical considerations, *Epilepsy Res.*, 2 (1988) 145–181.
52. McIntyre, D.C., Effect of focal vs. generalized kindled convulsions from anterior neocortex or amygdala on CER acquisition in rats, *Physiol. Behav.*, 23 (1979) 855–859.
53. McNamara, J.O., Bonhaus, D.W., Shin, C., Crain, B.J., Gellman, R.L. and Giacchino, J.L., The kindling model of epilepsy: a critical review, *CRC Crit. Rev. Clin. Neurobiol.*, 1 (1985) 341–391.
54. McNamara, R.K., Kirkby, R.D., dePape, G.E. and Corcoran, M.E., Limbic seizures, but not kindling, reversibly impair place learning in the Morris water maze, *Behav. Brain Research*, 50 (1992) 167–175.
55. McNamara, R.K., Kirkby, R.D., dePape, G.E., Skelton, R.W. and Corcoran, M.E., Differential effects of kindling and kindled seizures on place learning in the Morris water maze, *Hippocampus*, 3 (1993) 149–152.
56. Meyer, J.S., Shinohara, M., Kanda, T., Fukuuchi, Y., Ericson, A.D. and Kok, N.H., Diaschisis resulting from acute unilateral cerebral infarction, *Arch. Neurol.*, 23 (1970) 241–247.
57. Morimoto, K., Seizure-triggering mechanisms in the kindling model of epilepsy: collapse of GABA-mediated inhibition and activation of NMDA receptors, *Neurosci. Behav. Rev.*, 13 (1989) 253–260.
58. Pappius, H.M., Involvement of indoleamines in functional disturbances after brain injury, *Prog. Neuro-Psychopharmacol. & Biol Psychiat.*, 13 (1989) 353–61.

59. Paxinos, G. and Watson, C., *The Rat Brain in Stereotaxic Coordinates*, Academic Press, Sydney, 1986.
60. Peele, D.B. and Gilbert, M.E., Functional dissociation of acute and persistent cognitive deficits accompanying amygdala-kindled seizures, *Behav. Brain Research*, 48 (1992) 65–76.
61. Peterson, S.L. and Albertson, T.E., Neurotransmitter and neuromodulator function in the kindled seizure and state, *Prog. Neurobiol.*, 19 (1982) 237–270.
62. Racine, R.J., Modification of seizure activity by electrical stimulation: II. Motor seizure, *Electroenceph. Clin. Neurophysiol.*, 32 (1972) 281–294.
63. Rose, L., Bakal, D.A., Fung, T.S., Farn, P. and Weaver, L.E., Tactile extinction and functional status after stroke, *Stroke*, 25 (1994) 1973–1976.
64. Schallert, T., Hernandez, T.D. and Barth, T.M., Recovery of function after brain damage: severe and chronic disruption by diazepam, *Brain Res.*, 379 (1986) 104–111.
65. Schallert, T., Upchurch, M., Wilcox, R. and Vaughn, D.M., Posture independent sensorimotor analysis of inter-hemispheric receptor asymmetries in neostriatum, *Pharmacol. Biochem. Behav.*, 18 (1983) 753–759.
66. Schallert, T. and Whishaw, I.Q., Bilateral cutaneous stimulation of the somatosensory system in hemidecorticate rats, *Behav. Neurosci.*, 98 (1984) 518–540.
67. Schallert, T. and Wilcox, R.E., Neurotransmitter-selective brain lesions. In: A.A. Boulton and G.B. Baker (Eds.), *Neuromethods: Neurochemistry, General Techniques*, Humana Press, Clifton, N.J., 1985, 343–387.
68. Schwartz, A.S., Marchak, P.L., Kreinick, C.J. and Flynn, R.E., The asymmetric lateralization of the tactile extinction in patients with unilateral cerebral dysfunction, *Brain*, 102 (1979) 669–684.
69. Sosin, D.M., Sniezek, J.E. and Thurman, D.J., Incidence of mild and moderate brain injury in the United States, 1991, *Brain Injury*, 10 (1996) 47–54.
70. Sosin, D.M., Sniezek, J.E. and Waxweiler, R.J., Trends in death associated with traumatic brain injury, 1979–1992, *JAMA*, 273 (1995) 1778–1780.
71. von Monakow, C., *Die lokalisation im grosshim und der abbau der funktiondurch kortikale herde*, J.F. Bergman, Wiesbaden, 1914. Translated and excerpted by G. Harris, 1969. In: Moods, States and Mind. K.H. Pribram (Ed.), Penguin, London, 27–37.
72. Ward Jr., A.A. and Kennard, M.A., Effect of cholinergic drugs on recovery of function following lesions of the central nervous system in monkeys, *Yale J. Biol. Med.*, 15 (1942) 189–229.
73. Warner, L.A. and Hernandez, T.D., Amygdala kindling prior to brain lesion: impact on recovery from behavioral deficits, *Epilepsia*, 36 (1995) S121.
74. Watson, C.W. and Kennard, M.A., The effect of anticonvulsant drugs on recovery of function following cerebral cortical lesions, *J. Neurophysiol*, 8 (1945) 221–231.
75. Willmore, L.J., Sypert, G.W. and Munson, J.B., Recurrent seizures induced by cortical iron injection: a model of posttraumatic epilepsy, *Ann. Neurol.*, 4 (1978) 329–336.
76. Wolf, G. and DiCara, L.V., Progressive morphological changes in electrolytic brain lesions, *Exp. Neurol.*, 23 (1969) 529–536.

DISCUSSION OF THERESA HERNANDEZ'S PAPER

P. Engel: Could the effect you are measuring be due to the lesion, or might it have been due to the way their brains were wired from birth?

T. Hernandez: I'm not following your question.

K. Gale: I think that what Pete is saying that there might be some preexisting biological reason for the difference between animals.

T. Hernandez: No, it's an experimental difference. In the first two days of kindling, the stage 1 animals had two stimulations daily, then one stimulation daily for the rest of the time. The stage 0 animals had just one stimulation. I'm sorry I didn't make that clear.

J. McNamara: I was a bit puzzled by the fact that the ECS and pentylenetetrazol facilitated recovery but several class 5 seizures did not. How do you explain that and how the stage 1 vs. stage 0 seizures aid recovery?

T. Hernandez: I can't explain it but I can speculate for you. Things like pentylenetetrazol, ECS, and any sort of post injury activation theoretically facilitate recovery because they activate the brain when it is in a state of post-injury shock or metabolic depression. And the sooner the brain comes out of that state of shock, the sooner the animal can recover. There have been metabolic, bloodflow, and EEG correlates of this depressed function after brain injury in both humans and animals. The depressed function correlates with behavioral deficits as well. As the depressed function subsides, this correlates with recovery from some of those deficits. So that gets at the first part of the question. For the other part, my hypothesis relates to how epileptogenic a particular type of seizure is. For example, if we think of stage 1 as being more epileptogenic than stage 0, and if stage 1 seizure activity and its underlying transsynaptic changes are taking place in the brain at the same time as the recovery process, then there will be competition for resources. In the case of stage 1 seizure-induced epileptogenesis, this process will overshadow and interfere with that of recovery. Stage 5 seizures are the end product of epileptogenesis, and they may cause a lot of changes but are not bringing about the exact same changes as stage 1 seizures. They therefore are neutral in their impact on recovery, much like stage 0 seizures.

K. Gale: I think that it is very interesting that supposedly the stage 5 animals are already kindled and a stage 5 seizure should have the same promoting or trophic effect as pentylenetetrazol or ECS. I think that one big difference, however, especially with pentylenetetrazol, is the duration of the seizure activity or state. What we have found is that for the maximum induction of trophic factor you need recurrent seizures, as you would get with pentylenetetrazol or something that produces three or four seizure episodes within an hour. I would suggest that possibly if those stage 5 seizures were evoked three or four times a day over that 6 day period, it would be more similar to the pentylenetetrazol treatment and you might actually see a facilitation of recovery.

O. Lindvall: This is not actually related to this discussion. How many electroshocks or kindling stimulations did you give?

T. Hernandez: The electroshock was only a total of two. The pentylenetetrazol was 3 times a day for the first 3 days and twice a day for the next 18 days. So it was a lot, but it was a very low dose.

K. Gale: Right, so these were several episodes of seizures per day. Teri, did you do the ECS treatments?

T. Hernandez: No, that was Dennis Feeney's work.

O. Lindvall: How many seizures did he do?

T. Hernandez: Two. It's a motor cortex contusion model that has a very short window. The ECS studies were done with motor cortex lesion. Only two ECSs were given, in a very short period of time after the injury. The pentylenetetrazol was several times a day over 21 days after the lesion.

M. Gilbert: Did you include a group of animals that had been kindled and then not stimulated at stage 5 during that critical period?

T. Hernandez: Yes, and the recovery curves looked the same. We also did some non-kindled dual surgery just to see if the surgery itself had any effect, and they recover in the same way in 4 weeks.

P. Mohapel: You were talking about implications for the human clinical population, where the insult or the range of the insult is usually the cause of the epileptic-like seizures. In your model are you actually creating a focus?

T. Hernandez: We are not, that's right, and it is a definite limitation in this as a model. But it is a way to start to get at different types of seizure activity and how that influences recovery, and then I can move closer to the site of the injury and see what happens when seizures are generated from that focus.

27

KINDLING AND SPATIAL COGNITION

Michael E. Corcoran, Lisa L. Armitage, Trevor H. Gilbert, Darren K. Hannesson,* and Paul Mohapel*

Department of Psychology
University of Victoria
Victoria, British Columbia V8W 3P5, Canada

1. INTRODUCTION

If kindling involves a pathological modification or distortion of activity or connections in neural circuits that play a role in learning and memory under normal conditions, it is not unreasonable to expect that kindling should lead to alteration of the behaviors subserved by those circuits in animals tested after kindling or in the postictal period after a kindled seizure. This reasoning in part explains the long-standing interest in the effects of kindling on learning and memory.

One attractive paradigm for studying the effects of kindling on learning and memory involves various tasks that sample aspects of spatial cognition in rats. Leung and his colleagues[10–12] have reported that kindling with stimulation of hippocampal field CA1 produces deficits in working memory, a form of short-term memory that makes use of information that can change from trial to trial (i.e., trial-dependent memory), in the 8-arm radial arm maze. Using the radial arm maze, Lopes da Silva et al.[13] found that kindling of hippocampal field CA1 produces persistent deficits in reference memory, a form of long-term memory that makes use of information that is constant from trial to trial (i.e., trial-independent memory), but transient deficits in working memory during the kindling phase. Additional evidence[4] indicates that kindling of the dentate gyrus (DG) produced a marked increase in the number of errors in reference memory during the kindling period in rats tested in the radial arm maze. In contrast to these results, Robinson et al.[20] compared the transient and persistent effects of kindling the perforant path (PP) on the acquisition of two radial maze tasks. They found learning impairments only in a group of rats trained shortly after seizures, and suggested that the deficit is related to the transient aftereffects of seizures rather than to any persistent changes in neuronal firing associated with the kindled state.

* Now at Department of Psychology and Neuropsychiatry Research Unit, Department of Psychiatry, University of Saskatchewan, 9 Campus Drive, Saskatoon, SK, S7N 5A5, Canada.

Kindling 5, edited by Corcoran and Moshé.
Plenum Press, New York, 1998.

Over the past few years, we have been attempting to examine the effects of kindling different sites in the forebrain on spatial cognition and, more recently, other forms of learning. The strategy we evolved has been to compare the effects of kindling and kindled seizures triggered from different sites on acquisition and retention of spatial information in the Morris water maze. We have also begun to examine the effects of kindling on an object recognition task in a modified water maze. However, our initial research with a spatial task[3] was an attempt to ask a different question, whether amygdaloid kindling produces motivational effects (i.e., reward or punishment) that can be measured in a behavioral assay that measures a form of spatial cognition, the conditioned place preference/avoidance paradigm.

2. EFFECTS OF KINDLING ON MEMORY AND LEARNING

2.1. Conditioned Place Preference/Avoidance (CPP)

The CPP involves repeatedly exposing an organism to a distinctive environment while experiencing the effects of a particular treatment, for example, the effects of injection of a drug or vehicle solution. A testing apparatus with two distinctive chambers is used, differing in visual, tactile, and usually olfactory cues, which are separated by a removable barrier. Conditioning trials, in which the treatment is paired with one chamber, alternate with control trials, in which the control condition is experienced in the other chamber. After 4 conditioning trials, the barrier between the chambers is removed, the rats are given the opportunity to move freely between the chambers, and the amount of time spent in each is measured over a 10-min session. If the rats display a significant preference for the treatment chamber in the choice test it is concluded that the treatment associated with that chamber produced rewarding effects, whereas a preference for the control chamber (avoidance of the treatment chamber) indicates that the treatment produced punishing effects that are associated with the treatment chamber.

According to other research[19], kindling leads to an increase in defensive behavior in rats, a result that could be taken to suggest that kindling produces a punishing or aversive motivational state. On the other hand, we have never seen any active resistance to or escape from the kindling apparatus, as occurs with punishing peripheral footshock for example; and male rats occasionally display ejaculation during kindling, an event presumably associated with a rewarding state. We therefore predicted that kindling would be associated with rewarding effects, as measured in the CPP. In a distinctive chamber we[3] triggered either 4 nonconvulsive afterdischarges (AD) at the start of amygdaloid kindling or 4 generalized seizures kindled from the amygdala and confined the rats in the chamber for a short period of time after each kindling stimulation. Thus the rats had an opportunity to associate the features of the chamber with both the AD or seizure and any short-lived aftereffects of the AD or seizure, thereby maximizing the probability that an association would be formed.

Care had to be taken to adjust the duration of the conditioning sessions, during which time the rats were confined to the conditioning chamber. Once these parametric details were sorted out, we found that our prediction was only partially supported[3]. Contrary to expectations, generalized seizures failed to produce a significant CPP, suggesting that kindled seizures and their aftereffects are motivationally neutral. On the other hand, kindled AD produced a bidirectional effect: As shown in Figure 1, rats experiencing AD in the initially preferred chamber showed evidence of a conditioned avoidance response during the choice test, whereas rats experiencing AD in the initially nonpreferred chamber showed evidence of a conditioned preference response in the choice test.

Figure 1. Mean (±SEM) change in time spent in the conditioning chamber in the choice test by rats experiencing AD in conditioning sessions lasting 1 min in their initially preferred (AD1-P) or non-preferred (AD1-NP) chamber; rats experiencing AD in conditioning sessions lasting 5 min in their initially preferred (AD5-P) or nonpreferred (AD5-NP) chamber; or rats experiencing generalized seizures in their initially preferred (GEN-P) or nonpreferred (GEN-P) chamber. *Significantly different from pretest baseline, p<0.05. Modified from Corcoran et al.[3], © Elsevier Science B.V.

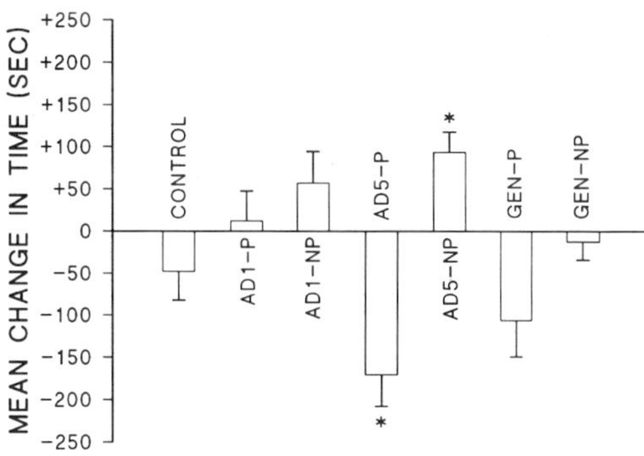

These results were taken to suggest[3] that the direction of the motivational effects of kindled AD are a function of the environmental context in which the AD is triggered. We also considered an alternative interpretation, however, that suggested some interesting additional experiments: Conceivably kindled AD and seizures produced both a motivational effect *and* an amnestic effect that interfered with spatial learning or memory. Since we had used a spatial task to measure the motivational effects of kindling, we came to recognize that the putative amnestic effects of the seizures might have interfered with accurate measurement of their motivational consequences. This in turn suggested that it would be informative to examine the possible effects of kindling and kindled seizures on spatial cognition in a paradigm in which any motivational effects of ictal activity could be avoided. We therefore turned to the Morris water maze.

2.2. The Morris Water Maze (MWM)

In our first experiments using the MWM[16], we compared the effects of kindling from the PP, amygdala, or septum on acquisition of spatial information in a conventional MWM, using a submerged platform. We also wished to compare the long-lasting effects of kindling on spatial cognition in this task vs. the short-lasting effects of kindled seizures. To test the effects of kindling per se, we kindled generalized seizures from the 3 sites in different groups of rats (*kindled* groups) and then began maze training 24 hr after the last seizure, at which point we arbitrarily assumed that short-term aftereffects of the seizures would have dissipated. To test the effects of kindled seizures, on the other hand, we triggered seizures 25 to 45 min before daily training in the maze during the acquisition period, so that acquisition occurred in the postictal period when short-lasting aftereffects of seizure might be present. All groups received 4 trials in the MWM daily for 8 days; each daily session lasted about 16 min. After the final trial on day 8 of acquisition, we gave a probe trial, in which the platform was removed and the rats' preference for the quadrants of the maze was measured over 60 sec. Probe trials are intended to measure memory unconfounded by ongoing learning. On the next day a visible platform (VP) task was conducted, to test for general motoric or motivational deficits. In subsequent sessions a reversal condition was imposed, in which the submerged platform was moved to a different quadrant and the rats had to learn the new location. In the reversal condition seizures were now triggered in the *kindled* groups shortly before training, whereas the *seizure* groups were now tested without seizures.

As shown in Figure 2, all *seizure* groups (PP, septum, amygdala) displayed significant deficits in the acquisition of spatial information, although the deficit was smaller in the amygdaloid kindled rats. The deficit in spatial learning was also evident in the probe

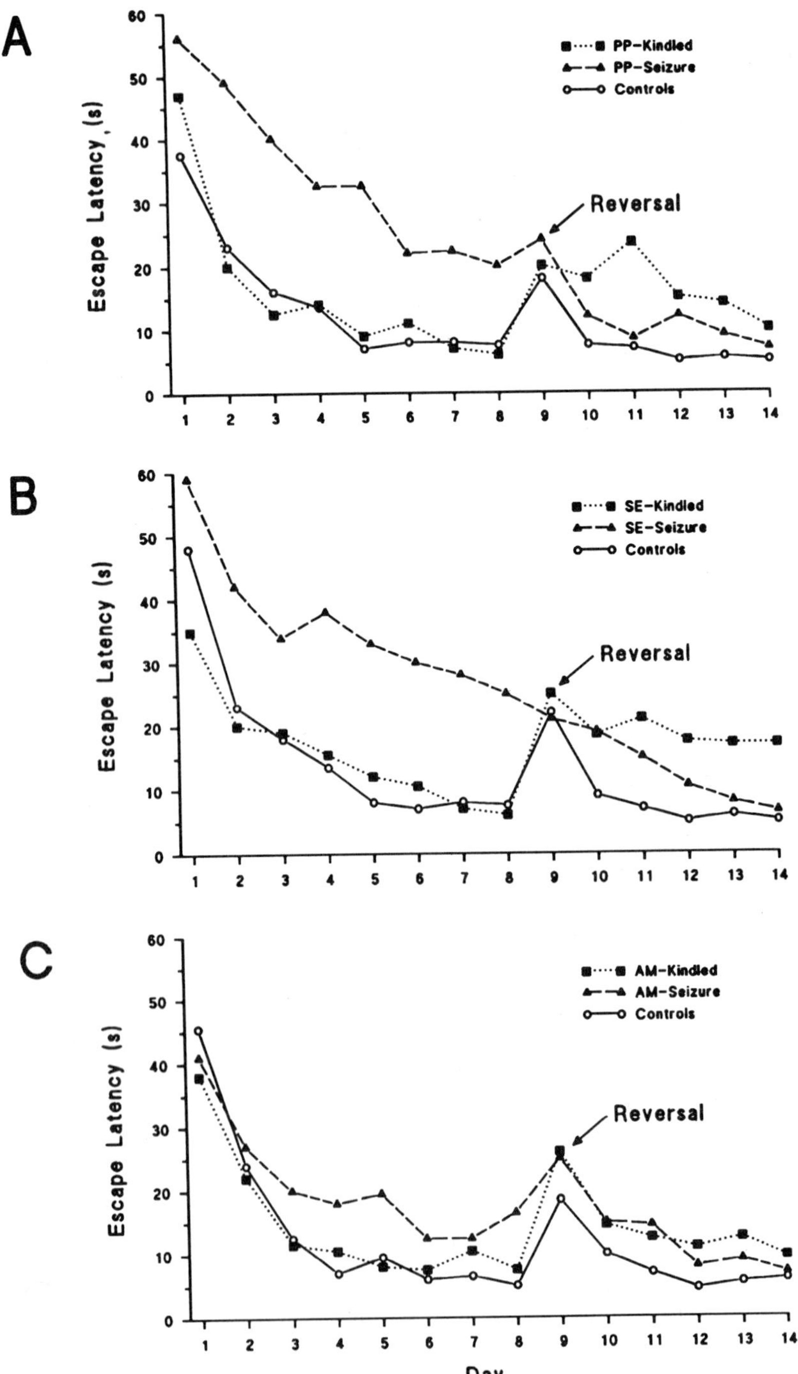

Figure 2. Mean escape latencies (in sec) during acquisition and reversal training after kindling (KINDLED groups) or pretraining seizures (SEIZURE groups) induced by stimulation of the medial PP (A), septum (B), or amygdala (C). Modified from McNamara et al.[16], © Elsevier Science B.V.

trials (data not shown; see ref. 16). However, there were no differences from controls in the VP task (data not shown; see ref. 16), suggesting that the deficits in spatial learning and memory were not secondary to motoric or motivational problems. When a new learning task was imposed in the reversal phase, a deficit was seen in the *kindled* groups, which were now learning in the postictal period, whereas behavior at control levels was seen in the *seizure* groups, which were now learning in the absence of pretrial seizures. In contrast to the deficits in spatial cognition produced by kindled seizures, no deficits were seen in the *kindled* groups during initial acquisition, although the PP group did display swim speeds on day 1 that were significantly slower than in controls.

Two general conclusions emerge from these studies. First, spatial cognition is disrupted by kindled limbic seizures, regardless of the site of stimulation, and this is likely an effect on learning or memory per se, not secondary to a general sensorimotor or motivational deficit. Second, spatial cognition is largely unaffected by kindling of the same sites, with kindling defined operationally as the state persisting for at least 24 hr after the last seizure. Although it was not unexpected that amygdaloid kindling was ineffective, given that amygdaloid lesions do not disrupt spatial learning[23], we were surprised at the ineffectiveness of PP and septal kindling, in light of evidence that lesions of these structures disrupt spatial learning[9,23]. One possible explanation is that kindled alterations of circuits in the stimulated sites may not act as a functional lesion, contrary to expectations. Another possibility is that sites have to be kindled bilaterally to produce a functional lesion. However, some rats in the *kindled* group were subjected to bilateral kindling of the PP, but still failed to show a deficit.

Another interesting aspect of this negative result is that it differs markedly from the disruptive effect of kindling on spatial cognition in the radial arm maze previously reported[4,10–13]. In considering this discrepancy, we noted that the other studies employed not only a different behavioral task, the radial arm maze rather than the MWM, but also stimulation within the hippocampal formation itself, rather than stimulation of sites anatomically connected to the hippocampus, as we had used. We therefore decided to hold constant the behavioral task (MWM) and examine the effects of kindling of field CA1 of the hippocampus.

2.3. CA1 Kindling and the MWM

As in our earlier studies[16], we compared the long-lasting effects of CA1 kindling on spatial cognition in the MWM vs. the short-lasting effects of kindled seizures. To test the effects of kindling per se[5], we kindled partial or generalized seizures with unilateral stimulation of field CA1 of dorsal hippocampus in different groups of rats (*kindled* groups) and then began maze training 24 hr after the last seizure, an interval that we assumed was sufficient to permit dissipation of the short-term aftereffects of the seizures. Training was given in 4 trials daily for 7 days. After the last trial of day 7, a probe trial was imposed. On day 8, the *reversal* phase began, wherein the submerged platform was moved to the opposite quadrant of the maze, with a probe trial on the last day of the phase. On day 15, the *seizure* phase began, wherein a seizure was triggered 25 to 45 min before each session in the maze, with the platform located in the same quadrant as during the reversal phase. A probe trial occurred on the last day of the seizure phase.

Figure 3 shows the effects of kindling of generalized (Figure 3A) or partial (Figure 3B) seizures on acquisition in the *kindled* groups. Kindling of generalized seizures from field CA1 led to a disruption in acquisition of spatial information, as indicated by the significant increases in distance swum by the generalized *kindled* group on days 3, 4, 5, and 7

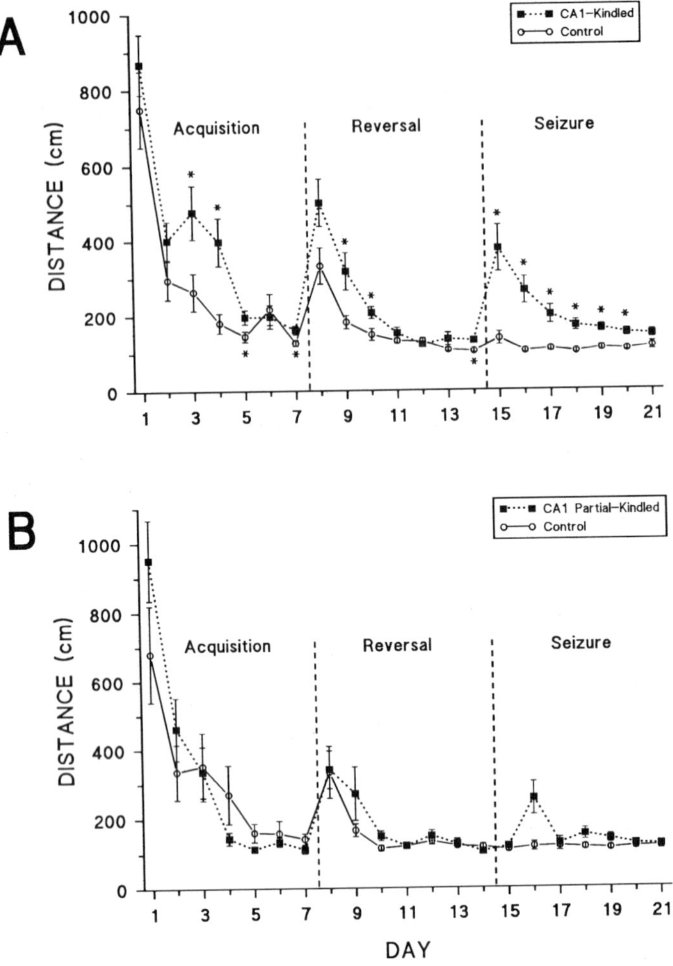

Figure 3. Effects of kindling of generalized (A) or partial (B) seizures from field CA1 on acquisition in the MWM, expressed as mean (± SEM) distance swum. *Significantly different from control, $p<0.05$. From Gilbert et al.[5], © Elsevier Science B.V.

(Figure 3A). By the last day of acquisition the generalized *kindled* rats were performing at a level near but somewhat worse than controls, and their accurate responses on the probe trial did not differ significantly from control (data not shown; see ref. 5). The generalized *kindled* rats also showed significant increases in distance swum on days 9, 10, and 14 of the reversal phase. Their performance by the end of reversal was not significantly different from control, as confirmed by their unimpaired performance on the probe trial. Triggering a generalized seizure before each session in the seizure phase resulted in significant impairments on all but the final days of the seizure phase. Spatial performance on the final day of the seizure phase did not differ from control, as was confirmed by the unimpaired performance of the *kindled* group in the probe trial.

In contrast to the disruptive effects of kindling of generalized seizures, kindling of partial seizures from field CA1 failed to affect acquisition of spatial information in any of the phases of the study (Figure 3B). The normal acquisition performance of the partial *kindled* group was mirrored in their accurate responses on the probe trials given at the end of each phase, which did not differ significantly from control (data not shown; see ref. 5).

A somewhat different picture emerged when we examined the effects of CA1 kindling on retention in the MWM. As shown in Figure 4A, kindling of generalized seizures from field CA1 produced an overall significant deficit in retention, with significant daily differences evident on days 2 to 4. Performance of rats in the *kindled* group was unimpaired during the reversal phase, although significant deficits appeared on the first two days of the seizure phase. In contrast to its lack of effect on acquisition, kindling of partial seizures produced an overall significant deficit in retention, evident on day 2 (Figure 4B). The performance of rats in the partial *kindled* group did not, however, differ significantly from control during either the reversal or seizure phases.

In contrast to the effects of kindling from other limbic sites, therefore, kindling of hippocampal field CA1 is associated with a significant deficit in acquisition of spatial information in the MWM. Our results indicate that the disruptive effects of CA1 kindling on

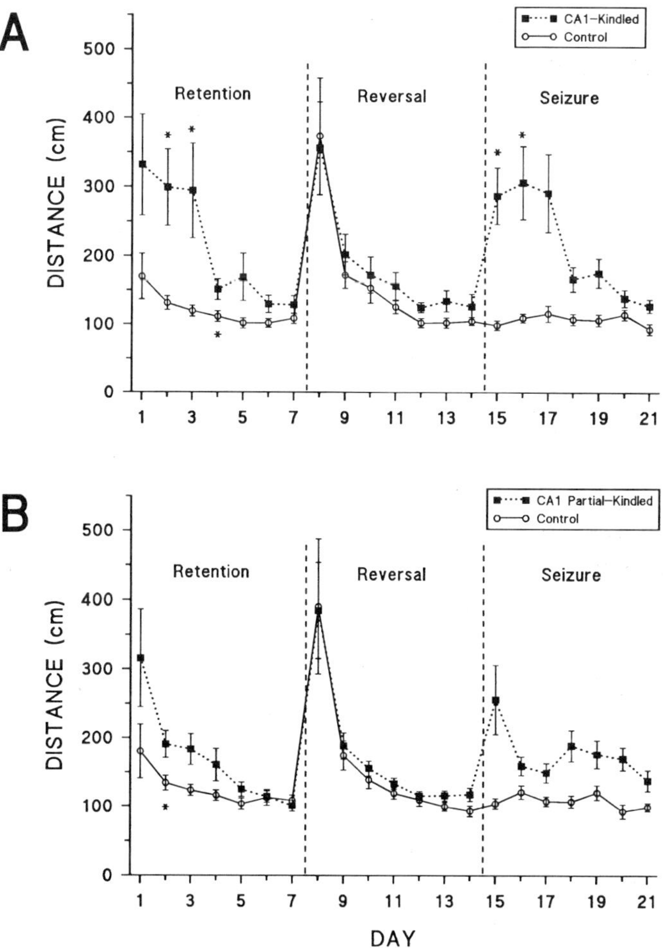

Figure 4. Effects of kindling of generalized (A) or partial (B) seizures from field CA1 on retention in the MWM, expressed as mean (±SEM) distance swum. *Significantly different from control, $p<0.05$. From Gilbert et al.[5], © Elsevier Science B.V.

spatial cognition extend to both the radial arm maze[10] and the MWM. Before discussing the significance of these results further, we should address the possibility that the observed deficits in spatial behavior in the MWM are due to general behavioral or motivational impairments, and not deficits in memory. We think this is unlikely for two reasons. First, performance in a VP task should also be impaired if the effects of kindling are due to a general deficit. As discussed below, however, we have found that triggering an AD or generalized seizure 25 to 45 min before a VP test does not affect escape[6], and it seems even more unlikely that a general deficit would affect behavior in kindled rats tested 24 or more hr after the last seizure. Second, swim speed in the VP task was not affected (data not shown; see Gilbert and Corcoran[6]), suggesting that motivation to escape was unimpaired.

Our results highlight one very significant difference between the effects of CA1 kindling in the radial arm maze and MWM: Although kindling of nonconvulsive or partial seizures is able to disrupt behavior in the radial arm maze[10–12], partial kindling is without effect in the MWM. A potential explanation for this discrepancy lies in the fact that we were examining the effects of CA1 kindling on *acquisition* of spatial information in the MWM, whereas other investigators examined the effects of CA1 kindling on *retention* of already learned information in the radial arm maze[4,10,13]. When we compared the effects of partial and generalized kindling on retention of spatial information in the MWM, we found that both produced a deficit in retention. Thus retention of spatial information in the MWM appears to be more vulnerable to the disruptive effects of CA1 kindling than is acquisition. Although the reasons for this are not immediately obvious, one possibility is that maze learning in naive control rats depends on the hippocampus, and the hippocampally mediated strategy employed in retention would be disrupted by CA1 kindling. When CA1 kindling is imposed before acquisition, however, disruption of hippocampal function could force the rats to employ strategies that are independent of the hippocampus, resulting in a gradual improvement in performance. Another possibility is that memory for the task is state dependent, and CA1 kindling interferes with retention by producing a state[14] that differs significantly from the state associated with memory.

Our results also suggest that an additional effect can be produced by triggering of kindled seizures from field CA1: During the seizure phase, triggering a seizure disrupted spatial behavior in the generalized *kindled* group but not in the partial *kindled* group (Figure 3A and 3B). By the time the seizure phase had been imposed, note that we were testing retention of a well-learned maze response. In view of the observation that triggering kindled seizures from the PP, septum, or amygdala can disrupt acquisition in the MWM[16], as can triggering of only AD from the PP,[2] we wondered whether acquisition of a maze response in the immediate postictal period would deviate from control.

We therefore examined other rats that were naive to the MWM, in which we induced a nonconvulsive AD or a generalized seizure 25 to 45 min before the rats' first daily training sessions in the maze[6]. Some *seizure* groups and some *AD* groups were tested during the acquisition period. Other *seizure* and *AD* groups were tested in *retention*: These rats were first trained in the maze, then seizures were kindled, and then maze testing resumed (mean interval of 52.5 d between end of initial training and start of retention testing), with retention testing occurring 25–45 min after the triggering of a seizure. The groups were given a VP task on the day after the completion of acquisition or retention, and then kindling stimulation was suspended for 7 days (*recovery* phase), during which time the rats received 4 trials in the MWM each day. Finally, the groups entered a *layoff* phase, in which kindling stimulation, handling, and maze training were suspended. This phase lasted for 7 days (*AD* groups) or 14 days (*seizure* groups), after which time testing resumed in the MWM for 4 trials daily for 5 days.

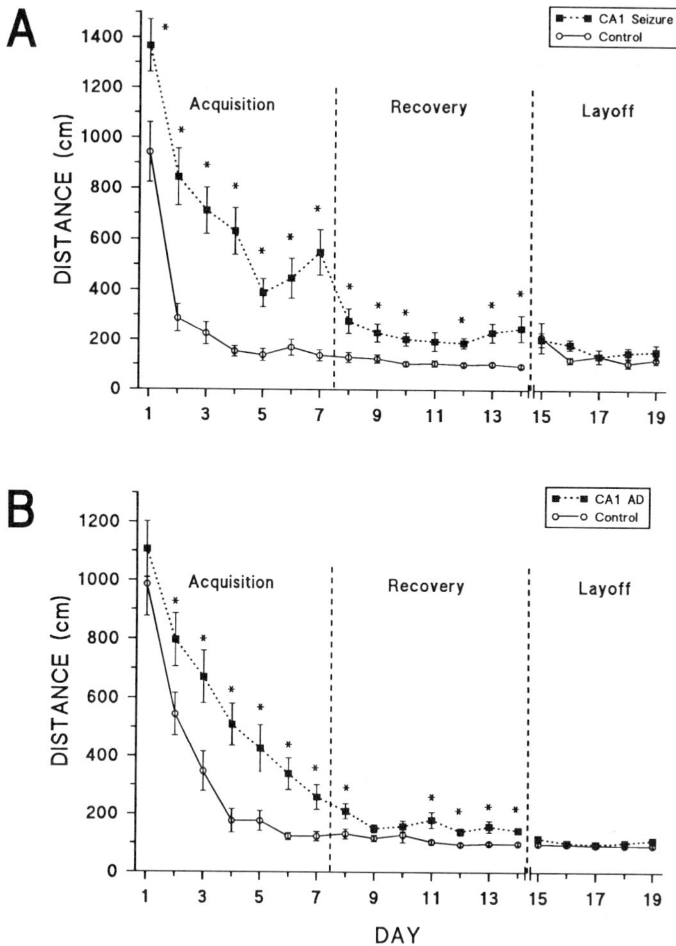

Figure 5. Effects of triggering a generalized seizure (A) or nonconvulsive AD (B) from field CA1 on acquisition in the MWM, expressed as mean (±SEM) distance swum. *Significantly different from control, $p<0.05$. From Gilbert and Corcoran[6].

Triggering either a generalized seizure (Figure 5A) or an AD (Figure 5B) from field CA1 resulted in a significant disruption of acquisition, evident on days 1 to 7 in the seizure group and on days 2 to 7 in the AD group. Rats in the seizure and AD groups displayed unimpaired behavior in the VP task imposed at the end of the acquisition phase, however, suggesting that they were not experiencing a generalized sensorimotor or motivational deficit. During the recovery phase, the seizure group's performance remained significantly impaired on all but day 11, and performance in the AD remained significantly impaired on all but days 9 and 10 in the recovery phase. By the layoff phase, however, behavior of the seizure group had recovered to control, and they displayed a bias for the target quadrant when tested on the final day in a probe trial that did not differ from control. Although the AD group's performance during layoff seems visibly similar to control (Figure 5B), statistically their overall performance was significantly worse than that of the control group's, and this was confirmed by the fact that the AD group spent significantly less dwell time in the target quadrant than controls on the probe trial.

In the retention groups, triggering either a generalized seizure (Figure 6A) or an AD (Figure 6B) from field CA1 resulted in a significant disruption in retention of a previously trained response, evident on days 3 and 4 in the seizure group and on days 2, 3, and 5 in the AD group. Again, rats in the seizure and AD groups displayed unimpaired behavior in the VP task imposed at the end of the retention phase. During the recovery phase, the seizure group's performance was significantly impaired on only day 11, and the performance of the AD group did not differ from control. Similarly, the seizure group's performance differed significantly from control only on day 15 of the layoff phase, and they displayed a bias for the target quadrant when tested on the final day in a probe trial that did not differ from control. The AD group's performance during the layoff phase and probe trial did not differ from control.

These results indicate that triggering kindled seizures from field CA1 can disrupt acquisition of spatial information, similar to the effects of seizures triggered from PP, septum, or amygdala[16]. Several aspects of the results seemingly rule out a sensorimotor or

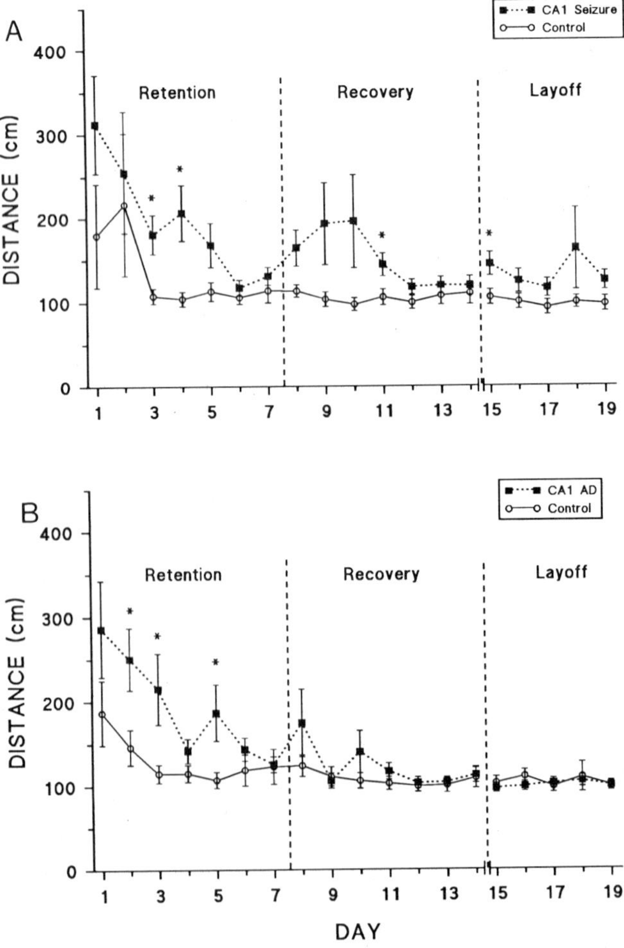

Figure 6. Effects of triggering a generalized seizure (A) or nonconvulsive AD (B) from field CA1 on retention in the MWM, expressed as mean (±SEM) distance swum. *Significantly different from control, $p<0.05$. From Gilbert and Corcoran[6].

motivational impairment as an explanation of the behavioral deficits: the absence of an effect of seizures on performance in the VP task; the persistence of the disruptive effect for several weeks in some groups (e.g., in the recovery phase in the acquisiton groups); and the disruption produced by triggering of AD alone, in the absence of convulsive seizures. Regardless of the site of initiation, therefore, limbic ictal activity can disrupt function in the neural circuits involved in acquisition and retention of spatial information. In this sense, kindling and kindled seizures produce a functional lesion.

2.4. Perirhinal Kindling and Varieties of Learning

The role of the perirhinal cortex (PRH) in epileptogenesis has recently become a topic of considerable interest, with evidence indicating that PRH is highly susceptible to kindling[15] and is a strongly dominant site in the kindling antagonism paradigm[17]. Other studies have examined the effects of PRH lesions in learning paradigms. Although PRH lesions do not have much effect on spatial cognition in the MWM[25], they do disrupt rats' ability to learn object discrimination in a delayed nonmatch to sample[18]. We wondered whether kindling of the PRH would affect either spatial cognition in the MWM or a simple object memory task in a modifed water maze (Hannesson, Mohapel, Armitage, and Corcoran, unpublished). Spatial learning and memory were tested using the conventional MWM task with a submerged platform, beginning 24 hr after the last kindled seizure. To facilitate initial learning of the escape response, rats received training with a VP for 6 trials on day 1. On day 2, we imposed massed training with 18 trials. Subsequently rats received 6 trials and a probe trial daily until they met a criterion for successful learning. Retention was measured 1 and 4 weeks after acquisition, with 3 submerged platform trials followed by a probe trial.

Following testing in the MWM, kindling stimulation resumed until 1 stage 5 seizure was triggered. We began training in object discrimination 24 hr after the seizure, in a modified water maze. The value of employing a modified water maze to test object memory is that it permitted us to hold constant the motivation for learning (escape from water) and as many features of the environment as possible, while at the same time varying the nature of the cognitive process employed (spatial cognition in the MWM vs. object memory in the modified maze). We therefore modified the MWM so that the surface of the water was divided into 3 wedge-shaped sections. Distinctive stimuli, such as a monochromatic circular object or a square with a cross drawn on it, were mounted on the wall above either corner in any section, with the submerged platform located consistently under one of the objects. We first shaped the rats' escape response in the new maze, with no objects present. For 2 days with 20 trials daily, a VP was inserted in a corner of a wedge, with the corner and wedge varying across trials. Then we began acquisition training with the objects and a submerged platform, involving 20 trials daily until the rats met a criterion for learning. Retention was measured at 1 and 4 weeks, with 5 trials each. During all phases of the study, we discouraged use of a spatial strategy by systematically varying the location of the objects in the maze from trial to trial.

We found no significant effect of PRH kindling on acquisition or retention of a spatial response in the MWM (Figure 7). Nor were there differences in the behavior of kindled and control rats on probe trials (data not shown). However, PRH kindling did affect object memory: Although there was no difference from control in acquisition of the object discrimination, kindled rats displayed a nonsignificant impairment in retention of the object discrimination at 1 week and much larger and statistically significant impairment at 4 weeks (Figure 8).

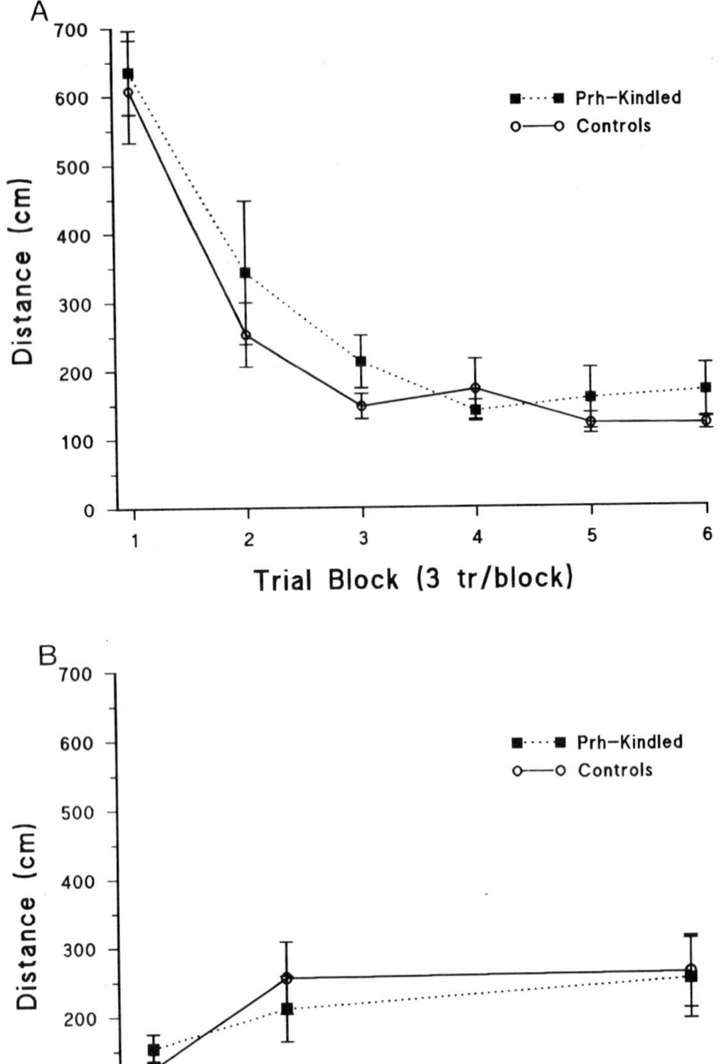

Figure 7. Effects of PRH kindling on acquisition (A) and retention (B) of a spatial response in the MWM, expressed as mean (±SEM) distance swum, in cm.

These results suggest that kindling the PRH produces a functional lesion. Similar to subtotal surgical lesions of the PRH[25], kindling had no effect on spatial performance in the MWM. PRH kindling had small disruptive effect on acquisition of an object discrimination, however, and an even larger disruptive effect on retention of an established response. Again, this effect of kindling resembles the effects of lesions of PRH on object memory[18]. To determine the anatomical specificity of the effect of kindling, it would be interesting to compare the effects of kindling of field CA1 on acquisition and retention of object discrimination.

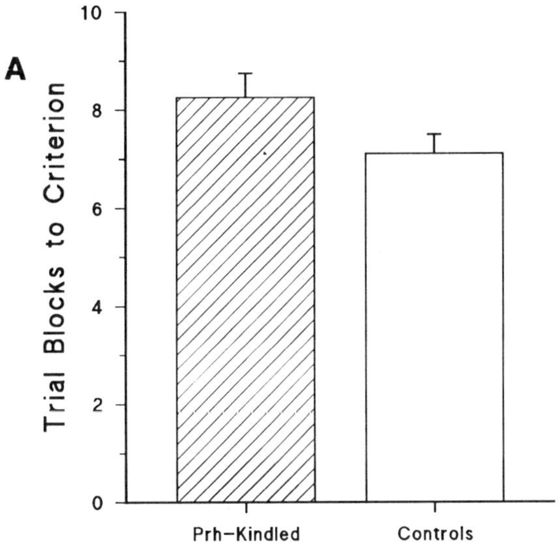

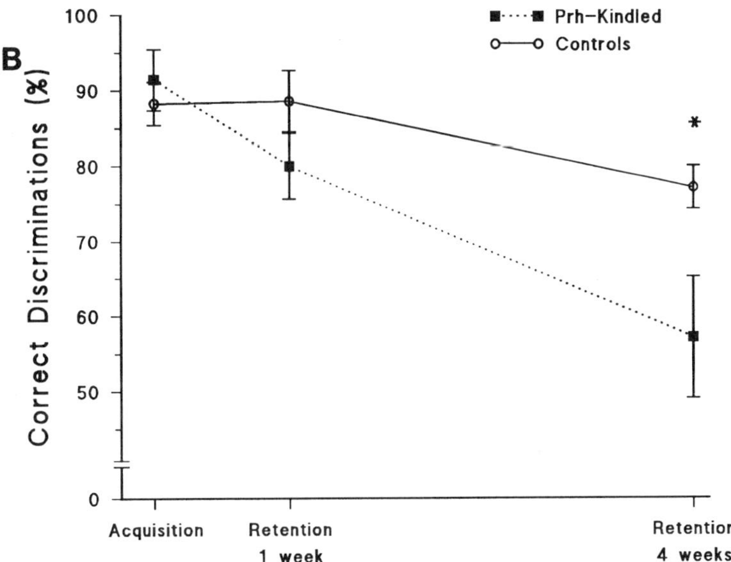

Figure 8. Effects of PRH kindling on mean (±SEM) trials to criterion (A) and percentage correct discriminations (B) for object discrimination. *Significantly different from control, $p<0.05$.

Such experiments are underway. It would also be worthwhile determining whether seizures triggered from field CA1 (or elsewhere) would affect an established object memory.

3. CONCLUSIONS

We have summarized a program of research that over the past few years has attempted to characterize the effects of kindling on spatial cognition and, more recently, another form of cognitive learning in rats. The results indicate that the effects of kindling on spatial cognition are regionally specific: Kindling of generalized seizures with stimulation of hippocampal field CA1 disrupts acquisition and retention in the MWM, whereas no effect is produced by kindling of PP, septal area, or amygdala. Kindling of even partial seizures from CA1 disrupts retention of an established spatial response in the MWM, suggesting either that retention is more vulnerable than acquisition to hippocampal ictal activity or that state dependent effects of hippocampal seizures are occurring that influence retention.

It is unclear why CA1 kindling affects spatial cognition but kindling of connected limbic sites is without effect. Possibly the other sites are too synaptically remote from the hippocampal circuitry that is critical for spatial learning. We note, however, that lesions of the PP do disrupt spatial learning[21], a finding that is inconsistent with this hypothesis. Spiller and Racine[22] have reported that PP kindling does not transfer to kindling of the DG, suggesting that PP kindling may not in fact activate the hippocampal circuits that participate in spatial cognition. But this hypothesis does not easily accommodate the seemingly incompatible observations that spatial learning is affected by lesions of the septum[9] but not septal kindling[16]. PP kindling and CA1 kindling do differ in electrophysiological correlates, and this could potentially explain their different effects on spatial learning. For example, CA1 kindling produces diminished inhibition in field CA1[8], whereas amygdaloid or PP kindling results in enhanced inhibition in the DG[24]. Whether these differences are responsible for the differing behavioral consequences of kindling the sites is not known at this time.

In contrast to the specificity of the effects of CA1 kindling, spatial cognition is disrupted by seizures triggered from PP, septum, or amygdala, as well as from CA1. If spatial learning and memory depend on a long-lasting alteration of synaptic strength similar to long-term potentiation (LTP), the disruptive effect of limbic seizures could be due to the ability of ictal discharge to transiently suppress LTP[1,7]. This hypothesis cannot account for the failure of PRH seizures to disrupt established object recognition, although we note that this paradigm has not yet been used to test the effects of seizures triggered from CA1, PP, septum, or amygdala. Conceivably the discrimination was established well enough that it would be resistant to the effects of the other seizures as well.

Kindling from several sites can affect the processes of several forms of cognitive learning in rats. These results are generally compatible with our working hypothesis that kindling can distort the activity of neural circuits involved in normal behavior, although some discrepancies must be resolved with further research. It is our hope that the approach followed here may generate insight into the functional anatomy of amnesia.

REFERENCES

1. Anwyl, R., Walshe, J. and Rowan, M., Electroconvulsive treatment reduces long-term potentiation in rat hippocampus, *Brain Res.*, 435 (1987) 377–379.
2. Cain, D.P., Hargreaves, E.L., Boon, F. and Dennison, Z., (1993). An examination of the relations between hippocampal long-term potentiation, kindling, afterdischarge, and place learning in the water maze, *Hippocampus*, 3 (1993) 153–164.
3. Corcoran, M.E., Lanius, R. and Duren, A., Reinforcing and punishing consequences of kindling, *Epilepsy Res.*, 13 (1992) 179–186.
4. Feasey-Truger, K.J., Kargl, L. and ten Bruggencate, G., Differential effects of dentate kindling on working and reference spatial memory in the rat, *Neurosci. Lett.*, 151 (1993) 25–28.
5. Gilbert, T.H., McNamara, R.K. and Corcoran, M.E., Kindling of hippocampal field CA1 impairs spatial learning and retention in the Morris water maze, *Behav. Brain Res.*, in press.

6. Gilbert, T.H. and Corcoran, M.E., Hippocampal kindled seizures impair spatial cognition in the Morris water maze, submitted for publication.
7. Hesse, G. and Teyler, T., Reversible loss of hippocmapal long-term potentiation following electroconvulsive seizures, *Nature*, 264 (1976) 562–564.
8. Kamphuis, W., Lopes da Silva, F. and Wadman, W.J., Changes in local evoked potentials in the rat hippocampus (CA1) during kindling epileptogenesis, *Brain Res.*, 440 (1988) 205–215.
9. Kelsey, J.E. and Landry, B.A., Medial septal lesions disrupt spatial mapping ability in rats, *Behav. Neurosci.*, 102 (1988) 289–293.
10. Leung, L.S., Boon, K.A., Kaibara, T. and Innis, N.K., Radial maze performance following hippocampal kindling, *Behav. Brain Res.*, 40 (1990) 119–129.
11. Leung, L.S. and Shen, B., Hippocampal CA1 evoked response and radial 8-arm maze performance after hippocampal kindling, *Brain Res.*, 555 (1991) 353–357.
12. Leung, L.S., Zhao, D. and Shen, B., Long-lasting effects of partial hippocampal kindling on hippocampal physiology and function, *Hippocampus*, 4 (1994) 696–704.
13. Lopes da Silva, F.H., Gorter, J.A. and Wadman, W.J., Kindling of the hippocampus induces spatial memory deficits in the rat, *Neurosci. Lett.*, 63 (1986) 115–120.
14. McIntyre, D.C., State-dependence learning in rats induced by kindled convulsions, *Physiol. Behav.*, 7 (1971) 15–20.
15. McIntyre, D.C., Kelly, M.E. and Armstrong, J.N., Kindling in the perirhinal cortex, *Brain Res.*. 615 (1993) 1–6.
16. McNamara, R.K., Kirkby, R.D., dePape, G.E. and Corcoran, M.E., Limbic seizures, but not kindling, reversibly impair place learning in the Morris water maze, *Behav. Brain Res.*, 50 (1992) 167–175.
17. Mohapel, P. and Corcoran, M.E., Kindling antagonism: Interactions of the amygdala with the piriform, perirhinal, and insular cortices, *Brain Res.*, in press.
18. Mumby, D.G. and Pinel, J.P.J., Rhinal cortex lesions and object discrimination in rats, *Behav.Neurosci.*, 108 (1994) 11–18.
19. Pinel, J.P.J., Long-term kindling and defensive behavior. This volume.
20. Robinson, G.B., McNeil, H.A. and Reed, G.D., Comparison of the short- and long-lasting effects of perforant path kindling on radial maze learning, *Behav. Neurosci.*, 106 (1993) 988–995.
21. Skelton, R.W. and McNamara, R.K., Bilateral knife cuts to the perforant path disrupt spatial learning in the Morris water maze, *Hippocampus*, 2 (1992) 73–80.
22. Spiller, A.E. and Racine, R.J., Transfer kindling between sites in the entorhinal cortex-perforant path-dentate gyrus system, *Brain Res.*, 635 (1994) 130–138.
23. Sutherland, R.J., Whishaw, I.Q., and Kolb, B., A behavioral analysis of spatial localization following elecrolytic, kainate- or colchicine-induced damage to the hippocampal formation in the rat, *Behav. Brain Res.*, 7 (1983) 133–153.
24. Tuff, L., Racine, R.J. and Adamec, R., The effects of kindling on GABA-mediated inhibition in the dentate gyrus of the rat. I. Paired-pulse depression. *Brain Res.*, 277 (1983) 79–90.
25. Wiig, K.A. and Bilkey, D.K., Subtotal perirhinal cortex lesions increase exploratory behavior in the rat without producing deficits in the Morris water maze, *Psychobiology*, 22 (1994) 195–202.

DISCUSSION OF MICHAEL CORCORAN'S PAPER

F. Lopes Da Silva: Very interesting data. I just wonder, if you stop the CA1 kindling procedure when you are looking at the effect on retention, how much time do you think that it takes to have recovery of the learned behaviour?

M. Corcoran: If we look at the slide with the acquisition results, what you can see here is that the performance of kindled rats that previously had generalized seizures eventually reached the levels of controls. I don't know whether that is because they eventually learned to overcome a deficit that the kindling produces or whether there is a recovery.

F. Lopes Da Silva: My question was on the retention.

M. Corcoran: We also don't know about retention. If we look at the slide with the retention results, again it's the same kind of thing, in that there is an initial deficit and then performance reaches control levels. I don't know whether that is reflecting decay of the disruption or whether it is just learning to overcome the handicap. The way to get at this, and we thought about doing it in either acquisition or retention, is to kindle stage 5 seizures and then wait 7 days or more before starting behavioral testing.

F. Lopes Da Silva: I asked this question because in the 8-arm maze when we do a similar type of experiment and then stop the stimulations, we see a recovery of the working memory component, not of the reference memory component. I was just wondering whether you can make a parallel with your paradigm. But I think it's difficult because you have a learning effect superimposed on memory.

S. Leung: Very nice data. I almost think I don't have to give my talk! Do you have any speculations on why perforant path kindling would have no effect compared to CA1 kindling? I know probably people around here swear that the effects, chemical or electrophysiological, are the same after both types of kindling, especially to the full kindling stage.

M. Corcoran: I don't know why they are different. The fact is that, as you know, perforant path kindling and CA1 kindling have different effects also in the 8-arm radial maze. Gil Robinson failed to get an effect of perforant path kindling, whereas we know that CA1 kindling is effective. So I don't know what the explanation is for that difference, but it is a consistent difference regardless of the task that one uses, I can say that. Uh oh, here comes Peter Cain, now I'm in trouble.

P. Cain: I was going to suggest a possible way to find out reasons for the differences between kindled and control rats. Did you observe details of behaviours like thigmotaxis or swimovers? What did they look like in retention? Did they show deflections from the platform?

M. Corcoran: That's an important question, and of course we'll want to look at that some more after hearing you. One thing our kindled rats do not do in the way that your drug treated rats do—I should explain that Peter gave a talk to my lab a few days ago, so we're referring back to the data he was discussing then—one thing our kindled rats do not do is to show the kind of deflections from the platform that your drugged rats do. So I don't think that's the explanation of what's going on here.

P. Cain: Do the CA1-kindled animals show thigmotaxis and excursions?

M. Corcoran: Well, you saw an example from the swim path I showed in one of my slides, which indicated that they do show some thigmotaxis but also show excursions into various quadrants of the maze; so they are not simply wall following.

J. McNamara: Mike, you might have said it but I missed it, with the visible platform, did the CA1 kindled rats get there just fine?

M. Corcoran: Yes, they did.

C. Applegate: For the retention data that you showed for the perirhinal kindled rats, what was the level of deficit? Fifty percent retention would of course indicate that they have forgotten entirely.

M. Corcoran: Darren Hannesson should answer that, since these are his data.

D. Hannesson: Yes, they were performing at a random level.

J. Wada: With the retention tests, was this unilateral kindling?

M. Corcoran: Yes.

J. Wada: Suppose if you did secondary site kindling, you might have a more persistent deficit that might tell us a story of where there the recovery is occurring, in terms of coping with the events in the kindled hemisphere.

M. Corcoran: That is an important point. We haven't done bilateral kindling with CA1 stimulation, but when you stimulate CA1 you see immediate propagation of afterdischarge to the contralateral hippocampus. So in a sense it is bilateral kindling, but of course not in the sense that you mean, that stimulation is applied bilaterally.

M. Gilbert: In response to that, your perforant path kindling is also giving you afterdischarge in CA1, and yet you got very different results with CA1 and perforant path kindling.

M. Corcoran: And what I didn't say about perforant path kindling is that Rob McNamara ran one group that he stimulated on both sides. He kindled for example the left hemisphere first and then kindled the right hemisphere, so that he had some rats that were bilaterally kindled, and it just didn't matter for spatial learning.

K. Gale: The task that you selected for the perirhinal kindled animals was not similar to Mumby's object recognition memory task—in fact is completely different, because it is a habit task. From what you describe, it is the same object repeatedly that they are looking for to associate with the platform. So my question is, have you tried using a task which you might suspect to test persistence of memory, like a match to sample or a delayed nonmatch to sample?

M. Corcoran: No. We haven't done that.

28

LONG-LASTING BEHAVIORAL AND ELECTROPHYSIOLOGICAL EFFECTS INDUCED BY PARTIAL HIPPOCAMPAL KINDLING

L. Stan Leung,* B. Shen, R. Sutherland, C. Wu, K. Wu, and D. Zhao

Department Physiology and Clinical Neurological Sciences
University of Western Ontario
London, Ontario N6A 5A5, Canada

1. INTRODUCTION

Partial epilepsy of temporal lobe origin, most commonly from the amygdala and the hippocampus, accounts for about one quarter of new epilepsy cases. Many epileptic patients are impaired in their memory and learning[52]. Relatively few studies have addressed the behavioral consequences of experimental seizures, and fewer yet have attempted to relate behavior and physiology.

We have used hippocampal kindling to study the long-lasting electrophysiological and behavioral changes caused by seizures. Kindling allows for a controlled evocation of electrographic seizures that progress toward generalized convulsions[14]. The hippocampus is selected for several reasons. First, it is an area where temporal lobe seizures often originate. Second, hippocampal physiology[32] is better understood than that of many other brain structures. The relatively simple hippocampal cortex simplifies the interpretation of extracellular potentials, and its lamellar organization preserves the main excitatory synapses in an in vitro 400-μm brain slice. Third, the functions of the hippocampus, while still debated, may be studied by well developed techniques such as the radial arm maze[44] and the Morris water maze[39].

Partial kindling refers to the repeated evocation of afterdischarges (ADs) to a stage before clinical convulsions. There are theoretical and practical reasons for using partial kindling. Theoretically, if seizure is regarded as an unstable, non-equilibrium state of the

* For correspondence: Dr. L. Stan Leung, Department Clinical Neurological Sciences, University Hospital, The University of Western Ontario, London, Canada N6A 5A5. (519) 663-3733; FAX (519) 661-3827. Email: sleung@julian.uwo.ca.

Kindling 5, edited by Corcoran and Moshé.
Plenum Press, New York, 1998.

brain, then the state of the brain after partial kindling is akin to a near-equilibrium state, which is more amendable to analysis[13]. Practically, partial kindling, like full kindling, induces a persistent change in seizure susceptibility[11]. About 40 ADs delivered to the dorsal hippocampal CA1 were needed to evoke fully generalized stage V convulsions[21]. Cell death and mossy fiber sprouting[6,7] were minimal after partial kindling. It appears that the changes of the brain after partial kindling could be better understood, because the effects are more localized and relatively limited. The spread of a hippocampal AD was limited to the hippocampus[34] and structures immediately connected to the hippocampus, such as the entorhinal cortex, amygdala and the nucleus accumbens. Independent lengthening of the AD in the entorhinal cortex was observed during partial hippocampal kindling, and behavioral hyperactivity after a hippocampal AD was blocked by infusion of dopamine D2 antagonist in the nucleus accumbens[35], confirming activation of the entorhinal cortex and nucleus accumbens during partial hippocampal kindling.

In the following, we shall review our work on the behavioral and physiological changes after hippocampal kindling. In all the studies, hippocampal AD was evoked by a 1-s train of 0.1 ms pulses, of 100–400 μA at 100–200 Hz delivered to dorsal hippocampal CA1 on one side (typically stratum radiatum and moleculare). ADs were evoked at a maximum of 5 times a day, at hourly intervals. As compared to daily kindling, hourly kindling required a similar number of ADs to reach the first stage V seizure but consistently evoking five stage V seizures during a day was difficult[31], likely because of the long 'refractory' period after an extended seizure. The increase in AD duration was an indication of the progression of kindling[30].

2. DISRUPTION OF SPATIAL PERFORMANCE AFTER HIPPOCAMPAL KINDLING

2.1. Performance on the Radial Arm Maze

Lopes da Silva et al.[33] demonstrated that hippocampal kindling disrupted spatial performance on the radial arm maze (RAM). However, rats were kindled and tested on the same day, likely confusing the effects of kindling on acquisition and retention, and RAM performance was only evaluated 1 day after the last AD[33]. Thus, we designed experiments that evaluated the long-lasting effects of kindling on acquisition and retention of the RAM.

In the first series of experiments, the effect of kindling on the retention of performance was studied using an open RAM with all 8 arms baited. The open RAM consisted of 8 arms radiating out from a central platform, and food was available at the ends of all 8 arms. A well-trained rat would run the RAM using extramaze, spatial cues, and it would typically enter each arm only once. A revisit of an arm was counted as an error. Rats were first trained on the RAM before full kindling[31], 35 hippocampal ADs[31], 21 ADs[25] or 15 ADs[30]. Full CA1 kindling (five stage V seizures) required 72.7 ± 10.4 ADs (N=9).[31] Kindled rats, either fully kindled or after 21–35 ADs, had more errors on the RAM for 3–4 weeks after kindling, as compared to a group of control rats which were run in the maze at the same time. The performance deficit in kindled rats, however, did not last 6 weeks after 15 ADs[30]. Since partial kindling of 15–21 ADs did not evoke any convulsions, the performance deficit of hippocampal kindled rats was not related to the evoked convulsions.

Subsequent experiments used the open RAM with only 4 of 8 arms baited. The advantage of the partially baited RAM is that stereotypic running patterns (like circling and entering sequential arm) are discouraged. Extramaze (spatial) information was used by the rat, and maze errors consisted of visits of non-baited arms (termed reference memory (RM) errors) or revisits (working memory (WM) errors) of baited or non-baited arms. Rats were trained on the RAM before 10 hippocampal ADs were evoked. After partial kindling, both RM and WM errors were significantly higher in kindled than control rats for 3 but not 6 weeks (not shown), with the RM deficit more robust than the WM deficit[28]. The sum of RM and WM errors is shown in Fig. 1A. Similar results were found after full kindling of the perforant path[12]. The disruption of both WM and RM scores is consistent with results in the all-arms-baited RAM, in which only WM can be scored. The effect of kindling may be interpreted as a disruption of spatial performance, without further interpretation of the meaning of WM and RM.

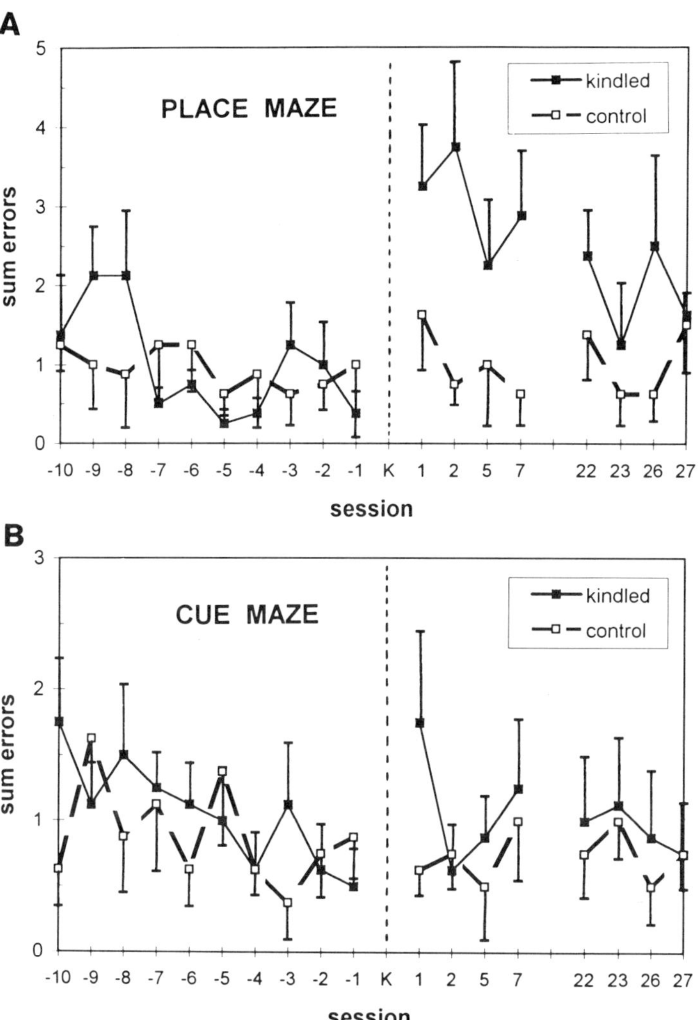

Figure 1. Total errors (sum of working memory and reference memory errors) on the (A) open radial arm maze (place maze) and (B) internal cue maze (cue maze) before and after partial hippocampal kindling (10ADs). Trials were performed once a day on both mazes. Error bar is the mean plus or minus one SEM. Abscissa labels: negative numbers are sessions before kindling (K) and positive numbers are day after kindling (last afterdischarge/low-frequency stimulation). Statistical difference was only found between kindled and control rats on the place maze and not the cue maze after kindling; no difference was found on either maze before kindling.

We have provided evidence that the retention deficit after partial kindling is specifically spatial in nature[28]. In this experiment, we trained rats in two types of RAMs before kindling: an open RAM with 4 of 8 arms baited (place maze) and an internal cue maze also with 4 of 8 arms baited (cue maze[15]). The cue maze was surrounded by a curtain and the 4 baited arms contained floor inserts (e.g. carpet, sandpaper, etc.) which were shuffled before each trial. After partial kindling (10 hippocampal ADs), rats showed maze errors only on the place (Fig. 1A) but not the cue maze (Fig. 1B)[28]. The specific deficit on the place maze is consistent with the view that the hippocampus is involved in spatial tasks[40]. The lack of deficit on WM in the cue maze suggests that the hippocampus is not involved with all types of WM[44]. Overall, the results strongly suggest that partial kindling exerts an effect directly on the hippocampus. The transient disruption of RM and WM on the place maze was similar to rats given partial lesion of the hippocampus, such as kainic acid lesion of CA3.[15] However, hippocampal cell loss is not detectable after partial kindling[7], and we suggest that the behavioral deficit is caused by a disruption of physiological function (below).

We have also reported that partially kindled rats acquired the open RAM at a rate similar to control rats[28]. Rats were first trained on a partially baited RAM (place task) in one room before kindling and on a new place task on the RAM in a different room using a different set of baited arms after kindling (Fig. 2). The initial training before kindling introduced the rat to the non-spatial requirements of the RAM. There was no difference in acquisition between kindled and control rats in the new room (Fig. 2). Subsequent test of retention of the RAM in the new room, after 11 day rest (layoff in Fig. 2), also did not show a significant difference between kindled and control rats. Thus, the acquisition of a new spatial task does not seem to depend on whether rats are partially kindled or not. Acquisition of the RAM was not affected by full kindling of the perforant path[48] but Sutula et al.[51] reported that fully kindled rats showed more difficulty in maintaining criterion performance on the RAM.

2.2. Performance on the Morris Water Maze

Kindled rats were reported to be not different from control rats in the acquisition or retention of a Morris water maze task, using a stationary hidden platform[5,36]. We con-

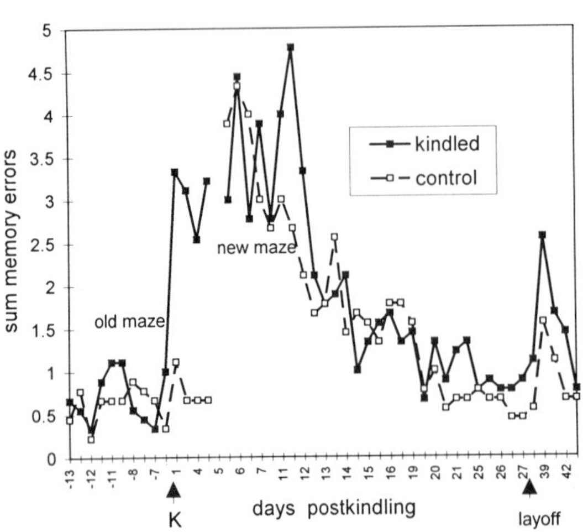

Figure 2. Sum errors immediately before and after kindling in an old maze (place) task in room A and acquisition of a new maze (place) task in room B. Partial hippocampal kindling (K) was 15 ADs over 3 days. Abscissa labels are days before (negative) and after (positive) kindling. Two trials were performed on each of the labeled days. Significant difference was found between the kindled and control groups of rats in retention of the old maze but no difference was found between the groups in acquisition of the new maze.

firmed this result in partially hippocampal kindled rats[50]. However, if the hidden platform was moved each day, partially kindled rats (after 20 hippocampal ADs) performed significantly worse than controls; both kindled and control rats were trained previously on the moving-platform task before kindling. The difference between controls and kindled rats was found 1 day and 1 week, but not 1 month, after partial hippocampal kindling[50]. These results support the hypothesis that spatial processing is disrupted in the partially kindled rats.

2.3. Summary of Spatial Deficits after Partial Kindling

In conclusion, full or partial kindling disrupted retention on a spatial RAM for up to 4 weeks, and on a moving platform water maze for up to 1 week. Retention on a non-spatial cue maze was not disrupted by partial kindling. Acquisition of a spatial RAM or the stationary-platform water maze was not disrupted by partial kindling. Why retention but not acquisition was affected by partial kindling can only be speculated about. Apparently, the spatial deficits after partial kindling are relatively mild. Perhaps acquisition of a spatial task after partial hippocampal kindling may use alternate strategies or alternate brain regions (outside of the hippocampus), although acquisition of a spatial task in the normal rat may depend critically on the hippocampus. Retrograde amnesia induced by kindling is unlikely since the temporal gradient of disruption had to extend 3 weeks before kindling, beyond the normal range of retrograde amnesia in rats[18]. Anterograde effects are likely induced by hippocampal kindling, perhaps by disrupting the spatial map in the hippocampus[40] or the neural circuitry responsible for the recall of spatial memory. The disruption of spatial map or memory may thus be manifested in the physiological changes after kindling.

3. PHYSIOLOGICAL CHANGES INDUCED BY PARTIAL HIPPOCAMPAL KINDLING

Two types of recordings have been used: field potentials in behaving rats in vivo and intracellular and field recordings in the hippocampal slice in vitro. In vivo recordings were done in a physiologically normal condition, as compared to in an isolated hippocampal slice preparation in vitro[49]. However, it is relatively easier to elucidate cellular mechanisms in vitro.

3.1. In Vivo Physiological Changes after Partial Hippocampal Kindling

Single-pulse stimulation of the electrode used for kindling in CA1 resulted in basal and apical dendritic excitation of the contralateral CA1.[29] The basal dendritic population excitatory postsynaptic potential (EPSP) in CA1 readily showed long-term potentiation (LTP) after a primed burst or a single AD.[29] After an AD, the commissural basal dendritic response was consistently enhanced in all rats for about a week (Fig. 3); the enhancement within 1 day may exceed 100%.[23] Repeated ADs apparently did not add much to this enhancement[23]. The apical dendritic population EPSP was more difficult to potentiate[29] and it was not consistently increased after a single or repeated ADs[23,27], though a small and persistent enhancement (up to 27 days) could sometimes be detected[25].

Recently, we have studied the changes in the perforant path responses following partial CA1 kindling (Leung and Shen, unpublished data). In 6 of 7 rats, the population spike

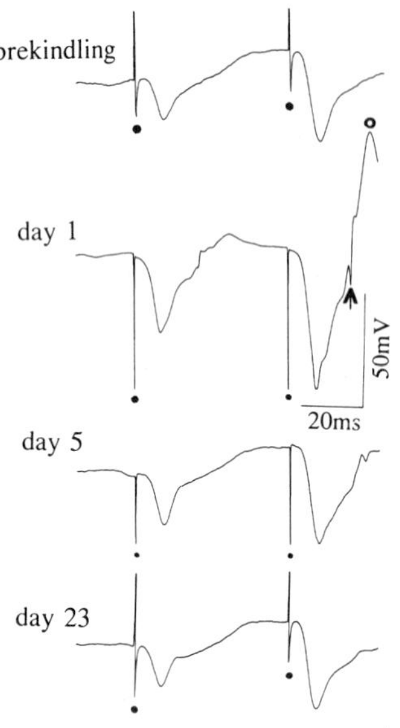

Figure 3. Potentiation of the basal dendritic EPSP and late potentials recording in the awake immobile rat before and on day 1, 5 and 23 after partial hippocampal kindling. Recording was in stratum radiatum of left CA1 and paired-pulses were delivered as 50 ms interpulse interval to the right CA1 alveus. The population EPSP and population spike were potentiated for 5 days. The late potential, arrow and open circle labeled in postkindling day 1 traces, was seen also for 5 days after kindling. The late potential was generated by the recurrent excitation of the hippocampus through the entorhinal cortex; the arrow indicates the population spike generated by dentate gyrus, and open circle the apical dendritic CA1 response. Negative is up.

evoked by the medial perforant path in the dentate gyrus was increased for up to 23–27 days after 15 ADs. No clear changes in the perforant path evoked population EPSP in the dentate gyrus were apparent, though in a few cases, an increase was found.

Long-latency events were readily detected in the single- or double-pulse evoked potentials evoked by CA1 (Fig. 3) or perforant path. These long-latency potentials typically started at about 20 ms after a pulse stimulus, and current source density analysis[55] revealed that they were generated by an entorhinal excitation that further re-excited the hippocampus[10], first at the medial perforant path synapses in the dentate gyrus (population spike in the dentate indicated by arrow in Fig. 3). The long-latency, recurrent entorhinal-hippocampal excitatory events were most salient immediately after an AD, and tended to disappear after 5 days.

Interictal spikes in the hippocampus were detected for several days after hippocampal kindling, with a decay time constant of about 1.5 days[22]. The generation of interictal spikes was apparently not disrupted by blockade of N-methyl-D-aspartate (NMDA) receptors or blockade of basal dendritic LTP in CA1.[23]

A weak sprouting of the mossy fibers may be detected within the most lateral 1 mm of the ventral blade of the dentate gyrus in rats 3 weeks after 15 hippocampal ADs, in agreement with Cavazos et al.[6] No abnormal physiology of the dentate gyrus following perforant path and CA3 stimulation could be attributed to these weakly sprouted mossy fibers (K. Wu and Leung, unpublished data).

In summary, partial hippocampal kindling was shown to affect many synapses in the hippocampus. LTP of the basal dendritic excitatory synapses in CA1 was induced for less than a week. LTP at the apical dendritic synapses in CA1 may sometimes be long-lasting but weak, and absent at other times. While not directly stimulated, the perforant path to dentate gyrus pathway showed a persistent increase in spike excitability. This is perhaps not unexpected, given that the dentate gyrus is often activated during an AD evoked by CA1 stimulation[17,21]. Multisynaptic pathway, particularly the hippocampal-entorhinal-hippocampal loop, was enhanced only for a few days after partial kindling, similar to the kindling-induced interictal spikes.

3.2. In Vitro Physiological Changes after Partial Hippocampal Kindling

3.2.1. Changes in Cellular Characteristics. We[60] found no change in resting membrane potential, input resistance, and spike threshold in CA1 cells in vitro after partial hippocampal kindling (15 ADs). This is in general agreement with the results after full kindling[37,45,57]. The number of action potentials in CA1 cells induced in the first 20 ms by a fixed depolarizing current was however increased on day 1–2 but not day 21–23 after partial kindling[57]; in some cells, this increase in spiking was clearly in a burst (cf. ref. 57). Bursting is consistent with a kindling-induced increase in Ca^{2+} currents in isolated CA1 cells[53].

3.2.2. Changes in Excitation in Vitro after Partial Kindling. The population EPSP (E1) and population spike (P1) in CA1 in vitro following single-pulse stimulation of the Schaffer collaterals were enhanced for 1–2 days after partial kindling[58]. In contrast, paired-pulse facilitation (PPF) of the EPSP and population spike in CA1 showed a persistent enhancement in partially kindled rats as compared to control rats (Fig. 4). PPF was found at interpulse intervals (IPIs) of 10–200 ms. PPF of the EPSPs in CA1 persisted up to 8 weeks after kindling, while PPF of the population spikes persisted for about 6 weeks[30]. The kindling-induced increase in PPF of the EPSPs in CA1 cells was robust when recorded intracellularly[60] and suggests an increase in presynaptic facilitation[24,56]. NMDA excitation in CA1 did not seem to be significantly enhanced after partial (Heale and Leung, unpublished data) or full hippocampal kindling[57], as compared to the change in dentate granule cells[38] and CA3 cells[19].

In CA3 in vitro, PPF of the population EPSPs and spikes following recurrent excitation by the Schaffer collaterals was enhanced for 3 weeks (but not 6 weeks) after partial kindling[30,59]. The facilitation appears to be similar to that in CA1. In contrast, paired-pulse depression (PPD) of the population spikes evoked by the medial perforant path was found in the dentate gyrus for 3 weeks (but not 6 weeks) after partial kindling[59]. The latter PPD in the dentate gyrus is consistent with the literature after full kindling of the amygdala, perforant path and commissural pathway[9,42]. Adamec[1] found PPD of the CA3 population spikes evoked by the perforant path, which may be caused by PPD in the dentate gyrus.

3.2.3. Changes in Inhibition in Vitro after Partial Kindling. There are few direct studies of inhibition in CA1 following kindling. Oliver and Miller[41] concluded that inhibition in CA1 was not changed after commissural kindling, but only 5 CA1 neurons were recorded. Kamphuis et al.[16] concluded that the ability of gamma-amino-butyric acid (GABA) to suppress glutamate-induced excitation in CA1 neurons was reduced persistently in fully kindled as compared to control rats. Here, we present data on the monosynaptic inhibition and PPD of the inhibitory postsynaptic currents (IPSCs) in CA1 cells after partial hippocampal kindling[54].

Monosynaptic IPSCs in CA1 cells were evoked by direct stimulation of the interneurons in stratum radiatum after excitation was blocked by the non-NMDA antagonist 6-cyano-7-nitroquinoxaline-2,3-dione (CNQX; 20μM) and the NMDA antagonist D-2-amino-5-phosphonovalerate (DAPV; 30μM). Sharp micropipettes of about 50 MΩ resistance, filled with 3M K acetate and 0.19M QX222 (to block Na spikes and $GABA_B$ IPSCs), were used for recordings in CA1 cells. Paired-pulse stimulations (100–500 ms IPIs) were delivered at 0.1 Hz. IPSCs were obtained using a single-electrode voltage

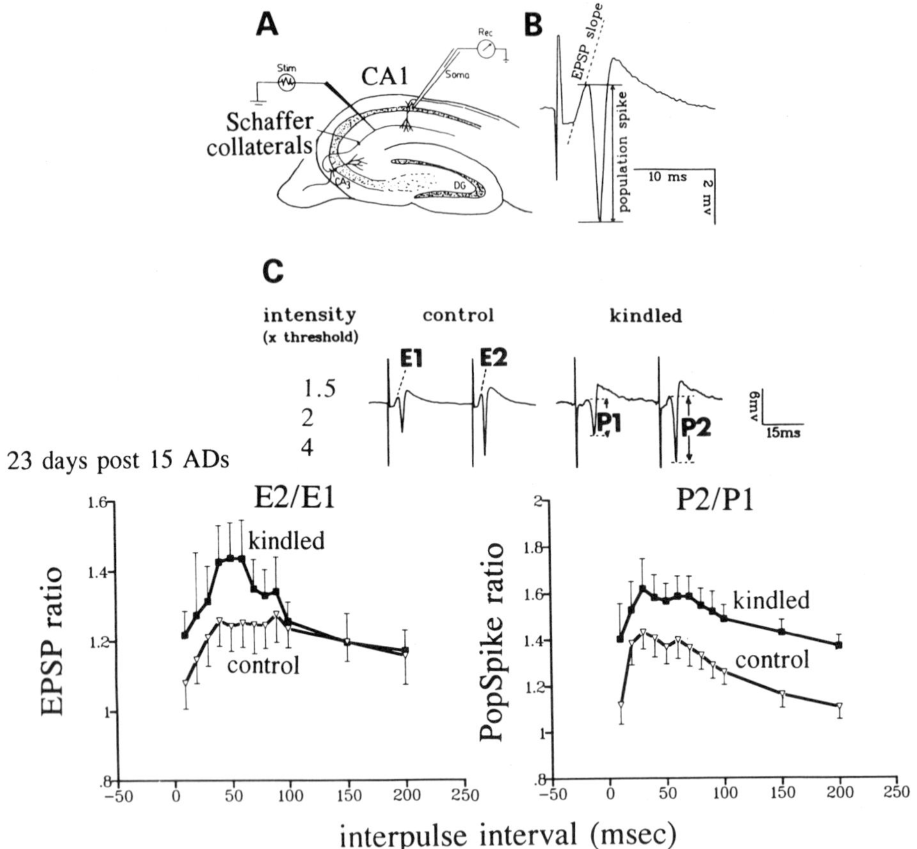

Figure 4. Paired-pulse facilitation (PPF) of the population EPSPs and population spikes in CA1 in vitro after partial hippocampal kindling (15 ADs). A. Schematic of stimulating and recording electrodes in the hippocampal slice in vitro. B. Illustration of the paired-pulse response (positive is up) and the measurement of the excitatory postsynaptic potential evoked by the first (E1) or second (E2) pulse, and the population spike evoked by the first (P1) and second (P2) pulse. Three stimulus intensities, 1.5, 2 and 4 times response threshold were used. C. When recorded in vitro at 23 days after kindling, PPF of the population EPSP (E2/E1) and population spike (P2/P1) was found at most interpulse intervals from 10 to 200 ms; stimulus intensity was 2 × response threshold.

clamp at a holding potential of −50 mV. In cells from control animals, IPSCs showed PPD[8,20,46]. When recorded in CA1 cells 1–2 days after partial kindling, the PPD was reduced significantly as compared to control cells (not shown). Using 2x threshold intensity Schaffer collateral pulses at 100 ms IPI, the paired-pulse ratio of IPSCs (IPSC2/IPSC1) was 0.69 ± 0.05 in control rats and 0.92 ± 0.03 in kindled rats ($P<0.01$, Wilcoxon, 13 cells in each group). The magnitude of the IPSC (IPSC1) evoked by the first pulse did not differ significantly between kindled and control rats. The reversal potential of the IPSC was not significantly different between cells from kindled and control rats. PPD of the IPSCs in control but not kindled slices was suppressed significantly by perfusing 1 mM CGP35348, a dose that blocked presynaptic (and postsynaptic) $GABA_B$ receptors; the IPSC2/IPSC1 ratio was not different between control and kindled rats (1–2 days after kindling) after perfusion of CGP35348. The latter result suggests that presynaptic $GABA_B$ receptors on $GABA_A$ terminals are blocked at 1–2 days after partial hippocampal kindling. No differences between PPD of IPSCs were detected at 21–22 days after partial kindling.

The result that partial hippocampal kindling induced a decrease of efficacy of presynaptic $GABA_B$ receptors on $GABA_A$ terminals is an original finding. Activity-dependent suppression of inhibition may be responsible for LTP and the onset of (electrographic) seizure activity. The relative lack of activity-dependent suppression of IPSCs after kindling will tend to make the hippocampal CA1 less susceptible to seizure and LTP. Thus, suppression of the PPD of IPSCs is functionally compensatory to the kindling-induced changes in excitation (PPF and LTP). Recently, Buhl et al.[4] reported a similar PPD of the monosynaptic IPSCs in dentate granule cells 1 day after full kindling. After non-convulsive limbic status epilepticus, Bekenstein and Lothman[3] found that monosynaptic IPSPs in CA1 cells (in DAPV and CNQX medium) were intact while disynaptic IPSPs were reduced. Thus far, we have no evidence that disynaptic IPSCs in CA1 were reduced after partial kindling, but the issue needs to be further evaluated.

The increase in PPD of the IPSCs in the dentate gyrus may be responsible for the increase in PPD of the population spike in the dentate in vitro (cf. ref. 43). We are not aware of studies on the persistence of the change in IPSCs in the dentate gyrus following hippocampal kindling.

3.2.4. Summary of in Vitro Results. The electrophysiological evidence in vitro indicated that there are persistent changes in various areas of the hippocampus following partial kindling of hippocampal CA1. It appears that the paired-pulse changes in CA1 and the dentate gyrus were among the most persistent changes. In CA1, PPF of the EPSPs and population spikes were found in vitro for more than 3 weeks. In the dentate gyrus, PPD of the population spikes was also found to last 3 weeks after partial kindling. A suppression of PPD of the IPSCs in CA1 cells by partial kindling was reported, but this was found 1–2 days but not 3 weeks after partial kindling.

4. RELATION BETWEEN PHYSIOLOGY AND SPATIAL PERFORMANCE

The effects of partial hippocampal kindling are many. Some physiological or morphological changes may underlie the changes in seizure susceptibility. Other changes may underlie the changes in behavioral function, such as performance on a spatial task. The physiological bases of seizure susceptibility and behavioral dysfunction need not be the same.

Since the effect on a spatial task (assumed to be caused by a hippocampal dysfunction) persisted for 1–4 weeks after partial kindling, only those electrophysiological changes that persisted to 3 weeks after partial kindling are considered likely candidates to cause the spatial task dysfunction. The list of physiological changes include (1) PPF of the EPSP and population spike in CA1 following Schaffer collateral (paired-pulse) stimulation. (2) PPD of the population spikes in the dentate gyrus following medial perforant path stimulation. (3) LTP of the population spike in the dentate gyrus evoked by the medial perforant path. Persistent LTP of the Schaffer collateral to CA1 synapses was not consistently found. In addition, the persistence of the PPF of the EPSPs in CA1 in vitro up to 8 weeks postkindling, at a time when RAM performance deficits have recovered[30], suggests that PPF of the EPSPs alone does not cause behavioral deficits. Further study of the persistence of the changes following partial hippocampal kindling will likely confirm and extend the list of physiological correlates that may account for the behavioral deficits. Other studies on molecular changes may elucidate the biochemical basis of the behavioral or physiological changes, but so far, only a few of these studies[17] (and this volume) address the persistence of the change after partial kindling.

There are problems in trying to go beyond correlation and explain the behavioral deficits by a change in physiology. The most disturbing one is that the mechanism whereby hippocampal physiology mediates spatial behavior is not known. Another problem is that the physiological measures may have nothing to do with how the brain works. The strength of a synapse is often expressed as the degree of LTP, without regard of the fact that synaptic transmission may also be modulated by behavior. The question whether LTP at the perforant path to dentate gyrus synapse is responsible for disruption of spatial learning is still unsettled[2,5,47]. Spatial behavior may be mediated by a neural circuit and not by a single cell or synapse, and it is possible that there is sufficient redundancy that alteration of a single pathway or structure would not disrupt behavioral functions (e.g., the perforant path also projects to CA3 and CA1). By inducing neural plasticity in a limited number of structures, partial kindling may offer a technique to study the difficult but overwhelmingly important question of how neural circuits mediate behavior.

5. SUMMARY

Partial kindling of the hippocampal CA1 area was used as a model of partial seizure of hippocampal origin. Experiments using pretraining on an open (spatial) radial arm maze and a moving-platform task on the Morris water maze indicated that spatial performance was disrupted for 1–4 weeks following partial hippocampal kindling (10 or more afterdischarges). Performance on a non-spatial cue radial arm maze and acquisition of a spatial maze was not affected by partial hippocampal kindling. It was postulated that persistent physiological changes in the hippocampus induced by partial kindling may underlie the deficit in spatial performance. Partial hippocampal kindling induced persistent enhancement effects (> 3 weeks) on the apical dendritic excitation in CA1 and the population spike in the dentate gyrus (evoked by the medial perforant path) in vivo, paired-pulse facilitation of excitatory postsynaptic potentials and population spikes in CA1 and CA3 in vitro, and paired-pulse depression of the population spike in the dentate gyrus in vitro. Less persistent effects of partial hippocampal kindling which persisted for a few days (but not 3 weeks) included a compensatory suppression of paired-pulse depression of inhibitory postsynaptic currents/potentials in CA1 in vitro, and an increase in interictal spikes, basal dendritic CA1 excitation and the hippocampal-entorhinal-hippocampal loop excitation in vivo. It is suggested that some of the long-lasting physiological changes in the hippocampus may be responsible for the disruption of the spatial tasks, but the nature and type of changes remain to be determined.

ACKNOWLEDGMENTS

This research was supported by grants from the National Institute of Neurological Diseases and Stroke NS-25383 and the Natural Sciences and Engineering Research Council.

REFERENCES

1. Adamec, R. E., Partial kindling of the ventral hippocampus: identification of changes in limbic physiology which accompany changes in feline aggression and defense, *Physiol. Behav.*, 49 (1991) 443–453.

2. Barnes, C.A., Jung, M.W., McNaughton, B.L., Korol, D.L., Andreasson, K., & Worley, P.F, LTP saturation and spatial learning disruption: Effects of task variables and saturation levels, *J. Neurosci.*, 14 (1994) 5793–5806.
3. Bekenstein, J.W. and Lothman, E.W., Dormancy of inhibitory interneurons in a model of temporal lobe epilepsy, *Science*, 259 (1993) 97–100.
4. Buhl, E.H., Otis, T.S. and Mody, I., Zinc-induced collapse of augmented inhibition by GABA in a temporal lobe epilepsy model, *Science*, 271 (1996) 369–373.
5. Cain, D. P., Hargreaves E.L. , Boon F. and Dennison, Z., An examination of the relations between hippocampal long term potentiation, kindling, afterdischarge, and place learning in the water maze, *Hippocampus*, 3 (1993) 153–164.
6. Cavazos, J.E., Golarai, G. and Sutula, T.P, Mossy fiber synaptic reorganization induced by kindling: time course of development, progression and permanence, *J. Neurosci.*, 11 (1991) 2795–2803.
7. Cavazos, J.E., Das, I. and Sutula, T.P., Neuronal loss induced in limbic pathways by kindling: evidence for induction of hippocampal sclerosis by repeated brief seizures, *J. Neurosci.*, 14 (1994) 3106–3121.
8. Davies, C.H., Davies, S.N. and Collingridge, G.L., Paired-pulse depression of monosynaptic GABA-mediated inhibitory postsynaptic responses in rat hippocampus, *J. Physiol.*, 424 (1990) 513–531.
9. de Jonge, M. and Racine, R.J., The development and decay of kindling-induced increases in pair-pulse depression in the dentate gyrus, *Brain Res.*, 412 (1987) 318–328.
10. Deadwyler, S.A., West, J.R., Cotman, C.W. and Lynch, G., Physiological connections between the hippocampus and the entorhinal cortex, *Exp.Neurol.*, 49 (1975) 35–56.
11. Dennison, A. Teskey, G.C. and Cain, D.P., Persistence of kindling: effect of partial kindling, retention interval, kindling site, and stimulation parameters, *Epilepsy Res.*, 21 (1995) 171–182.
12. Feasey-Truger, K.J., Kargl L. and ten Bruggencate, G., Differential effects of dentate kindling on working and reference spatial memory in the rat, *Neurosci. Letts.*, 151 (1993) 25–28.
13. Glansdorff, P. and Prigogine, I. *Thermodynamic theory of structure, stability and fluctuations.* Wiley, London, 1971.
14. Goddard, G.V., McIntyre, D.C. and Leech, C.K., A permanent change in brain function resulting from daily electrical stimulation, *Exp. Neurol.*, 25 (1969) 295–330.
15. Jarrard, L.E., Selective hippocampal lesions and behavior: implications for current research and theorizing. In R.L. Isaacson & K.H. Pribram (Eds.), *The Hippocampus, Vol. 4*, Plenum Press, New York, 1986, pp. 83–126.
16. Kamphuis, W., Gorter, J.A., and Lopes da Silva, F.H., A long-lasting decrease in the inhibitory effect of GABA on glutamate responses of hippocampal pyramidal neurons induced by kindling epileptogenesis, *Neurosci.*, 41 (1991) 425–431.
17. Kamphuis, W., De Rijk, T.C., Talamini, L.M. and Lopes da Silva, F.H., Rat hippocampal kindling induces changes in the glutamate receptor mRNA expression patterns in dentate granule neurons, *Eur. J. Neurosci.*, 6 (1994) 1119–1127.
18. Kesner, R.P. and Wilburn, M.W., A review of electrical stimulation of the brain in context of learning and retention, *Behav. Biol.*, 10 (1974) 259–293.
19. Kraus, J.E., Yeh, G., Bonhaus, D.W., Nadler, J.V. and McNamara, J.O., Kindling induces the long-lasting expression of a novel population of NMDA receptors in hippocampal region CA3, *J. Neurosci.*, 14 (1994) 4196–4205.
20. Lambert, N.A. and Wilson, W.A., Temporally distinct mechanisms of use-dependent depression at inhibitory synapses in rat hippocampus in vitro, *J. Neurophysiol.*, 72 (1994) 121–30.
21. Leung, L.S., Hippocampal electrical activity following local tetanization. I. Afterdischarges, *Brain Res.*, 419 (1987) 173–187.
22. Leung, L.S., Spontaneous hippocampal interictal spikes following local kindling: time-course of change and relation to behavioral seizures, *Brain Res.*, 513 (1990) 308–314.
23. Leung, L.S., Evaluation of the hypothesis that interictal spikes are caused by long-term potentiation, *Epilepsia*, 35 (1994) 785–794.
24. Leung, L. S. and Fu, X.-W., Factors affecting paired-pulse facilitation in CA1 neurons in vitro, *Brain Res.*, 650 (1994) 75–84.
25. Leung, L.S. and Shen, B., Hippocampal CA1 evoked response and radial 8-arm maze performance after hippocampal kindling, *Brain Res.*, 555 (1991) 353–357.
26. Leung, L.S. and Shen, B., Long-term potentiation in hippocampal CA1: Effects of afterdischarges, NMDA antagonists and anti-convulsants, *Expt. Neurol.*, 119 (1993) 205–214.
27. Leung, L.S. and Shen, B., Long-term potentiation at the apical and basal dendritic synapses of CA1 following local stimulation in behaving rats, *J. Neurophysiol.*, 73 (1995) 1938–1946.
28. Leung, L.S., Brzozowski, D. and Shen, B., Partial hippocampal kindling affects retention but not acquisition, place but not cue task on the radial arm maze, *Behav. Neurosci.*, in press.

29. Leung, L.S., Shen, B. and Kaibara, T., Long-term potentiation induced by patterned stimulation of the commissural pathway to hippocampal CA1 region in freely moving rats, *Neurosci.*, 48 (1992) 63–74.
30. Leung, L.S., Zhao D. and Shen, B., Long-lasting effects of partial hippocampal kindling on hippocampal physiology and function, *Hippocampus*, 4 (1994) 696–704.
31. Leung, L.S., Boon, K.A., Kaibara, T. and Innis, N.K., Radial maze performance following hippocampal kindling, *Behav Brain Res.*, 40 (1990) 119–129.
32. Lopes da Silva, F.H., Witter, M.P., Boeijinga, P. and Lohman, A.H.M., Anatomical organization and physiology of the limbic cortex, *Physiol. Rev.*, 70 (1990) 453–511
33. Lopes da Silva, F.H., Gorter, J.A. and Wadman, W.J., Kindling of the hippocampal induces spatial memory deficits in the rat, *Neurosci. Lett.*, 63 (1986) 115–120.
34. Lothman, E.W., Hatlelid, J.M. and Zorumski, C.F., Functional mapping of limbic seizures originating in the hippocampus: a combined 2-deoxyglucose and electrophysiological study, *Brain Res..*, 360 (1985) 92–100.
35. Ma, J., Brudzynski, S.M. and Leung, L. S., Involvement of the nucleus accumbens-ventral pallidal pathway in postictal behavior induced by a hippocampal afterdischarge in rats, *Brain Res.*, in press.
36. McNamara, R.K., R.D. Kirkby, G.E. dePape, G.E., R.W. Skelton and Corcoran, M.E., Differential effects of kindling and kindled seizures on place learning in the Morris water maze, *Hippocampus*, 3 (1993) 149–152.
37. Mody, I and Staley, K.J., Cell properties in the epileptic hippocampus, *Hippocampus*, 4 (1994) 275–280.
38. Mody, I., Stanton, P.K. and Heinemann, U., Activation of N-methyl-D-aspartate receptors parallels changes in cellular and synaptic properties of dentate gyrus granule cells after kindling, *J. Neurophysiol.*, 59 (1988) 1033–1054.
39. Morris, R.G.M., Schenk, F., Tweedie, F. and Jarrard, L.E., Ibotenate lesions of hippocampus and/or subiculum: dissociating components of allocentric spatial learning, *Eur. J. Neurosci.*, 2 (1991) 1016–1028.
40. O'Keefe, J. and Nadel, L., *Hippocampus as a cognitive map*, Oxford University Press, London, 1978.
41. Oliver, M.W. and Miller, J.J., Inhibitory processes of hippocampal CA1 pyramidal neurons following kindling-induced epilepsy in the rat, *Can. J. Physiol. Pharmacol.*, 63 (1985) 313–878.
42. Oliver, M.W. and Miller, J.J., Alterations of inhibitory processes in the dentate gyrus following kindling-induced epilepsy, *Exp. Brain Res.*, 57 (1985) 443–447.
43. Otis, T.S., de Koninck, Y. and Mody, I., Lasting potentiation of inhibition is associated with an increased number of gamma-aminobutyric acid type A receptors activated during miniature inhibitory postsynaptic currents, *Proc. Natl. Acad. Sci. (USA)*, 91 (1994) 7698–7702.
44. Olton, D.S., Becker, J.T. and Handelman, G.E., Hippocampus, space, and memory, *Behav. Brain Sci.*, 2 (1979) 313–322.
45. Racine, R. Burnham, W.M., Gilbert, M. and Kairiss, E.W., Kindling mechanisms: I. Electrophysiological Studies. In *Kindling 3*, Wada, J.A. (Ed.), Raven Press, New York, 1986, pp. 263–279.
46. Roepstorff, A. and Lambert, J.D.C., Factors contributing to the decay of the stimulus-evoked IPSC in rat hippocampal CA1 neurons, *J. Neurophysiol.*, 72 (1994) 2911–2926.
47. Robinson, G.B., Maintained saturation of hippocampal long-term potentiation does not disrupt acquisition of the 8-arm radial maze, *Hippocampus*, 2 (1992) 389–395.
48. Robinson, G.B., McNeil, H.A. and Reed, R.D., Comparison of short- and long-lasting effects of perforant path kindling on radial maze learning, *Behav. Neurosci.*, 6 (1993) 1–8.
49. Schwartzkroin, P.A., To slice or not to slice. In G.A. Kerkut and H.V. Wheal (Eds.), *Electrophysiology of isolated mammalian CNS preparations*, Academic Press, New York, 1981, pp. 15–50.
50. Sutherland, R.J., Leung, L.S., Weisend, M.P. and McDonald, R.J., An evaluation of the effect of partial hippocampal kindling on place navigation by rats in the Morris water task. In revision, Psychobiology.
51. Sutula, T., Lauersdorf, S. Lynch, M., Jurgella, C. and Woodard, A., Deficits in radial arm maze performance in kindled rats: evidence for long-lasing memory dysfunction induced by repeated brief seizures, *J. Neurosci.*, 15 (1995) 8295–8301.
52. Thompson, P.J., Memory function in patients with epilepsy. In D.B. Smith, D.M. Treiman, M.R. Trimble (Eds.), *Neurobehavioral Problems in Epilepsy, Advances in Neurology, Vol. 55*, Raven Press, New York, 1991, pp. 369–384.
53. Vreugdenhil, M. and Wadman, W.J., Kindling-induced long-lasting enhancement of calcium current in hippocampal CA1 area of the rat, *Neurosci.*, 59 (1994) 105–114.
54. Wu, C. and Leung, L.S., Suppression of paired-pulse depression of monosynaptic inhibitory postsynaptic currents (IPSCs) in CA1 neurons by partial hippocampal kindling, *Neurosci. Abstr.*, 22 (1996), in press.
55. Wu, K. and Leung, L.S., Field responses in dentate gyrus and CA1 following CA3b stimulation, *Neurosci. Abstr.*, 20 (1994) 340.
56. Wu, L.G. and Saggau, P., Presynaptic calcium Is increased during normal synaptic transmission and paired-pulse facilitation, but not in long-term potentiation in area CA1 of hippocampus, *J. Neurosci.*, 14 (1994) 645–654.

57. Yamada, N. and Bilkey, D.K., Kindling-induced persistent alterations in the membrane and synaptic properties of CA1 pyramidal cells, *Brain Res.*, 561 (1991) 324–331.
58. Zhao, D. and Leung, L.S., Effects of hippocampal kindling on paired-pulse response in CA1 in vitro, *Brain Res.*, 564 (1991) 220–229.
59. Zhao, D. and Leung, L.S., Hippocampal kindling induced paired-pulse depression in the dentate gyrus and paired-pulse facilitation in CA3, *Brain Res.*, 582 (1992) 163–167.
60. Zhao, D. and Leung, L.S., Partial hippocampal kindling increases paired-pulse facilitation and burst frequency in hippocampal CA1 neurons, *Neurosci. Lett.*, 154 (1993) 191–194.

DISCUSSION OF STAN LEUNG'S PAPER

M. Burnham: I think it would be fun to run this experiment again using subthreshold stimulation. Racine showed that you can get threshold drop without having afterdischarge. I wonder if you do subthreshold stimulation whether you would see threshold drop as well.

S. Leung: Yes, thank you for your suggestions, both of which we have tried to do. First we actually had a batch of rats in which we did long-term potentiation. I can't say that the parameters are the same, because we used different paradigms for stimulation. We had no effect on retention in the same behavioral situation.

F. Lopes Da Silva: About your GABA-B experiment, I think that it is interesting to have done it in this way, but I just wonder about what you think the contribution of GABA-A and the complex inhibition that you have at the same time in the same duration. Your interval was how many msec?

S. Leung: The paired-pulse interval is 100 msec, and we also did some with 500 msec.

F. Lopes Da Silva: Is there a GABA-A effect?

S. Leung: We look at the first response, that is a GABA-A effect. The cells were impaled with QX314 in the pipette so GABA-B postsynaptic response is blocked and presumably we are only looking at a GABA-A response. The first response was not changed significantly. It is actually slightly decreased in the kindled animals but it is not significant. The other thing you are wondering about is the inter-pulse intervals? To get good statistics we mainly look at 100 msec, but preliminary results suggest that other intervals are also affected. But the suppression is higher at about 100 or 150 msec; that seems to be the most sensitive one.

K. Gale: Talking about your behavioural studies, in your 8-arm radial maze, you said that you were looking at the re-entering of the unbaited arms. Are you getting similar effects on working and reference memory? This was unclear from the data you presented.

S. Leung: Yes, it's the same result. Using this task, we could not distinguish a differential effect after kindling. In fact this might be different from Fernando's results, which showed differential effects on reference and working memory. So we just thought that this is some sort of spatial disruption without trying to infer more about what reference memory and working memory are.

K. Gale: The second question I had is about the study where you did the 4 trials a day in the Morris water maze with a hidden platform. On the first trial they have had no experience with that position of the platform, but that's the one on which you found the biggest difference between kindled animals and controls. Doesn't this mean that it had to have been a difference in swim speed, because they didn't have any differential information to start out with?

S. Leung: I don't know. You could say that maybe just before hand the kindled rats were more confused, and they just don't go anywhere.

K. Gale: But what was the reason for the difference on the first trial—clearly it can't be memory.

S. Leung: I don't know. Maybe Rob Sutherland would have a better idea. It could be some sort of confusion effect, perhaps not so specific as to spatial location.

I. Mody: For a while I thought that perhaps the enhancement of the paired-pulse inhibition in the dentate may be due to a reduced autoinhibition of the GABA receptors. But now I'm confused, because you see the same thing in CA1 where there is no reduction of paired-pulse inhibition. Do you have evidence for how much presynaptic GABA-B receptors participate in the field recordings in CA1?

S. Leung: Well there are two types of effects in CA1, at least in vitro. One is that there is a paired-pulse facilitation of the EPSP, presumably a presynaptic facilitation that has nothing to do with the spike. Now the way we measure paired-pulse pop-spike response would always confuse inhibition with facilitation of excitation; so that is one complication there. Two other comments: One is that this effect that we see did not persist—so far we only took it to 21 days, where there is a trend but it is not significant. So we probably could not explain any effect on paired-pulse response after the first week at least, I would think.

R. Racine: I just have one more question for Corcoran. On your schedule it says 3:30 pm Break and on the next page it says Drugs, but it doesn't have a room number and I'd like to know where to go.

29

PROTECTIVE EFFECTS OF BRAIN-DERIVED NEUROTROPHIC FACTOR IN HIPPOCAMPAL KINDLING

Sophie Reibel,[1] Yves Larmet,[2] Josette Carnahan,[3] Bich-Thuy Lê,[1] Christian Marescaux,[1] and Antoine Depaulis[1]

[1]Unité INSERM 398, Université Louis Pasteur
11 rue Humann, Strasbourg, France
[2]URA 1446 CNRS
Université Louis Pasteur
21 rue René Descartes, Strasbourg, France
[3]Amgen Center, Thousand Oaks
1840 DeHavilland Drive, Thousand Oaks, California

1. INTRODUCTION

Several reports have suggested the involvement of different growth factors in the cascade of events that underlies epileptogenesis. Among these, nerve-growth factor (NGF) and brain-derived neurotrophic factor (BDNF) from the neurotrophin family appear to play a critical role [16]. These neurotrophins are involved in the development of the central nervous system as well as in adult brain plasticity [38, 24]. Neurotrophins bind to receptors of the tyrosine kinase family, and the high affinity receptors for NGF and BDNF are TrkA and TrkB respectively [17]. Expression of both NGF and BDNF and their high affinity receptor messenger RNAs increases in the hippocampus, amygdala and cortex after different forms of convulsive seizures in the rat [4, 3, 14, 19, 18, 28, 34, 12]. In the kindling model of epilepsy, the first electrical stimulation of the hippocampus induces a rapid increase of BDNF mRNA expression in the granule cells of the dentate gyrus, in both the stimulated and the non-stimulated sides [14] (see Lindvall et al., chapter 22 in this volume). After several stage 5 seizures, BDNF mRNA expression is also increased throughout CA1-CA3 pyramidal layer, the hilar region of the dentate gyrus, the amygdala, parietal and piriform cortex [14, 3]. During kindling, a parallel increase of BDNF and *trkB* mRNAs occurs in the dentate granule cells and suggests an autocrine or paracrine action of BDNF in the hippocampus [3]. However, the physiological significance of the increased expression of neurotrophins remains to be determined and BDNF and NGF could

Kindling 5, edited by Corcoran and Moshé.
Plenum Press, New York, 1998.

be involved in the neuroplastic processes that either facilitate or inhibit the development of seizures. Recent studies (see Racine et al., chapter 15 in this volume) suggest that overexpression of NGF could promote the occurrence of seizures. In our laboratory, we have investigated the effects of BDNF on epileptogenesis by examining the effects of chronic intracerebral perfusions of recombinant human BDNF on the development of seizures in the kindling model in the rat [23]. In the conditions used in the present study, this model is not associated with neuronal death [5], thus allowing us to dissociate the effects of BDNF on seizures from effects on neuronal survival. In order to apply the neurotrophin on the same neuronal population that is activated by the electrical stimulation, we used a combined electrode/cannula implanted in the structure to be kindled. This methodology was designed to exaggerate the increase of BDNF observed during the development of kindling. Animals were perfused with BDNF during the first week of the kindling protocol and kindling development was evaluated on the basis of behavioral and electroencephalographic parameters. Our results show that application of exogenous BDNF exerts protective effects during hippocampal kindling.

2. MATERIALS AND METHODS

2.1. Animals

Adult male Wistar rats (320–350 g) were selected from a non epileptic strain bred in our laboratory. Once weaned, they were raised in groups of 8–12 males until surgery. After surgery, they were placed in individual plexiglass cages and received food and water *ad libitum*. All animal experiments were carried out in accordance with the EC Council Directive of 24 November 1986 (86/609/EEC).

2.2. Surgery and Kindling Procedure

Rats were premedicated with valium (4 mg/kg, i.p.) and anaesthetized with ketamine (100 mg/kg, i.p.) and placed in a stereotaxic frame. Unilateral or bilateral stainless steel cannulae (o.d., 0.5 mm; i.d., 0.4 mm) were implanted in the dorsal hippocampus (A/P: 4.0 mm; M/L: 2.0 mm; D/V: 4.0 mm, with lambda as reference, flat skull position) or the basolateral nucleus of the amygdala (A/P: 1.8 mm; M/L: 4.5 mm; D/V: 9 mm, with bregma as reference, flat skull position). A bipolar electrode formed of two enamel-insulated wires (0.18 mm) was glued with cyanolate on the right-hand side cannula so that the distal tip was located 1.0 mm below the tip of the cannula. In addition, the animals were equipped with two monopolar electrodes fixed in the skull over the controlateral fronto-parietal cortex. The electrodes were connected to a female connector placed over the rat's head and secured with acrylic cement. A stainless steel stylet (o.d., 0.38 mm) was inserted into the cannula to keep its patency. The animals were allowed a week for recovery during which time they were handled daily for habituation.

During the kindling protocol, the animals were stimulated through the bipolar electrode using a monophasic square wave current (frequency = 50 Hz; duration = 2 s; pulse = 1 ms) with current set at twice the threshold for inducing an afterdischarge. In the hippocampal kindling paradigm, electrical stimulations were applied once daily during the first week and then twice daily for the remaining two weeks. In the amygdala kindling protocol, the animals were stimulated once daily for two weeks. After each electrical stimulation, the duration of cortical and hippocampal or amygdala afterdischarges was measured on the EEG recording and behavioral seizures were scored as described previously [30].

2.3. BDNF Perfusion

Mini-osmotic pumps (Alzet, model 2001) were filled with phosphate-buffered saline (PBS) or with a freshly prepared solution of recombinant human brain-derived neurotrophic factor (BDNF; Amgen, USA) in PBS, and incubated overnight in 0.9% saline at 37°C. The next day, animals were implanted under light anaesthesia with one or two mini-osmotic pumps placed subcutaneously between the shoulder blades. The osmotic pumps were connected to the cannulae after removal of the stylet via a catheter threaded under the skin. The mini-osmotic pumps delivered 1 μl/h of solution. On the seventh day of perfusion, the pumps were disconnected by sectioning the catheter and the stylets were replaced in the cannulae. According to the experiments carried out, different concentrations of BDNF were used: 0.25, 0.5, 2 or 5 μg/μl, corresponding to 6, 12, 48 or 120 μg daily infusions.

2.4. Histological Control

On completion of the experiments, the animals were killed with an overdose of nembutal (100 mg/kg). Their brain was removed, frozen in isopentane at –30°C and cut in 20 μm sections mounted on gelatin-coated slides. These sections were later stained with cresyl violet. Only animals with correct location of the bipolar electrode in the dorsal hippocampus or the basolateral nucleus of the amygdala were used for the analysis.

For Timm's staining [8], 3 rats from the PBS group and 3 from the BDNF group (unilateral perfusion at 5 μg/h) were killed with an overdose of nembutal (100 mg/kg) and then perfused transcardially with 300 ml of a 0.37% solution of sodium sulfide followed by 300 ml of a 4% paraformaldehyde solution in 0.4 M phosphate buffer. Additional animals which received PBS (n=3) and BDNF (n=3) in the same conditions but without kindling were perfused using the same protocol. The brains were then removed and postfixed for three hours in paraformaldehyde 4%. Forty μm thick free-floating sections were collected in 60 mM phosphate buffer on a vibratome. The sections were mounted on gelatin-coated slides, dried and processed for Timm's staining within 48 hours. Sections were dehydrated in ethanol and developed in the dark for 60 minutes in a solution of arabic gum (50%), citrate buffer (0.05 M) and hydroquinone (6%) with silver nitrate at 26°C. The slides were then rapidly washed under tap water, dehydrated and mounted using a standard procedure.

Quantification of fiber sprouting was carried out for each rat on one section corresponding to the 5.7 AP level in the atlas of Paxinos and Watson [29]. Using a camera lucida, the tip of the hilus of the dentate gyrus ipsilateral to the cannula/electrode was delimited in a frame so that the counting surface was equivalent for each section. The Timm stained fibres were then drawn on an individual transparent sheet and were counted, whatever their length, by a blind experimenter.

2.5. Statistical Analysis

Afterdischarge durations (s), epileptic scores and anatomical data were expressed as means ± SEM and were compared using non parametric tests for independent samples (Kruskal Wallis and Mann Whitney tests).

3. RESULTS

3.1. Effect of a Perfusion of BDNF on Hippocampal Kindling

3.1.1. Unilateral Perfusion of BDNF. BDNF applied unilaterally at the dose of 12 or 120 μg/day during the first week of kindling stimulations significantly reduced the development of seizures. In control rats, the duration of hippocampal and cortical afterdischarges as well as seizure scoring increased progressively throughout the experiment (Figure 1). In rats treated with BDNF at 12 or 120 μg/day, the duration of hippocampal

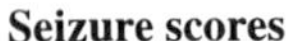

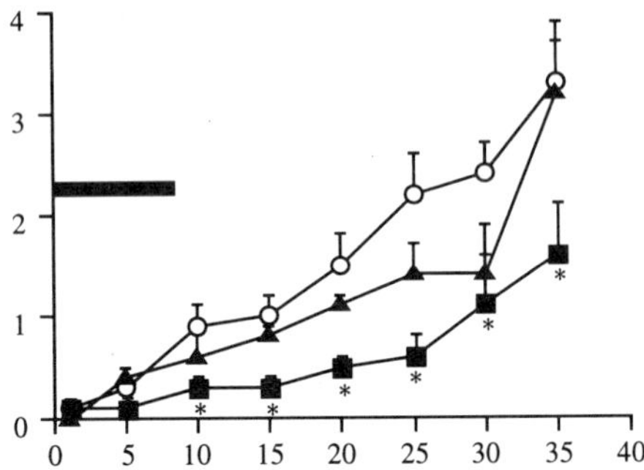

Hippocampal afterdischarges (s)

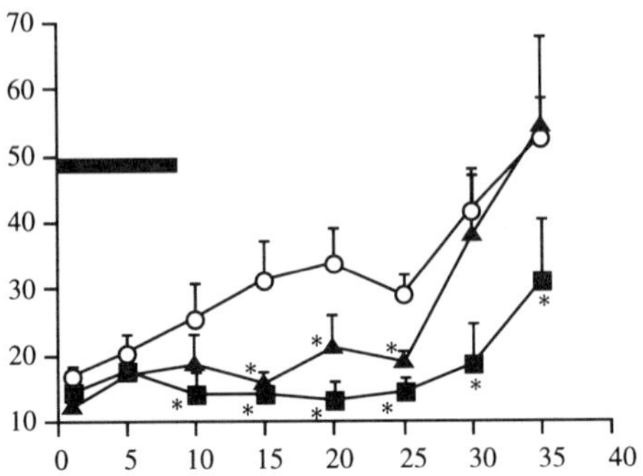

Cortical afterdischarges (s)

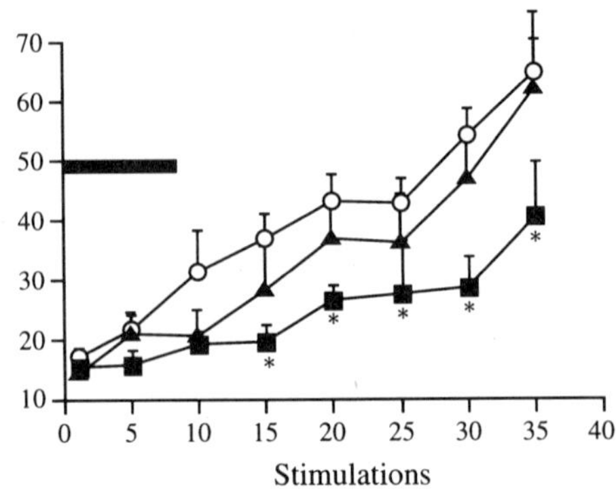

Figure 1. Effects of a unilateral perfusion of BDNF on hippocampal kindling. ■ = BDNF 120 μg/day (n = 9); ▲ = BDNF 12 μg/day (n = 8); ○ = PBS (n = 20). Solid bar: perfusion period. *p < 0.05 vs. PBS (Mann-Whitney test).

afterdischarges remained at initial values until the 25th and 30th stimulation respectively, i.e., 9 and 12 days after the end of the perfusion, before increasing. Rats treated with the highest dose of BDNF also displayed significantly reduced cortical afterdischarges compared to control animals, which was not the case at the dose of 12 μg/day. Furthermore, in rats perfused with BDNF 120 μg/day, stimulations were only followed by a behavioral arrest with no other signs of limbic seizures up to the 25th stimulation. A perfusion of BDNF 12 μg/day led to lower seizure scores compared to control animals. Finally, a unilateral perfusion of BDNF at the dose of 6 μg/day did not modify the development of hippocampal kindling compared to PBS-treated animals (data not shown).

3.1.2. Bilateral Perfusion of BDNF. Bilateral perfusion of BDNF at the dose of 12 μg/side/day resulted in a significant reduction of both seizure scores and hippocampal and cortical afterdischarges, close to that obtained by unilateral perfusion of BDNF at the dose of 120 μg/day and with a similar time course (Figure 2). The suppressive effects of BDNF on hippocampal kindling can also be evidenced when considering the number of stimulations necessary to reach a seizure score of 2 (i.e., chewing and head nodding; Figure 3). The dose-dependent effects of a perfusion of BDNF on hippocampal kindling and the greater effectiveness of bilateral versus unilateral perfusion for a given BDNF concentration are demonstrated by a significantly increased number of stimulations necessary to induce stage 2 seizures.

During the kindling experiments, animals displayed no motor impairment and background EEG activity was not modified (data not shown). Histological examination of the dorsal hippocampus of BDNF-treated rats (cresyl staining) did not reveal any cell body degeneration or glial cell proliferation around the tip of the cannula/electrode, as compared to control rats.

3.2. Effect of a Unilateral Perfusion of BDNF on Amygdala Kindling

The effects of BDNF at the dose of 48 μg/day on amygdala kindling were less pronounced than those observed in the hippocampus after unilateral perfusion at 12 and 120 μg/day (Figure 4). Increase of amygdala afterdischarge durations was delayed compared to the control animals. Cortical afterdischarge durations (data not shown) and seizure scores were not significantly different in the two groups, although behavioral seizures tended to aggravate less rapidly in the BDNF-treated animals.

3.3. Effect of a Unilateral Perfusion of BDNF (120 μG/Day) on Dentate Mossy Fiber Sprouting

Using the Timm's technique to stain mossy fiber terminals, we observed a two-fold increase of axonal sprouting in the dentate gyrus of kindled as compared to non-kindled animals (Figure 5). However, no significant differences were observed between BDNF-treated animals and the controls, whether kindled or not.

4. DISCUSSION

These results show that a chronic perfusion of BDNF during the first week of hippocampal kindling significantly suppressed epileptogenesis. Both behavioral and EEG signs of the seizures were reduced by BDNF in a dose-dependent manner, but this effect was not

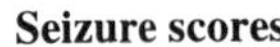

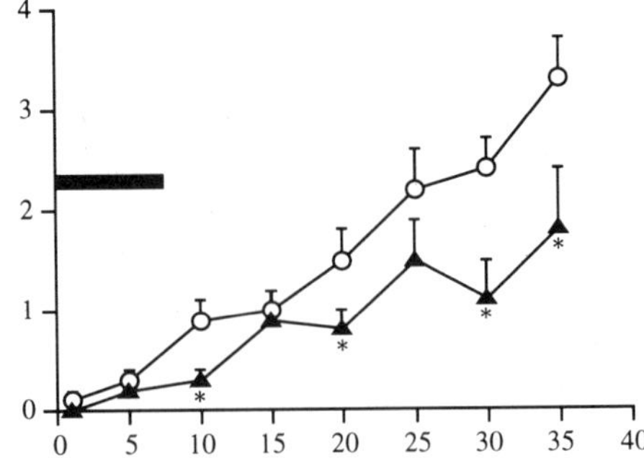

Hippocampal afterdischarges (s)

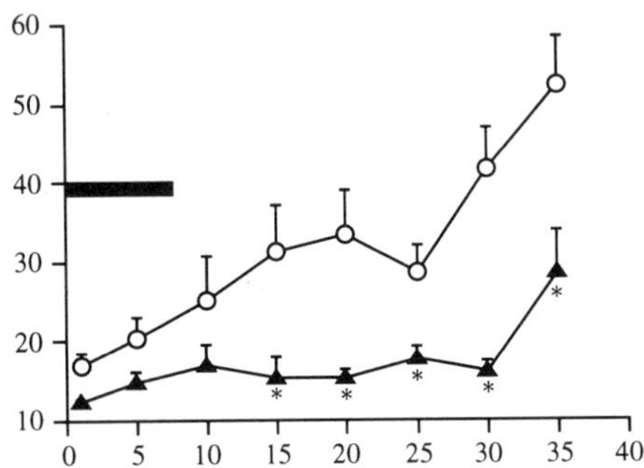

Cortical afterdischarges (s)

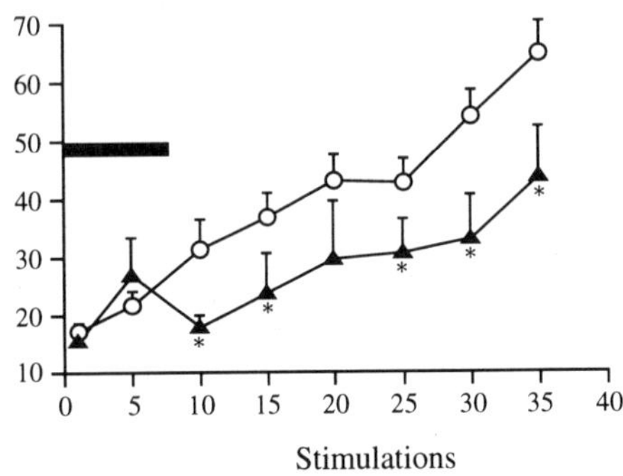

Stimulations

Figure 2. Effects of a bilateral perfusion of BDNF on hippocampal kindling. ▲ = BDNF 12 μg/day (n = 6); ○ = PBS (n = 20). Solid bar: perfusion period. *p < 0.05 vs. PBS (Mann-Whitney test).

secondary to any modifications of the background EEG activity nor to motor impairments. Although further controls are required to rule out a possible cell toxicity, no gross histological lesions could account for these suppressive effects of BDNF, even at the highest dose (120 μg/day). At the dose of 12 μg/day, bilateral perfusion of BDNF resulted in a greater protective effect than unilateral perfusion. During unilateral hippocampal kindling stimulations, c-Fos protein immunoreactivity is increased bilaterally in the hippocampus, suggesting the involvement of both hippocampi in kindling development [11] (personal observation). This could explain our observation that bilateral perfusion confers increased protection compared to unilateral perfusion at the dose of 12 μg/day. It has been shown

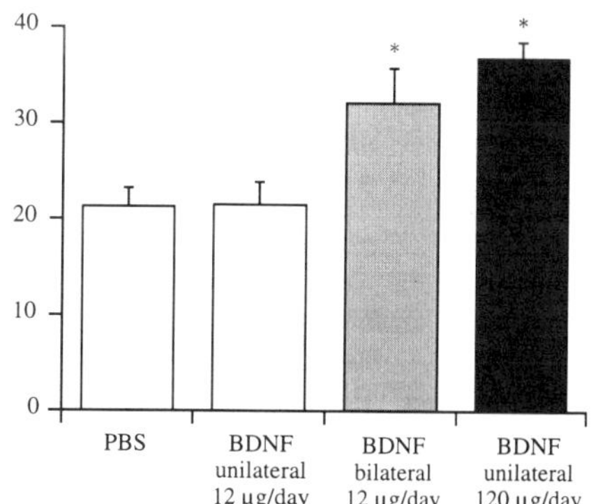

Figure 3. Number of stimulations necessary to reach seizure score 2. *p < 0.05 vs. PBS (Mann-Whitney test).

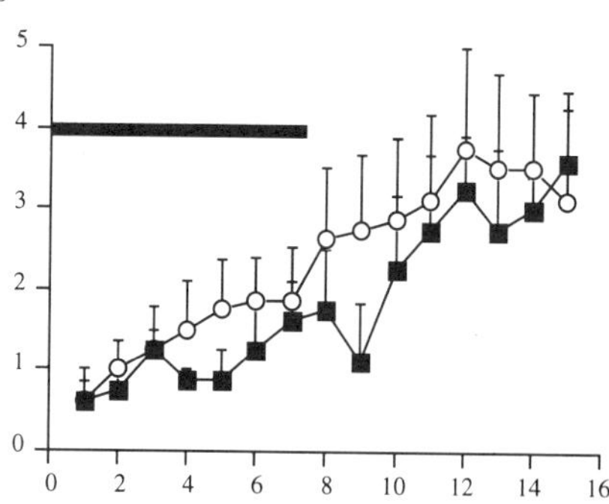

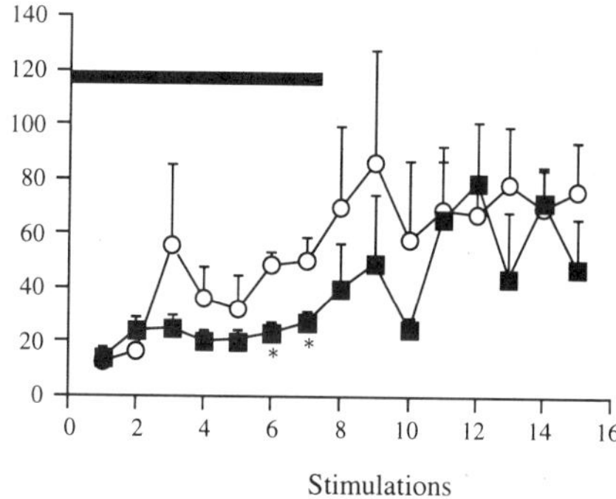

Figure 4. Effect of a unilateral perfusion of BDNF on amygdala kindling. ■ = BDNF 48 µg/day (n = 4); ○ = PBS (n = 4). Solid bar: perfusion period. *p < 0.05 vs. PBS (Mann-Whitney test).

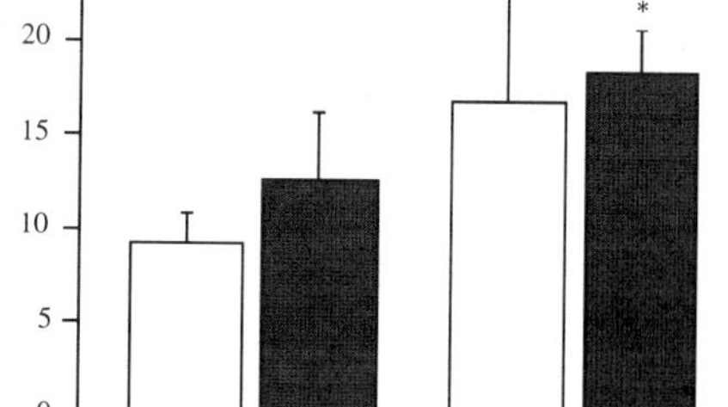

Figure 5. Effect of a perfusion of BDNF on dentate mossy fiber sprouting. ▓ = BDNF 120 µg/day (n = 3); □ = PBS (n = 3). *p < 0.05 vs. PBS (Mann-Whitney test).

that BDNF perfused unilaterally in the hippocampus can be retrogradely transported to the contralateral dentate gyrus [1, 10]. This could account for the protection induced by a high dose (120 µg/day) of BDNF applied unilaterally. Our preliminary results on amygdala kindling show that a unilateral perfusion of BDNF in the basolateral nucleus of the amygdala does not lead to a suppressive effect as strong as that observed in the hippocampal kindling experiments. Differing experimental conditions (BDNF concentration and unilateral or bilateral perfusions) used in the hippocampal and amygdala kindling protocols could account for this difference. However, following seizures induced by amygdala or hippocampal kindling, increased levels of *trkB* mRNA are confined to the dentate gyrus and are not reported in the amygdala [3]. If BDNF exerts its protective effects by triggering a cascade of genomic events through binding to its high affinity receptor, this modulation of *trkB* mRNA expression specific to the hippocampus could explain the lower effects of BDNF in the amygdala.

One of the most striking characteristics of the protective effects of exogenous BDNF on hippocampal kindling is the long-lasting suppression of kindling development. Indeed, in animals treated with BDNF unilaterally at 120 µg/day or bilaterally at 12 µg/day, the suppressive effect of BDNF was still present at least one week after the end of the perfusion, which suggests that BDNF impaired the development of seizures through long term genomic changes. It is established that BDNF is increased for several days after convulsive seizures in structures which are critical in the development of epilepsy [16]. In addition, it is generally thought that effects of BDNF on neuronal survival require the presence of target cells or chronic *in vitro* BDNF addition [2] . In this respect, the chronic perfusion technique used in the present study exaggerated the BDNF increase induced by seizures and may have amplified the related neuronal responses. Since BDNF has been shown to regulate genomic expression in CNS neurons [25], it may be involved in the neuroplasticity phenomena which accompany epileptogenesis [27]. The seizure-induced synthesis of this neurotrophin may trigger and amplify, through an autocrine or paracrine mechanism, a cascade of molecular events involved in neuronal plasticity and leading to the protective effects observed in our experiments. Among these possible events, we investigated the effects of BDNF on sprouting of the mossy fibers of the dentate gyrus. Sprouting of mossy fibers in the supragranular molecular layer of the dentate gyrus has been reported following perforant path kindling and has been suggested to participate in the increase of excitability of the hippocampal cells [36, 35, 37]. One way of visualizing this sprouting is by staining of heavy metal grains which are abundant in processes of mossy fibers [8]. In the present study, a significant difference in the number of stained fibers was observed in the hilus between non-kindled and kindled animals in agreement with previous reports [35, 37]. However, no significant difference was found between PBS and BDNF-treated rats whether they were kindled or non-kindled. Although further experiments using other ways of visualizing the sprouting of mossy fibers are needed to confirm these findings, our data suggest that BDNF-induced blockade of hippocampal kindling is not associated with a modification of mossy fiber sprouting. The protective effects of BDNF on hippocampal kindling described here could also result from long term changes in the expression of proteins involved in kindling epileptogenesis. One hypothesis which we are currently investigating concerns the implication of neuropeptide Y (NPY) in the protective effects of BDNF. Several lines of evidence suggest that NPY neurotransmission could be involved in the control of epileptic seizures. NPY expression is increased after generalized convulsive seizures [32]. Following amygdala or hippocampal kindling, the levels of NPY mRNA and immunoreactivity are significantly increased in the granule cell layer and in the hilar cells of the dentate gyrus [33, 39]. Moreover, it has been shown that NPY can reduce neuronal excitability and prevent seizure-like activity in hippocampal slices [6]. Mice lacking NPY have been reported to be more susceptible to seizures induced by a GABA antagonist and occasionally display spontaneous seizures [13]. Finally, BDNF induces a long-lasting increase in NPY expression in interneurons of the hippocampus *in vivo* and *in vitro* [7, 26]. Hence, chronic application of BDNF could increase NPY levels in the hippocampus, which in turn could lead to protective effects by an inhibitory action of NPY.

The effects of BDNF on hippocampal kindling and mossy fiber sprouting reported here appear to be different from those of NGF. It has been described that intracerebroventricular injections of antibodies directed against NGF inhibit amygdaloid kindling and kindling-induced mossy fiber sprouting [15, 40]. Furthermore, intraventricular infusion of a peptide which prevents binding of NGF to its high affinity receptors retards seizure development and inhibits mossy fiber sprouting in amygdala kindling [31]. These reports suggest that NGF could facilitate amygdala kindling and induce mossy fiber sprouting. Several findings can be put forward to explain the discrepancies between the effects of BDNF and NGF. These two neurotrophins appear to act through specific high affinity receptors, TrkA and TrkB for NGF and BDNF respectively [17]. Moreover, they have been shown to be differently regulated during kindling [3]. A seizure promoting effect of BDNF, similar to NGF, has been suggested by data collected in heterozygous mutant mice with a deletion of the gene coding for BDNF. In these animals (see Lindvall, this volume), a greater number of electrical stimulations is required to induce amygdala kindling, suggesting that lower levels of BDNF retard the kindling process [21]. However, the hippocampal neuronal excitability of these mutant animals is very likely modified. In particular, long term potentiation has been shown to be significantly reduced [22]. The suppression of seizure development observed in BDNF mutant mice may thus be related to a modification of neuronal properties. Moreover, BDNF is necessary for normal neuronal differentiation and cytoarchitecture [9, 20] and reduced levels of this neurotrophin during development may impair the establishment of normal synaptic connections in mutant animals. Finally, data obtained in BDNF mutant mice were obtained by kindling the amygdala, and our present results suggest that this structure is less sensitive to BDNF protective effects. Although further research is required to clarify the role of endogenous BDNF in epileptogenesis, our current data are in agreement with the wealth of recent reports indicating that BDNF plays a critical role in the neuroprotection of adult CNS [24] and suggest that this neurotrophin may be involved in endogenous control mechanisms aimed at limiting the consequences of epileptic seizures.

ACKNOWLEDGMENTS

We thank Thomas Boone, Randy Hecht and Jeff Hogan (Amgen Center, Thousand Oaks, USA) for providing us with recombinant BDNF. This work was supported by INSERM and the Ligue Française Contre l'Epilepsie.

REFERENCES

1. Anderson, K.D., Alderson, R.F., Altar, C.A., Distefano, P.S., Corcoran, T.L., Lindsay, R.M. and Wiegand, S.J., Differential distribution of exogenous BDNF, NGF, and NT-3 in the brain corresponds to the relative abundance and distribution of high-affinity and low-affinity neurotrophin receptors, *J Comp Neurol*, 357 (1995) 296–317.
2. Barde, Y.A., Trophic factors and neuronal survival, *Neuron*, 2 (1989) 1525–1534.

3. Bengzon, J., Kokaia, Z., Ernfors, P., Kokaia, M., Leanza, G., Nilsson, O.G., Persson, H. and Lindvall, O., Regulation of neurotrophin and trkA, trkB and trkC tyrosine kinase receptor messenger RNA expression in kindling, *Neurosci*, 53 (1993) 433–446.
4. Bengzon, J., Söderström, S., Kokaia, M., Ernfors, P., Persson, H., Ebendal, T. and Lindvall, O., Widespread increase of nerve growth factor protein in the rat forebrain after kindling-induced seizures, *Brain Res*, 587 (1992) 338–342.
5. Cavazos, J.E. and Sutula, T.P., Progressive neuronal loss induced by kindling: A possible mechanism for mossy fiber synaptic reorganization and hippocampal sclerosis, *Brain Res.*, 527 (1990) 1–6.
6. Colmers, W.F. and Bleakman, D., Effects of neuropeptide Y on the electrical properties of neurons, *Trends Neurosci*, 17 (1994) 373–379.
7. Croll, S.D., Wiegand, S.J., Anderson, K.D., Lindsay, R.M. and Nawa, H., Regulation of neuropeptides in adult rat forebrain by the neurotrophins BDNF and NGF, *Eur J Neurosci*, 6 (1994) 1343–1353.
8. Danscher, G., Histochemical demonstration of heavy metals. A revised version of the sulphide silver method suitable for both light and electron microscopy, *Histochemistry*, 71 (1981) 1–16.
9. Davies, A.M., The role of neurotrophins in the developing nervous system, *J Neurobiol*, 25 (1994) 1334–1348.
10. DiStefano, P.S., Friedman, B., Radziejewski, C., Alexander, C., Boland, P., Schick, C.M., Lindsay, R.M. and Wiegand, S.J., The neurotrophins BDNF, NT-3, and NGF display distinct patterns of retrograde axonal transport in peripheral and central neurons, *Neuron*, 8 (1992) 983–993.
11. Dragunow, M., Robertson, H.A., Kindling stimulation induces c-fos protein (s) in granule cells of the rat dentate gyrus, *Nature*, 329, (1987) 441–442.
12. Elmer, E., Kokaia, M., Kokaia, Z., Ferencz, I. and Lindvall, O., Delayed kindling development after rapidly recurring seizures: Relation to mossy fiber sprouting and neurotrophin, GAP-43 and dynorphin gene expression, *Brain Res*, 712 (1996) 19–34.
13. Erickson, J.C., Clegg, K.E. and Palmiter, R.D., Sensitivity to leptin and susceptibility to seizures of mice lacking neuropeptide Y, *Nature*, 381 (1996) 415–418.
14. Ernfors, P., Bengzon, J., Kokaia, Z., Persson, H. and Lindvall, O., Increased levels of messengers RNAs for neurotrophic factors in the brain during kindling epileptogenesis, *Neuron*, 7 (1991) 165–176.
15. Funabashi, T., Sasaki, H. and Kimura, F., Intraventricular injection of antiserum to nerve growth factor delays the development of amygdaloid kindling, *Brain Res*, 458 (1988) 132–136.
16. Gall, C., Seizure-induced changes in neurotrophin expression: implications for epilepsy, *Experimental Neurology*, 124 (1993) 150–166.
17. Glass, D.J. and Yancopoulos, G.D., The neurotrophins and their receptors, *Trends in cell biology*, 3 (1993) 262–268.
18. Humpel, C., Ebdendal, T., Cao, Y. and Olson, L., Pentylenetetrazol seizures increase pro-nerve growth factor-like immunoreactivity in the reticular thalamic nucleus and nerve growth factor mRNA in the dentate gyrus, *J Neurosci Res*, 35 (1993) 419–427.
19. Humpel, C., Wetmore, C. and Olson, L., Regulation of brain-derived neurotrophic factor messenger RNA and protein at the cellular level in pentylenetetrazol-induced epileptic seizures, *Neurosci*, 53 (1993) 909–918.
20. Jones, K.R., Farinas, I., Backus, C. and Reichardt, L.F., Targeted disruption of the BDNF gene perturbs brain and sensory neuron development but not motor neuron development, *Cell*, 76 (1994) 989–999.
21. Kokaia, M., Ernfors, P., Kokaia, Z., Elmer, E., Jaenisch, R. and Lindvall, O., Suppressed epileptogenesis in BDNF mutant mice, *Exp Neurol*, 133 (1995) 215–224.
22. Korte, M., Carroll, P., Wolf, E., Brem, G., Thoenen, H. and Bonhoeffer, T., Hippocampal long-term potentiation is impaired in mice lacking brain-derived neurotrophic factor, *Proc Natl Acad Sci USA*, 92 (1995) 8856–8860.
23. Larmet, Y., Reibel, S., Carnahan, J., Nawa, H., Marescaux, C. and Depaulis, A., Protective effects of brain-derived neurotrophic factor on the development of hippocampal kindling in the rat, *Neuroreport*, 6 (1995) 1937–1941.
24. Lindvall, O., Kokaia, Z., Bengzon, J., Elmér, E. and Kokaia, M., Neurotrophins and brain insults, *Trends Neurosci*, 17 (1994) 490–496.
25. Marsh, H.N., Scholz, W.K., Lamballe, F., Klein, R., Nanduri, V., Barbacid, M. and Palfrey, H.C., Signal transduction events mediated by the BDNF receptor gp145trkB in primary hippocampal pyramidal cell culture, *Journal of neuroscience*, 13 (1993) 4281–4292.
26. Marty, S., Carroll, P., Cellerino, A., Castren, E., Staiger, V., Thoenen, H. and Lindholm, D., Brain-derived neurotrophic factor promotes the differentiation of various hippocampal nonpyramidal neurons, including Cajal-Retzius cells, in organotypic slice cultures, *J Neurosci*, 16 (1996) 675–687.
27. McNamara, J.O., Cellular and molecular basis of epilepsy, *J Neurosci*, 14 (1994) 3413–3425.

28. Merlio, J.P., Ernfors, P., Kokaia, Z., Middlemas, D.S., Bengzon, J., Kokaia, M., Smith, M.L., Siesjö, B.K., Hunter, T., Lindvall, O. and Persson, H., Increased production of TrkB protein tyrosine kinase receptor after brain insults, *Neuron*, 10 (1993) 151–164.
29. Paxinos, G. and Watson, C., The rat brain in stereotaxic coordinates, Academic Press, Sydney, 1986, pages.
30. Racine, R.J., Modification of seizure activity by electrical stimulation: II. Motor seizure, *Electroencephalogr Clin Neurophysiol*, 32 (1972) 281–294.
31. Rashid, K., Van der Zee, C.E.E.M., Ross, G.M., Chapman, C.A., Stanisz, J., Riopelle, R.J., Racine, R.J. and Fahnestock, M., A nerve growth factor peptide retards seizure development and inhibits neuronal sprouting in a rat model of epilepsy, *Proc Natl Acad Sci USA*, 92 (1995) 9495–9499.
32. Rizzi, M., Monno, A., Samanin, R., Sperk, G. and Vezzani, A., Electrical kindling of the hippocampus is associated with functional activation of neuropeptide Y-containing neurons, *Eur J Neurosci*, 5 (1993) 1534–1538.
33. Rosen, J.B., Kim, S.Y. and Post, R.M., Differential regional and time course increases in thyrotropin-releasing hormone, neuropeptide Y and enkephalin mRNAs following an amygdala kindled seizure, *Mol Brain Res*, 27 (1994) 71–80.
34. Sato, K., Kashihara, K., Morimoto, K. and Hayabara, T., Regional increases in brain-derived neurotrophic factor and nerve growth factor mRNAs during amygdaloid kindling, but not in acidic and basic fibroblast growth factor mRNAs, *Epilepsia*, 37 (1996) 6–14.
35. Sutula, T., Cascino, G., Cavazos, J., Parada, I. and Ramirez, L., Mossy fiber synaptic reorganization in the epileptic human temporal lobe, *Ann Neurol*, 26 (1989) 321–330.
36. Sutula, T., Xiao-Xian, H., Cavazos, J. and Scott, G., Synaptic reorganization in the hippocampus induced by abnormal functional activity, *Science*, 239 (1988) 1147–1150.
37. Tauck, D.L. and Nadler, J.V., Evidence of functional mossy fiber sprouting in hippocampal formation of kainic acid-treated rats, *Journal of Neuroscience*, 5 (1985) 1016–1022.
38. Thoenen, H., Neurotrophins and neuronal plasticity, *Science*, 270 (1995) 593–598.
39. Tønder, N., Kragh, J., Finsen, B.R., Bolwig, T.G. and Zimmer, J., Kindling induces transient changes in neuronal expression of somatostatin, neuropeptide Y, and calbindin in adult rat hippocampus and fascia dentata, *Epilepsia*, 35 (1994) 1299–1308.
40. Van der Zee, C.E.E.M., Rashid, K., Le, K., Moore, K.A., Stanisz, J., Diamond, J., Racine, R.J. and Fahnestock, M., Intraventricular administration of antibodies to nerve growth factor retards kindling and blocks mossy fiber sprouting in adult rats, *J Neurosci*, 15 (1995) 5316–5323.

DISCUSSION OF ANTOINE DEPAULIS'S PAPER

C. Wasterlain: First, could your infusions of BDNF be decreasing sensitivity of the trkB receptors? Second, there is some evidence from Thoenen's group that injection of BDNF into the hippocampus will give rise to epileptiform activity. Did you see any epileptiform activity?

A. Depaulis: We very carefully checked the animal during the first day of perfusion and we checked that very late at night by doing EEG monitoring almost 24 hr a day. We didn't see any epileptic discharges in these animals; so that is a little bit different than what is reported by the group of Thoenen. Thoenen injected BDNF at once, within a few minutes. In the hippocampus, I am always a bit sceptical, because the hippocampus is a very ticklish structure, as you know. To answer your first point, I think that is a very good possibility, and something that we plan to check, that the trkB receptor may be down-regulated by the perfusion of BDNF. The other important point is about the physiological role of BDNF, and of course the obvious experiment to do is to block the expression of BDNF during kindling, using for instance oligonucleotides. We have tried already with natural oligos, but as you know these oligos are rapidly degraded; so we are currently developing a technique that will protect the oligos and we'll know in a few months whether it is more effective to block the expression of BDNF.

K. Gale: Since you're using pharmacologic doses of BDNF, what are your controls? Have you tried any inactive fragments or digestive materials or something like that, because obviously saline is not an adequate control.

A. Depaulis: We used PBS as everyone else does, but I agree that's not the best control. In one experiment I didn't show we compared the effects of BDNF with the effect of PBS, and we found that PBS in fact has the opposite effect. It facilitates kindling. In this experiment we used denatured NGF, and the kindling was like in controls. We also control a PBS perfused animal against a non-perfused animal and don't find much of a difference.

G. Rondouin: I have two questions for Antoine or Sophie Reybiel. The first, did you look very carefully for lesions around the canula in the two groups, for example using immunoreactivity for GABA? The second question, what happens if you continue to stimulate animals after they have had the perfusion?

S. Reybiel: We've looked for lesions in cresyl stained sections, and we could not see obvious difference between BDNF treated and PBS treated animals, whether they've kindled or not kindled. We also used GFAP immunocytochemistry to see whether there was increased gliosis between the four groups, and we couldn't see any difference between the BDNF and the PBS animals. Obviously there are other cell markers that we should use, and we are at the moment developing apoptosis markers to see whether there is a difference between the BDNF and PBS treated animals.

C. Wasterlain: What is the biological basis of this phenomenon? Do you have a reduction in LTP? Do you have a change in transmitter release or postsynaptic effects?

A. Depaulis: Unfortunately, I can't answer the question right now, but we have several hypotheses. One hyposthesis is based on the well known observation that BDNF increases NPY expression both in vitro and in vivo. Sophie has obtained data recently using our experimental parameters showing that after perfusion of BDNF there is a huge increase of NPY expression, especially in the hilus of the dentate gyrus. Knowing the inhibitory effects of NPY on neuronal excitability in the hippocampus, that may be one possibility; especially it will fit pretty well with the time course of BDNF suppressive effect. Another possibility is that it may up-regulate calbindin, which is down-regulated during kindling. There are invitro data showing that BDNF increases the expression of calbindin. So that is also a hypothesis that we will investigate but there may be other possibilities of course.

J. McNamara: I realize the lesions aren't any different between the control and experimental rats, but what kind of lesion does 24 microliters injected into a hippocampus for a day make?

A. Depaulis: I was very concerned about that because I have done a lot of acute injections, and in fact the lesions are much less after a chronic perfusion than after an acute injection. I think that it is a question of speed and ratio of volume per time. I was very surprised, when I first did the first chronic perfusion, that the lesions are much less than after 1 or 2 acute injections.

30

PERFORANT PATH KINDLING, NMDA ANTAGONISM, AND LATE PAIRED PULSE DEPRESSION

Mary E. Gilbert*

National Research Council
Neurotoxicology Division, US Environmental Protection Agency
Research Triangle Park, North Carolina
Department of Psychology
University of North Carolina, Chapel Hill, North Carolina

The N-methyl-d-aspartate (NMDA) subtype of the glutamate receptor has been strongly implicated in the development of limbic kindling[9,14,18,20,25,27,33]. Antagonists of NMDA have been reported to increase afterdischarge (AD) thresholds and retard the development of motor seizures. In the amygdala, the development of electrographic as well as behavioral seizures is profoundly reduced by the noncompetitive NMDA antagonist, MK-801. Paradoxically, an augmentation rather than a retardation in AD duration is evident in animals kindled in the perforant path following treatment with MK-801[15,16,18].

Kindling potentiates excitatory and inhibitory synaptic transmission in the dentate gyrus[1,11,15,18,23,24,26,30,31,36]. The integrity of inhibitory systems can be assessed in vivo by stimulating the perforant path with pairs of stimulus pulses separated by varying interpulse intervals (IPI). If the second pulse of the pair falls within the period of activation of inhibitory currents, the population spike amplitude of the test pulse is reduced. At brief IPIs (< 40 msec), a strong suppression of test population spike amplitude reflects recurrent feedback inhibition of granule cells from activation of GABAergic interneurons. Early paired pulse depression is mediated by a chloride conductance that follows $GABA_A$ receptor activation[1,36]. Late paired pulse depression occurs at IPIs of 150 msec or more, is modest in comparison the depression recorded at briefer intervals, and most likely represents inhibition that is feedforward rather than feedback in nature[2,6]. Suppression of the dentate gyrus population spike at these longer IPIs reflects the activation of a number of potassium currents of both synaptic and nonsynaptic origins. The synaptic component of late

* Address correspondence to: M.E. Gilbert, PhD, Neurotoxicology Division (MD-74B), Health Effects Research Laboratory, U.S. Environmental Protection Agency, Research Triangle Park, NC 27711. Phone: (919) 541-4394; Fax: (919) 541-4849; E-mail: gilbert@herl45.herl.epa.gov

Kindling 5, edited by Corcoran and Moshé.
Plenum Press, New York, 1998.

paired pulse depression may be mediated by activation of $GABA_B$ receptors, whereas a calcium dependent afterhyperpolarization (AHP) contributes nonsynaptically to currents summating to depress field potentials at long intervals[2,21,29,35].

As suggested by Maru and Goddard[24] and deJonge and Racine[11], kindling-induced increases in paired pulse depression may reflect potentiation of synaptic transmission of inhibitory neurons, akin to long-term potentiation (LTP). This conclusion was supported by the observation that LTP and kindling-induced potentiation of inhibitory processes are reduced by the NMDA antagonist, MK-801[15,18,30]. However, the block of potentiation of inhibitory neurotransmission is limited to late paired pulse depression, suggesting independent populations of interneurons control early and late paired pulse depression and potentiation of only one of these populations is NMDA sensitive[15].

Coincident with a blockade of potentiation of late paired pulse depression and suppression of motor seizure development, MK-801 increased the duration of evoked ADs[15,16,18]. The increase in AD duration associated with perforant path kindling was attributable to increases in the incidence and duration of secondary ADs. Leung[22] proposed that secondary ADs following dorsal hippocampal kindling originated in the entorhinal cortex and reflected activation of reverberatory activity in the parahippocampal loop. Depth electrode analysis indicated local generation of secondary ADs within the hippocampus which was reduced in duration or abolished by entorhinal cortex lesions. A delayed onset secondary AD has also been reported in a combined entorhinal cortex/hippocampal slice preparation following dorsal hippocampal stimulation[28]. It is possible that the relative decrement of inhibitory tone in the dentate gyrus in MK-801 treated animals due to their failure to exhibit potentiation of late paired pulse depression may facilitate the transmission of secondary ADs from the entorhinal cortex to the dentate gyrus. To examine further the relationship between potentiation of late paired pulse depression and secondary AD generation, we employed a crossover design in which animals were stimulated for a number of sessions in the presence or absence of MK-801, followed by a series of sessions in which the dose groups were reversed. Behavioral and electrographic seizure indices were recorded and late paired pulse depression was monitored intermittently throughout the study.

CROSSOVER STUDY WITH MK-801

Three groups of animals were prepared with electrodes in the perforant path and dentate gyrus for perforant path kindling. The perforant path was stimulated once daily (800 μA, 2 sec) for 10 consecutive days followed by a 10 day rest period. A subset of each group (n=7–9/group) were monitored for alterations in paired pulse depression before and 18–24 hours after 1, 4, 7 and 10 evoked ADs. The degree of paired pulse depression and paired pulse facilitation was compared to prekindling baseline levels. Two groups of animals received saline prior to each daily stimulation (groups Control-Control, CC, and Control-Drugged, CD). The third group was administered 1.0 mg/kg MK-801, ip, 30 min prior to each daily stimulation. After the rest period, two of the dose groups were reversed, group CD was administered MK-801, DC was administered saline, and group CC continued to receive saline injections prior to stimulation for the next 10 consecutive days.

As we had previously observed[15,18], seizure development was suppressed and AD duration prolonged by MK-801 (Group DC) in the first phase of the study. After the rest period, AD duration was reduced in group DC now stimulated under saline and duration was increased in Group CD treated with MK-801 in the second phase of the study (Figure 1a).

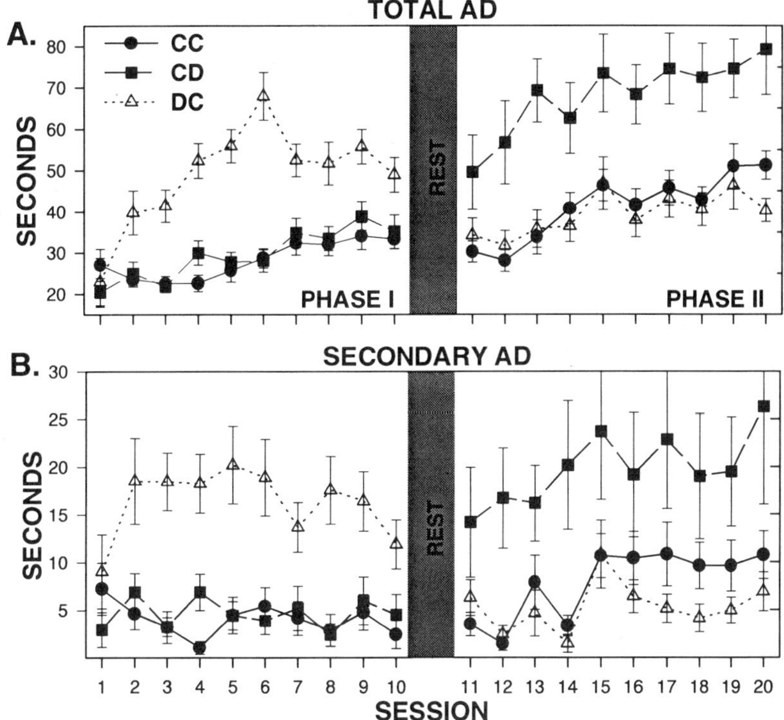

Figure 1. Mean (±SEM) total (A) and secondary (B) afterdischarge (AD) duration recorded in the dentate gyrus of perforant path kindled animals. MK-801 (1.0 mg/kg/, ip) augmented total AD in group DC in Phase 1 of the study. Post-rest reversal of the dose groups revealed increases in AD duration in MK-801 treated animals previously stimulated under saline (Group CD). Conversely, reductions in AD duration to control levels (Group CC) were evident in the post rest phase of the study in animals stimulated in the drug-free state (Group DC). Mean secondary AD duration (B) is doubled in animals tested under the influence of MK-801 in Phase 1 (Group DC) and Phase 2 (Group CD) of study and contributes significantly to the increases in total AD of Figure 1A. Adapted from Gilbert[16].

Consistent with earlier findings, secondary ADs were prolonged by MK-801, irrespective of phase of the study or stage of seizure development (Figure 1b)[16].

Potentiation of early paired pulse depression and a reduction in paired pulse facilitation were evident in all groups (CC, CD and DC) in Phase I of the study (Figure 2a). Saline-treated animals (Groups CC and CD) also displayed augmentation in the magnitude of late paired pulse depression. No change in the amplitude of late paired pulse depression was observed over the first 10 sessions of Phase I in MK-801 treated animals (Group DC). During the 10-day rest period that followed the completion of Phase I of the study, some decay in the potentiation of paired pulse functions occurred (compare AD10 Figure 2a vs Rest Figure 2b). When kindling resumed and the dose conditions were reversed, animals that were previously treated with MK-801 and had failed to exhibit increases in late paired pulse depression, now displayed an enhancement (group DC, bottom panel Figure 2b). Group CC showed further increments in late paired pulse depression, whereas Group CD failed to demonstrate any change in the magnitude of late paired pulse depression (middle panel Figure 2b). These data demonstrate the selective effects of MK-801 in preventing potentiation of late paired pulse depression. The findings are consistent with the notion that an MK-801 induced block of potentiated late paired pulse depression may contribute to the expression of longer secondary ADs in the dentate gyrus.

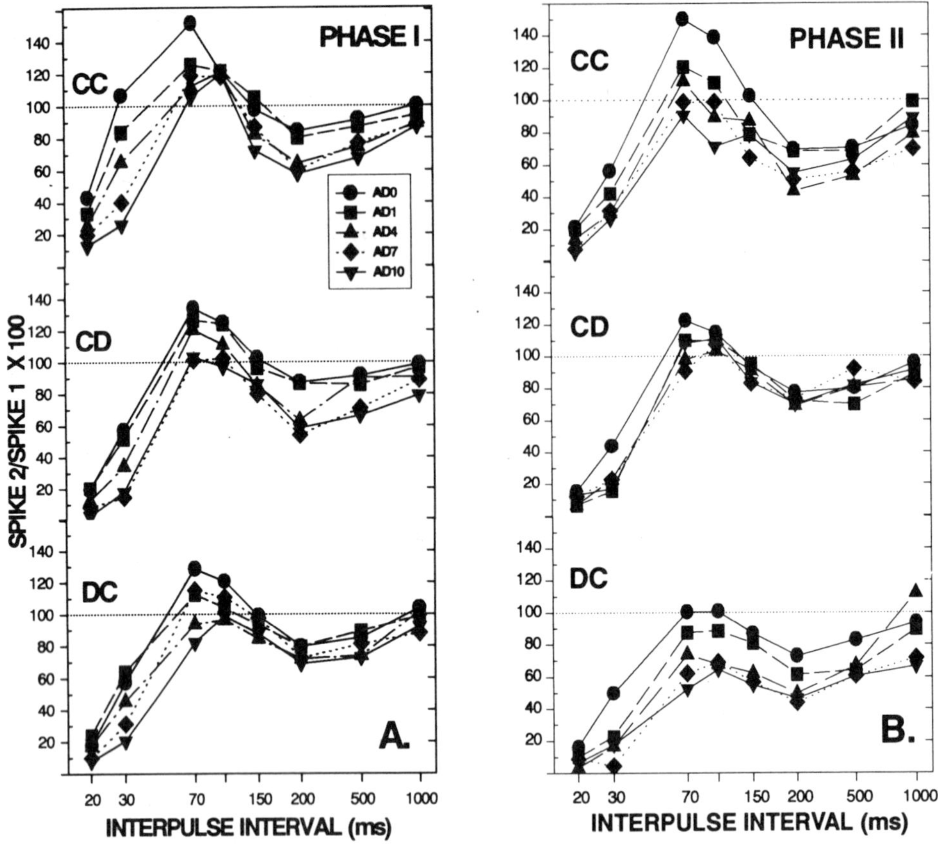

Figure 2. Paired pulse depression in saline (CC, top and CD, center) treated animals before (AD0) and 18–24 hours after one (AD1), four (AD4), seven (AD7), and ten (AD10) ADs evoked by perforant path stimulation (2 sec train, 1.0 ms pulse width, 800 μA). Baseline responses to pairs of stimulus pulses of equal intensity were collected at an intensity yielding a population spike 80% of maximal prior to kindling (AD0). Stimulus intensity was adjusted thereafter to match population spike amplitudes of the conditioning pulse to prekindling levels. Kindling stimulation produced an increase in early (20–30 msec) and late (150–500 msec) paired pulse depression, and a reduction of paired pulse facilitation (70–100 msec). (B) Resumption of kindling stimulation following a 10-day rest period further potentiated early and late paired pulse depression in the group of control animals continued on saline treatment (CC, top). Animals previously stimulated under saline conditions and now kindled with MK-801 (1.0 mg/kg, ip) failed to show increases in late paired pulse depression (150–500 msec intervals). In comparison, previously drugged animals (DC, bottom), who had failed to demonstrate potentiated late paired pulse depression in Phase 1 (compare bottom graphs of Figures 2 and 3), now revealed enhanced depression at long IPIs when tested drug-free.

A regression analysis revealed a negative correlation (r=-0.62) between increases in late paired pulse depression and AD duration (Figure 3). Although highly significant, the strength of the correlation indicated that the strength of late paired pulse depression accounted for approximately 20% (AD4 through AD10) to 40% (AD10 only) of the variance in AD duration (Figure 3). Clearly, other factors contribute to the expression of secondary ADs in perforant path kindling. This led to a more detailed analysis of the characteristics of secondary ADs. Additionally, in the described experiments, late paired pulse depression was always monitored in a drug-free state, the day following an evoked AD. Noncompetitive NMDA antagonists including MK-801 and phencyclidine have been reported to block

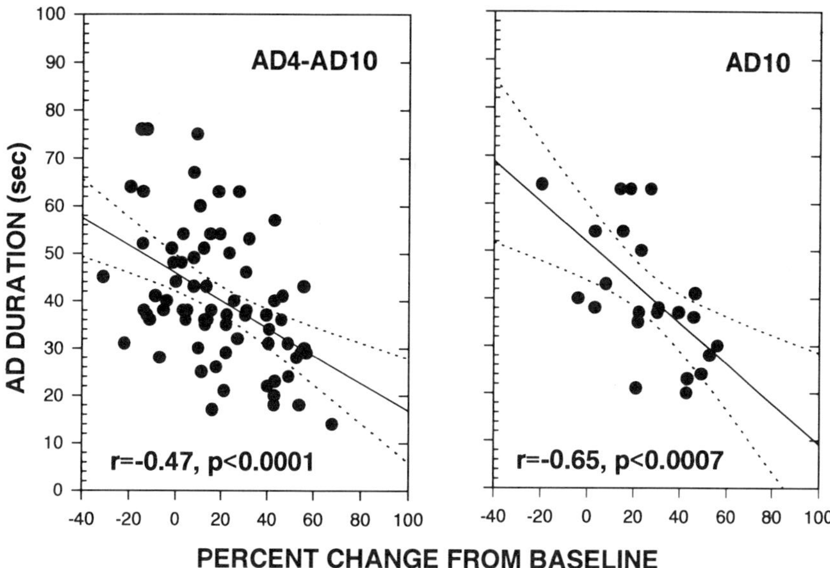

Figure 3. Regression analysis for AD duration and percent increase above prekindling baseline levels of late paired pulse depression for AD4 through AD10 in Phase 1, or for the final AD in Phase 1 (AD10). A significant negative correlation exists between AD duration and potentiation of late paired pulse depression, but accounts for less than 50% of the variance.

potassium currents in cultured hippocampal neurons[12,13,32] and may decrease potassium currents that contribute to late paired pulse depression in the dentate gyrus in vivo, and it is possible that MK-801 may also reduce late paired pulse depression. A block in the potentiation of late paired pulse depression coupled with an acute pharmacological reduction in late paired pulse depression may further promote the expression of secondary AD. This possibility was explored by examining the effects of MK-801 on late paired pulse depression in naive and kindled animals.

ACUTE EFFECTS OF MK-801 ON LATE PAIRED PULSE DEPRESSION

Late paired pulse depression was assessed in a group of naive animals before and after administration of saline (n=12) or MK-801 (n=11). Contrary to expectations, an increase in late paired pulse depression by MK-801 was observed. MK-801 had no effect on early inhibitory or facilitation processes (Figure 4a). Similar increases were observed with a lower dose of MK-801 (0.25 mg/kg)[17] and pretreatment with saline was without effect (Figure 4b). In contrast to the effects in naive animals, challenging fully kindled animals with MK-801 failed to alter late paired pulse depression (Figure 5). As these measures were obtained within 24 hours of a generalized convulsion in well kindled animals, the loss of efficacy of MK-801 on late paired pulse depression may reflect a ceiling effect, i.e., a fully potentiated inhibitory system may exist in well kindled animals that cannot be further augmented by MK-801 administration. However, in the crossover study, animals were challenged with MK-801 during the 10-day rest period that followed Phase I. Late paired pulse depression in partially-kindled animals was enhanced by MK-801, but to a

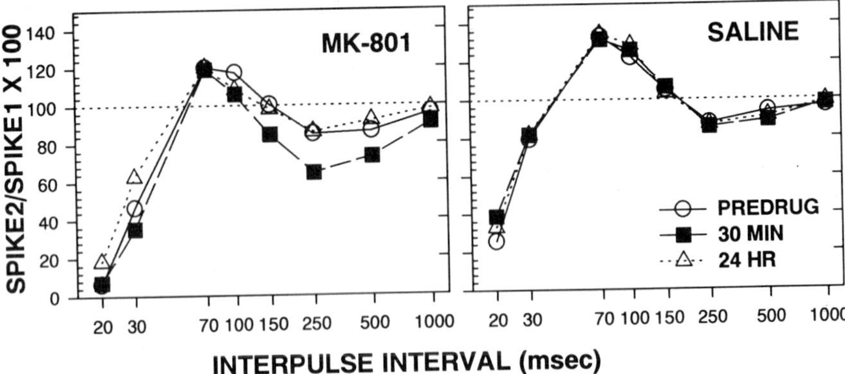

Figure 4. Paired pulse functions in naive animals following administration of MK-801. Mean (±SEM) percent change in test relative to conditioning population spike amplitude across a range of interpulse intervals before, 30 minutes, and 24 hours after ip injection of 1.0 mg/kg MK-801 (A) or saline (B). MK-801 selectively increased late paired pulse depression. Portions adapted from Gilbert and Burdette[17].

lesser degree than that observed in these subjects prior to kindling (Figure 5). This occurred in groups of animals having demonstrated some augmentation in late paired pulse depression (CC and CD) and in group DC which had failed to exhibit potentiation of late paired pulse depression. Furthermore, the potentiation of late paired pulse depression that had occurred in the two saline-treated groups of Phase 1 (CC and CD) had declined appreciably during the rest period prior to the MK-801 challenge. These data suggest that the kindling process per se alters the response of inhibitory systems that comprise late paired pulse depression to this NMDA antagonist.

LATE PAIRED PULSE DEPRESSION AND AD THRESHOLD

Although a decrease in early inhibition has long been associated with AD initiation[3], the influence of late inhibition on seizure susceptibility has received less attention. Burdette et al.[8] recently have reported that a loss of late paired pulse depression may contribute to initiation of an AD triggered by low frequency stimulation of the perforant path. At

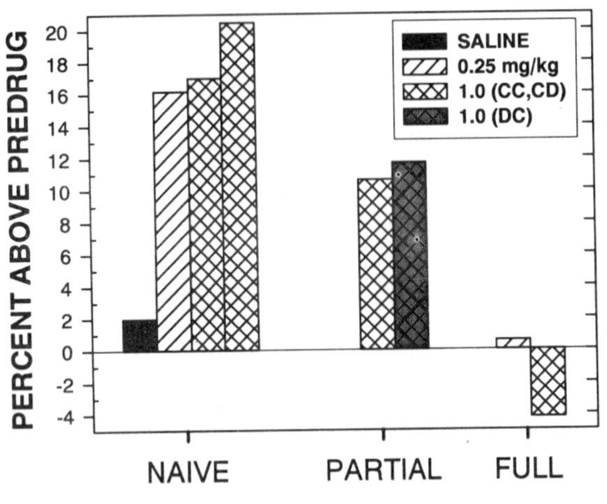

Figure 5. Percent change from predrug levels of late paired pulse depression prior to kindling (Naive, left), and in partially (center) and fully kindled rats (right) challenged with MK-801. Potentiation of late paired pulse depression had occurred in groups CC and CD (see Figure 2), but had partially decayed 4–7 days after the 10th evoked AD when these animals were challenged with MK-801. MK-801 did not produce as large an increase in late paired pulse depression (IPIs=200–250 msec) in partially-kindled rats relative to a naive control group or this same group of animals tested prior to kindling. MK-801 failed to enhance late paired pulse depression in fully kindled animals. Portions adapted from Gilbert and Burdette[17].

stimulation frequencies of 1 and 5 Hz, within the range of late paired pulse depression, the population spike was decreased when train parameters were below threshold for evoking an AD[7,8]. The authors suggest that the depression in the population spike during low frequency stimulation may reflect the accumulation of late paired pulse depression with successive pulses in the train. When the intensity of 5 Hz trains was increased to exceed AD threshold, late paired pulse depression was lost by the middle of the train and eventually was followed by multiple population spikes, signifying the onset of the AD (Figure 6a). On trials failing to produce an AD, a fairly stable level of late paired pulse depression was maintained throughout the train (Figure 6b). These data suggest that a failure of late paired pulse depression may be a precipitating event in AD initiation triggered by low frequency stimulation of the perforant path.

NMDA antagonists have been consistently reported to increase AD thresholds in both the amygdala and perforant path in response to traditional kindling stimuli (60 Hz, 1.0 msec pulse width, 1–2 sec trains)[14–18]. With low frequency stimulation (5 Hz, 0.1 msec pulse width, 15 sec trains), MK-801 also increased the threshold for AD initiation[8]. Consistent with an increase in late paired pulse depression by MK-801 (see above), the depression in population spike amplitudes was more pronounced and was maintained throughout 5 Hz trains that failed to trigger an AD in the drug condition (Figure 6c). When train parameters were adjusted to compensate for the higher AD thresholds present with MK-801, a loss of late paired pulse depression was observed prior to AD initiation (Figure 6d). These findings suggest that the anticonvulsant properties of MK-801 may be explained by its enhancement of late paired pulse depression[8].

CHARACTERISTICS OF SECONDARY AFTERDISCHARGES

In the crossover study, a subset of animals for which clear identification of the onset of secondary ADs could be made were selected from each of the dose groups, and EEG records examined across the 20 stimulation sessions comprising Phase I and Phase II. Secondary ADs, although varying slightly from animal to animal, were characterized by consistency in morphology, duration, and latency to onset. There was little change in these parameters as a function of kindling (e.g. Figure 1b and Figure 7a). Under control conditions, secondary AD of 1–2 Hz occurred on about 40% of the trials and appeared out of a background of suppressed EEG, 1–2 minutes after termination of the primary AD (e.g. Figure 7a). Background EEG remained suppressed for a period following the termination of the secondary AD (Figure 7). Treatment with MK-801 increased the incidence of secondary AD from approximately 40% to 70%, doubled the duration from 10 to 25 sec, and reduced the mean latency to onset from 80 sec to 45 sec[16]. In the combined entorhinal cortex/hippocampal slice preparation, the NMDA antagonist APV also increased the duration of secondary AD and decreased the latency to onset[28].

MK-801 AND POSTICTAL DEPRESSION

In control subjects, strong postictal depression (PID) of baseline electrographic seizure record (EEG) follows the termination of the primary AD and extends beyond the secondary AD episode in control animals (Figure 7a, 7b top). When tested under MK-801, suppression of the EEG following the primary ictal event is not as apparent. As exemplified in Figure 7b (bottom) and 7c (top), low amplitude spiking often tailed the primary

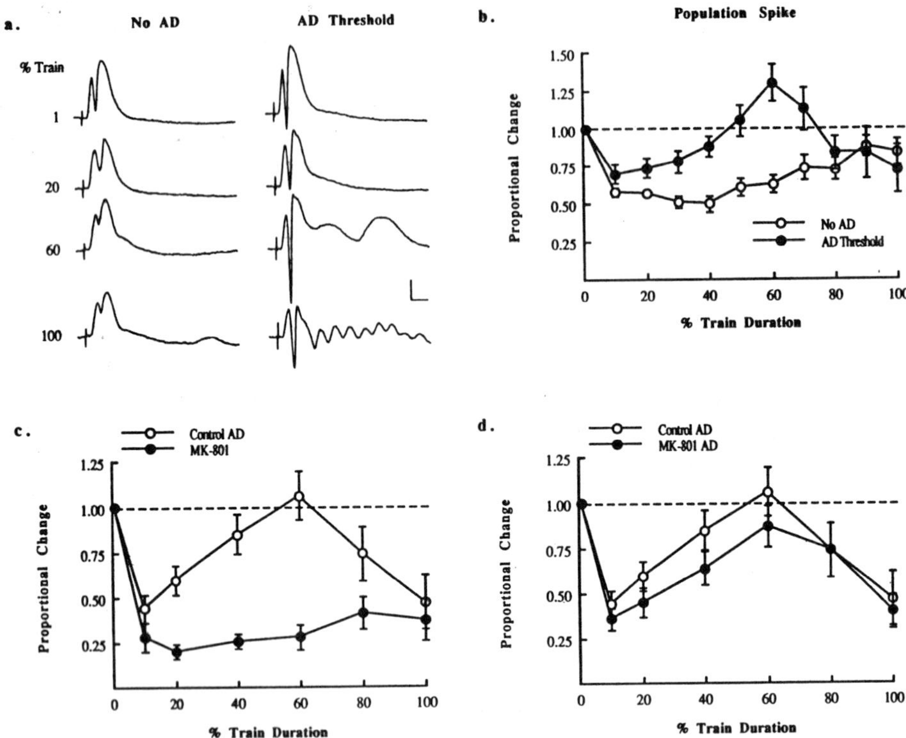

Figure 6. Changes in dentate granule cell field potentials during delivery of a 5 Hz train of stimulus pulses (0.1 msec pulse duration) in naive animals. (A) Representative waveforms illustrate that the depression in population spike amplitude (i.e. late paired pulse depression) persists throughout the 5 Hz train delivered at a stimulus intensity below the threshold for evoking an AD (No AD). A higher stimulus intensity (AD Threshold) produces an initial depression in population spike amplitude (i.e. late paired pulse depression), followed by an increase to above pretrain amplitudes (i.e. weakening and eventual loss of late paired pulse depression). Population spike amplitudes peaked at mid-train then steadily declined until multiple population spikes (AD initiation) occurred. (B) Population spike amplitudes during 5 Hz trains expressed relative to the first response in the train. Depression in population spike amplitude during low frequency stimulation reflects the cumulative influences of late paired pulse depression generated by the previous response in the train. When 5 Hz trains were below AD threshold, the population spike was initially depressed and later began to recover to pre-train values. When intensity was increased sufficiently to elicit an AD, the initial depression was followed by an increase in population spike amplitude to above pretrain values, signifying a loss of late paired pulse depression. (C) Population spike amplitudes in MK-801 treated animals (0.25 mg/kg, ip) were significantly depressed throughout 5 Hz trains that under control conditions triggered an AD, but that were below AD threshold following MK-801 administration. The anticonvulsant properties of MK-801 may be attributed, in part, to its augmentation of late paired pulse depression during low frequency stimulation. (D) In contrast, a loss of late paired pulse depression preceded AD initiation in control and MK-801 treated rats when train parameters were increased to compensate for the elevation in AD threshold in the drug condition. Taken from Burdette et al.[7]

AD, increased in amplitude, and eventually merged with the pattern of EEG activity characteristic of secondary AD. In direct contrast to the pattern seen in controls, recovery of the background EEG to prestimulation amplitude was evident upon termination of secondary ADs in these samples from treated animals (e.g Figure 7b bottom, 7c top, 7d middle). Under saline conditions in the same animal, strong PID was prominent prior to and following the cessation of secondary AD (e.g. Figure 7a, 7b top).

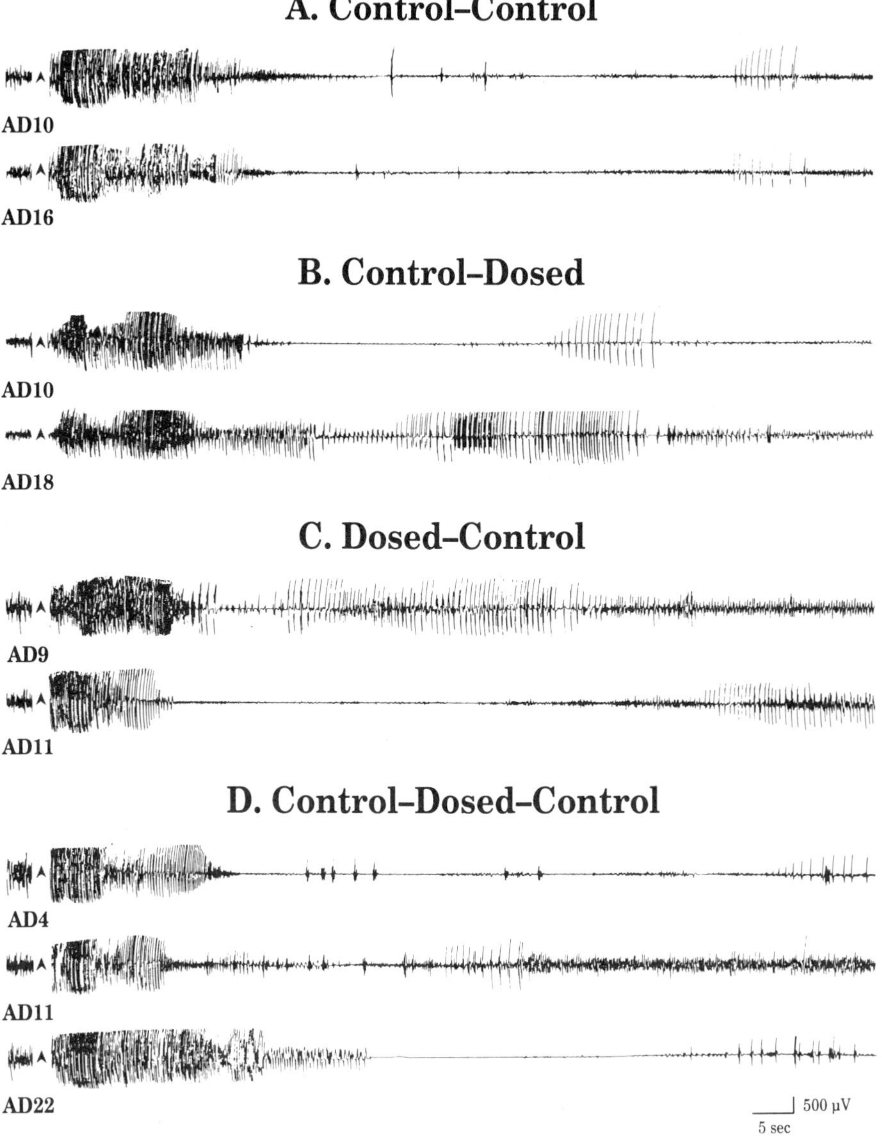

Figure 7. Pairs of sample records from 4 different animals stimulated under saline (A), saline followed by MK-801 (B), MK-801 followed by saline (C), or saline, MK-801, and saline (D). A 2 sec train of 60 Hz pulses at an intensity of 800 μA was delivered at the arrowhead. Differences in secondary AD characteristics and postictal depression cannot be accounted for by seizure severity or primary AD durations. Focal seizures were observed in both sessions of A and C. Both sessions in B were accompanied by generalized seizures. In (D) focal seizures were evoked with AD4 and AD11, and AD22 produced a Stage 5 generalized convulsion. Taken from Gilbert[16].

The effects of MK-801 on the PID and the pattern of secondary AD expression in Figure 7 also appeared to be independent of the severity of the preceding motor seizure. Each pair of EEG records in Figure 7 is from the same animal. Focal seizures were recorded in both saline sessions depicted in Figure 7a and the saline (top) and MK-801 (bottom) sessions of Figure 7b. Generalized seizures occurred in the MK-801 (top) and saline (bottom) sessions of Figure 7c. Within animal comparisons revealed that following either focal or generalized seizures, PID was less prevalent and secondary AD was augmented under drugged conditions.

In the dorsal hippocampus, PID is a consequence of an ictal event. MK-801 may reduce PID and in this manner increase the probability of occurrence and facilitate early onset of secondary AD propagated from entorhinal cortex. Berman and his colleagues[4,37] have suggested that adenosine, an endogenous neuromodulator which is released during seizure activity, may be responsible for the profound PID seen following primary AD in kindled animals. One of the primary actions of adenosine is to block neurotransmission by presynaptic inhibition of transmitter release[34]. The molecular layer of the dentate gyrus is rich in adenosine receptors[34] and in vivo release of adenosine in hippocampus is induced by perfusion with NMDA, and is blocked by NMDA antagonists[10]. If PID normally suppresses the expression of secondary AD, then by analogy, adenosine antagonists might be expected to increase secondary AD duration. With dorsal hippocampal stimulation, Burdette and Dyer[5] reported more than a doubling of the duration of secondary AD following administration of 75 mg/kg of caffeine, a potent adenosine antagonist. As was observed in the present study, no change in the duration of primary AD was detected. Future research examining PID, secondary ADs, and late paired pulse depression may begin to clarify the interrelationship among these systems and their roles in kindling epileptogenesis.

SUMMARY

In summary, the NMDA antagonist MK-801 selectively blocks the potentiation of late paired pulse depression during kindling. This relative reduction in inhibitory tone may contribute in part to the longer and more frequent induction of secondary ADs in the dentate gyrus in response to perforant path stimulation. In direct contrast to the ability of MK-801 to block kindling-induced potentiation of late paired pulse depression, MK-801 selectively augments late paired pulse depression in naive rats. Increases in late paired pulse depression by MK-801 treatment may contribute to the threshold increases for AD initiation observed by NMDA antagonists. As kindling proceeds, however, the efficacy with which MK-801 enhances late paired pulse depression is reduced. These two actions of MK-801 in perforant path kindling, i.e., selective block of potentiation of inhibition and reduced efficacy to increase late paired pulse depression over the course of kindling, may culminate in longer electrographic seizures. Alternatively, MK-801 may enhance electrographic seizure expression by interfering with the processes responsible for postictal depression. NMDA antagonists may reduce the degree of postictal depression that follows primary evoked ADs, thereby creating a more permissive environment for the propagation of secondary ADs from the entorhinal cortex to the dorsal hippocampus.

ACKNOWLEDGMENTS

The significant contribution of Cina Mack to the experiments described is most gratefully acknowledged. This work was supported by the U.S. Environmental Protection Agency, through contract #68-02-4450 to ManTech Environmental Technology Services Inc., and the National Research Council. The manuscript has been reviewed by the National Health Effects and Environmental Research Laboratory, U.S. EPA, and approved for publication.

REFERENCES

1. Adamec, R.E., McNaughton, B., Racine, R.J. and Livingston, K.E., Effects of diazepam on hippocampal excitability in the rat: Action in the dentate area. Epilepsia, 22(1981)205–215.
2. Alger, B. E., Characteristics of a slow hyperpolarizing synaptic potential in rat hippocampal pyramidal cells in vitro. J. Neurophysiol., 52(1984)892–910.
3. Ben-Ari, Y., Krnjevic, K. And Reinhardt, W., Hippocampal seizures and failure of inhibition. Can. J. Physiol. Pharmacol., 57(1979)1462–1466.
4. Berman, R.F., Jarvis, M.F. and Lupica, C.R., Adenosine involvement in kindled seizures. In J. Wada (Ed), Kindling 4, Plenum Press:New York(1990)423–435.
5. Burdette, L.J. and Dyer, R.S., Differential effects of caffeine, picrotoxin and pentylenetetrazol on hippocampal afterdischarge activity and wet dog shakes. Exper. Neurol., 96(1987)381–392.
6. Burdette, L.J. and Gilbert, M.E., Stimulus parameters affecting paired pulse depression of dentate gyrus granule cell field potentials: I. Stimulus Intensity. Brain Research, 680(1995)53–62.
7. Burdette, L.J. and Masukawa, L.M., Stimulus parameters affecting paired pulse depression of dentate granule cell field responses. II. Low frequency stimulation. Brain Res., 680(1995)63–72.
8. Burdette, L.J., Hart, G., and Masukawa, L.M., Changes in dentate granule cell field potentials during afterdischarge initiation triggered by 5 Hz perforant path stimulation. Brain Research, in press.
9. Cain, D.P. , Desborough, K. And McKitrick, D., Retardation of amygdala kindling by antagonism of NMD-aspartate and muscarinic cholinergic receptors: Evidence for the summation of excitatory mechanisms of kindling. Exp. Neurol., 100(1988)179–187.
10. Chen, Y., Graham, D.I. and Stone, T.W., Release of endogenous adenosine and its metabolites by the activation of NMDA receptors in the rat hippocampus in vivo. Br. J. Pharmacol., 106(1992)632–638.
11. deJonge, M. and Racine, R.J., The development and decay of kindling-induced increases in paired pulse depression in the dentate gyrus. Brain Research, 412(1986)318–328.
12. Ffrench-Mullen, J.M.H. and Rogawski, M.A., Interaction of phencyclidine with voltage-dependent potassium channels in cultured rat hippocampal neurons: Comparison with block of the NMDA receptor-ionophore complex. J. Neurosci., 9(1989)4051–4061.
13. Ffrench-Mullen, J.M.H. and Rogawski, M.A. and Barker, J.L., Phencyclidine at low concentrations selectively blocks the sustained but not the transient voltage-dependent potassium current in cultured hippocampal neurons. Neurosci. Lett., 88(1991)325–330.
14. Gilbert, M.E., The NMDA-receptor antagonist, MK-801, suppresses limbic kindling and kindled seizures. Brain Res., 463(1988)90–99.
15. Gilbert, M.E., Potentiation of inhibition with perforant path kindling: An NMDA-dependent process. Brain Research, 564(1991)109–116.
16. Gilbert, M.E., The NMDA antagonist, MK-801 suppresses behavioral seizures, augments afterdischarges, but does not block development of perforant path kindling. Epilepsy Research, 17(1994)145–156.
17. Gilbert, M.E. and Burdette, L.J., Enhancement of paired pulse depression in the dentate gyrus in vivo by the NMDA antagonist, MK-801, and electrical kindling. Brain Res., in press.
18. Gilbert, M.E. and Mack, C.M., The NMDA-receptor antagonist, MK-801, suppressed long-term potentiation, kindling, and kindling-induced potentiation in the perforant path of the unanesthetized rat. Brain Research, 519(1990)89–96.
19. Heinemann, U., Beck, H., Drier, J.P., Ficker, E., Stabel, J. And Zhang, C.L., The dentate gyrus as a regulated gate for the propagation of epileptiform activity. In C.E. Ribak, C.M. Gall and I. Mody (Eds.), The Dentate Gyrus and Its Role in Seizures, Epilepsy Res. Suppl., 7(1992)272–280.
20. Holmes, K.H., Bilkey, D.K., Laverty, R. And Goddard, G.V., The N-methyl-d-aspartate antagonists aminophophonovalerate and carboxypiperazinephosphonate retard the development and expression of kindled seizures. Brain Res., 506(1990)227–235.
21. Lancaster, B., Nicoll, R.A. and Perkel, D.J., Calcium activates two types of potassium channels in rat hippocampal neurons in culture. J. Neurosci., 11(1991)23–30.
22. Leung, K-W. S., Hippocampal electrical activity following local tetanization. I. Afterdischarges. Brain Research, 419(1987)173–187.
23. Maru, E. and Goddard, G., Alteration in dentate neuronal activities associated with perforant path kindling. I. Long-term potentiation of excitatory synaptic transmission. Experimental Neurol., 96(1987)19–32.
24. Maru, E. and Goddard, G., Alteration in dentate neuronal activities associated with perforant path kindling. III. Enhancement of synaptic inhibition. Experimental Neurol., 96(1987)46–60.
25. McNamara, J.O., Russell, R.D. , Rigsbee, L. And Bonhaus, D.W., Anticonvulsant and antiepileptogenic actions of MK-801 in the kindling and electroshock models. Neuropharmacol., 27(1988)563–568.

26. Milgram, N.W., Michael, M., Cammisuli, S., Head, E., Ferbinteanu, J., Reid, C., Murphy, M.P. and Racine, R.J. Development of spontaneous seizures over extended electrical kindling. II. Persistence of dentate inhibitory suppression. Brain Res., 670(1995)112–120.
27. Morimoto, K., Katayama, K., Inoue, K. And Sato, K., Effects of competitive and noncompetitive NMDA receptor antagonists on kindling and LTP. Pharmacol. Biochem. Behav., 40(1991)893–899.
28. Rafiq, A., DeLorenzo, R.J. and Coulter, D., Generation and propagation of epileptiform discharges in a combined entorhinal cortex/hippocampal slice. J. Neurophysiol., 70(1993)1962–1974.
29. Rausche, G., Sarvey, J.H. and Heinemann, U.. Slow synaptic inhibition in relation to frequency habituation in dentate granule cells of rat hippocampal slices. Experimental Brain Res., 78(1989)233–242.
30. Robinson, G.B., Kindling-induced potentiation of excitatory and inhibitory inputs to hippocampal dentate granule cells. II. Effects of the NMDA antagonist MK-801. Brain Res., 562(1991)26–33.
31. Robinson, G.B., Sclabassi, R.J. and Berger, T.W., Kindling-induced potentiation of excitatory and inhibitory inputs to hippocampal dentate granule cells. I. Effects on linear and nonlinear response characteristics. Brain Res., 562(1991)17–25.
32. Rothman, S., Noncompetitive N-methyl-d-aspartate antagonists affect multiple ionic currents. J. Pharmacol. Exp. Ther., 246(1988)137–142.
33. Sato, K., Morimoto, K. And Okamoto, M., Anticonvulsant action of a noncompetitive antagonist of NMDA receptors (MK-801) in the kindling model of epilepsy. Brain Res., 463(1988)12–20.
34. Synder, S.H., Adenosine as a neuromodulator. Ann. Rev. Neurosci., 8(1985)103–124.
35. Thalmann, R.H. and Ayala, G.F., A late increase in potassium conductance follows synaptic stimulation of granule neurons of the dentate gyrus. Neurosci. Lett., 29(1982)243–248.
36. Tuff, L.P., Racine, R.J. and Adamec, R., The effects of kindling on GABA-mediated inhibition in the dentate gyrus of the rat. I. Paired pulse depression. Brain Res., 277(1983)79–90.
37. Whitcomb, K., Lupica, C.R., Rosen, J.B. and Berman, R.F., Adenosine involvement in postictal events in amygdala kindled rats. Epilepsy Res., 6(1990)171–179.

DISCUSSION OF MARY GILBERT'S PAPER

S. Leung: Those are quite interesting results. My first question is, did you record from the entorhinal cortex or anywhere there?

M. Gilbert: No.

S. Leung: O.K., so possibly the afterdischarge there may be changed as well. My second question is more of a comment: Does quenching occur with a natural afterdischarge? This secondary afterdischarge has the characteristics of 1–3 Hz, and what you show seems to be that it has some sort of depotentiation effect. If this afterdischarge is long enough then you can block the increase in the late paired-pulse depression.

M. Gilbert: That's an interesting observation, and I hadn't put those two together. Thank you.

F. Lopes da Silva: I wonder whether you have recorded also with the very long time constant. If you record at DC, with the development of afterdischarge you have a DC shift that is sometimes even very pronounced, and if you stimulate strong enough can even give rise to a spreading depression due to a change in potassium in the tissue. I wonder, also considering that MK-801 is affecting all the potassium currents, whether you are not looking here at an effect on the potassium current that you could perhaps come to some idea about using some antagonist or just to record in another way with a DC recording.

M. Gilbert: Well, the easy answer is no. We haven't done any other recordings than what I have shown you. We actually discovered this quite by accident, and we're just using the

EEG to count the duration of the evoked afterdischarge. I think that it is quite likely that we are affecting a potassium current with MK-801.

R. Racine: Just to comment, I suspect that part of what turns off a seizure and accounts for the depression after the discharge depends on the strength of the discharge. I don't mean the duration, I mean the burst activity in the cells—how strong those might be. If MK-801 is producing a weaker burst response in the cells it may not have that much effect on the EEG measure of the afterdischarge, but the weaker discharge may be more prolonged because its not shutting itself off as quickly.

M. Gilbert: We often saw examples where the primary afterdischarge was terminated, and then the secondary afterdischarge still came on but at an earlier time point and lasted longer. So what you are suggesting is going to be more applicable to a change in the primary afterdischarge and not necessarily the onset of the secondary.

Ulrich Ebert: Have you ever tried to record bilaterally from the other hippocampus as well. This is because we also tried to record secondary afterdischarges after amygdala kindling but not hippocampal kindling systematically. What we found was that sometimes especially after inducing generalized seizures the epileptic activity spreads to the other hippocampus and then from the contralateral hippocampal loop there the secondary afterdischarge is generated. This can cause such an effect that the secondary afterdischarge is not very separated by this post-ictal depression but gives effects like the ones you showed. It just starts right with the primary afterdischarge in the ipsilateral hippocampus.

M. Gilbert: I think just because we are using an NMDA antagonist that is blocking the development of kindling, you would really expect that you would see less evidence of that in animals that were not progressing as quickly and also should have more focally contained afterdischarges. In the saline treated animals you would expect to see more discharge propagating to the contralateral hippocampus, rather than in the treated animals, which is counter to what we saw.

31

PHARMACOLOGY OF GLUTAMATE RECEPTOR ANTAGONISTS IN THE KINDLING MODEL

Wolfgang Löscher

Department of Pharmacology, Toxicology and Pharmacy
School of Veterinary Medicine
D-30559 Hannover, Germany

1. INTRODUCTION

Both decrease in GABAergic inhibition and increase in glutamatergic excitation are thought to be critically involved in the cellular mechanisms underlying the initiation and spread of epileptic seizures and the processes that lead to epileptogenesis and, as a consequence, chronic epilepsy.[3,7,8,17,18,31,34] The kindling model of temporal lobe epilepsy has been particularly helpful in elucidating the important roles of inhibitory and excitatory synaptic function in the development and spread of epileptic activity.[34] Based on findings in the kindling and other models of epilepsy, increasing GABAergic transmission and decreasing glutamatergic transmission have been proposed as promising antiepileptic strategies with potential advantages compared with current therapies.[17,31] Various drugs which selectively potentiate GABAergic transmission have been developed over the last three to four decades and some of them, e.g. vigabatrin, have recently been marketed for treatment of epilepsy.[29] In contrast to the long history of the "GABA hypothesis of epilepsy" and GABAergic drugs developed because of this hypothesis,[17] it was not until the development in the early 1980s of subtype-selective excitatory amino acid (EAA) receptor agonists and antagonists that the role of EAA receptor systems in the generation of epileptic activity was fully recognized.[34] This initiated an enormous interest in the potential therapeutic use of EAA receptor antagonists in epilepsy and other brain disorders for which an involvement of glutamatergic transmission has been suggested. However, it took several years before systemically active compounds (i.e., compounds which pass the blood-brain-barrier after systemic administration) became available. Furthermore, the vast majority of studies on anticonvulsant effects of such compounds was done in experimental models of acute seizures, while until recently no systematic drug evaluation in chronic models of epilepsy such as kindling was reported. This prompted us to carry out a large series of experiments on different categories of glutamate receptor antagonists, which was started in 1989 and is still continued today. In the following, the most important findings from these experiments with glutamate receptor antagonists in the kindling model will be reviewed.

Kindling 5, edited by Corcoran and Moshé.
Plenum Press, New York, 1998.

2. GLUTAMATE RECEPTORS

EAA receptors using glutamate (and in part aspartate) as endogenous transmitters consist of at least three ionotropic subtypes which incorporate an ion channel within the receptor complex, and one metabotropic receptor subtype.[6] Ionotropic glutamate receptors can be distinguished pharmacologically be specific binding of the agonists N-methyl-D-aspartate (NMDA), kainic acid (KA), and a-amino-3-hydroxy-5-methyl-4-isoxazole (AMPA) and include receptors that gate both voltage-dependent and voltage-independent currents carried by Na^+, K^+, and, in some cases, Ca^{2+}.[6] Of these ionotropic receptors it is the NMDA receptor which has been most extensively studied in epilepsy research. The activity of this receptor subtype is highly regulated via several allosteric regulatory binding sites on the receptor/channel complex, thus allowing complex possibilities to pharmacologically manipulate NMDA receptor function. At a single brain synapse, NMDA receptors usually coexist with either AMPA or KA receptors and are thought to be involved in amplification of the glutamate signal.[6] At resting potentials, NMDA channels are normally blocked by Mg^{2+} and there must be sufficient concurrent depolarization of the postsynaptic neuronal membrane before the Mg^{2+} block is relieved and the NMDA channel can contribute to the electrical response of the cell. The level of concurrent depolarization depends on AMPA/KA activation and/or other modulatory postsynaptic signals controlling depolarization. Activation of the NMDA receptor and concurrent depolarization result in the development of a relatively slow-rising, long-lasting current mediated primarily by the influx of Ca^{2+}.[6] In experiments on the role of NMDA and AMPA receptors in seizures and burst-firing in the hippocampus, it was shown that synaptic activation of AMPA receptors triggers burst initiation, whereas NMDA receptors become active after the initial AMPA receptor-meditated depolarization has caused Mg^{2+} to dissociate from the NMDA channel.[8] Both NMDA and AMPA receptors contribute to seizure elaboration[8] so that pharmacological strategies inhibiting both glutamate receptor subtypes might be particularly promising (see below).

Precise modulation of NMDA channel activity is required for normal neuronal function, and there are several regulatory sites in addition to the agonist (glutamate or NMDA) recognition site on the NMDA receptor channel which control NMDA-mediated activity further.[6] The binding of glycine to a strychnine-insensitive glycine site on the receptor/channel complex increases the frequency of agonist-induced channel opening. Glycine binding to this site appears to be an absolute requirement for NMDA channel activation, so that drugs inhibiting the binding of glycine to this site (noncompetitive NMDA receptor antagonists) are an effective means of blocking NMDA receptor function.[4] In addition to the agonist recognition site (to which competitive antagonists bind) and the glycine site on the NMDA receptor/channel complex, there is a distinct site within the channel (the "PCP site") which binds "uncompetitive" NMDA receptor antagonists such as MK-801 (dizocilpine) and phencyclidine (PCP) inhibiting channel opening. There are several other regulatory sites which will not be further discussed here because as yet they are not major targets for development of novel anticonvulsant drugs. Furthermore, although subtypes of NMDA receptors (NR-1 and NR-2) have been identified, which opens the possibility of developing subtype selective ligands, the currently available antagonists are not able to distinguish readily and consistently between the two NMDA receptor subtypes[36] so that this issue has as yet no relevance for the topic of this review.

Non-NMDA receptors (AMPA and KA) mediate fast excitatory synaptic transmission and are associated primarily with voltage-independent channels which gate a depolarizing current primarily carried by an influx of Na^+ ions. The pharmacologies of KA and AMPA receptors are similar, so that they are more often distinguished by the relative rank order of potencies of a series of agonists rather than by the selective action of a single compound. Similarly, there are currently no antagonists which can differentiate with sufficient selectivity between the two types of non-NMDA receptors. Of the currently available drugs, the quinoxalinedione NBQX (2,3-dihydroxy<-6-nitro-7-sulfamoyl-benzo[F]quinoxaline) appears to exhibit the greatest selectivity for AMPA receptors, while highly selective KA antagonists are not yet available.

3. GLUTAMATE RECEPTOR ANTAGONISTS EVALUATED IN THE KINDLING MODEL

In our experiments in fully kindled rats, the following drugs were evaluated:

1. NMDA receptor antagonists: (a) competitive NMDA receptor antagonists, i.e. CPP (3-(2-carboxypiperazin-4-yl)propyl-1-phosphonic acid), CGP 37849 (DL-[E]-2-amino-4-methyl-5-phosphono-3-pentenoic acid) and its ethyl ester CGP 39551; (b) the high-affinity uncompetitive NMDA antagonist MK-801; (c) the low-affinity uncompetitive NMDA antagonists memantine, dextrorphan and dextromethorphan; (d) noncompetitive (i.e., glycine/NMDA site) NMDA receptor ligands, i.e. the glycine site antagonist 7-chlorokynurenic acid, the low efficacy glycine partial agonist (+)-HA-966 (R-(+)-3-amino-1-hydroxypyrrolid-2-one), which has less than 8% of the efficacy of glycine at the strychnine-insensitive glycine/NMDA site, the high efficacy glycine partial agonist D-cycloserine, which has about 40–70% of the efficacy of glycine, and the full glycine site agonist D-serine.
2. non-NMDA (AMPA/KA) receptor antagonists: (a) the AMPA antagonist NBQX; (b) several novel non-NMDA antagonists that differentially block AMPA receptors and KA receptor subtypes.
3. Combinations of NMDA and non-NMDA antagonists.
4. Combinations of NMDA antagonists and standard antiepileptic drugs.

For comparison with glutamate receptor antagonists, standard antiepileptics were used. Except for some experiments with glycine site ligands, all glutamate receptor ligands and antiepileptic drugs were administered intraperitoneally. Not all doses and pretreatment times tested will be described here.

For characterizing the anticonvulsant effect of the various glutamate receptor antagonists in kindled rats, the following parameters were determined after vehicle or drug treatment in fully (amygdala-) kindled rats: (a) the focal seizure threshold (i.e., the electrical current inducing afterdischarges in the amygdala; afterdischarge threshold; ADT) as a means of evaluating anticonvulsant action on seizure initiation in the focus, and (b) severity of behavioral seizures recorded at ADT current as a means of evaluating drug action on seizure propagation from the focus. The duration of seizures and focal afterdischarges was also recorded, but will not be described here.

In addition to anticonvulsant activities on seizure initiation and spread, the adverse behavioral effects of the various drugs were determined in kindled rats in the open field. Behavioral alterations and ataxia were quantitated by a score system as described previously.[21] Furthermore, motor impairment was assessed by the rotarod test.[22] Adverse effects induced by glutamate receptor antagonists in kindled rats were compared with respective effects in nonkindled rats in order to examine if kindling alters the adverse effect potential of these drugs. If not otherwise indicated, all experiments were done in female Wistar rats.

3.1. Reference Drugs

Antiepileptic drugs clinically used in treatment of temporal lobe epilepsy are effective in the kindling model at doses below those inducing any marked adverse behavioral effects or motor impairment. As shown in Fig. 1A, carbamazepine, phenobarbital, and valproate both increase the focal seizure threshold (ADT) and reduce severity of seizures recorded at ADT, thus indicating that these drugs affect both initiation and propagation of seizures. Phenytoin, on the other hand, increases focal seizure threshold but does not reduce seizure severity, clearly separating this drug from the other substances. It should be considered that stimulation of the rats at individual ADT or 20% above threshold (as used by several other groups) would have resulted in total blockade of focal and secondarily generalized seizures at the doses of drugs shown in Fig. 1A. Since kindling is generally thought to be the most useful model of temporal lobe epilepsy, i.e. the most common and difficult-to-treat type of epilepsy, novel anticonvulsant drugs should be at least as effective as standard antiepileptics in this model.[28]

3.2. NMDA Receptor Antagonists

In contrast to clinically used antiepileptics, the competitive NMDA antagonists CGP 39551 and CGP 37849 did not induce any marked effects on focal seizure threshold (ADT), although the drugs were administered up to doses inducing marked adverse effects (see below). The only significant effect on ADT was observed after 30 mg/kg CGP 39551, which, however, was associated with severe motor impairment (see Fig. 2A). Some reduction in seizure severity was observed with CGP 39551 and CGP 37849, indicating that these drugs attenuate seizure propagation (Fig. 1B). CPP, however, did not exert any effect on seizure severity, which might be due to the fact that the drug was tested at only one fixed current (500 μA) instead of ADT (which is in the range of about 50–150 μA in amygdala-kindled rats).

As shown in Fig. 1C, the uncompetitive NMDA antagonists MK-801 and memantine neither increased ADT nor decreased seizure severity in kindled rats although both drugs were tested up to doses inducing marked adverse effects (see below). Memantine, 10 mg/kg, even increased seizure severity (Fig. 1C) and, at 20 mg/kg, induced prolonged paroxysmal activity in the recordings from the amygdala and spontaneous motor seizures, indicating that the drug was proconvulsant rather than anticonvulsant in kindled rats (no seizures were induced in non-kindled rats). In contrast, significant anticonvulsant activity was obtained with dextromethorphan, which increased ADT but did not affect seizure severity (Fig. 1C). Dextrorphan, the major active metabolite of dextromethorphan, was effective on both seizure parameters only at the highest dose tested. As shown in Fig. 2A, this dose (30 mg/kg) induced marked motor impairment in both open field and rotarod test. Motor impairment was also seen with all other uncompetitive and competitive NMDA receptor antagonists except dextromethorphan. The latter drug was therefore the only drug of this series which exerted anticonvulsant activity in the kindling model without concomitantly impairing motor function. In this respect, however, it is important to note that dextromethorphan, in addition to blocking NMDA receptor channels, is a potent blocker of voltage-gated calcium and sodium currents, which might explain its relatively high potency in the kindling model.[23] This is also indicated by the observation that dextromethorphan, in contrast to dextrorphan, did not induce any PCP-like behavioral effects at anticonvulsant doses.[23]

In addition to motor impairment, most competitive and uncompetitive NMDA receptor antagonists examined induced signs of central stimulation, such as hyperlocomotion and stereotypies (e.g., head weaving) in kindled rats. In comparison to age-matched non-kindled

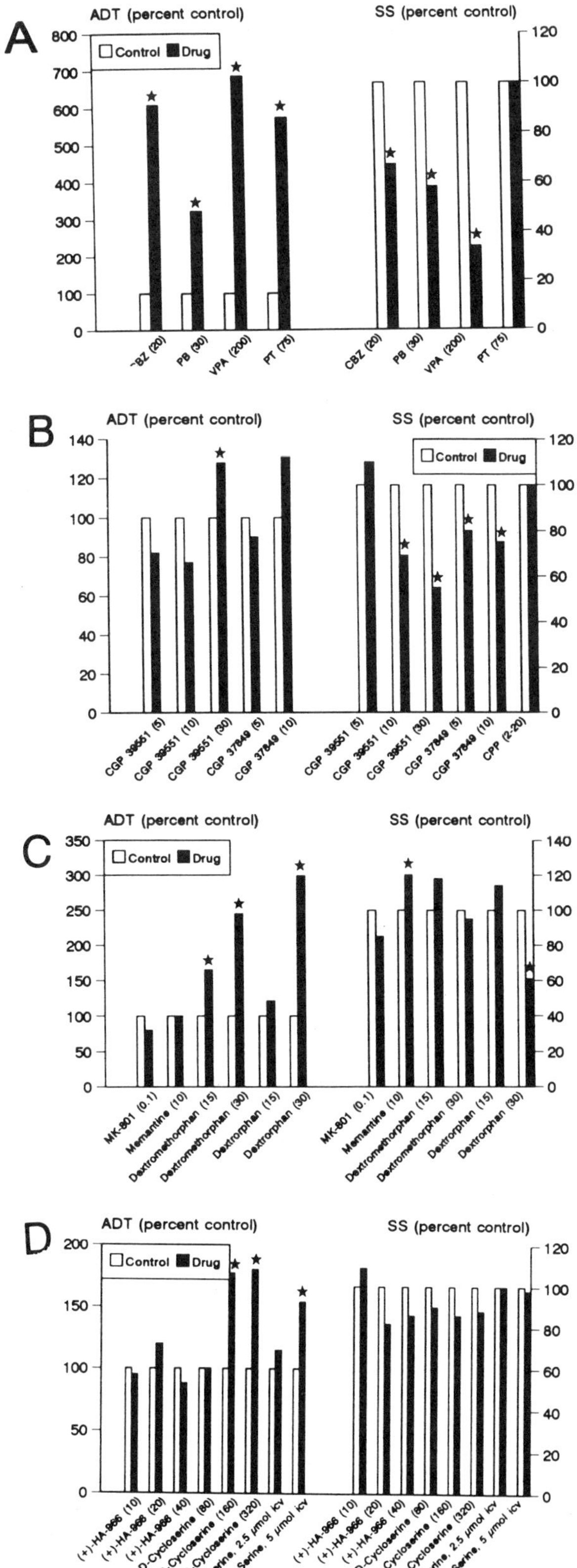

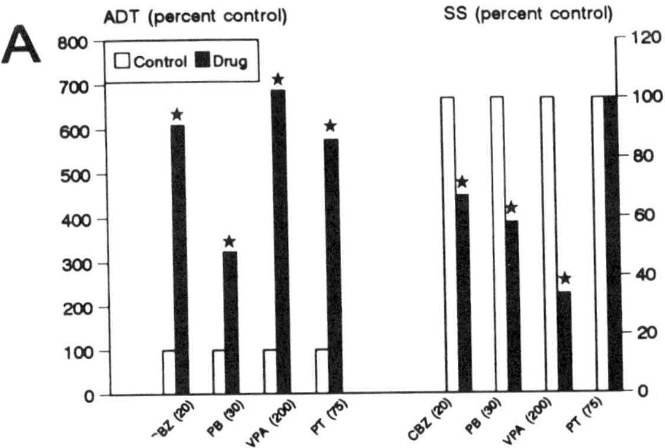

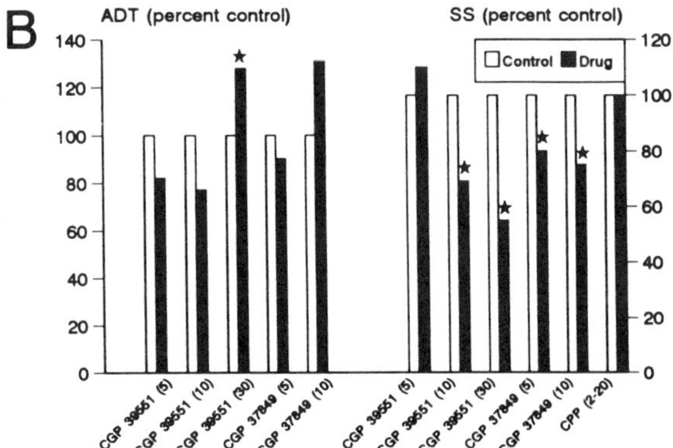

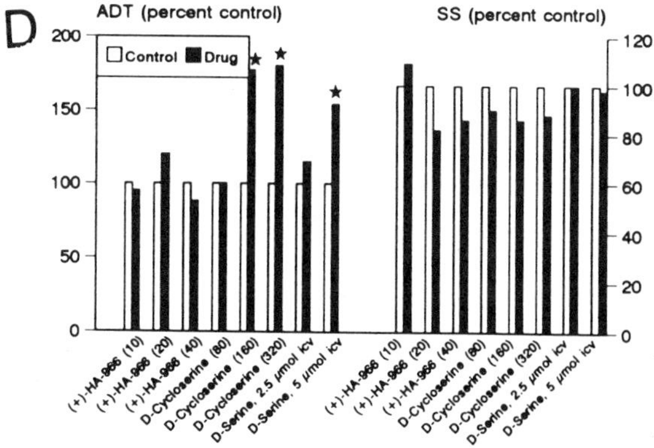

Figure 1. Effects of standard antiepileptic drugs (A), competitive NMDA receptor antagonists (B), uncompetitive NMDA receptor antagonists (C), and glycine site ligands (D) on focal seizure threshold (ADT) and seizure severity (SS) recorded at ADT in amygdala-kindled rats. In B, CPP was tested only at one suprathreshold current (500 μA) instead of ADT. The data are means of 8–12 rats per group and are shown as percent of individual vehicle control data which were determined in the same rats 2–3 days before drug administration. Control ADTs were in the range of about 50–150 μA in the individual animals; seizure severity at ADT current was stage 4–5 (i.e., focal plus secondarily generalized seizures) in most rats. Significant differences from controls are indicated by stars (P at least <0.05). All drugs were administered by the i.p. route except D-serine, which was injected intracerebroventricularly (i.c.v.). The doses of drugs are given together with drug names in mg/kg (D-serine μmol per rat). Depending on the individual time of peak drug effect, drug administration was 0.25–4 h before amygdala stimulation. Abbreviations used for standard antiepileptic drugs are CBZ (carbamazepine), PB (phenobarbital), VPA (valproate), and PT (phenytoin). Data are from Rundfeldt et al.,[35] Löscher and Hönack,[22,23] Löscher et al.,[26,27,30] and unpublished experiments.

rats, kindled rats proved to be much more sensitive to induction of such stimulatory adverse effects (Fig. 2B), indicating that kindling-induced epileptogenesis had altered susceptibility of the brain to such adverse effects. As a consequence, competitive NMDA antagonists such as CGP 37849 behaved like PCP-like uncompetitive NMDA receptor antagonists in kindled rats. Furthermore, with several NMDA antagonists, e.g. dextrorphan, motor impairment in kindled rats was much more severe compared to nonkindled rats. From these observations, we predicted that epileptic patients will exhibit more severe adverse effects in response to competitive NMDA receptor antagonists than non-epileptic individuals,[20] which was subsequently substantiated in clinical studies. Thus, in the first clinical study with a competitive NMDA antagonist (D-CPP-ene) in epileptic patients, the drug was not anticonvulsant, but induced severe adverse effects (including confusion, gait ataxia, and sedation) in all patients, requiring hospitalization of most patients and premature termination of the trial.[37] In contrast to the epileptic patients, the drug had been well tolerated in volunteers during phase I studies. Similar disappointing clinical experience was obtained with MK-801 in epileptic patients.[29] Based on these data, clinical development of other competitive or uncompetitive NMDA antagonists for treatment of epilepsy was suspended.

During our experiments with NMDA receptor antagonists in kindled rats, we also compared adverse behavioral effects in female and male animals. Female rats were much

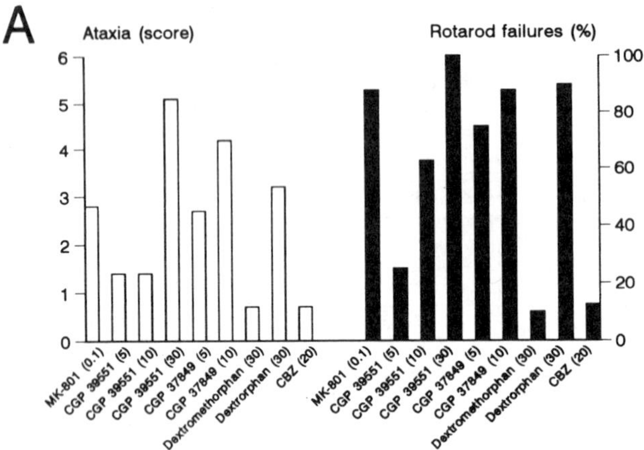

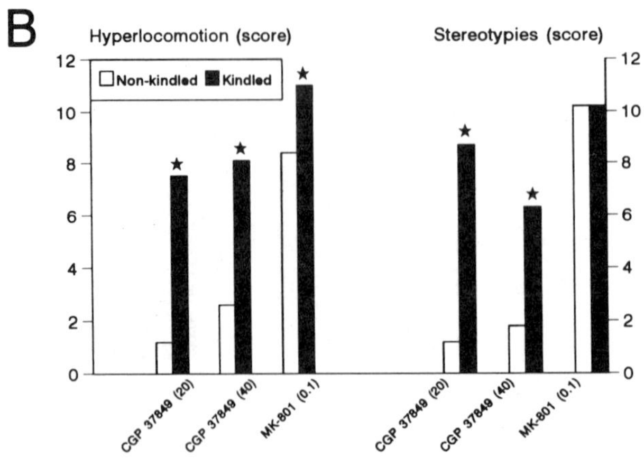

Figure 2. Adverse effects of some competitive and uncompetitive NMDA receptor antagonists and carbamazepine (CBZ) in kindled (A) and kindled versus nonkindled (B) rats. In A, ataxia and rotarod failures were determined immediately before testing anticonvulsant activity as shown in Fig. 1, while data in B are cumulative scores for hyperlocomotion and head weaving determined 30, 45, 60 and 75 min after drug injection. Data are means of 8–12 rats per group. Doses of drugs in mg/kg i.p. are indicated in brackets. For further details see Fig. 1 legend. Data are from Löscher and Hönack[21–23] and Löscher et al.[27]

more susceptible than male rats to induction of PCP-like behavioral alterations, suggesting sex related differences in the endogenous modulation of the NMDA receptor.[11]

In contrast to the disappointing data from experiments with competitive or uncompetitive NMDA receptor antagonists in the kindling model, the glycine/NMDA site partial agonist D-cycloserine markedly increased the focal seizure threshold in kindled rats (Fig. 1D) at doses that did not induce any adverse behavioral or motor impairing effects. In contrast, (+)-HA-966 did not alter the ADT or seizure recordings at ADT after systemic administration (Fig. 1D), although the drug was given up to doses inducing motor impairment. Subsequent studies showed that (+)-HA-966, but not D-cycloserine, induce paroxysmal activity in limbic brain regions of kindled rats, which was almost absent in nonkindled rats, again demonstrating that kindling changes the adverse effect potential of some NMDA receptor ligands.[39] Proconvulsant effects such as observed with (+)-HA-966 have also been reported for "silent" glycine site antagonists such as 7-chlorokynurenic acid[15,16] and for several uncompetitive NMDA receptor antagonists, including PCP, ketamine, tiletamine, memantine and dextrorphan (cf. [39]). For instance, in epileptic patients, ketamine has been used for activation of epileptic discharge as a means of localization of epileptic foci during surgical treatment of epilepsy.[1] As suggested by our data on memantine in kindled versus non-kindled rats, epileptogenesis appears to decrease the threshold for induction of proconvulsant activity in response to NMDA antagonists.[19] One explanation for such proconvulsant effects of NMDA antagonists might be reduction of GABA release in response to complete blockade of NMDA receptor-mediated glutamatergic transmission,[5,10,32] which is less likely to occur with partial agonists. In summary, our data in kindled rats cast doubt on the assumption that glycine site antagonists or low-efficacy partial agonists such as (+)-HA-966 may have a larger therapeutic window as anticonvulsants than other types of NMDA antagonists.[4,14] On the other hand, in line with recent data on the high-efficacy glycine partial agonist 1-aminocyclopropanecarboxylic acid (ACPC),[29] the data on D-cycloserine indicate that glycine partial agonists with high efficacy (> 50%) might have advantages over low-efficacy or silent glycine ligands and over competitive and uncompetitive NMDA antagonists. Whether such high-efficacy glycine ligands act as functional antagonists or by reversibly desensitizing NMDA receptors is not clear at present. Interestingly, anticonvulsant activity in the kindling model was also obtained by intracerebroventricular injection of the glycine site agonist D-serine (Fig. 1D), which seems to argue against receptor desensitization as the responsible mechanism for anticonvulsant effects of high-efficacy partial agonists such as D-cycloserine.

3.3. Non-NMDA Receptor Antagonists and Coadministration of NMDA and Non-NMDA Antagonists

NBQX was used as a prototype antagonist of non-NMDA receptors with high affinity for the AMPA subtype.[6] An added advantage of this compound compared to other dihydroxyquinoxaline derivatives is that NBQX is almost devoid of affinity for the glycine site of NMDA receptors (see below). In kindled rats, NBQX potently increased the focal seizure threshold and decreased seizure severity at ADT (Fig. 3A). The magnitude of these effects was similar to that obtained with standard antiepileptics (Fig. 1A). At anticonvulsant doses, NBQX induced only slight ataxia and no rotarod failures (Fig. 1D) or PCP-like behavioral effects. These data thus demonstrate that an AMPA antagonist is a much more effective means of blocking seizure initiation and spread in the kindling model than NMDA receptor antagonists. However, low doses of competitive or uncompetitive NMDA antagonists synergistically increased the anticonvulsant effect of NBQX in the kindling

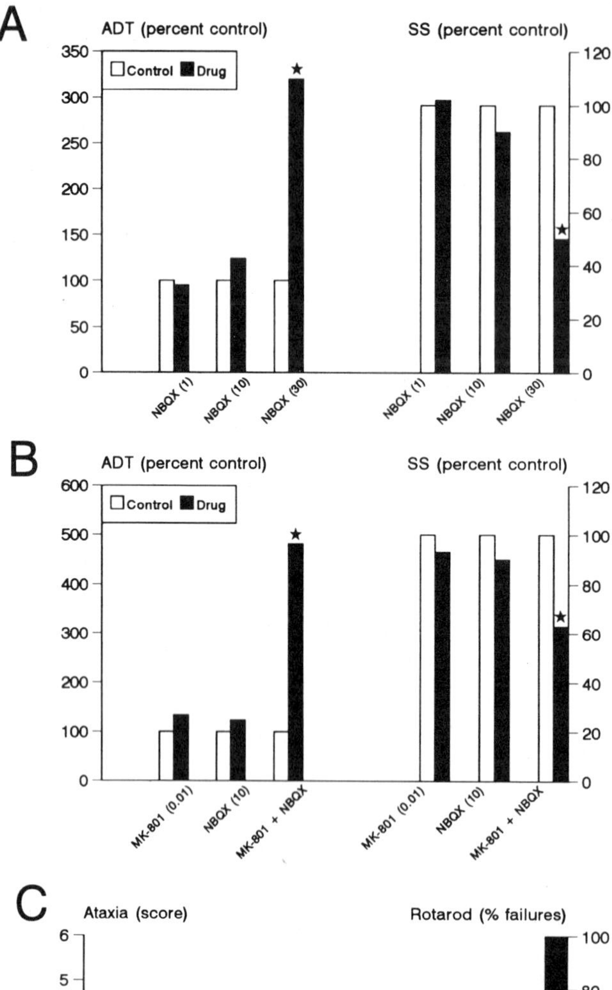

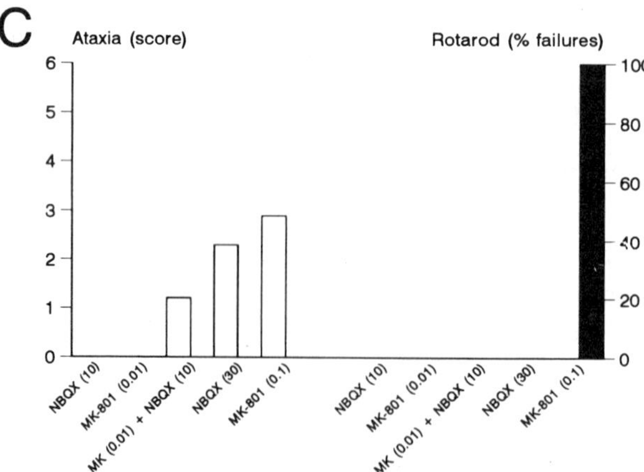

Figure 3. Effects of the AMPA receptor antagonist NBQX alone (A) or in combination with the NMDA antagonist MK-801 (B) on focal seizure threshold (ADT) and seizure severity (A,B) as well as in the open field and rotarod test (C) in kindled rats. Pretreatment times were 2.5 h for MK-801 and 0.5 h for NBQX. For further details see Fig. 1 legend. The absence of bars in C indicates that no adverse effects were observed at this dose. Data are from Löscher et al.[27]

model (Fig. 3B, Fig. 4A, Fig. 4B), indicating that both non-NMDA and NMDA receptors are critically involved in the kindled state.[27] As shown in Fig. 3C, the synergistic increase in anticonvulsant activity was not parallelled by any marked increase in adverse effects, suggesting that combinations of AMPA and NMDA receptor antagonists provide a new strategy for treatment of epileptic seizures. Interestingly, with MK-801 a synergistic effect was only obtained when the drug was administered at very low doses (the maximum effect

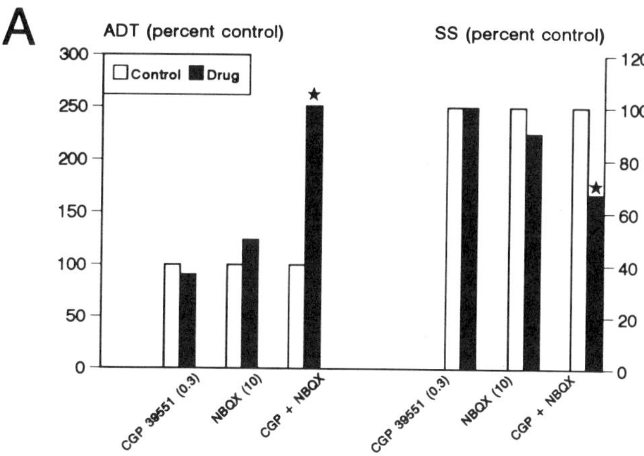

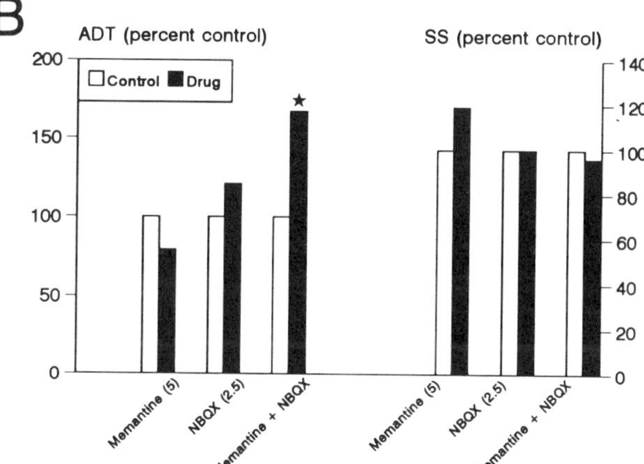

Figure 4. Effects of NBQX alone or in combination with the NMDA receptor antagonists CGP 39551 (A) or memantine (B) on focal seizure threshold (ADT) and seizure severity (SS) in kindled rats. Pretreatment times were 4 h for CGP 39551, and 0.5 h for memantine and NBQX. For further details see Fig. 1 legend. Data are from Löscher et al.[27] and Löscher and Hönack.[25]

being reached at 0.01 mg/kg) several hours before NBQX, while concomitant treatment or use of higher doses reduced or prevented a synergistic interaction.[27] The long pretreatment time could be explained by the slow onset of NMDA receptor blockade with high-affinity antagonists such as MK-801.[33] In order to test this possibility, we used the low-affinity uncompetitive NMDA antagonist memantine, which exhibits a faster apparent rate of block and unblock.[33] With this drug, concomitant administration with NBQX led to synergistic increases in anticonvulsant activity (Fig. 4B).

4. COADMINISTRATION OF NMDA ANTAGONISTS AND STANDARD ANTIEPILEPTIC DRUGS

Stimulated by the promising findings from coadministration of NMDA and non-NMDA antagonists, we undertook a series of experiments in which we coadministered NMDA antagonists and the antiepileptic valproate. From various dose combinations, only those resulting in synergistic interactions are shown in Fig. 5. In contrast to the findings with NBQX, where very low doses of MK-801 or CGP 39551 were maximally effective to synergistically increase anticonvulsant activity (i.e., doses far below the doses of these NMDA antagonists needed to induce anticonvulsant or other pharmacodynamic effects when given alone), much higher doses of NMDA antagonists were needed to increase the anticonvulsant activity of valproate. Furthermore, such an interaction was only seen at anticonvulsant doses of valproate (80–100 mg/kg), while in case of NBQX synergistic interactions were obtained with a dose of NBQX that was ineffective when given alone (Fig. 3). However, the most important difference to the experiments with NBQX was that coadministration of NMDA antagonists markedly increased the severity of adverse effects compared to single drug treatment (Fig. 5C, Fig. 5D). Thus, an increase of the dose of valproate to 200 mg/kg resulted in a more marked anticonvulsant effect than combined treatment with lower doses of valproate and NMDA antagonists, but the severity of adverse effects obtained with 200 mg/kg was clearly below that obtained with the combined treatments, thus resulting in considerable reduction of the therapeutic index of the combined treatment compared to valproate alone. Interestingly, nonkindled rats were much less sensitive to induction of adverse effects by combined treatment with valproate and NMDA antagonists than kindled rats, again demonstrating the altered susceptibility to NMDA antagonists induced by kindling.[9,24] In summary, these data indicate that add-on treatment of epileptic patients with NMDA antagonists might decrease the tolerability of the standard medication.

5. NOVEL NON-NMDA RECEPTOR ANTAGONISTS

Molecular biology studies on the non-NMDA receptors have not only confirmed the existence of the KA and AMPA classes, but also indicated that the potential heterogeneity within these receptor families reveals a remarkable degree of complexity.[2,6,13] AMPA receptor channels can be formed by reconstituting one or any two of four subunits (GluR1-GluR4), while the KA subclass of receptors includes GluR5-GluR7 and KA-1-KA-2.[2,6,13] GluR5-GluR7 correspond to the previously described low-affinity KA site, while KA-1-KA-2 correspond to the high-affinity KA site. The only currently available non-NMDA antagonist that displays some selectivity for KA receptors is NS-102 (5-nitro-6,7,8,9-tetrahydrobenzo[G]indole-2,3-dione-3-oxime), which has been reported to competitively antagonize low-affinity KA binding with a K_i of 600 nM.[12] More recent experiments with recombinant KA receptor subunits expressed in fibroblasts showed that NS-102 reduced currents mediated by GluR-6 receptors.[38] The heterogeneity of non-NMDA receptors has stimulated the pharmaceutical industry to develop novel antagonists which differentially block specific subunit combinations. A number of such drugs has been tested by us in the kindling model (Fig. 6). Like NBQX, these compounds are pyrrolyl-quinoxaline-diones, which, however, markedly differ in their AMPA and KA affinities from NBQX (Fig. 6A). Thus, while NBQX essentially does not bind to KA receptors at relevant concentrations (Fig. 6A), several of the novel compounds shown in Fig. 6 exhibit relevant affinity to KA receptors in addition to AMPA receptors, and some of the compounds show some selectivity for KA receptor subtypes. For instance, compound D-2 binds to native high affinity KA receptors and GLuR5-GluR7 subunits with much higher affinities than to AMPA receptors (Fig. 6A).

Although all of these novel non-NMDA receptor antagonists exerted anticonvulsant effects in the kindling model, they markedly differed in anticonvulsant potency and adverse effects (Fig. 6A, Fig. 6B). For instance, compound D-6 induced marked increases in ADT and decreases in seizure severity without inducing any significant motor impairment, while compound D-1 induced comparable anticonvulsant effects only at motor impairing doses. To our knowledge, these data are the first evidence that non-NMDA receptor subtype selectivity has a striking influence on therapeutic index of non-NMDA receptor antagonists.

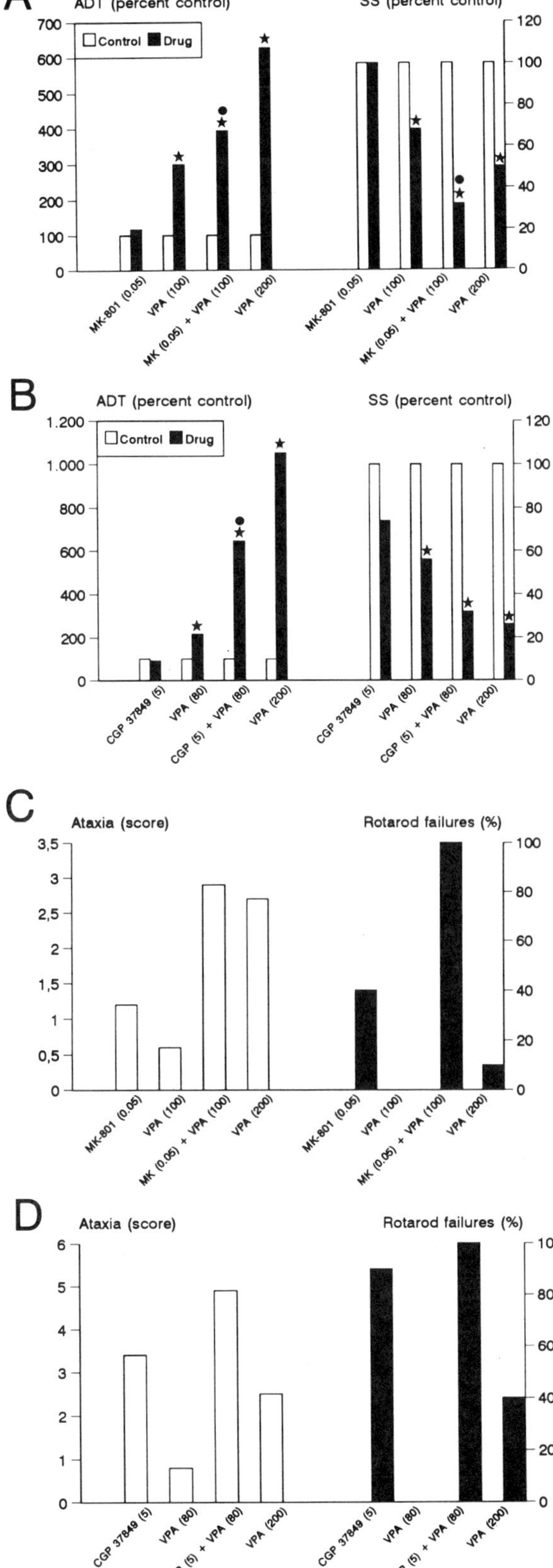

Figure 5. Effects of valproate (VPA) alone or in combination with the NMDA antagonists MK-801 or CGP 37849 on focal seizure threshold (ADT) and seizure severity (A,B) as well as in the open field and rotarod test (C,D) in kindled rats. Pretreatment times were 2.5 h for MK-801, 2 h for CGP 37849 and 0.25 h for valproate. For further details see Fig. 1 legend. The absence of bars in C indicates that no adverse effects were observed at this dose. Data are from Dziki et al.[9] and Löscher and Hönack.[24]

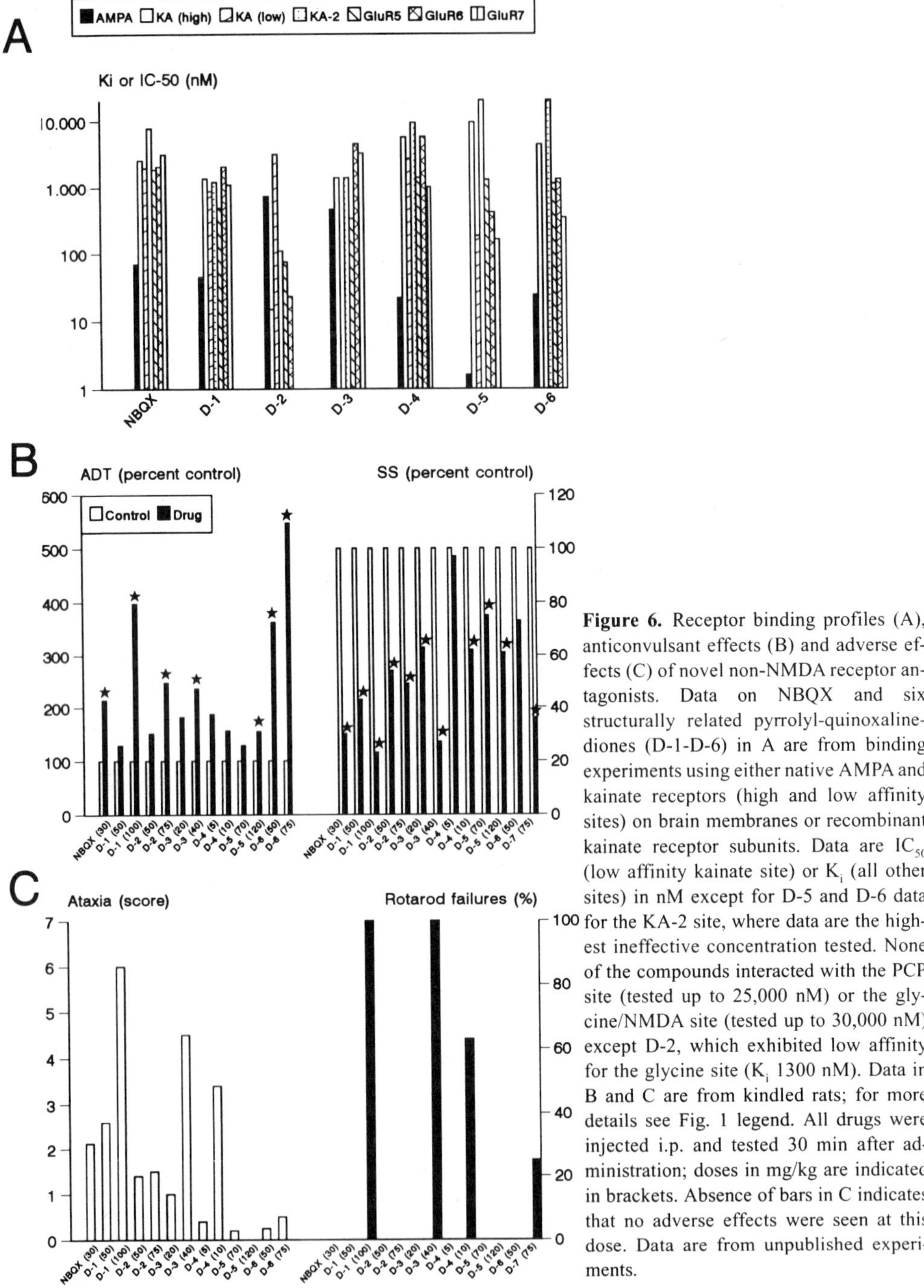

Figure 6. Receptor binding profiles (A), anticonvulsant effects (B) and adverse effects (C) of novel non-NMDA receptor antagonists. Data on NBQX and six structurally related pyrrolyl-quinoxalinediones (D-1–D-6) in A are from binding experiments using either native AMPA and kainate receptors (high and low affinity sites) on brain membranes or recombinant kainate receptor subunits. Data are IC_{50} (low affinity kainate site) or K_i (all other sites) in nM except for D-5 and D-6 data for the KA-2 site, where data are the highest ineffective concentration tested. None of the compounds interacted with the PCP site (tested up to 25,000 nM) or the glycine/NMDA site (tested up to 30,000 nM) except D-2, which exhibited low affinity for the glycine site (K_i 1300 nM). Data in B and C are from kindled rats; for more details see Fig. 1 legend. All drugs were injected i.p. and tested 30 min after administration; doses in mg/kg are indicated in brackets. Absence of bars in C indicates that no adverse effects were seen at this dose. Data are from unpublished experiments.

6. CONCLUSIONS

Although several lines of evidence have implicated enhanced NMDA receptor-mediated neurotransmission in the cellular basis of the increased neuronal excitability in kindling,[34] the present data on NMDA receptor antagonists indicate that, once kindling is established, NMDA receptors are not critical for the expression of fully kindled seizures. In contrast, non-NMDA receptor antagonists exerted potent anticonvulsant effects on both initiation and propagation of kindled seizures, substantiating recent findings that enhanced expression of specific non-NMDA receptor subunit mRNAs in the dentate gyrus and other brain regions of kindled rats might be critically involved in the development *and* expression of kindling.[34] Furthermore, combinations of an AMPA antagonist with very low doses of NMDA antagonists proved to be an effective means of inducing marked anticonvulsant activity in the kindling model, thus indicating that optimal treatment of partial and secondarily generalized seizures may require combined use of both non-NMDA and NMDA antagonists. A further important finding of the studies described in this review is the enhanced susceptibility of kindled rats to PCP-like adverse effects of competitive and uncompetitive NMDA receptor antagonists, indicating that chronic epilepsy models such as kindling are more predictive in terms of therapeutic efficacy in epilepsy than acute seizure models with normal (non-epileptic) animals. The finding that such drugs are clearly less effective as anticonvulsants in the kindling model than in acute models of generalized seizures (e.g., electroshock-induced tonic seizures) but more potent to induce adverse effects in kindled rats corresponds to the disappointing clinical findings with NMDA antagonists in patients with temporal lobe epilepsy. The possibility that glycine site partial agonists such as D-cycloserine or ACPC have advantages in this respect has to await clinical studies.

ACKNOWLEDGMENTS

We wish to acknowledge the following persons for their assistance in the experiments described in this review: Dr. Dagmar Hönack, Dr. Björn Nolting, Dr. Chris Rundfeldt, Dr. Holger Lehmann, Dr. Piotr Wlaz, Dr. Marek Dziki, Dr. Halina Baran, Doris Pieper, and Christiane Bartling. We appreciate Dr. Ulrich Ebert's help during preparation of the manuscript. The studies were supported by grants from the Deutsche Forschungsgemeinschaft.

REFERENCES

1. Bacia, T., Szpiro-Zurkowska, A., Bidzinski, J. and Czarkwiani, L. Use of ketamine for activation of EEG and electrocorticographic records in patients with epilepsy, *Epilepsia*, 30 (1989) 642
2. Bettler, B. and Mulle, C. Neurotransmitter receptors II: AMPA and kainate receptors, *Neuropharmacology*, 34 (1995) 123–139.
3. Bradford, H.F. Glutamate, GABA and epilepsy, *Progr. Neurobiol.* 47 (1995)
4. Carter, A.J. Glycine antagonists: regulation of the NMDA receptor-channel complex by the strychnine-insensitive glycine site, *Drugs Future*, 17 (1992) 595–613.
5. Carter, A.J. Antagonists of the NMDA receptor-channel complex and motor coordination, *Life Sci.* 57 (1995) 917–929.
6. Cotman, C.W., Kahle, J.S., Miller, S.E., Ulas, J. and Bridges, R.J. Excitatory amino acid neurotransmission. In F.E. Bloom and D.J. Kupfer (Eds.) *Psychopharmacology. The fourth generation of progress*, Raven Press, New York, 1995, pp. 75–85.
7. Dichter, M.A. Cellular mechanisms of epilepsy and potential new treatment strategies, *Epilepsia*, 30 (Suppl. 1) (1989) S12
8. Dingledine, R., McBain, C.J. and McNamara, J.O. Excitatory amino acid receptors in epilepsy, *Trends Pharmacol. Sci.* 11 (1990) 334–338.
9. Dziki, M., Hönack, D. and Löscher, W. Kindled rats are more sensitive than non-kindled rats to the behavioural effects of combined treatment with MK-801 and valproate, *Eur. J. Pharmacol.* 222 (1992) 273–278.
10. Garcia, Y., Ibarra, C. and Jaffe, E.H. NMDA and non-NMDA receptor-mediated release of [H-3]GABA from granule cell dendrites of rat olfactory bulb, *J. Neurochem*, 64 (1995) 662–669.

11. Hönack, D. and Löscher, W. Sex differences in NMDA receptor mediated responses in rats, *Brain Res.* 620 (1993) 167–170.
12. Johansen, T.H., Drejer, J., Watjen, F. and Nielsen, E.O. A novel non-NMDA receptor antagonist shows selective displacement of low-affinity [^{3}H]kainate binding, *Eur. J. Pharmacol.* 246 (1993) 195
13. Jorgensen, M., Tygesen, C.K. and Andersen, P.H. Ionotropic glutamate receptors—focus on non-NMDA receptors, *Pharmacol. Toxicol.* 76 (1995) 312–319.
14. Kemp, J.A. and Leeson, P.D. The glycine site of the NMDA receptor—five years on, *Trends Pharmacol. Sci.* 14 (1994) 20–25.
15. Koek, W. and Colpaert, F.C. Selective blockade of N-methyl-D-aspartate (NMDA)-induced convulsions by NMDA antagonists and putative glycine antagonists: relationship with phencyclidine-like behavioral effects, *J. Pharmacol. Exp. Ther.* 252 (1990) 349–357.
16. Lapin, I.P., Prakhie, I.B. and Kiseleva, I.P. Excitatory effects of kynurenine and its metabolites, amino acids and convulsants administered into brain ventricles: differences between rats and mice, *J. Neural Trans.* 54 (1982) 229–238.
17. Löscher, W. GABA and the epilepsies. Experimental and clinical considerations. In N.G. Bowery and G. Nisticò (Eds.) *GABA. Basic research and clinical applications*, Pythagora Press, Rome, 1989, pp. 260–300.
18. Löscher, W. Basic aspects of epilepsy, *Curr. Opin. Neurol. Neurosurg.* 6 (1993) 223–232.
19. Löscher, W. and Hönack, D. High doses of memantine (1-amino-3,5-dimethyladamantane) induce seizures in kindled but not in non-kindled rats, *Naunyn-Schmiedeberg's Arch. Pharmacol.* 341 (1990) 476–481.
20. Löscher, W. and Hönack, D. Responses to NMDA receptor antagonists altered by epileptogenesis, *Trends Pharmacol. Sci.* 12 (1991) 52
21. Löscher, W. and Hönack, D. The novel competitive N-methyl-D-aspartate (NMDA) antagonist CGP 37849 preferentially induces phencyclidine-like behavioral effects in kindled rats: attenuation by manipulation of dopamine, *alpha*-1 and serotonin$_{1A}$ receptors, *J. Pharmacol. Exp. Ther.* 257 (1991) 1146–1153.
22. Löscher, W. and Hönack, D. Anticonvulsant and behavioral effects of two novel competitive N-methyl-D-aspartic acid receptor antagonists, CGP 37849 and CGP 39551, in the kindling model of epilepsy. Comparison with MK-801 and carbamazepine, *J. Pharmacol. Exp. Ther.* 256 (1991) 432–440.
23. Löscher, W. and Hönack, D. Differences in anticonvulsant potency and adverse effects between dextromethorphan and dextrorphan in amygdala-kindled and non-kindled rats, *Eur. J. Pharmacol.* 238 (1993) 191–200.
24. Löscher, W. and Hönack, D. Effects of the competitive NMDA receptor antagonist, CGP 37849, on anticonvulsant activity and adverse effects of valproate in amygdala-kindled rats, *Eur. J. Pharmacol.* 234 (1993) 237–245.
25. Löscher, W. and Hönack, D. Over-additive anticonvulsant effect of memantine and NBQX in kindled rats, *Eur. J. Pharmacol.* 259 (1994) R3-R5.
26. Löscher, W., Nolting, B. and Hönack, D. Evaluation of CPP, a selective NMDA antagonist, in various rodent models of epilepsy. Comparison with other NMDA antagonists, and with diazepam and phenobarbital, *Eur. J. Pharmacol.* 152 (1988) 9–17.
27. Löscher, W., Rundfeldt, C. and Hönack, D. Low doses of NMDA receptor antagonists synergistically increase the anticonvulsant effect of the AMPA receptor antagonist NBQX in the kindling model of epilepsy, *Eur. J. Neurosci.* 5 (1993) 1545–1550.
28. Löscher, W. and Schmidt, D. Which animal models should be used in the search for new antiepileptic drugs? A proposal based on experimental and clinical considerations, *Epilepsy Res.* 2 (1988) 145–181.
29. Löscher, W. and Schmidt, D. Strategies in antiepileptic drug development: is rational drug design superior to random screening and structural variation? *Epilepsy Res.* 17 (1994) 95–134.
30. Löscher, W., Wlaz, P., Rundfeldt, C., Baran, H. and Hönack, D. Anticonvulsant effects of the glycine/NMDA receptor ligands D-cycloserine and D-serine but not R-(+)-HA-966 in amygdala-kindled rats, *Brit. J. Pharmacol.* 112 (1994) 97–106.
31. Meldrum, B.S. Excitatory amino acids in epilepsy and potential novel therapies, *Epilepsy Res.* 12 (1992) 189–196.
32. Perouansky, M. and Grantyn, R. Is GABA release modulated by presynaptic excitatory amino acid receptors? *Neurosci. Lett.* 113 (1990) 292–297.
33. Rogawski, M.A. Therapeutic potential of excitatory amino acid antagonists: channel blockers and 2,3-benzodiazepines, *Trends Pharmacol. Sci.* 14 (1993) 325–331.
34. Rogawski, M.A. Excitatory amino acids and seizures. In T.W. Stone (Ed.) *CNS neurotransmitters and neuromodulators: glutamate*, CRC Press, Boca Raton, 1995, pp. 219–237.
35. Rundfeldt, C., Hönack, D. and Löscher, W. Phenytoin potently increases the threshold for focal seizures in amygdala-kindled rats, *Neuropharmacology*, 29 (1990) 845–851.
36. Stone, T.W. Subtypes of NMDA receptors, *Gen. Pharmacol.* (1993) 825–832.

37. Sveinsbjornsdottir, S., Sander, J.W.A.S., Upton, D., Thompson, P.J., Patsalos, P.N., Hirt, D., Emre, M., Lowe, D. and Duncan, J.S. The excitatory amino acid antagonist D-CPP-ene (SDZ EAA-494) in patients with epilepsy, *Epilepsy Res.* 16 (1993) 165–174.
38. Verdoorn, T.A., Johansen, T.H., Drejer, J. and Nielsen, E.O. Selective block of recombinant glur6 receptors by NS-102, a novel non-NMDA receptor antagonist, *Eur. J. Pharmacol.* 269 (1994) 43–49.
39. Wlaz, P., Ebert, U. and Löscher, W. Low doses of the glycine/NMDA receptor antagonist R-(+)-HA-966 but not D-cycloserine induce paroxysmal activity in limbic brain regions of kindled rats, *Eur. J. Neurosci.* 6 (1994) 1710–1719.

DISCUSSION OF WOLFGANG LÖSCHER'S PAPER

K. Morimoto: Your result with NBQX is very similar to our previous results in 1993. My question is, did you see the effects of NBQX on hippocampal kindling, since in human temporal lobe epilepsy the epileptic focus often resides in the hippocampus? In your report there is also some discrepancy between the amygdala kindled seizure and the hippocampal seizure. I think the potency in the hippocampus was less than in the amygdala. Did you see the effect in the hippocampus?

W. Löscher: No, we didn't do any hippocampal kindling.

A. Fernandez-Guardiola: Did you measure any sleep disorder provoked by this antagonist? It is important because many anticonvulsants produce a disturbance of sleep.

W. Löscher: No, we did not do that, but just one more piece of information: We looked at sex differences, and most of the data which I showed you were from female rats. So we are one of few groups using females, and of course people ask us about the effects on males. So we did a study on both males and females and we found that the males tend to be less sensitive by an effect of 3 to 5 in terms of doses to induction of seizure adverse effects. So there seem to be sex differences, but we did not study any sleep disturbances.

P. Mohapel: I noticed that a couple of your graphs had metabotropic glutamate receptors presented, but you never talked about them. I'm just curious whether you have explored any metabotropic antagonists and their effects on kindling and thresholds?

W. Löscher: No, at the time when we started, in 1988–89, there were no selective ligands for this receptor and we did so many other studies that we have had no time to start the metabotropic since then. We have no data on that.

32

INTERACTIONS BETWEEN CONVULSANTS AT LOW-DOSE AND PHENOBARBITAL IN THE HIPPOCAMPAL SLICE PREPARATION

Larry G. Stark,[1] R. M. Joy,[2,*] W. F. Walby,[3] and T. E. Albertson[3]

[1]Department of Medical Pharmacology and Toxicology
School of Medicine, University of California, Davis, California, 95616
[2]Department of Molecular Biosciences, School of Veterinary Medicine
University of California, Davis, California, 95616
[3]Division of Pulmonary Medicine, Department of Internal Medicine
School of Medicine, University of California, Davis, California, 95616

1. INTRODUCTION

Our laboratory has had a sustained interest in development and use of animal models of epilepsy, and some of our previous studies were included in the proceedings of the Kindling 4 conference[17]. One of the reasons the kindling model has been of special interest is because the slow development of the electroencephalographic and behavioral events associated with it provide us with the opportunity to study the transitional events leading to the final kindled state. We have exploited the model from both the pharmacological and the toxicological point of view. On the pharmacological side, we have studied many conventional and novel compounds for their effects on retardation of kindling development, or on fully kindled seizures[1,2,11,13]. On the toxicological side, we have reported the proconvulsant effects of a number of compounds, including lindane[12–14], a chlorinated hydrocarbon insecticide which was previously broadly used throughout the world and is still the principal ingredient in a medicated shampoo. The work to be described is a direct outgrowth and extension of studies previously reported on lindane, and we have sought to compare it with several other convulsants known to interact with the GABA-A receptor-chloride ionophore complex by examining the electrophyiological consequences of exposing hippocampal slices to each of them.

Since many of the effects of lindane on intact animals being kindled have been expressed at doses which do not provoke overt seizures, we have focused the current studies on sub-convulsant doses of lindane, picrotoxin and pentylenetetrazol. In particular, we

* Deceased, November 1995.

Kindling 5, edited by Corcoran and Moshé.
Plenum Press, New York, 1998.

were interested in neurophysiological differences among the effects of these agents with respect to potential changes in synaptic pharmacology as they might be expressed in the hippocampal slice. It seemed to us that, just as in the case of intact preparations, the transitional events, e.g., changes in electrical activity short of intermittent or sustained high-frequency bursting, should be studied if epileptogenic rather than fully-epileptic events were of particular interest.

2. BACKGROUND

There is ample evidence that lindane induces epileptogenic responses in both whole animals[9] and in other neurophysiological preparations[9,10] Lindane, in a dose-related manner, facilitates the acquisition of electrically kindled responses from both the amygdala and the hippocampus[12]. The rate of kindling was considerably slower for the hippocampal site. These effects have been shown to last for at least two months[16] beyond the last dose and the last kindled seizure in the case of the amygdala site. Maternal or neonatal exposure to the drug induced a greater susceptibility to kindling of the amygdala after the exposed offspring became adults[2]. Not all of the isomers of lindane possess convulsant properties and one of them[15] has been shown to be anticonvulsant during electrical kindling acquisition. In addition, the effects of lindane seem to be somewhat specific for the acquisition stages of kindling since the drug, in the doses used for kindling, did not potentiate the expression of seizures in previously kindled animals.

More recently, Gilbert[9] and her colleagues have extended our findings with lindane and have demonstrated that the drug itself can act as a chemical kindling agent for both behavioral and EEG events even in the absence of electrical stimulation. These effects also lasted for more than one month after the last dose of the drug. Many similar studies have shown that pentylenetetrazol and picrotoxin can also act as either facilitators of electrical kindling acquisition or directly as chemical kindling agents. Pentylenetetrazol and picrotoxin are routinely used within the pharmaceutical industry as screening tools during the discovery and study of new, potentially clinically useful antiepileptic drugs. The convulsant effects of these compounds have also been studied in hippocampal slice preparations taken from both normal[8],[19] and kindled rats[6]. Slices with fully-developed epileptiform spikes and bursts have been used as a test system to evaluate whether drugs can decrease the overall spike frequency after a set time of exposure[8].

The hippocampal slice preparation has not been extensively studied with respect to the interactions between subconvulsant doses of these compounds and classical anticonvulsant drugs, but there have been reports on the effects of receptor-specific antagonists following exposure to some of them[18]. Fisher has reviewed[7] the advantages and disadvantages of many animal models of epilepsy, including the hippocampal slice preparation. The advantages include extensive knowledge of the anatomical interconnections, ease of study and the opportunity to directly expose the tissue to drugs. We have found that disadvantages from a pharmacological point of view include practical problems of drug solubility in artificial cerebral spinal fluid used as the perfusion medium and professional disagreements over exposure levels and dose equivalency in relation to intact preparations. Nevertheless, we have shown that our slice preparations are sensitive to both GABA-A agonists such as propofol[5] and that lindane can induce changes in CA1 pyramidal cell excitability and recurrent inhibition at doses that do not cause the preparation to exhibit overt seizure activity[14]. Some of these effects indicated that transitional events occurring at approximately 100 msec after the first response to a paired-pulse stimulus[14] might be worthy of further examination in our attempts to understand steps involved in epileptogenesis. Since our previous work in intact animals involved the effects of both lindane and anticonvulsants on the acquisition stages of kindling, we included both convulsants and anticonvulsants in our experimental designs for the slice prepartation and quantified the effects using several distinct endpoints. We conducted feasibility studies with these compounds which we report on here as we continue to plan for further work involving slices to be taken from additional control and kindled animals.

3. METHODS

This study protocol was approved by the Animal Studies Committee of the University of California, Davis, and all of the work was carried out in accordance with established guidelines. The basic methods we employed for studies on the hippocampal slice have been published in detail elsewhere[14].

3.1. Slice Preparation

Male Sprague-Dawley rats (185–250 g) were decapitated and the brains were rapidly removed and chilled in an artificial cerebral spinal fluid (ACSF) medium. The hippocampi were dissected free and cut into 400 μm slices with a Brinkman Instruments tissue slicer. The slices were immediately transferred to a Hass-type interface chamber (Medical Systems, Inc.) and placed on nylon netting. Perfusion with the medium at 22°C was maintained at a flow rate of 4ml/minute. A cover was kept over the slices at all times and they were gassed with humidified 95% O_2/5% CO_2. After 20 minutes the medium was warmed to and maintained at 35°C by a temperature controller heating unit (Medical Systems Corporation, TC-102) for the duration of the experiment. Two hours of perfusion and recovery elapsed before initiation of all subsequent experimental procedures.

3.2. Electrophysiological Stimulation and Recording

After perfusion and recovery, a bipolar electrode was placed through an opening in the cover over the slices to the surface of the stratum radiatum of area CA1 to orthodromically stimulate Schaffer collateral/commissural (SC/C) fibers. A glass microelectrode filled with ACSF (resistance 4mOhms) was placed 1–2mm from the stimulating electrode into the stratum pyramidale to record population spikes (PS) in response to varying stimulus intensities.

Stimuli were constant-curent, square-wave pulses formed by a WPI Model 1800 stimulator and delivered through a WPI Model 1800 isolation unit. Pulses were 0.02–0.04 msec in duration and were delivered at a rate of 0.067 Hz (1/15 sec.). Paired pulses of equal intensity were delivered at either a 15msec or 100msec interpulse interval (IPI).

The evoked responses were amplified using an AM Systems Model 1800 amplifiers with high and low cutoff frequencies at 1 Hz and 10 Khz and were viewed on a Tektronic Model 201 oscilloscope. Responses were also digitized and stored using a Keithly DAS Series 570 analog-to-digital converter coupled to an IBM PC computer. The conversion rate was 10 Khz.

3.3. Analysis of Responses

Responses were gathered in groups of 3, averaged and stored as a single record prior to analysis. The evoked potential recorded from the stratum pyramidale consisted of a slow wave (field EPSP) interrupted at higher stimulation currents by a prominent population spike (PS) wave. Computer analyses of the PS waveforms followed closely those previously reported. PS amplitudes were measured from the extrapolated EPSP baseline to the peak of the PS. In addition to measuring the amplitude of the first PS (R1) as a function of stimulation intensity, ratios of second/first responses (R2/R1) were calculated and used as a measure of pyramidal cell excitability at the time of the second stimulus. As a measure of pyramidal cell hyperexcitability, the area under the curve for the second response at the 100 msec IPI was determined under both control and experimental conditions.

3.4. Experimental Procedures

3.4.1. Effects of Convulsants on Measures of CA1 Pyramidal Cell Excitability, Recurrent Collateral Inhibition and Hyperexcitability. Slices were selected that exhibited robust recurrent collateral inhibition at a 15 msec IPI and no hyperexcitability at the 100 msec IPI under control conditions. After final electrode placement, one or more control series of recordings at 15 msec and 100 msec IPIs were collected using a varying set of stimulus intensities from subthreshold to supramaximal levels with respect to evoked PS amplitude. A stimulus intensity which evoked an 80% maximal response at 15 msec IPI was noted and visually saved on the oscilloscope screen so that all subsequent recordings could be done at stimulus intensities which included one capable of evoking a PS response of equal amplitude for meaningful comparisons to the control conditions. Following control (ACSF) perfusion and baseline recordings, the perfusion medium was changed to include a fixed concentration of convulsant drug contained in ACSF. Additional recordings were made at 10, 30, 40 and 60 min. intervals after the perfusion with the convulsant had begun. All effects noted were corrected for changes occurring with ACSF perfusion alone.

3.4.2. Effects of Phenobarbital on Convulsant-Induced Changes in CA1 Pyramidal Cell Excitability, Recurrent Collateral Inhibition and Hyperexcitability. Phenobarbital is a standard antiepileptic drug known to affect electrically kindled seizures[4,3] and several types of human epileptic seizures. We determined the ability of phenobarbital to antagonize the effects of the convulant drugs on the slice preparation by adding it to the combined ACSF/convulsant perfusion mixture after the first 30 min. period of perfusion with the convulsant alone. Subsequent recordings were obtained at the 40 and 60 min. interval as before. Preliminary studies (unpublished) were used to determine an effective dose for phenobarbital in these preparations.

3.4.3. Drugs. The convulsants were dissolved in ACSF and delivered to the slices at the following levels of exposure: lindane (50 μM, LIN), pentylenetetrazol (4 mM, PTZ) and picrotoxin (1 μm, PIC). Phenobarbital (80ug/ml) was delivered in combination with these exposure levels of convulsants for the anticonvulsant studies.

4. RESULTS

The results of preliminary experiments (unpublished) were used to determine the appropriate doses which produced roughly equivalent amounts of hyperexcitability in the slice. These doses were chosen for further study using the endpoints described above and for studies on phenobarbital as a prototypic anticonvulsant drug. All comparisons between treatments were done on responses that had been adjusted so that the first response under the treatment condition matched the 80% of maximum PS height obtained during control recordings made while perfusing with ACSF.

4.1. Effects of Subconvulsant Doses of Drugs on Pyramidal Cell Excitability as Measured by the Amplitude of the First Response (R1)

Lindane increased the excitability of pyramidal cells as evidenced by shifts to the left in responses to each increase in stimulus intensity (Fig. 1). The effects were evident by 30 min. of exposure to the 50 μM dose and became more pronounced with time (Fig. 1).

Picrotoxin (1 μM) produced similar shifts in responsiveness of the pyramidal cells, although the effects were less pronounced at the highest stimulus intensities (Fig. 2).

Pentylenetetrazol (4 mM) had less extensive effects than the other two convulsants on the amplitude of the first response with time (Fig. 3). The effects were most pronounced at intermediate stimulus intensities (Fig. 3).

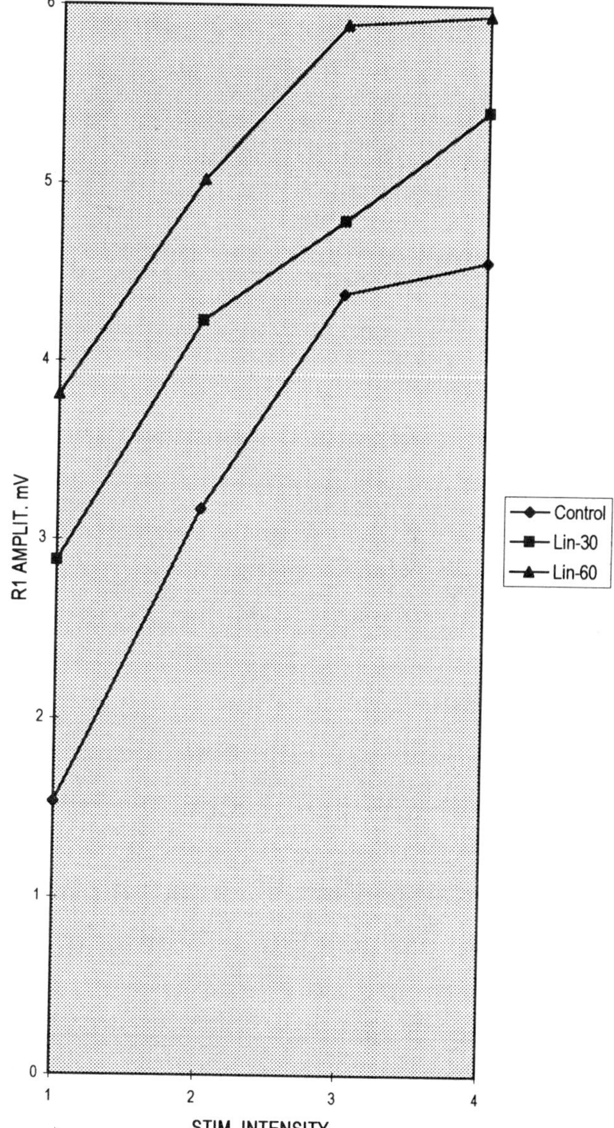

Figure 1. Lindane I/O relationships. The amplitude of the response to the first of two stimuli of a pair is shown at identical stimulus intensities over time. A time-dependent increase in the amplitude of the response is seen following exposure of the slice to lindane (50 μM) in the perfusion fluid.

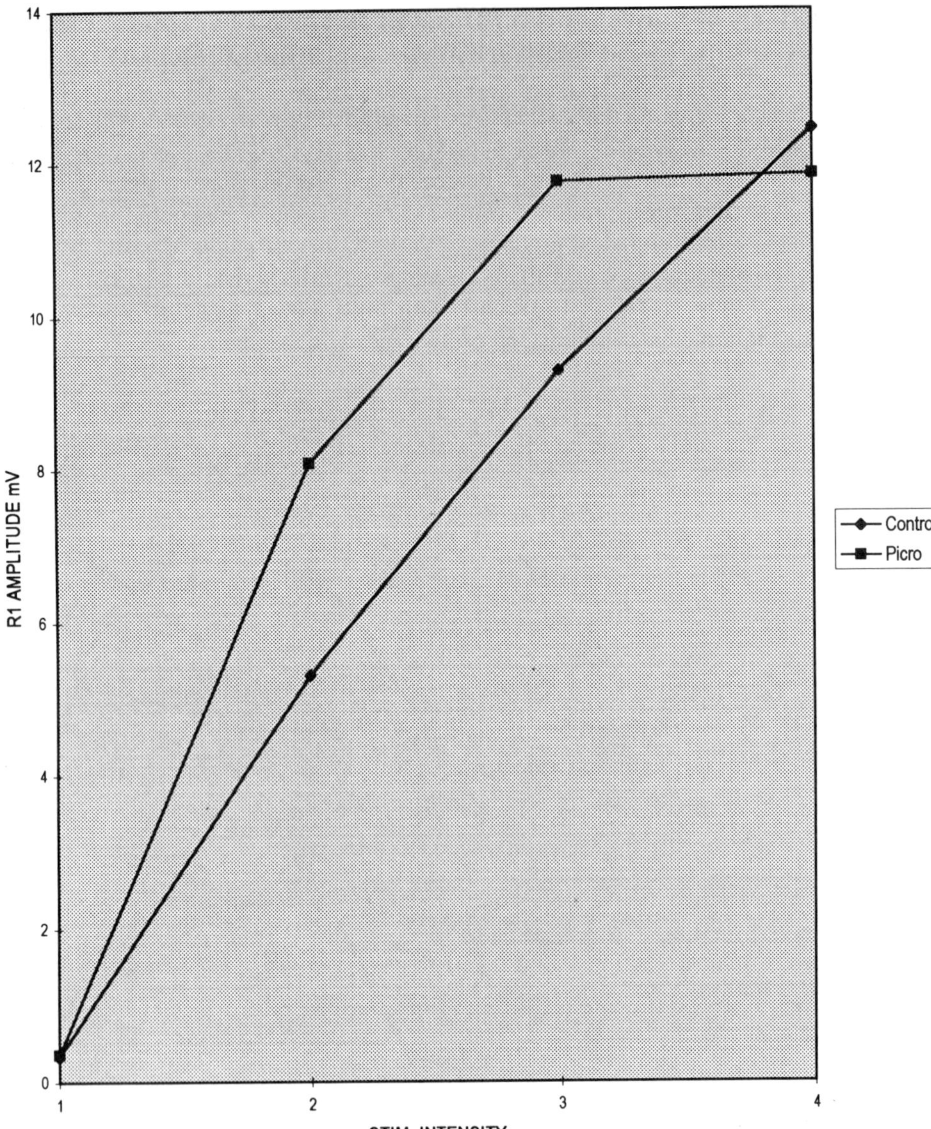

Figure 2. Picrotoxin I/O relationships. The amplitude of the response to the first of two stimuli of a pair is shown at identical stimulus intensities over time. An increase in the amplitude of the response is seen following exposure of the slice to picrotoxin (1 μM) in the perfusion fluid.

4.2. Effects of Subconvulsant Doses of Drugs on Pyramidal Cell Hyperexcitability

Each of the convulsant drugs in the doses used produced similar increases in the hyperexcitability of the pyramidal cells as evidenced by the increasing number of additional population spikes, occasionally on the first response, but particulary following the second stimulus in the 100 msec IPI pair. Figure 4 shows the changes in waveforms obtained following 30 min of exposure to lindane (50 μM). In contrast to our published findings using

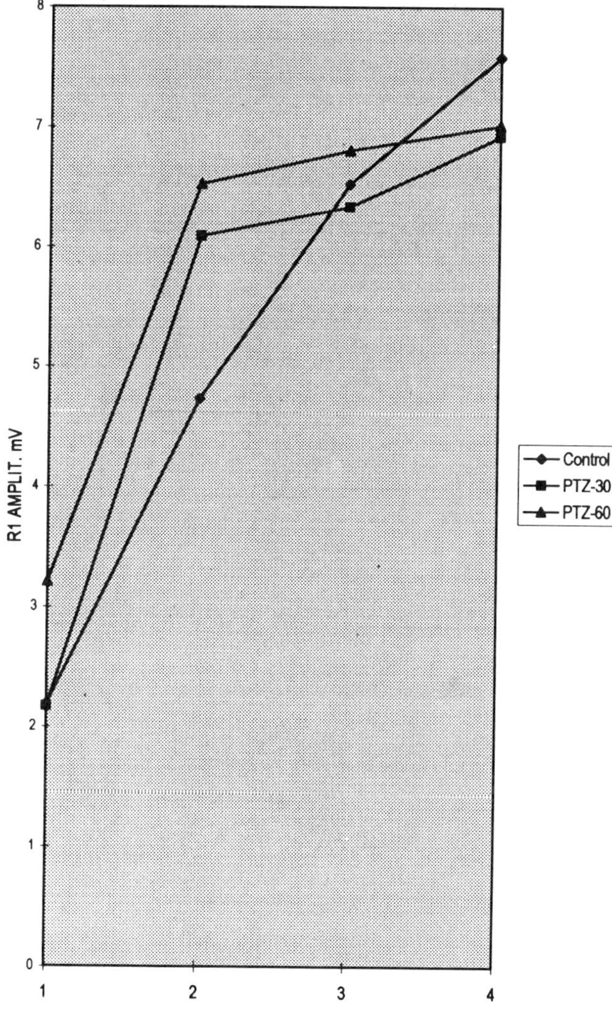

Figure 3. Pentylenetetrazol I/O relationships. The amplitude of the response to the first of two stimuli of a pair is shown at identical stimulus intensities over time. A modest time-dependent increase in the amplitude of the response is seen at low stimulus intensities following exposure of the slice to pentylenetetrazol (4 mM) in the perfusion fluid.

lower doses of lindane (25 μM), the appearance of the secondary PS seemed to occur at about the same time after exposure as did the loss of recurrent inhibition (see below).

Picrotoxin (1 μM) produced similar changes in waveforms at 30 min. as shown in Figure 5. Like lindane, picrotoxin tended to produce multiple PS at each stimulus after 30 min., but the effect was most pronounced on the second response in the 100 msec IPI pair (Fig. 5).

The effects of pentylenetetrazol (4 μM) with respect to induction of hyperexcitability are shown in Figure 6. In the example shown, PTZ increased the amplitude of the first response after 30 min of exposure, but did not produce multiple PS on the initial response of the pair. Two and three additional spikes on the second response were quite common (Fig. 6).

We did not quantify the increases in excitability evident in the first response following drug exposure in these studies, but the time course and extent of hyperexcitability of the second response are shown in Figure 7 as a comparison for all three drugs. The increases following lindane exposure were somewhat slower to develop (Fig. 7), but the overall degree of hyperexcitability produced by the three convulsants was nearly the same by 60 min. (Fig. 7).

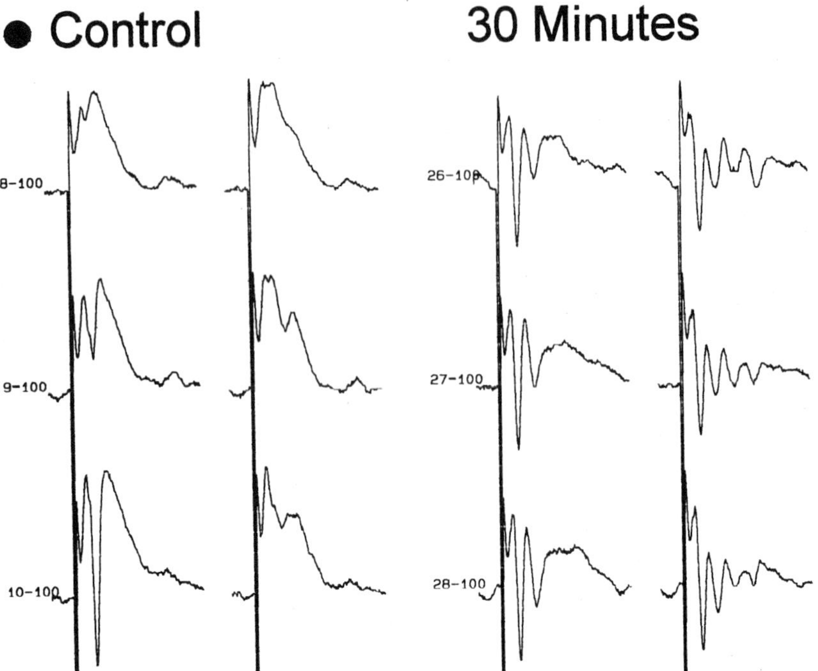

Figure 4. Lindane and hyperexcitability waveforms. Responses to the first stimulus of a pair is shown in the first and third panels while the responses to the second stimulus delivered 100 msec later is shown in the second and fourth panels. Under control conditions, the slice shows considerable inhibition while after 30 minutes of exposure to lindane (50 μM) both the first and second responses show increasing complexity.

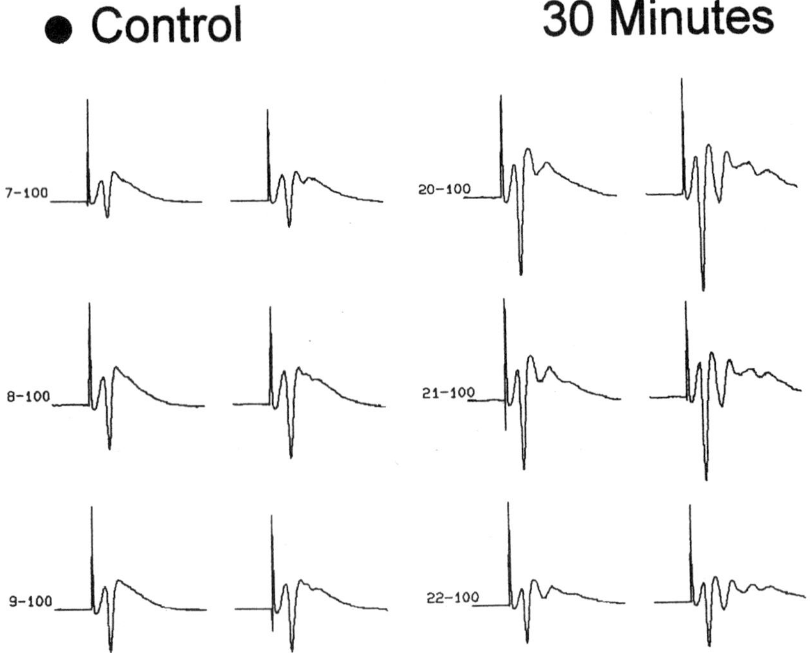

Figure 5. Picrotoxin and hyperexcitability waveforms. Responses to the first stimulus of a pair is shown in the first and third panels while the responses to the second stimulus delivered 100 msec later is shown in the second and fourth panels. Under control conditions, the slice shows minimal facilitation at 100 msec while after 30 minutes of exposure to picrotoxin (1 μM) both the first and second responses show increasing complexity.

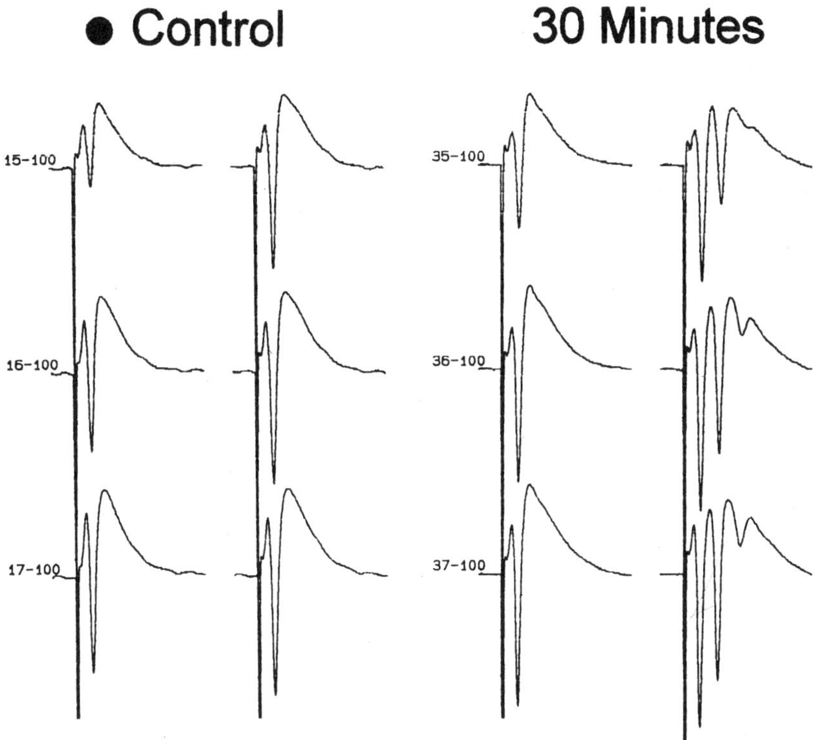

Figure 6. Pentylenetetrazol and hyperexcitability waveforms. Response to the first stimulus of a pair is shown in the first and third panels while the response to the second stimulus delivered 100 msec later is shown in the second and fourth panels. Under control conditions, the slice shows some potentiation at 100 msec while after 30 minutes of exposure to pentylenetetrazol (4 mM) the second response shows increasing complexity without much change in the first.

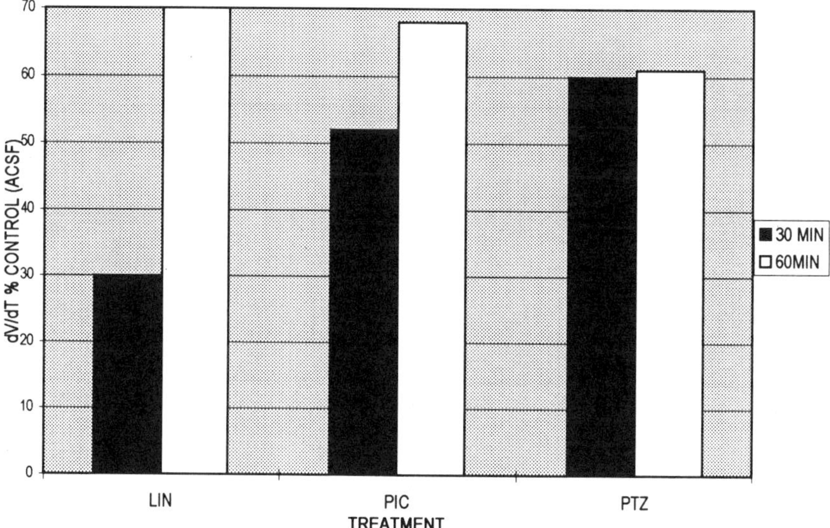

Figure 7. Convulsants and hyperexcitability. The increasing amount of hyperactivity in the second response at 100 msec is quantified and graphed to show changes during a total of 60 min exposure of the slice to each of the convulsant drugs. Each of the drugs increased the excitability of the response more than 60% over control values obtained with perfusions of ACSF.

4.3. Effects of Subconvulsant Doses of Drugs on Pyramidal Cell Recurrent Collateral Inhibition

The results and comparisons shown here for the effects of the drugs on recurrent collateral inhibition were done after establishing the doses required to produce similar amounts of hyperexcitability in the slice as evidenced by the development of additional PS responses at 100 msec. As shown in the comparisons in Figure 8, lindane had more profound effects on recurrent collateral inhibition than did either picrotoxin or pentylenetetrazol. While the loss of some recurrent inhibition was evident for all drugs at 30 min, only lindane had more pronounced effects at 60 min at the dose levels being compared here (Fig. 8).

4.4. Phenobarbital and Antagonism of Drug Effects on Recurrent Inhibition and Hyperexcitability

We have only had limited opportunities to compare the endpoints following convulsant exposure to those obtained following co-exposure of the slices to convulsants combined with phenobarbital. Preliminary results obtained with phenobarbital perfusion and its effects on changes in recurrent inhibition produced by lindane and pentylenetetrzol are shown Figure 9. Phenobarbital was able to diminish the effects of both convulsants on recurrent inhibition following 30 min. of exposure, perhaps showing somewhat greater activity against pentylenetetrazol (Fig. 9) than against lindane.

Figure 10 shows the effects of phenobarbital against lindane and pentylenetetrazol using the measure of hyperexcitability. The levels of hyperexcitability induced without phenobarbital are shown at 30 min, followed by the effects of 30 min exposure to the anticonvulsant (Fig. 10, 60 min).

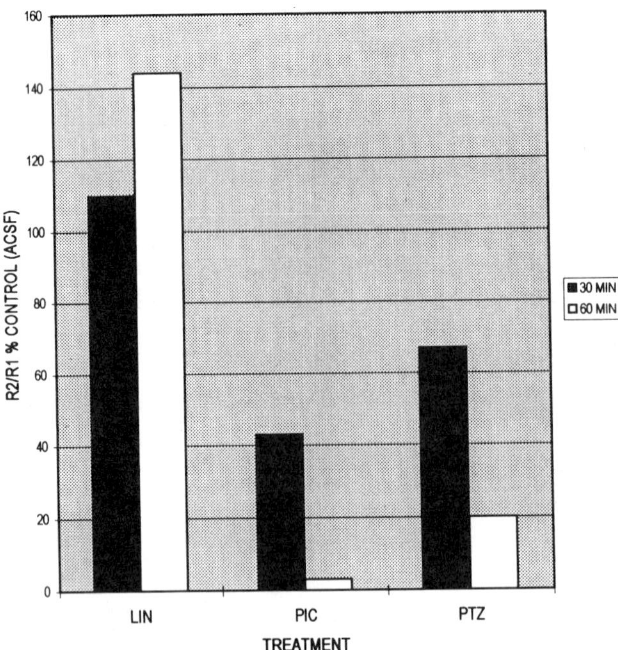

Figure 8. Recurrent inhibition. The amplitude of the second response (R2) as a ratio to the amplitude of the first response (R1) of a stimulus pair delivered 15 msec apart is shown as a function of time of exposure to each of the convulsant drugs. Decreases in the amount of recurrent inhibition observed under control conditions are shown as increases in the relative size of the second response. Each convulsant was tested at doses which produced relatively the same amount of hyperexcitability (see Fig. 7).

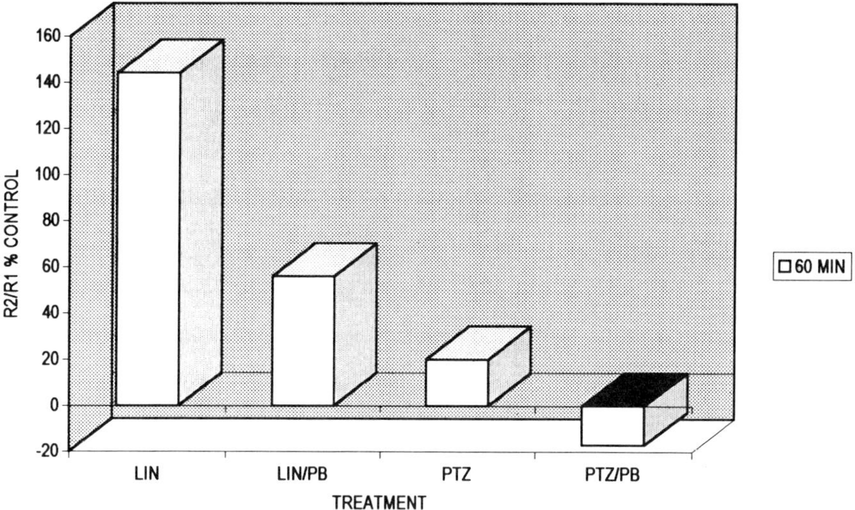

Figure 9. Phenobarbital and recurrent inhibition. The first and third columns in the figure show the relative loss of recurrent inhibition induced by either lindane (50 μM) or pentylenetetrazol (4 mM) while the second and fourth columns depict the effect of phenobarbital (80 μg/ml) in the slice after 60 minutes of exposure to the convulsant, but with 30 min of exposure to convulsant + phenobarbital.

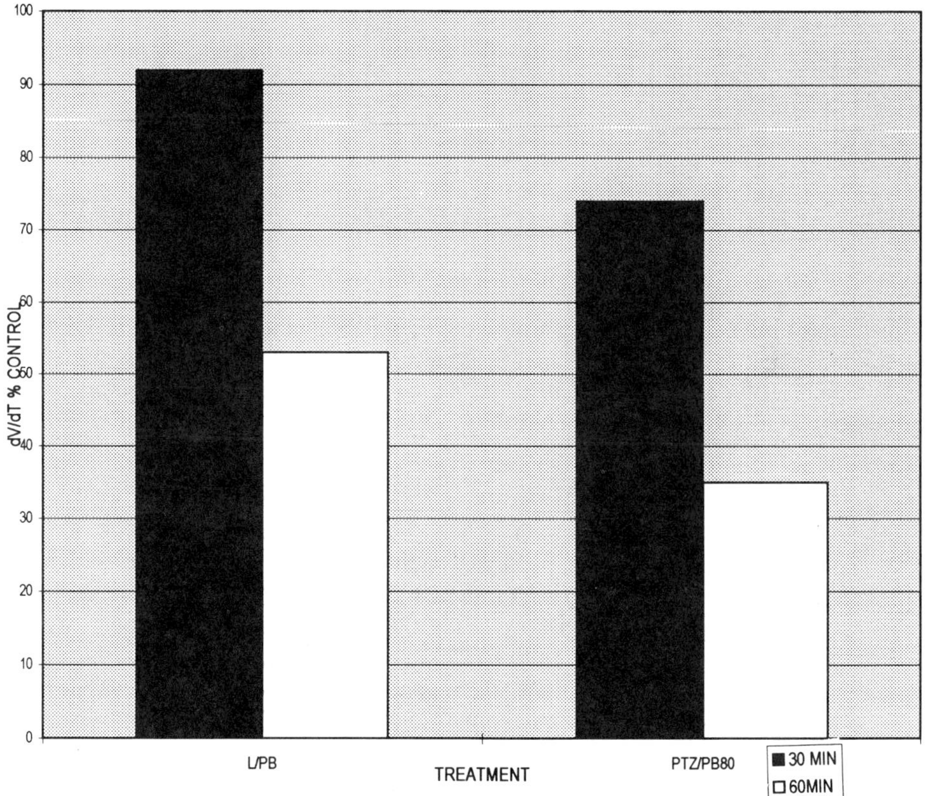

Figure 10. Phenobarbital and hyperexcitability. The amount of hyperexcitability observed after 30 min of exposure to the convulsant is shown in the two dark columns while the effects of 30 min of exposure to convulsant + phenobarbital is shown in the while columns.

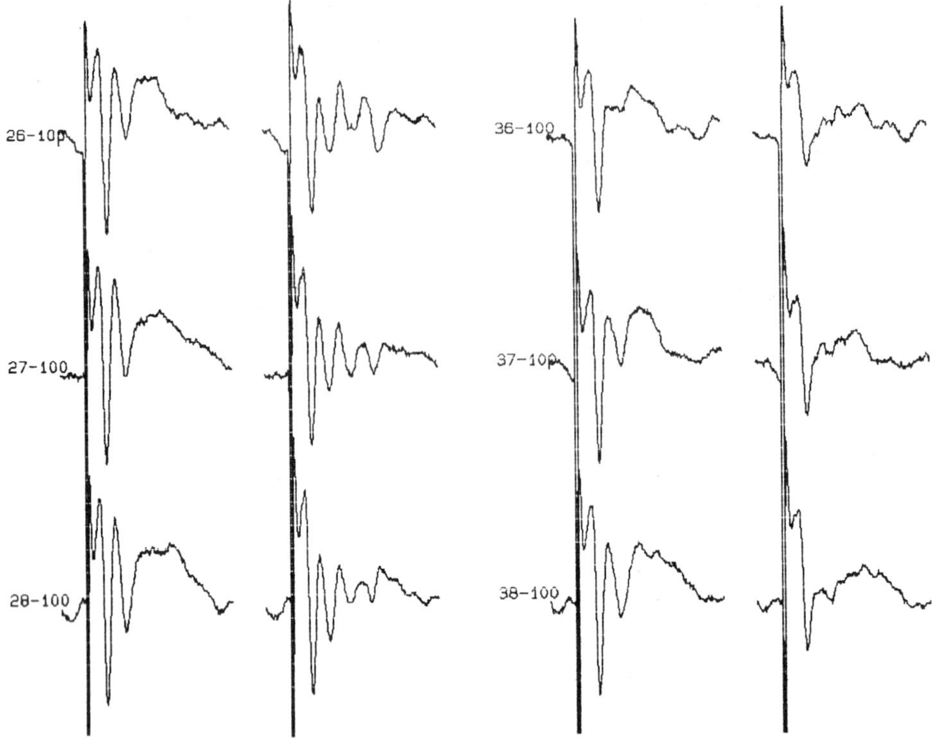

Figure 11. The changes in the complexity of the waveforms following exposure to lindane followed by exposure to lindane + phenobarbital are shown. Phenobarbital appeared to affect the second response at 100 msec after the first within the first 10 min. Note the relative lack of effect of phenobarbital on the first response.

Inspection of the actual waveforms obtained with lindane treatment followed by phenobarbital exposure reveal that the anticonvulsant may be able to decrease hyperexcitability in the slice before it has any influence on the amount of decreased recurrent collateral inhibition induced by lindane (Figure 11).

5. DISCUSSION

The purpose of these experiments in the hippocampal slice was to establish whether or not it might serve as a suitable model in which to study further the effects of lindane and similar convulsants as well as prototypic anticonvulsants. The results, taken together with recently published work, make it clear that the paired-pulse technique used in combination with drug exposure can reveal systematic changes in pyramidal cell excitability as a function of the duration of exposure to convulsants. These effects were demonstrated to occur at doses that did not evoke spontaneous spiking or discharge bursts in the slice. Changes in recurrent collateral inhibition were obtained, and these either preceded or were accompanied by changes in hyperexcitability of the cells at 100 msec following the first stimulus. This change in hyperexcitability suggests that new indices of excitability, not routinely studied at this time, can be measured and quantified as the cells become more synchronous in their firing patterns. We have also demonstrated that a prototypic anticonvulsant, phenobarbital, can diminish these proconvulsant effects, perhaps in a selective way, affecting the cellular properties responsible for late hyperexitability before antagonizing effects on recurrent collateral inhibition induced by the convulsants. Many of these findings are preliminary and must be replicated and expanded before definitive statements can be made about the comparisons between the individual convulsants or the effects of phenobarbital, since it was studied at only one dose in the current protocol.

Now that the feasibility studies are finished, our plan will be to complete more systematic control and anticonvulsant experiments with other drugs known to influence kindling acquisition to establish baseline data against which to judge the effects of similar treatments on slices to be taken from animals previously kindled to various stages. The neurophysiological and neuropharmacological responses of hippocampal slices taken from the kindled animals may provide additional clues to the mechanisms responsible for the facilitation of electrical kindling acquisition by lindane and similar compounds.

REFERENCES

1. Albertson T.E., Joy R.M., Stark L.G., A pharmacological study in the kindling model of epilepsy. *Neuropharmacology,* 23 (1984) 1117–23.
2. Albertson T.E., Joy R.M., Stark L.G., Facilitation of kindling in adult rats following neonatal exposure to lindane. *Brain Res,* 349 (1985) 263–6.
3. Albertson T.E., Peterson S.L., Stark L.G., Anticonvulsant drugs and their antagonism of kindled amydgaloid seizures in rats. *Neuropharmacology,* 19 (1980) 643–652.
4. Albertson T.E., Peterson S.L., Stark L.G., Effects of phenobarbital and SC-13504 on partially kindled hippocampal seizures in rats. *Exp Neurol,* 61 (1978) 270–80.
5. Albertson T.E., Walby W.F., Stark L.G., Joy R.M., The effect of propofol on CA1 pyramidal cell excitability and GABA-A-mediated inhibition in the rat hippocampal slice. *Life Sci,* 58 (1996) 2397–2407.
6. Corda M.G., Orlandi M., Lecca D., Carboni G., Frau V., Giorgi O., Pentylenetetrazol-induced kindling in rats: effect of GABA function inhibitors. *Pharmacol Biochem Behav,* 40 (1991) 329–33.
7. Fisher RS.,Animal models of the epilepsies. *Brain Res Rev,* 14(1989)245–78
8. Garske GE, Palmer GC, Napier JJ, et al.,Preclinical profile of the anticonvulsant remacemide and its enantiomers in the rat.*Epilepsy Res,* 9(1991)161–74
9. Gilbert M.E., Repeated exposure to lindane leads to behavioral sensitization and facilitates electrical kindling. *Neurotoxicol Teratol,* 17 (1995) 131–41.
10. Joy R.M., Albertson T.E., Lindane and limbic system excitability. *Neurotoxicology,* 6 (1985) 193–214.
11. Joy R.M., Albertson T.E., Stark L.G., An analysis of the actions of progabide, a specific GABA receptor agonist, on kindling and kindled seizures. *Exp Neurol,* 83 (1984) 144–54.
12. Joy R.M., Stark L.G., Albertson T.E., Proconvulsant action of lindane compared at two different kindling sites in the rat—amygdala and hippocampus. *Neurobehav Toxicol Teratol,* 5 (1983) 465–8.
13. Joy R.M., Stark L.G., Albertson T.E., Proconvulsant actions of lindane: effects on afterdischarge thresholds and durations during amygdaloid kindling in rats. *Neurotoxicology,* 4 (1983) 211–9.
14. Joy R.M., Walby W.F., Stark L.G., Albertson T.E., Lindane blocks GABAA-mediated inhibition and modulates pyramidal cell excitability in the rat hippocampal slice. *Neurotoxicology,* 16 (1995) 217–28.
15. Stark L.G., Albertson T.E., Joy R.M., Effects of hexachlorocyclohexane isomers on the acquisition of kindled seizures. *Neurobehav Toxicol Teratol,* 8 (1986) 487–91.
16. Stark L.G., Joy R.M., Albertson T.E., The persistence of kindled amygdaloid seizures in rats exposed to lindane. *Neurotoxicology,* 4 (1983) 221–5.
17. Stark. L.G., Peterson SL, Albertson TE , Pharmacological and Toxicological Evaluation of Potential Antiepileptic Drugs in the Kindling Model of Epilepsy. In: In J.A. Wada (Ed.), *Kindling 4,* Plenum, New York, 1990, pp. 267–281.
18. Wigstrom H., Gustafsson B., Facilitation of hippocampal long-lasting potentiation by GABA antagonists. *Acta Physiol Scand,* 125 (1985) 159–72.
19. Zhao D., Leung L.S., Boon F., Cain D.P., Persistent physiological effects caused by a single pentylenetetrazol induced seizure in neonatal rats. *Brain Res Dev Brain Res,* 80 (1994) 190–8.

DISCUSSION OF LARRY STARK'S PAPER

B. Adamec: Very nice talk. Do you have some ideas about the mechanisms of action of lindane and blocking inhibition?

L. Stark: I think that the data are pretty good with the other work that has been done with lindane that it does interfere with recurrent inhibition by binding in the chloride channel and so on. That diminishes recurrent inhibition, just as we've seen. One of the things that I should have pointed out, just in terms of methodology, was that Stan Leung earlier mentioned the notion that it is sometimes hard to separate what is going on with recurrent inhibition if you are also seeing facilitation. The way that we chose to address that was each time we did a determination to include an intensity of stimulation that would produce on the first spike 80% of the maximum, so that as we entered into each one of these measurements we compensated for whatever degree of recurrent inhibition or rise in that first spike had occurred by just diminishing the amount of stimulation. Then we still saw the facilitation in other things, in more or less pure form. It is sort of a constant amplitude kind of response, as opposed to a constant stimulus response. Dr. Joy and Dr. Albertson worked that out previously in the intact hippocampus, looking at the dentate gyrus. Its of interest actually that lindane is a compound which will produce a loss of recurrent inhibition in both the dentate and in CA1, and it may be a useful tool for some of you who are seeing some of these kind of odd reversals and things.

S. Leung: One thing that I did not mention just now in answer to a question is that we did perfuse this GABA-B antagonist in the slice. If you do it in CA1 with paired pulses at a high intensitym what will happen is the P2 over P1, in terms of the first pop-spike, that ratio is not changed. But because you block the presynaptic GABA-B receptors you have a burst of spikes with the second pulse, and that seems to be some of the data that you showed with lindane or maybe some other compounds, in that you have many spikes with your second pulse. I wonder if maybe there is a way you can perfuse a GABA-B antagonist and see if that effect still persists.

L. Stark: I think that is a very good suggestion. This whole study was undertaken from a different bias than trying to sort these things out, and so your suggestion is well received. I think that that is the kind of thing we need to start looking at now that we have seen some of these changes at 100 milliseconds.

G. Ronduin: Do you know if repeated exposure to subconvulsive doses of lindane can lead to chemical kindling?

L. Stark: Mary Gilbert actually reported that last year, yes.

GENERAL DISCUSSION 5

G. Ronduin: Dr. Löscher, I agree with you that NMDA antagonists usually have no anticonvulsant activity if you give them before the seizure. However, there is at least one report where administration of a compound, a small dose over 13 minutes, was reported to be able to block seizures and to reduce normal damage. It was TCP, a derivative of phencyclidine. Do you have a comment about this discrepancy?

W. Löscher: No.

C. Wasterlain: My comment is for Dr. Löscher. I was happy to see your results, but I'm not surprised because seven years ago we had a bright idea since Tortella and Musaccio had reported the potentiation of phenytoin by dextromethorphan. We tried to do a combination and found out that they are highly epileptogenic and facilitate kindling. Bob Fisher tried that combination in patients, and actually there was an increase in seizure frequency, although the report simply concluded that there was no improvement with the combination.

W. Löscher: Of course, I know that study, but it has to be criticized because it was a relatively small sample of patients and he tested only one dose. It was claimed by several people that he should have used a higher dose, but then there are problems because of anecdotal reports that dextromethorphan produces psychotic behaviour, which is not that unexpected. But an interesting thing that I did not mention was that not all the rats in our experiments behaved the same to dextrorphan. About 10% of them showed spontaneous seizures in response to dextromethorphan, and the other 80 to 90% exhibited anticonvulsant effects. I don't know what is the reason, but if this is similar in patients then some patients might react to these drugs just in the opposite way to other patients. This will of course destroy the use of records of any clinical trial with a small number of patients. This is just a speculation, but this is one of the problems of such trials, that they use 8 or 10 patients, and even patients of the same seizure type might be dramatically different. Then if you use such a small sample the outcome might be difficult to interpret.

C. Wasterlain: Actually they did observe a significant increase in number of seizures. The other comment I have is on the toxicity of the combination of NMDA and non-NMDA antagonists. I can tell you with rat pups the combination of low doses of MK-801 and NBQX is immediately fatal, by depressing the respiratory center.

W. Löscher: What we did was like homeopathy -- we used very low doses, much lower than other groups have used with MK-801, and only with these very low doses we found synergism. When we increased the dose of MK-801 to the usual 0.1 mg, there was no synergism anymore. So this might be the reason why at this very low doses we did not observe any toxicity. But these were adult rats. In other studies with such combinations using higher doses of the two compounds in cats, combining MK-801 and NBQX, you can induce respiratory failures. So these combinations may be really toxic, but my impression is that this depends on the dose range that you use.

J. Wada: To Dr. Löscher: In your first slide I think you showed the effect of phenytoin, which elevates threshold but left the seizure unchanged. Is it correct that when the seizure threshold is elevated, you increase the stimulation intentionally and induce seizure, and then seizure is as before? Does that mean that the phenytoin does act on local site to elevate threshold but does not interfere with propagation?

W. Löscher: That was my interpretation in this model. These were group mean data of course, but if you look at individual animals, there were animals in which there was no increase in threshold but even an increase in the duration of the behavioural seizures recorded at threshold. So there could be a proconvulsant effect at the same dose which in other animals does the things that you saw in my slide. We reported a couple of years ago that if you use very large populations of kindled rats, 100 kindled rats or something like that, then you can select subpopulations of these animals and some of these, about 20% of these animals, react all the time with anticonvulsant effects and another subpopulation never reacts with anticonvulsant effects to phenytoin, at the same doses. So again, even if all the rats were amygdala kindled, there were no differences between the subgroups in terms of the location of the kindling electrode, but there seems to be a genetic background that might explain this difference to phenytoin. The next step was that we used these subpopulations and look at whether these differences in phenytoin extend to other antiepileptic drugs and found the same difference with phenobarb. So in those rats which did not react to phenytoin there was a very low frequency of response with phenobarb, and visa versa with the other subgroup. The only exception to that was with carbamazepine, which showed the same effect in both subgroups. This for me was one hint that the mechanisms operating with these two drugs, carbamazepine and phenytoin, are different, must be different because phenytoin non-responders reacted to carbamazepine. Anyhow, my impression is that there is much more genetics behind what we see with anticonvulsant drugs in the kindling model even the same rat strain.

J. Wada: I have to agree, because when we did a number of years ago a systematic of antiepileptic compounds for therapeutic capability against prophylactic capability, phenytoin did not affect threshold in our preparation of primates. It did have a wonderful anticonvulsant effect, but no prophylactic effect. I imagine our population is small and if we increased our population there would be a spectrum of different responses to the outcome. I have another question for Peter Cain. I think in your second group of knock-out mice kindling was rapid but the afterdischarge duration was prolonged. How do interpret that discrepancy?

P. Cain: You're asking about the cam-kinase II transgenics, the group that had the shift toward long-term depression at low frequencies of tetanization. They kindled at a normal rate, but the afterdischarge was prolonged as you said. One thing that I forgot to say was that they had more severe seizures, they had running fits actually, in contrast to controls, which did not. It is an apparent dissociation between afterdischarge strength and convulsion development, and I have wondered about this and have tried to come an explanation. But that is a long way to say that I don't know the answer to your question.

J. Wada: I recall when we began to do bisection studies. In the monkey it takes a long time to kindle, as you know, but when the anterior commissure is bisected they kindle fast, in terms of number of stimulations, but afterdischarge duration increases more slowly than in the control group, indicating possibly that the propagation of seizure is much slower although the final outcome is faster kindling.

P. Cain: Sure, we are at a great disadvantage with mice, because they are so small we are lucky to have one electrode in them. In the case of your primates, if I recall, there were routinely a dozen recording sites and you get a great deal of information about propagation. We did have contralateral placements in the mice, but we really need to get more information about propagation.

C. Wasterlain: In the C-K II knockouts, as I remember, Jim McNamara found accelerated kindling. How do your mutants differ from the C-K II knockouts?

P. Cain: The knock-out that you are talking about is a true cam-kinase knockout, I believe, ours is a transgenic actually. The mutation involved the replacement at the 286 locus of threonine with aspartate. So they still had cam-kinase but it was a version that autophosphorylated so that was different from the knock-out that you mentioned. They were calcium independent.

33

THE SYNDROME OF MESIAL TEMPORAL LOBE EPILEPSY

A Role for Kindling

Jerome Engel, Jr.

Departments of Neurology and Neurobiology
and the Brain Research Institute
UCLA School of Medicine
Los Angeles, California

For almost three decades kindling has been a popular experimental tool for investigating enduring changes in neuronal excitability that presumably utilize natural mechanisms underlying normal as well as abnormal behaviors. The most common rationale for its use has been its presumed relevance to human epileptogenesis, and it has been referred to by many as "the kindling model of epilepsy." Strictly speaking, however, routine kindling is not a model for epilepsy, because animals do not experience spontaneous seizures. Nevertheless, changes clearly occur that increasingly dispose specific brain regions to generate epileptic seizures, given an appropriate stimulus.

Kindling is clearly not a singular phenomenon, but a series of phenomena that develop over time [15]. For instance, with amygdala kindling, there is first a decrease in the threshold for afterdischarge such that subthreshold stimulation, when repeated, will eventually result in the appearance of afterdischarge [46]. This change clearly involves neuronal elements in the immediate vicinity of the stimulating electrode. When continued, the same stimulus produces longer and longer afterdischarges, which eventually are associated with behavioral signs [47]. These events reflect transsynaptic mechanisms which recruit distant structures into the epileptogenic process. The appearance of stage 5 convulsions is most likely an extension of this recruitment; however, some innate generalized seizure-generating system, involving subcortical as well as cortical structures, must become engaged [22]. In addition, a variety of both positive and negative transfer effects has been demonstrated which represent enduring transsynaptic inhibitory, as well as excitatory, changes, with widespread involvement of both hemispheres of the brain. Whether kindling induces persistent excitation or inhibition depends upon multiple factors, including the pathways involved, the timing of the events, and the relationship between multiple

Kindling 5, edited by Corcoran and Moshé.
Plenum Press, New York, 1998.

epileptogenic regions [18]. Finally, if kindling is continued for prolonged periods, spontaneous seizures will occur as a result of transynaptic epileptogenesis [45].

Many morphological, biochemical and electrophysiological changes have been identified to result from kindling, and some which persist for a long time following the last kindled seizure could underlie the enduring epileptogenicity exhibited by kindled animals. Apart from an intrinsic interest in understanding the fundamental mechanisms of such kindling phenomena, the intention of using this experimental model to elucidate the neuronal basis of human epilepsy requires a concerted effort to determine relevance. This does not merely mean establishing a relationship between kindling per se and a type of human epilepsy or seizure, for instance temporal lobe epilepsy or a temporal lobe seizure. Rather, it is necessary to consider the various component parts of human epileptic events or disorders, and determine their possible relationship to the various phenomena encountered during the process of kindling. It might be a profitable exercise to perform this comparison between limbic kindling in the rat and what is likely to be the most common human epileptic disorder, mesial temporal lobe epilepsy (MTLE).

1. MESIAL TEMPORAL LOBE EPILEPSY

MTLE is that form of human temporal lobe epilepsy that is associated with hippocampal sclerosis [9,20,60,62]. Hippocampal sclerosis is the most common pathological substrate for complex partial seizures in the human [2], which in turn are the most common seizure type experienced by patients with chronic epilepsy [24]. Recent work from several epilepsy surgery centers suggests that MTLE represents a specific syndrome, if not a disease, with features that distinguish it from epilepsy due to other types of lesions in the temporal lobe [9,20,60,62]. Table 1 characterizes this syndrome. It can be seen from this table that there are several aspects of the condition that appear to involve progressive processes, and that both epileptiform and nonepileptiform abnormalities eventually appear at considerable distances from the sclerotic hippocampus. Each of these disturbances represents an opportunity to invoke mechanisms similar to some aspect of kindling.

1.1. Anatomical Substrates

The cause of hippocampal sclerosis remains a mystery; however, the pathophysiology of this condition is the most studied of all human epileptogenic lesions, due to the abundance of mesial temporal brain tissue made available as a result of surgical treatment [54]. There is a characteristic pattern of cell loss, with the greatest reduction in principal neurons found in the dentate hilar and CA1 regions and the least in the CA2 region [2,7]. There is also a specific loss of somatostatin and neuropeptide Y-containing neurons in the dentate hilus, and sprouting of mossy fiber axons which appear to make synaptic contact on the areas of dentate granule cell proximal dendrites vacated by their usual hilar cell input [3,7,27,57]. Inhibitory interneurons appear to be relatively preserved, and there may also be sprouting of inhibitory terminals [1]. Pyramidal and granule cells reveal a variety of degenerative changes ranging from loss of dendritic spines through beading of the dendrites and reduction and eventual loss of the dendritic domain, suggesting an ongoing progressive process [53]. Undoubtedly, many of the surviving neurons will exhibit sprouting and participate in new circuit formation, although this can not be easily demonstrated outside the mossy fiber system using present morphological techniques. A current hypothesis for epileptogenesis in MTLE is that an initial insult causes cell loss, which is then fol-

Table 1. The syndrome of mesial temporal lobe epilepsy (MTLE)

A. History
 1. Increased incidence of complicated febrile convulsions or other predisposing insults within first five years of life.
 2. Increased incidence of a family history of epilepsy.
 3. Onset in latter half of first decade of life.
 4. Auras common and occur in isolation.
 5. Secondarily generalized seizures occur infrequently.
 6. Seizures often remit for several years until adolescence or early adulthood.
 7. Seizures often become medically intractable.
 8. Interictal behavioral disturbances can occur (most commonly depression).

B. Clinical seizure
 1. *Aura* is usually present - most common is epigastric rising, often other autonomic or psychic symptoms, with emotion (e.g., fear), can be olfactory or gustatory sensation (several seconds).
 2. *Complex partial seizure* - often begins with arrest and stare, oroalimentary automatisms and complex automatisms common. Posturing of one upper extremity may occur contralateral to the ictal discharge (one to two minutes).
 3. *Postictal phase* - usually includes disorientation, recent memory deficit, amnesia for the event, and dysphasia if seizures begin in the language dominant hemisphere (several minutes).

C. Neurological examination
 1. Usually normal.
 2. May have recent memory deficit.

D. EEG
 1. Unilateral or bilateral independent anterior temporal spikes, maximum amplitude in basal electrodes.
 2. May be intermittent or continuous rhythmic slowing in one mesial temporal area.
 3. Extracranial ictal activity appears only with complex partial symptoms, usually initial or delayed focal onset pattern of 5–7/sec rhythmic activity, maximum amplitude in one basal temporal derivation.
 4. Depth electrode ictal onset most often high amplitude rhythmic spikes or sharp waves, less commonly low voltage fast or suppression.
 5. Propagation to contralateral side is slow (> 5 sec, but may be minutes), or does not occur at all.

E. Focal functional deficits
 1. Usually unilateral temporal lobe hypometabolism on interictal FDG-PET, often involves ipsilateral thalamus and basal ganglia.
 2. Usually unilateral temporal lobe hypoperfusion on interictal SPECT and characteristic pattern of hyper- and hypoperfusion on ictal SPECT.
 3. Usually material specific memory disturbances on neuropsychological testing and amnesia with contralateral intracarotid sodium amobarbital injection.
 4. Mesial temporal EEG slowing and attenuation of normal rhythms on one side can be seen with scalp/sphenoidal electrodes, but more common with depth electrodes; exacerbated by iv pentothal test.

F. Structural imaging
 1. Usually unilateral hippocampal atrophy on T_1-weighted MRI scan.
 2. Usually unilateral increased mesial temporal signal on T_2-weighted MRI scan.
 3. May have enlarged temporal horn on one side.

G. Pathophysiology
 1. Hippocampal sclerosis (> 30% cell loss with specific patterns).
 2. Sprouting of dentate granule cell mossy fibers.
 3. Selective loss of certain hilar neurons (somatostatin and NPY-containing cells).
 4. Hamartomas and heterotopias may occur as “dual pathology”.
 5. Microdysgenesis common.
 6. Seizures may originate in sclerotic hippocampus but much larger area appears to be included in the epileptogenic region.

From Ref. 11, with permission.

lowed by extensive neuronal reorganization, abnormally strengthening both excitatory and inhibitory circuits, which then predispose to hypersynchronous discharges [16].

It is uncertain to what extent the pathophysiological disturbances exhibited by the sclerotic hippocampus in patients with medically refractory MTLE represent the cause of spontaneous seizures, or the result of frequently occurring ictal events. Most likely both conditions apply. Whereas kindling, as an example of seizure-induced changes in neuronal integration, may not cause significant cell loss, this experimental procedure does result in axonal sprouting and synaptic reorganization similar to that seen in hippocampal sclerosis [58; See also other chapters in this volume]. Other changes at the membrane and channel level may also be similar between kindling and hippocampal sclerosis, suggesting that at least some of these disturbances encountered in the human condition are at least exacerbated by recurrent epileptic seizures (see Mody et al., this volume).

An intriguing pathological aspect of hippocampal sclerosis is its coexistence in 10 to 20 percent of patients with other pathological lesions [34]. This so-called dual pathology is of mechanistic interest because the second lesion is usually dysgenetic (e.g., heterotopias and hamartomas). Gliomas are rarely seen in association with hippocampal sclerosis unless they are located in, or very near, the hippocampus itself [21]. This suggests a congenital disturbance in cortical development that might predispose to the later appearance of hippocampal sclerosis. The report of laminar dispersion within the dentate gyrus of the sclerotic hippocampus suggests congenital dysgenesis of this structure as well [28]; however, a similar anatomical defect can be produced by recurrent seizures in adult animals [40]. There is also an increased incidence of family history of epilepsy among people with mesial temporal lobe epilepsy [19], suggesting that there may also be a genetic contribution to the factors that lead to the appearance of hippocampal sclerosis later in life.

The role of the amygdala in MTLE is uncertain. Amygdala, as well as hippocampal, atrophy has been documented on MRI volumetry [5], but detailed histopathological studies have not been carried out on amygdala tissue resected from patients with intractable MTLE, in part because of the difficulty in en bloc removal of this structure. Depth electrode recordings demonstrate that electrographic seizures rarely, if ever, begin in the amygdala alone, although it is usually involved early in the course of the seizure and is clearly important for many of the behavioral manifestations [59]. Although well-defined morphological changes in temporal lobe neocortex have not been identified in MTLE, evidence for the importance of adjacent neocortex in habitual seizure generation comes from surgical studies. In patients undergoing amygdalohippocampectomy, oucome with respect to seizures depends more on the amount of parahippocampal gyrus received than in the volume of amygdala or hippocampal resection [55]. The parahippocampal gyrus in humans may represent the areas of entorhinal and perirhinal cortex in the rat that are crucial to kindling, as discussed in several other chapters in this volume.

1.2. Physiological Substrates

It is assumed, although not definitively proven, that hippocampal sclerosis appears some time after birth, presumably as a result of some insult. Most patients with hippocampal sclerosis have a history of complicated febrile convulsions or some other event, such as head trauma or encephalitis within the first four or five years of life [19,38], which could conceivably cause some degree of brain damage. The current view, therefore, is that such initial predisposing insults in a susceptible individual will result in loss of hippocampal neurons, which then causes synaptic reorganization and other changes within the damaged areas, eventually leading to the appearance of hypersynchronous epileptiform discharges. Why this sclerotic structure eventually develops the potential for spontaneous paroxysmal activity (what Penfield and Jasper referred to as "ripening of the scar" [44]) is unknown, and this process could involve mechanisms similar to the early local phenomena of kindling. More likely, however, is that the morphological changes within the reorganized hippocampus cause intermittent hypersynchronous events merely as a property of the newly formed circuits, but that the resultant discharge then acts as an electrical kindling stimulus which initiates transynaptic epileptogenesis.

In vitro studies of slices from human sclerotic hippocampus have revealed enhanced NMDA-mediated excitation [30,36], as has been reported in kindling [41]. GABA-mediated inhibition appears to be preserved in the dentate gyrus; however, its strength is reduced by NMDA-mediated excitation [29]. Electrophysiological evidence for enhanced inhibition in MTLE has been obtained from bilateral depth electrode recordings of mesial temporal structures during presurgical evaluation. On the side of habitual seizure generation, paired pulse suppression is a predominant feature of the interictal state, particularly in the perforant path, although paired pulse facilitation occurs with stimulation of association pathways within the hippocampus itself [64]; these results are identical to those obtained in kindling [32]. This inhibition could represent natural mechanisms to maintain the interictal state, or it could contribute to the appearance of hypersynchronous discharges. *In vivo* microelectrode recordings of single units in the hippocampus where seizures originate have demonstrated enhanced synchronous firing between cells with strong post stimulus inhibition, compared with those showing weak post stimulus inhibition, supporting the view that enhanced inhibition acts to promote hypersynchronous activity [31]. Bursting neurons, however, do not appear to be a feature of the human epileptic hippocampus [6], a state which resembles kindling more than acute models of epileptic seizures [42,48].

It is well known from depth electrode recordings of patients with MTLE that prolonged afterdischarge in the hippocampus is often unaccompanied by ictal signs or symptoms [56]. The manifestation of simple and complex partial seizures which characterize MTLE, appears to require propagation of this discharge to distant structures. The classical electrographic ictal onset pattern from direct brain recording is a recruiting rhythm consisting of a buildup of low voltage fast activity. More commonly in MTLE, however, electrodes within the sclerotic hippocampus reveal the initial pattern to be hypersynchronous, which usually persists for some period of time without clinical signs or symptoms, or is associated with the habitual aura [8,10]. If the event is to become a more clinically apparent seizure, transition to low voltage fast activity usually appears at the time of propagation to ipsilateral and contralateral structures. In most patients studied with depth electrodes, this transition corresponds to the onset of impaired consciousness, which heralds the complex partial seizure. It is reasonable to assume, therefore, that whatever changes take place in the damaged hippocampus early in life manifests as clinical seizures only after some distant structures can be recruited into the electrographic ictal event. This process would seem to involve enduring transsynaptic changes, which resemble phenomena encountered in the kindling model.

1.3. Progression of Epileptogenesis

Although patients may have complicated febrile convulsions within the first few years of life, the habitual ictal events do not occur until somewhat later in childhood. The initial episode may be a partial or secondarily generalized seizure, which usually responds readily to treatment with appropriate antiepileptic drugs. Typically, seizures are controlled by pharmacotherapy for several years and patients may even be able to discontinue medication. It is not known how often control can be maintained through adolescence and into adulthood because patients who are no longer having seizures do not come to the attention of epilepsy specialists. For many, however, seizures eventually return at some time after puberty and ultimately become refractory to antiepileptic drugs. This suggests that the condition is progressive, even during the time when clinical seizures are not apparent. If some kindling-like mechanism is responsible for increasing epileptogenicity in distant structures in order for clinical seizures to manifest initially, it is reasonable to assume that this process continues after clinical seizures occur, so that seizures become more severe and less responsive to medical therapy [17]. Additional evidence for continuing progression of the epileptogenic process comes from results of surgical treatment; anterior temporal lobectomy performed within ten years of onset of habitual ictal events is more likely to eliminate all seizures than later surgery, which is more likely to be associated with residual auras or even occasional complex partial seizures [15]. It is, therefore, reasonable to assume that mechanisms similar to some kindling phenomena accompany the active phase of MTLE.

The typical ictal events in MTLE begin with an aura (simple partial seizure), usually consisting of psychic and autonomic signs and symptoms that reflect the projection areas of the sclerotic hippocampus and amygdala. Auras almost always occur in isolation, as well as before a complex partial event, most likely due to the fact that hippocampal commissural connections are poor or nonexistent in the human [63]; thus ictal discharges remain isolated for long periods of time and may never propagate to the contralateral hemisphere or other structures responsible for impairment of consciousness. Common features of the complex partial seizure include arrest of motion, a blank stare and oroalimentary automatisms. The anatomical substrates of these clinical behaviors are also the projection fields of the amygdala and hippocampus, and may be similar to those areas of the rat brain which give rise to stage 1 through 3 of amygdala kindled seizures. The complex partial seizures of mesial temporal lobe epilepsy can go on for a minute or more and often include complicated spontaneous and reactive automatic behaviors. These automatisms can reflect both ictal and postictal disturbances in conscious cortical control of ongoing activities.

Unlike amygdala kindling, where the end result in a fully kindled animal is a stage 5 seizure, generalized seizures rarely occur in MTLE. The reduced propensity for secondary generalization can be attributed to the fact that patients are invariably on antiepileptic medications, which are much more effective in controlling convulsive ictal events than they are in controlling limbic simple and complex partial seizures. This differential therapeutic effect supports the view that the fundamental neuronal mechanisms of limbic seizures and generalized convulsions are not the same, and underlines the need for better methods of screening new potentially antiepileptic compounds with animal models that utilize mechanisms relevant to human temporal lobe seizures. Screening with maximal electroshock and subcutaneous metrazol, which reproduce mechanisms more relevant to generalized convulsions and absences, results in the marketing of more drugs for seizure types that are already easy to control, while drugs that would be effective against MTLE might only be identified using models like amygdala kindling (see chapter by Loscher in this volume).

1.4. Progression of Other Dysfunction

There are many lines of evidence documenting persistent widespread disturbances in cerebral function in patients with unilateral hippocampal sclerosis. On depth electrode EEG recordings, interictal spikes are commonly seen to occur independently from both mesial and lateral temporal regions, ipsilateral and contralateral to the site of ictal onset [35]. Interictal positron emission tomography with ^{18}F-fluorodeoxyglucose (FDG-PET) reveals widespread temporal hypometabolism on the side of seizure generation in 80 to 90 percent of patients with hippocampal sclerosis, and this often also includes ipsilateral thalamus, basal ganglia and other adjacent neocortical areas [26]. Similar observations have been made with respect to hypoperfusion on interictal single photon emission computed tomography (SPECT) [43], and μ opiate binding is increased in lateral temporal neocortex, as measured by PET with the opiate ligand carfentanil [23]. Neuropsychological testing in these patients reveals deficits, particularly in verbal memory and learning, when seizures originate in the dominant hemisphere [49]. Such diffuse changes should not be consequences of any initial insult, and although clear progression has not been documented over long periods of time in this patient population, it is likely that these disturbances reflect enduring transsynaptic seizure induced neuronal dysfunction, both epileptiform and nonepileptiform. Further supporting this view is the fact that the extensive hypometabolism can resolve following amygdalohippocampectomy that eliminates habitual seizures [61], and that cognitive function, particularly memory function that is material-specific for the contralateral temporal lobe, improves after successful anterior temporal lobe resection [50].

Much has been written about the increased incidence of interictal behavioral disturbances in patients with temporal lobe epilepsy, particularly of the type with seizures that begin in mesial temporal structures. Although it remains controversial whether patients with MTLE are more likely to develop specific interictal personality disturbances and late onset schizophrenia or schizophreniform psychosis, there seems to be consistent documentation for an increased association with depression [14]. Certainly patients with MTLE who have medically refractory seizures have increasing difficulty in psychosocial adaptation which to large extent can be attributed to environmental factors, particularly the limitations placed on their activity by society and the consequences of stigmatization. There is animal evidence, however, that some of these behavioral disturbances could represent the neurobiological effects of recurrent seizures [25; see also chapter by Adamec in this volume]. These effects might employ mechanisms similar to kindled epileptogenesis per se, or to the associated persistent changes in excitation and inhibition that give rise to positive and negative transfer effects in kindling [39]. Some of these may represent natural homeostatic mechanisms which develop in response to repeated epileptic seizures in order to maintain the interictal state. Of particular interest is the evidence for disturbances in endogenous opioid activity in kindling [4,51,52] and in MTLE [23], in view of the role this peptide might have in mediating pleasure and depression [33].

2. SUMMARY AND CONCLUSIONS

From the preceding discussion, at least four component parts of MTLE could involve phenomena that contribute to the development of kindled seizures in animals. These concern: 1) the initial development of clinical seizures; 2) the progressive nature of seizures with ultimate medical intractability; 3) the existence of wide areas of dysfunction and the appearance of interictal behavioral disturbances; and 4) the persistent nature of some features and reversibility of others following surgical treatment.

1. The first habitual seizure occurs several years after the putative predisposing insult (e.g., febrile convulsion, infection, trauma). The insult induces neuronal re-

organization within the sclerotic hippocampus which takes place over a period of time, resulting in the development of intermittent hypersynchronous discharges. Although mechanisms similar to those of subthreshold kindling might be involved, the creation of new local circuitry might be sufficient to cause these paroxysms. However, the epileptiform discharges could then act as kindling stimuli to recruit distant structures into the epileptogenic process, an apparently necessary factor in the ultimate manifestation of clinical seizures.
2. Habitual seizures typically respond to antiepileptic drugs when they first appear, but after many years they may become intractable to pharmacotherapy. Continuing reorganization within the primary epileptogenic region may result in stronger seizure-generating mechanisms. Structural and functional changes induced in projection areas by kindling-like mechanisms would make seizures more severe and more difficult to stop.
3. When the condition of intractable seizures persists, dysfunction in relatively large brain areas can be demonstrated with EEG, functional imaging, and neuropsychological tests. These can be associated with interictal behavioral disturbances. Three possible explanations might be offered. Distant areas recruited into the epileptogenic process by kindling-like mechanisms may mediate behavioral disturbances. Widespread homeostatic mechanisms that arise naturally to suppress spontaneous seizures and maintain the interictal state, similar to negative transfer phenomena in kindling, may interfere with normal behavior. Recurrent seizures might actually be associated with structural changes in secondary epileptogenic areas that alter their function, a phenomenon that has not yet been demonstrated in either the kindling model or in MTLE.
4. Patients often have persistent auras following surgical removal of the sclerotic hippocampus where seizures originate, even when other mesial and lateral temporal lobe tissue is resected as well, demonstrating that brain areas distant from the primary lesion have developed the capacity to generate spontaneous ictal events. This strongly suggests a form of secondary epileptogenesis, perhaps similar to the process that occurs when kindling is continued in animals until spontaneous seizures appear.

The fact that postoperative persistence of auras and occasional seizures is more likely when the duration of illness is longer, and the fact that certain interictal behavioral disturbances can be reversed by surgical resection that is successful in eliminating habitual seizures, indicates that these phenomena result from a progressive epileptogenic process, and are not due to the initial insult. The most important clinical lesson to be learned from these observations, as well as the overwhelming evidence that kindling-like phenomena do occur in MTLE, is that early surgical intervention provides the best opportunity for complete elimination of disabling seizures and satisfactory psychosocial rehabilitation [12].

3. POSTSCRIPT

Kindling remains an important investigational tool for studying the various progressive epileptogenic and nonepileptogenic disturbances associated with human epilepsy, particularly the syndrome of MTLE. In order to take greatest advantage of the kindling model, however, it is necessary to carry out parallel *in vivo* and *in vitro* studies in patients with MTLE, which can now be accomplished in the setting of an epilepsy surgery program [13].

These parallel studies should be aimed at identifying those component parts of MTLE which might resemble various kindling-induced phenomena, in order to dissect out fundamental mechanisms using electrophysiological, morphological, neurochemical, and molecular biological techniques. A possibly important adjunct to this experimental strategy would be the use of an additional experimental animal model of chronic temporal lobe seizures induced by intrahippocampal injection of kainic acid in rats [37]. This procedure creates a hippocampal lesion that has many of the morphological features of hippocampal sclerosis, and is associated with progressive electroclinical disturbances, which resemble the chronic human condition of MTLE. Parallel studies in this animal model, therefore, will permit research to be carried out that cannot be pursued in patients for ethical or technical reasons. Close comparisons between the various epileptogenic and nonepileptogenic changes that occur over time in limbic kindling and the intrahippocampal kainic acid model will greatly facilitate development of hypotheses which can then be tested in patients.

ACKNOWLEDGMENTS

Original research reported by the author was supported in part by Grants NS-02808, NS-15654, NS-33310, and GM-24839, from the National Institutes of Health, and Contract DE-AC03-76-SF00012 from the Department of Energy.

REFERENCES

1. Babb, T.L., GABA neurons, synapses and inhibition in human hippocampal epilepsy. In E.-J. Speckmann and M.J. Gutnick (Eds.), *Epilepsy and Inhibition*, Urban and Schwarzenberg Press, München, 1992, pp. 375–397.
2. Babb, T.L. and Brown, W.J., Pathological findings in epilepsy. In J. Engel Jr. (Ed.), *Surgical Treatment of the Epilepsies*, Raven Press, New York, 1987, pp. 511–540.
3. Babb, T.L., Kupfer, W.R., Pretorius, J.K., Crandall, P.H. and Levesque, M.F., Synaptic reorganization by mossy fibers in human epileptic fascia dentata, *Neuroscience*, 42 (1991) 351–363.
4. Caldecott-Hazard, S. and Engel, J. Jr., Limbic postictal events: Anatomical substrates and opioid receptor involvement, *Prog. Neuropsychopharmacol. Biol. Psychiat.*, 11 (1987) 389–418.
5. Cendes, F., Andermann, F., Gloor, P., Evans, A., Jones-Gotman, M., Watson, C., Melanson, D., Olivier, A., Peters, T., Lopes-Cendes, I., et al., MRI volumetric measurement of amygdala and hippocampus in temporal lobe epilepsy, *Neurology*, 43 (1993) 719–725.
6. Colder, B.W., Frysinger, R.C., Wilson, C.L., Harper, R.M. and Engel, J. JR., Decreased neuronal burst discharge near site of seizure onset in epileptic human temporal lobes, *Epilepsia*, 37 (1996) 113–121.
7. DeLanerolle, N.C., Brines, M.L., Kim, J.H., Williamson, A., Philips, M.F. and Spencer, D.D., Neurochemical remodeling of the hippocampus in human temporal lobe epilepsy. In J. Engel, Jr., C. Wasterlain, E.A. Cavalheiro, U. Heinemann and G. Avanzini (Eds.), *Molecular Neurobiology of Epilepsy* (Epilepsy Research, Suppl. 9), Elsevier, Amsterdam, 1992, pp. 205–220.
8. Engel, J. Jr., Brain metabolism and pathophysiology of human epilepsy. In M. Dichter (Ed.), *Mechanisms of Epileptogenesis: Transition to Seizure*, Plenum Press, New York, 1988, pp. 1–15.
9. Engel, J. Jr., Recent advances in surgical treatment of temporal lobe epilepsy, *Acta Neurol. Scand.*, 86(Suppl 5) (1992) 71–80.
10. Engel, J. Jr., Intracerebral recordings: Organization of the human epileptogenic region, *J. Clin. Neurophysiol.*, 10 (1993a) 90–98.
11. Engel, J. Jr., Update on surgical treatment of the epilepsies, *Neurology*, 43 (1993b) 1612–1617.
12. Engel, J. Jr., Current concepts: Surgery for seizures, *N. Engl. J. Med.*, 334 (1996) 647–652.
13. Engel, J. Jr., Babb, T.L. and Crandall, P.H., Surgical treatment of epilepsy: Opportunities for research into basic mechanisms of human brain function, *Acta Neurochirugica* (Suppl.), 46 (1989) 3–8.
14. Engel, J. Jr., Bandler, R., Griffith, N.C. and Caldecott-Hazard, S., Neurobiological evidence for epilepsy-induced interictal disturbances. In D. Smith, D. Treiman and M. Trimble (Eds.), *Advances in Neurology, Vol. 55*, Raven Press, New York, 1991, pp. 97–111.

15. Engel, J. Jr. and Cahan, L., Potential relevance of kindling to human partial epilepsy. In J. Wada (Ed.), *Kindling 3*, Raven Press, New York, 1986, pp. 37–51.
16. Engel, J. Jr., Dichter, M. and Schwartzkroin, P., Basic mechanisms of human epilepsy. In J. Engel, Jr. and T. Pedley (Eds.), *Epilepsy: A Comprehensive Textbook*, Lippincott-Raven, New York (in press).
17. Engel, J. Jr. and Shewmon, D.A., Impact of the kindling phenomenon on clinical epileptology. In F. Morrell (Ed.), *Kindling and Synaptic Plasticity: The Legacy of Graham Goddard*, Birkhäuser Boston, Cambridge, Mass., 1991, pp. 195–210.
18. Engel, J. Jr. and Wilson, C.L., Evidence for enhanced synaptic inhibition in epilepsy. In G. Nisticò, P.L. Morselli, K.G. Lloyd, R.G. Fariello and J. Engel, Jr. (Eds.), *Neurotransmitters, Seizures and Epilepsy, III*, Raven Press, New York, 1986, pp. 1–13.
19. Falconer, M.A., Genetic and related aetiological factors in temporal lobe epilepsy: A review, *Epilepsia*, 12 (1971) 13–31.
20. French, J.A., Williamson, P.D., Thadani, V.M., Darcey, T.M., Mattson, R.H., Spencer, S.S. and Spencer, D.D., Characteristics of medial temporal lobe epilesy: I. Results of history and physical examination, *Ann. Neurol.*, 34 (1993) 774–780.
21. Fried, I., Kim, J. and Spencer, D.D., Hippocampal pathology in patients with intractable seizures and temporal lobe masses, *J. Neurosurg.*, 76 (1992) 735–740.
22. Fromm, G.H., The brain-stem and seizures: Summary and synthesis. In G.H. Fromm, C.L. Faingold, R.L. Browning and W.M. Burnham (Eds.), *Epilepsy and the Reticular Formation: The Role of the Reticular Core in Convulsive Seizures*, Alan R. Liss, New York, 1987, pp. 203–218.
23. Frost, J.J., Mayberg, H.S., Fisher, R.S., Douglass, K.H., Dannals, R.F., Links, J.M., Wilson, A.A., Ravert, H.T., Rosenbaum, A.E., Snyder, S.H. and Wagner, H.N., Mu-opiate receptors measured by positron emission tomography are increased in temporal lobe epilepsy, *Ann. Neurol.*, 23 (1988) 231–237.
24. Gastaut, H., Gastaut, J.L., Goncalves e Silva, G.E. and Fernandez-Sanchez, G.R., Relative frequency of different types of epilepsy: A study employing the classification of the International League Against Epilepsy, *Epilepsia*, 16 (1975) 457–461.
25. Griffith, N., Engel, J. Jr. and Bandler, R., Ictal and enduring interictal disturbances in emotional behaviour in an animal model of temporal lobe epilepsy, *Brain Res.*, 400 (1987) 360–364.
26. Henry, T.R., Mazziotta, J.C. and Engel, J. Jr., Interictal metabolic anatomy of limbic temporal lobe epilepsy, *Arch. Neurol.*, 50 (1993) 582–589.
27. Houser, C.R., Miyashiro, J.E., Swartz, B.E., Walsh, G.O., Rich, J.R. and Delgado-Escueta, A.V., Altered patterns of dynorphin immunoreactivity suggest mossy fiber reorganization in human hippocampal epilepsy, *J. Neurosci.*, 10 (1990) 267–282.
28. Houser, C.R., Swartz, B.E., Walsh, G.O. and Delgado-Escueta, A.V., Granule cell disorganization in the dentate gyrus: Possible alterations of neuronal migration in human temporal lobe epilepsy. In J. Engel, Jr., C. Wasterlain, E.A. Cavalheiro, U. Heinemann and G. Avanzini (Eds.), *Molecular Neurobiology of Epilepsy*, Elsevier, Amsterdam, 1992 pp. 41–49.
29. Isokawa, M., Decrement of $GABA_A$ receptor-mediated inhibitory postsynaptic currents in dentate granule cells in epileptic hippocampus, *J. Neurophysiol.*, 75 (1996) 1901–1908.
30. Isokawa, M., Levesque, M.F., Babb, T.L. and Engel, J. Jr., Single mossy fibre axonal systems of human dentate granule cells studied in hippocampal slices from patients with temporal lobe epilepsy, *J. Neurosci.*, 13 (1993) 1511–1522.
31. Isokawa-Akesson, M., Wilson, C.L. and Babb, T.L., Prolonged inhibition in synchronously firing human hippocampal neurons, *Epilepsy Res.*, 3 (1989) 236–247.
32. Kamphuis, W., Gorter, J.A., Wytse, J.W. and Lopes da Silva, F.H., Hippocampal kindling leads to different changes in paired-pulse depression of local evoked field potentials in CA1 area and in fascia dentata, *Neurosci Letters*, 141 (1992) 101–105.
33. Kline, N.S., Li, C.H., Lehman, H.E., Lajtha, A., Laski, E. and Cooper, T., Beta-endorphine-induced changes in schizophrenic and depressed patients, *Arch. Gen. Psychiat.*, 34 (1977) 1111–1113.
34. Levesque, M.F., Nakasato, N., Vinters, H.V. and Babb, T.L., Surgical treatment of limbic epilepsy associated with extrahippocampal lesions: The problem of dual pathology, *J. Neurosurg.*, 75 (1991) 364–370.
35. Lieb, J.P., Engel, J. Jr., Gevins, A.S. and Crandall, P.H., Surface and deep EEG correlates of surgical outcome in temporal lobe epilepsy, *Epilepsia*, 22 (1981) 515–538.
36. Masukawa, L.M., Higashima, M., Kim, J.H. and Spencer, D.D., Epileptiform discharges evoked in hippocampal brain slices from epileptic patients, *Brain Res.*, 493 (1989) 168–174.
37. Mathern, G.W., Cifuentes, F., Leite, J.P., Pretorius, J.K. and Babb, T.L., Hippocampal EEG excitability and chronic spontaneous seizures are associated with aberrant synaptic reorganization in the rat kainate model, *Electroencephalogr. Clin. Neurophysiol.*, 87 (1993) 326–339.

38. Mathern, G.W., Pretorius, J.K. and Babb, T.L., Influence of the type of initial precipitating injury and at what age it occurs on course and outcome in patients with temporal lobe seizures, *J. Neurosurg.*, 82 (1995) 220–227.
39. McIntyre, D.C., Split brain rat: Transfer and interference of kindled amygdala convulsions, *Can. J. Neurol. Sci.*, 2 (1975) 429–437.
40. Mello, L.E.A.M., Cavalheiro, E.A., Tan, A.M., Pretorius, J.K., Babb, T.L. and Finch, D.M., Granule cell dispersion in relation to mossy fiber sprouting, hippocampal cell loss, silent period and seizure frequency in the pilocarpine model of epilepsy. In J. Engel, Jr., C. Wasterlain, E.A. Cavalheiro, U. Heinemann and G. Avanzini (Eds.), *Molecular Neurobiology of Epilepsy*, Elsevier, Amsterdam, 1992, pp. 51–60.
41. Mody, I. and Staley, K.J., Cell properties in the epileptic hippocampus, *Hippocampus*, 4 (1994) 275–280.
42. Mody, I. and Heinemann, U., NMDA receptors of dentate gyrus granule cells participate in synaptic transmission following kindling, *Nature Lond.*, 326 (1987) 701–704.
43. Newton, M.R., Berkovic, S.F., Austin, M.C., Rowe, C.C., McKay, W.J. and Bladin, P.F., SPECT in the localisation of extratemporal and temporal seizure foci, *J Neurol. Neurosurg. Psychiatry*, 59 (1995) 26–30.
44. Penfield, W. and Jasper, H., *Epilepsy and the Functional Anatomy of the Human Brain*, Little, Brown & Co., Boston, 1954.
45. Pinel, J.P.J. and Rovner, L.I., Experimental epileptogenesis: Kindling-induced epilepsy in rats, *Exp. Neurol.*, 58 (1978) 190–202.
46. Racine, R.J., Modification of seizure activity by electrical stimulation. I. Afterdischarge threshold, *Electroencephalogr. Clin. Neurophysiol.*, 32 (1972a) 269–279.
47. Racine, R.J., Modification of seizure activity by electrical stimulation. II. Motor seizure, *Electroencephalogr. Clin. Neurophysiol.*, 32 (1972b) 281–294.
48. Racine, R., Kairiss, E. and Smith, G., Kindling mechanisms: The evaluation of the burst response versus enhancement. In J.A. Wada (Ed.), *Kindling 2*, Raven Press, New York, 1981, pp. 15–29.
49. Rausch, R., Psychological evaluation. In J. Engel, Jr. (Ed.), *Surgical Treatment of the Epilepsies*, Raven Press, New York, 1987, pp. 181–195.
50. Rausch, R. and Crandell, P.H., Psychological status related to surgical control of temporal lobe seizures, *Epilepsia*, 23 (1982) 191–202.
51. Rocha, L.L., Maidment, N.T., Evans, C.J., Ackermann, R.F. and Engel, J. Jr., Opioid peptide release and mu receptor binding during amygdala kindling in rats: Regional discordances, *Epilepsy Research* (in press).
52. Rocha, L., Maidment, N.T., Evans, C.J., Ackermann, R.F. and Engel, J. Jr., Microdialysis reveals changes in extracellular opioid peptide levels in the amygdala induced by amygdaloid kindling stimulation, *Exp. Neurol.*, 126 (1994) 277–283.
53. Scheibel, M.E., Crandall, P.H. and Scheibel, A.B., The hippocampal-dentate complex in temporal lobe epilepsy, *Epilepsia*, 15 (1974) 55–80.
54. Schwartzkroin, P.A., Basic research in the setting of an epilepsy surgery center. In J. Engel, Jr. (Ed.), *Surgical Treatment of the Epilepsies, 2nd Edition*, Raven Press, New York, 1993, pp. 755–773.
55. Siegel, A.M. Wieser, H.G., Wichmann, W. and Yasargil, G.M., Relationships between MR-imaged total amount of tissue removed, resection scores of specific mesiobasal limbic subcompartments and clinical outcome following selective amygdalohippocampectomy, *Epilepsy Research*, 6 (1990) 56–65.
56. Sperling, M.R. and O'Connor, M.J., Auras and subclinical seizures: Characteristics and prognostic significance, *Ann. Neurol.*, 28 (1990) 320–328.
57. Sutula, T., Cascino, G., Cavazos, J., Parada, I. and Ramirez, L., Mossy fiber synaptic reorganization in the epileptic human temporal lobe, *Ann. Neurol.*, 26 (1989) 321–330.
58. Sutula, T., He, X.-X., Cavazos, J. and Scott, G., Synaptic reorganization in the hippocampus induced by abnormal functional activity, *Science*, 239 (1988) 1147–1150.
59. Wieser, H.G., *Electroclinical Features of the Psychomotor Seizure: A Stereoelectroencephalographic Study of Ictal Symptoms and Chronotographical Seizure Patterns Including Clinical Effects of Intracerebral Stimulation*, Butterworth's, London, 1983.
60. Wieser, H.G., Engel, J. Jr., Williamson, P.D., Babb, T.L. and Gloor, P., Surgically remediable temporal lobe syndromes. In J. Engel, Jr., (Ed.), *Surgical Treatment of the Epilepsies, 2nd Edition*, Raven Press, New York, 1993, pp. 49–63.
61. Wieser, H.G., Hajek, M., Siegel, A.M., Witztum, A. and Leenders, K.L., PET findings before and after selective amygdalohippocampectomy, *Neurologia et Psychiatria*, 14(Suppl 1) (1992) 55–58.
62. Williamson, P.D., French, J.A., Thadani, V.M., Kim, J.H., Novelly, R.A., Spencer, S.S., Spencer, D.D. and Mattson, R.H., Characteristics of medial temporal lobe epilepsy: II. Interictal and ictal scalp electroencephalopathy, neuropsychological testing, neuroimaging, surgical results and pathology, *Ann. Neurol.*, 34 (1993) 781–787.

63. Wilson, C.L., Isokawa-Akesson, M., Babb, T.L., Engel, J. Jr., Cahan, L.D. and Crandall, P.H., A comparative view of local and interhemispheric limbic pathways in humans: An evoked potential analysis. In J. Engel, Jr., G.A. Ojemann, H.O. Lüders and P.D. Williamson (Eds.), *Fundamental Mechanisms of Human Brain Function*, Raven Press, New York, 1987, pp. 27–38.
64. Wilson, C., Khan, S.U., Engel, J. Jr., Isokawa, M., Babb, T.L. and Behnke, E.J. Paired pulse inhibition and facilitation in human epileptogenic hippocampal formation (submitted).

DISCUSSION OF PETER ENGEL'S PAPER

J. Pinel: I have always been puzzled by the role of sclerosis in the epilepsy, and you seem to talk about it as if it was the cause. The thing that puzzled me many years ago, when I was kindling spontaneous seizures in rats and sending some of the brains to Arnold Schiebel and other people that work with epileptic human tissue, was that despite the fact that these animals were having spontaneous seizures they were not showing the expected hippocampal sclerosis. So I have always thought as a result that the sclerosis was probably epiphenomenal and was a progressive consequence of lesions or seizures but was not the critical change that was making these individuals epileptic.

P. Engel: I would interpret your data the other way around. I think that if they are the consequence of seizures you ought to see them when you produce these seizures over and over again. If you don't see them, then it means that there is more than one way to trigger that hypersynchronous discharge. When you do trigger it with kindling, it is different from the way nature does it when the discharges produce hippocampal sclerosis. I think that the evidence is better that this is a cause of epilepsy, although it may continue to get worse over time as a result of recurrent seizures. The fact that you remove it and the seizures go away is interesting. One of the things that is very confusing about human temporal lobe epilepsy is that PET scan shows that the area of hypometabolism in this disorder is very large. It involves the entire temporal lobe usually, it involves ipsilateral thalamus often, it may involve adjacent neocortex like frontal neocortex, and yet patients continue to have auras. When you localize the seizures to one hippocampus and you do even a radical anterior temporal lobectomy, most or many patients will continue to have some auras. Where are they coming from? I think it means that the area of the brain capable of generating seizures is much more than the hippocampal sclerosis, but I still think that's where it is initiated.

J. Burchfiel: A point that you really need to emphasize is that from a surgical point of view, no one has ever cured temporal lobe epilepsy by removing hippocampus. You need to remove substantial amounts of all the mesial structures, and even when you do that, patients can continue to have either auras or sometimes complex partial seizures which don't necessarily come from the other side. Its much more of an expanded syndrome than simply involving the hippocampus.

P. Engel: And an interesting thing that we saw that we reported at one of the kindling symposia is that the percentage of patients that have auras depends on how long they've had seizures before they were operated on; so the longer you have seizures before you are operated on the more likely you are to have persistent auras.

P. Schinnick-Gallagher: You said that 40% of all epilepsies are complex partial seizures. Are they all mesial temporal lobe seizures with sclerosis?

P. Engel: I have no idea. That was an epidemiological study that was done by Gastaut a long time ago, and there was no way to make that diagnosis. So there are other types of epilepsy that produce complex partial or temporal lobe seizures, and clearly they are not all involving hippocampal sclerosis.

J. Wada: I would like you to comment on the potential mechanism of the post-ictal psychiatric condition, the emergence of psychiatric problems after you have successfully removed the epileptic focus, and the relationship to the hippocampal sclerosis or the hypometabolic region of the focus.

P. Engel: This would take more than the time than we have allotted. Just to make it very simple, one interesting hypothesis is that people who have epilepsy are giving themselves ECT on a regular basis. Our hypothesis is that this has something to do with endogenous opiates that are released during seizures and when they stop having seizures suddenly, a reasonable percentage of them over the first year will develop depression, some of them serious depression that requires treatment. That may be a withdrawal phenomenon, perhaps related to the release of the endogenous opiates.

M. Burnham: This is really kind of a general discussion question: We come here to these kindling meetings and we hear Bob Adamec and John Pinel talk about these personality changes and we hear Stan Leung and Mike Corcoran talk about learning changes, and I get evoked potential changes and Ron Racine sees them all over. I think that we are all convinced that repeated seizure activity is changing the brain in a significant functional way, and when I work with parents they tell me that their children are changing cognitively and they are changing emotionally. Then when I go to clinical meetings I don't hear anything about this, nobody seems to be dealing with it. Do we have a duty to try to push the clinical world to begin to recognize this and to be very aggressive with seizures?

P. Engel: There is no doubt that there are problems that are psychosocial and those are acknowledged and dealt with all the time—and with drugs. But the concept that seizures themselves may be progressive and produce problems is something that has been resisted by the clinical community and by the patient advocacy groups, because the problem with having epilepsy or the stigma associated with epilepsy is so severe already, for parents to believe that there is some continuing process that's going to drag their children down is considered to be too much for them to bear. I think that you have to be careful because not all epilepsy is like that. Most types of epilepsy doesn't seem to have the type of progression that we see in this disorder, but I think that we really do need to make the point that there are some that are progressive and that it is very important to understand why and to deal with that process.

S. Moshe: I would like to make a comment because of this argument. There are two different aspects: You can have seizures, and they do not necessarily get progressively worse. That's not all the bad seizures that sometimes you see. Some of the conditions that Pete describes are relatively rarer, and we see that in the more advanced epilepsy centers. But the majority of kids who have seizures will do all right because their immature brains seem to respond to seizures and to environmental stimuli that otherwise the adults cannot tolerate. Now the other point that I would like to bring out is that Pete is discussing the concept of a familial tendency in people with temporal lobe epilepsy, and that means that the brain of these people may be slightly different from the brains of normal people who happen to have a seizure for other causes. And we are studying animals that are normal and then we find some kind of changes and will produce a lot of seizures and we think that this will happen in everybody. It turns out that a lot of people with seizures have an underlying disease that can create other deficits and has nothing to do with the seizures. So you cannot take that as all or none. The other thing that you mentioned is about the possibility of getting infections. That's another reason why the brain can be injured and I think one of the questions that I am trying to wrestle with, and Claude Wasterlain is wrestling at the same time also, is what is the type of seizure that is more dangerous in the mature brain and what are the predisposing factors that makes these seizures progressively worse and permit the kindling phenomenon to occur? Because it does not occur in most of the patients that we see.

F. Lopes Da Silva: I would like to come back to this question about what you do with these patients with temporal lobe epilepsy and what are you really doing when you do surgery. And one of the things that comes to mind is that in fact what you do by removal of the hippocampus and adjacent cortex, you change an intractable form of epilepsy into a form of epilepsy that you can control with medication. Most of these patients still need medication and will keep on medication for a long time, and if you reduce it they will have seizures again. I would like to know what is your experience on medication postsurgery and whether this view makes some sense to you.

P. Engel: That is something that nobody knows, because the problem is that patients don't want to go off their medication. Most patients that have had successful surgery and are seizure-free are still on medication. The reason for that is that we wait 2 years before we say that they are seizure-free and then offer them withdrawal from medication, and by that time they are driving for the first time in their lives. When we say, "We'll take you off medication but you'll have to stop driving for 6 months," and they're going to lose their job or their girlfriend or whatever else, they don't do it. And that is the main reason why they do not come off the medication. When patients agree to go off medication, we usually get them off with no problem. But you are right, there are a significant number of patients who are seizure-free who can't go off the medication and what we have done is reduced this from an intractable to a tractable problem. May I remind you that most patients who have hippocampal sclerosis have some degree of bilateral damage and that there may also be contributions from the other side. There is some feeling that if we do early intervention, which is what we are getting at now, we will be more likely to stop the seizures completely and get them off the medication. It will be interesting to see if that is the case.

C. Wasterlain: Well I think that it is a very important question. When pursuing the same line of thought, I'm a disciple of the Goddard–McIntyre principles and I think that that means that probably kindling and epilepsy use the natural memory mechanisms to spread disease. I mean that it has to use biochemical mechanisms that are in the brain to do its deed. If you think about memories, they are initially processed through the hippocampus and then they are transferred through multiple neocortical sites over a period of many years, not weeks or days or months. Over a period of many years there is transfer to multiple neocortical sites, and once there they are very difficult to erase. I think that if we think of epilepsy and the fact that you just outlined, in that light it makes sense that perhaps epilepsies are first associated with mesial temporal sclerosis within the hippocampus but probably go to hippocampal structures and then to multiple neocortical sites. There are strange facts like frequently when you do successful surgery for temporal lobe epilepsy you end up with a patient still having auras but no generalized seizures. Now how can you explain that if you have removed the focus and the aura is simply a manifestation of turning on the part of the brain where the focus is? You can explain it if that property is transferred as a memory to multiple neocortical sites that were not removed. However, the facilitation of spread, which the hippocampus does so well, is removed by the surgery; and therefore you still have the focus with no organized spread. I think that you mentioned that earlier surgeries are more successful than late surgery, and so on. I think that finding fits fairly well into the general concept.

P. Engel: I think the hologram concept of brain function may be true to a certain extent, but it doesn't get you anywhere because it's impossible to really study it. I think there is something in temporal lobe epilepsy and probably in memory as well that is much more specific than that. I think that because the PET scans show you such a characteristic of hypometabolism that involves ipsilateral structures that are in the projection fields of the mesial temporal area. It is so consistent from one patient to another, and it isn't seen in neocortical epilepsy at all. It suggests that there is something about this area that progressively recruits other areas of the brain it projects to specifically into some kind of enduring dysfunction that is there even when the patient is not having seizures. It may predispose not only to recurrent spontaneous seizures but also to behavioral disturbances, and what we need to understand is how does it do that and where does it do that. I think that the message that I want to give you as kindlers is that it would be nice if you could also look at animal models of spontaneous seizures to try to identify kindling-like phenomena that are occurring spontaneously, not just from the stimulation that you are doing—where you can find parallels would be of great clinical value.

B. Adamec: My question actually relates back to the behavior issue. I was interested in your comment about auras growing in incidence and perhaps frequency and the intensity the longer the epilepsy is there. In the 80's and early 90's two laboratories, Hermann's and ours, reported an association between aura intensity and frequency of aura types that indicated sub-cortical activation, a close association between that and psychopathology was much better than diagnosis or focus location. Depression, anxiety and mood lability were the patterns that were apparently accentuated in these patients. I was wondering whether you had seen anything like that in your center.

P. Engel: Yes, I'm familiar with your work and Bruce Hermann's, but we just haven't looked at that.

B. Adamec: I encourage you to try it because it is an interesting contact point between kindling and psychopathology.

P. Engel: Yes, absolutely.

CONTRIBUTIONS OF KINDLING TO CLINICAL EPILEPTOLOGY

Kiyoshi Morimoto,[1] Hitoshi Sato,[1] Mariko Osawa,[2] and Mitsumoto Sato[2]

[1]Department of Neuropsychiatry
Faculty of Medicine, Kagawa Medical University
Kagawa, 761-07 Japan
[2]Department of Psychiatry
Tohoku University School of Medicine
Sendai, 980-77 Japan

1. INTRODUCTION

Regarding the involvement of kindling in clinical epilepsy (Table 1) as reviewed previously [1], the discussion herein is focused on two issues: the neuromechanisms of repeated brief seizures (RBS)-induced epileptogenesis and the neuropharmacology of antiepileptics. The former is related to the refractoriness in some types of epilepsy, and the latter may be important to the developent of new antiepileptics able to alleviate the epileptic disorders of Engel [2]. Results of our recent studies on these central problems of epilepsy are presented.

2. REPEATED BRIEF SEIZURE-INDUCED EPILEPTOGENESIS AND MORPHOLOGIGAL ALTERATION IN THE DENTATE GYRUS

Kindling is an ideal model of epilepsy in which recurrent spontaneous epileptic seizures can be produced [3]. Kindling-induced epileptogenesis has been regarded to persist for a considerable time without induction of gross tissue damage in the brain. Recently, however, it has been demonstrated that morphological alterations induced by kindling include progressive neuronal loss in the hilus of the dentate gyrus (DG) [4] and synaptic reorganization of the mossy fiber pathway from granule cells [5]. Mossy fiber sprouting and neuronal loss in the DG, CA1, and CA3 have been also reported in both the kainate-treated animal model of epilepsy and human temporal lobe epilepsy. Cavazos et al. [6] reported that mossy fiber synaptic terminals developed in the supragranular regions of the DG by 4 days after initiation of kindling stimulation in a time course compatible with axon sprouting. They reported a strong correlation between mossy fiber synaptic reorganization and the

Kindling 5, edited by Corcoran and Moshé.
Plenum Press, New York, 1998.

Table 1. Kindling model of epilepsy and human epilepsy

Kindling model	vs	Human epilepsy
Limbic kindling		Temporal lobe epilepsy
Kindling seizure development		Development of partial seizure to secondary generalized seizures
Kindled seizure		"Epileptiform" seizures partially due to epileptogenesis induced by RBS
Persistence of kindled events		Acquired epileptogenesis induced by RBS (refractoriness of seizures)
Lasting interictal spikes		Interictal epileptic discharge in clinical EEG
Spontaneous seizures		"Epileptic seizures" fully depended upon acquired epileptogenesis
Postictal and interictal behavior disorders		Postictal and interictal psychoses
Morphological alterations in the hippocampus		Mesial temporal sclerosis
Pharmacology		
Kindling development		Treatment of epileptogenesis (antiepileptics)
Kindled seizures		Treatment of epileptic seizures (anticonvulsants)

development, progression, and permanence of the kindling phenomenon, and suggested that axonal sprouting and the resultant synaptic reorganization in limbic pathways may contribute to the development of kindling. It has also been reported that RBSs evoked by kindling stimuli induce neuronal loss in the hilus of the DG, which is accompanied by sprouting and permanent reorganization of the synaptic connections of the mossy fiber pathways [7]. However, it has been not distinguished whether sprouting with synaptic reorganization of the mossy fiber pathway is a cause or effect of neuronal loss of the DG.

To investigate the role of afterdischarges (ADs) in the induction of these morphological alterations and the relationship of neuronal loss in the DG to mossy fiber sprouting, we first examined the neuronal density and Timm scores in an unstimulated control, in a control stimulated with low frequency stimuli without induction of ADs, and in standard kindling groups stimulated with high frequency stimuli sufficient to produce ADs. We then examined the progression of the neuronal loss and Timm scores during repetition of ADs induced by different numbers of daily amygdala stimulations.

2.1. Materials and Methods

2.1.1. Kindling Procedures. Forty-three male Sprague-Dawley rats weighing 280–330 g at the time of surgery were used. A twisted tripolar nichrome electrode was implanted stereotaxically into the left basolateral nucleus of the amygdala under pentobarbital anesthesia. After a recovery period of one week, each rat was subjected to a kindling stimulus (a 1-second train of 60-Hz sine wave pulses at 200 μA) or a low frequency stimulus (a 1-second train of 3-Hz sine wave pulses at 200 μA). The development of AM seizures was assessed according to the 5 stages of Racine's classification [8].

2.1.2. Histology. The kindled rats were divided into 4 groups according to the number of total ADs: AD-6, AD-11, AD-18 and AD-27. Two weeks after the last seizure except in the unstimulated control group, all rats were anesthetized and perfused transcardially with 0.1 M phosphate buffer with 0.16% (w/v) Na_2 followed by 3% glutalaldehyde, and subsequently with 0.1 M phosphate buffer with 15% sucrose. The brains were removed and fixed for 2 hours in 0.1 M phosphate buffer with 15% sucrose. Horizontal 20-μm frozen sections were cut with a microtome and developed in the dark for 30–60 min in a mixture of gum arabic, frozen hydroquinon, and citric acid-sodium citrate buffer with silver nitrate solution for Timm histochemistry. Alternate sections were stained with Cresyl violet for neuron counting.

Mossy fiber reorganization was evaluated by rating the distribution of Timm granules in the supragranular layer of the DG on a scale of 0–5, using the method of Cavazos et al. [6]: (0) no granules between the tips and crest of the DG, (1) more numerous granules in the supragranular region in a patchy distribution between the tips and crest of the DG, (2) more numerous granules in the supragranular region in a continuous distribution between the tips and crest of the DG, (3) prominent granules in the supragranular region in a continuous pattern between the tip and the crest, with occasional patches of confluent granules between the tips and crest of the DG, (4) prominent granules in the supragranular region that form a confluent, dense and laminar band between the tips and the crest, and (5) confluent, dense, and laminar band of granules in the inner molecular layer.

Neurons in the hilar polymorphic region were counted by the method of Cavazos and Sutula [4]. The differences in mean neuronal densities were expressed as neurons per mm^3 and mean scores of the Timm granules were statistically analyzed with one-way ANOVA or Kruskal-Wallis, followed by Fisher's PLDS or the Mann-Whitney U test.

2.2. Results and Discussion

There was no difference in cell counts and Timm scores between the unstimulated controls and controls stimulated with 3-Hz stimuli without induction of ADs (Fig. 1, Fig. 2). In the rats which received 60-Hz stimuli with induction of ADs, a significant decrease of neuronal density was found bilaterally in the hilar region after induction of 11, 18, and 29 ADs. There was no change in the neuronal density after induction of 6 ADs, when 4 of 8 rats had developed stage 5 seizures. In the supragranular layer of the dentate gyrus, there was a significant increase in the Timm score in the stimulated side only after 29 ADs, as compared with the stimulated control group. These results indicate that neither neuronal loss nor mossy fiber sprouting appears merely due to electrical stimuli with the same current as the kindling stimuli. It is suggested that recurrence of brief seizures is a necessary condition for production of the morphological alterations in kindling.

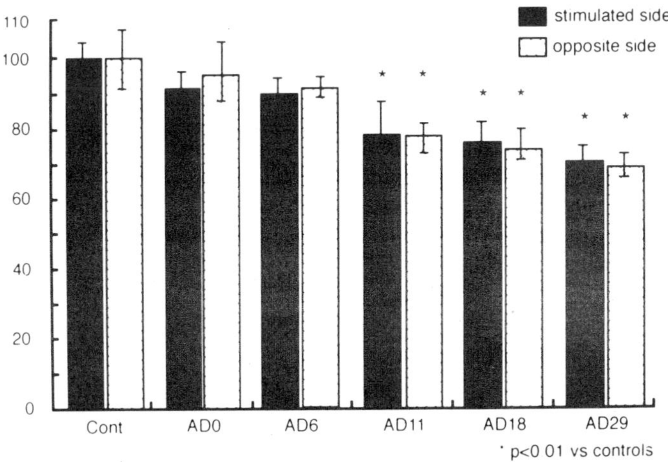

Figure 1. Decreased neuronal densities in the DG after repeated ADs. Please note a progressive decrease in neuronal densities bilaterally after repetition of more than 11 ADs.

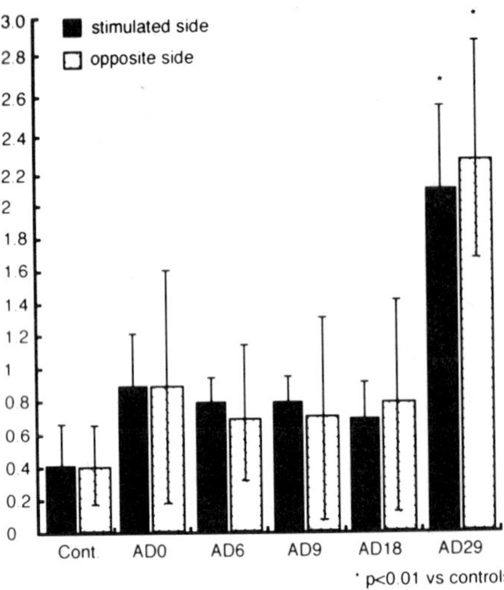

Figure 2. Increased Timm scores in the DG after repeated ADs. Increased Timm score was found after repetition of 29 ADs that occurred later than significant decrease in neuronal densities (Fig. 1).

This finding is also important in the investigation of the cause of mesial temporal lobe sclerosis that is a common lesion found in 50–70% of temporal lobe specimens resected in patients with interactable epileptic seizures. The absence of morphological change in the rats that developed kindled seizures confirmed our previous report that amygdala kindling can develop without evidence of decreased neuronal densities or increased Timm scores [9]. This finding did not confirm the report of Cavazos et al. [6] suggesting that axonal sprouting and the resultant synaptic reorganization in DG may contribute to the development of kindling.

In the hilus of the DG ipsilateral to the stimulated amygdala, we found 16.0%, 18.3% and 23.2% decreases in the number of cells as compared with controls after 11 ADs, 18 ADs, and 29 ADs, respectively. In the hilus opposite the stimulated amygdala, there were 20.5%, 22.0%, and 28.8% decreases after 11 ADs, 18 ADs, and 29 ADs, respectively. There was no difference in the stimulated and unstimulated sides. These results indicate that neuronal loss in the bilateral DG becomes evident after development of the stage 5 seizures but prior to mossy fiber sprouting. Neuronal loss was progressive along with additional induction of ADs with stage 5 seizures. These results are partially consistent with earlier reports by others. Spillar and Racine [10] reported a decrease in the number of cells in the hilus of the DG following kindling. They reported an 11.5% decrease in the number of cells following the induction of 4 stage-5 seizures and a 15.2% decrease following an additional 40 stage-5 seizures. This reduction, as well as our finding, was not as large as that reported by Cavazos and Sutula [4], who found a 12.7% decrease after 3 stage-5 seizures and a 40.1% decrease following 30 stage-5 seizures.

In addition, Cavazos et al. [7] examined the distribution and time course of neuronal loss induced by 3, 30, and 150 stage-5 seizures in hippocampal, limbic, and neocortical pathways. They found neuronal loss in the DG (20%) and CA1 (18%) after 3 stage-5 seizures, the loss at thee sites progressing to 37% and 32% after 30 stage-5 seizures, and 49% and 44% of controls after 150 stage-5 seizures. Neuronal loss was also observed in CA3, the entorhinal cortex, and the rostral endopyriform nucleus after 30 seizures, and was detected in the granule cell layer and CA2 after 150 seizures, while no evidence of neuronal loss was found in the somatosensory cortex. Since the mossy fiber normally establishes synaptic contacts with polymorphic neurons in the hilus of DG, and with pyramidal neurons in the CA3 and CA3c regions of the hippocampus, they suggested that kindling induces alterations in neural circuitry at a variety of locations in the limbic system.

In this study, there was a significant correlation between the decrease in neuronal density number of ADs ($p<0.001$), cumulative AD duration (data shown: $p<0.01$) and number of stage-5 seizures (data not shown: $p<0.01$). These results strongly suggest that neuronal loss appeared prior to mossy fiber sprouting, and became progressively evident due to repetition of kindled convulsions after kindling ("over-kindling"). As spontaneous epileptic seizures have been reported to appear in about 50% of amygdala kindled rats after 150 daily stimulations with induction of ADs, progressive neuronal loss in the DG with subsequent appearance of mossy fiber synaptic reorganization may be related to the "true" epileptogenesis that may cause recurrent spontaneous epileptic seizures.

In summary, we conclude that 1) amygdala kindling may develop without evidence of neuronal loss in the hilar region of the DG, 2) repetition of ADs, but not the electrical stimuli themselves, produces morphological alterations in the DG, 3) neuronal loss in the DG may be observed prior to the evidence of increased Timm scores in the supragranular layer of the DG, and 4) neuronal loss with subsequent mossy fiber sprouting may progress parallel with an increase in the number of kindled seizures, which may eventually be related to the emergence of spontaneous epileptic seizures. More information on firing of the sprouted neurons and of synaptic activity in the over-kindled rats needed to delineate the clinical implications of the morphological alterations in the hippocampus.

3. KINDLING AND DEVELOPMENT OF NEW ANTIEPILEPTIC DRUGS

Since the clinical introduction of phenobarbital in 1912, a number of antiepileptic drugs (AEDs) have been developed and drug control of epilepsy has clearly been improved. However, even recently, more than 30% of epilepsy cases are drug-resistant and, in adult epilepsy, complex partial seizures (temporal lobe epilepsy: TLE) are indicated to be the most refractory to AED therapy. For these reasons, further development of AEDs is required.

The kindling model is well accepted as the best model of TLE. Using this model, two important aspects of the development of new AEDs have been highlighted. First, new types of AEDs which selectively act on the neuronal mechanisms underlying kindling have been produced. For instance, a series of selective GABA enhancers, such as a direct GABA receptor agonist (e.g., progabide), a GABA-degrading enzyme inhibitor (e.g., vigabatrin) and a GABA uptake inhibitor (e.g., tiagabine), have been developed [11]. These agents are expected to enhance inhibitory neurotransmission, which is presumed to be impaired in the kindled brain. Another instance is the recent pharmacological development of various antagonists of glutamate systems as prospective AEDs.

Second, the kindling model is essential for preclinical screening tests of new AEDs to obtain antiepileptic profiles and determine the existence of any adverse effects. In kindled seizures, epileptogenic foci are precisely located, and the effects of drugs on focal seizures with secondary generalization can be clearly observed.

3.1. Selective GABA Uptake Inhibitors

A variety of clinical and experimental evidence has implicated the functional impairment of GABA-ergic systems as a basic mechanism in epilepsy. Recent clinical studies in

TLE patients have demonstrated the disturbed rise of extracellular GABA concentration in the epileptogenic hippocampus during seizures [12]. The impaired GABA release is suggested to be due to a decrease of glutamate-induced, calcium-independent GABA release, and is associated with a significant reduction in the number of GABA transporters [13].

We have recently examined regional changes in mRNA of GABA transporters after amygdala-kindled generalized seizures in rats [24]. GAT1 mRNA significantly increased (111–118%) in the DG at 1 hour and in the CA1 region of the ipsilateral hippocampus at 4 hours after kindled seizures, but it recovered to the control level at 24 hours (Fig. 3). In contrast, GAT3 mRNA was significantly increased bilaterally in the amygdala and in the contralateral pyriform cortex and cerebral cortex 1 hour after seizure. These increases in mRNA of GABA transporters may reflect alterations of GABA-ergic neurotransmission in the hippocampus during kindled generalized seizures.

Two types of GABA uptake inhibitors, tiagabine (nipecotic acid derivative) and NNC-711 (guvacine derivative), have recently been developed as a new AED. These agents selectively block the GAT1 subtype of GABA transporters and increase the GABA concentration in the synaptic cleft [14]. We have analyzed the antiepileptic profile and adverse effects of tiagabine and NNC-711 in the rat amygdala and hippocampal kindling model and compared findings with those for conventional AEDs, valproate, and carbamazepine [15]. Tiagabine (2.5–40 mg/kg, i.p.) and NNC-711 (2.5–20 mg/kg, i.p.) showed potent and dose-dependent anticonvulsant effects against both amygdala- and hippocampal-kindled seizures (Fig. 4). The anticonvulsant efficacy of NNC-711 was more potent than that of tiagabine, which was related to the potency of in vitro GABA uptake. Adverse effects of tiagabine on motor systems (sedation, ataxia and muscle hypotonus) were significantly less, compared with those of valproate and carbamazepine (Table 2). Toxic high doses of these GABA uptake inhibitors, however, often causes EEG paroxysm and myoclonus. These results indicate the clinical usefulness of tiagabine in drug-resistant TLE.

3.2. Glutamate Antagonists

3.2.1. Inhibitors of Excessive Glutamate Release. In human epilepsy [12] or animal models of epilepsy [16], excessive release of glutamate was demonstrated, suggesting it to be a cause of epileptic activity and brain damage such as hippocampal cell loss.

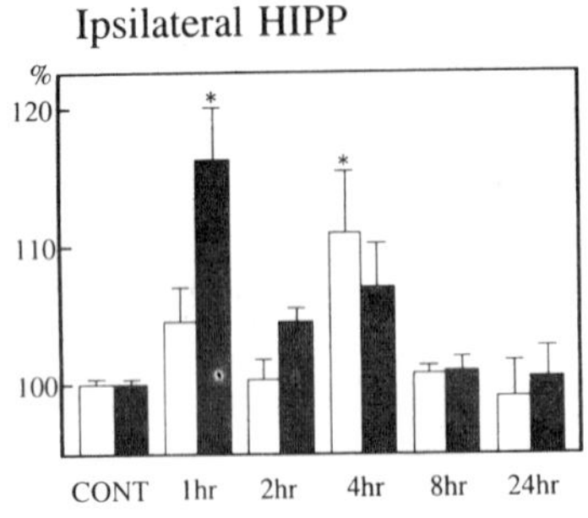

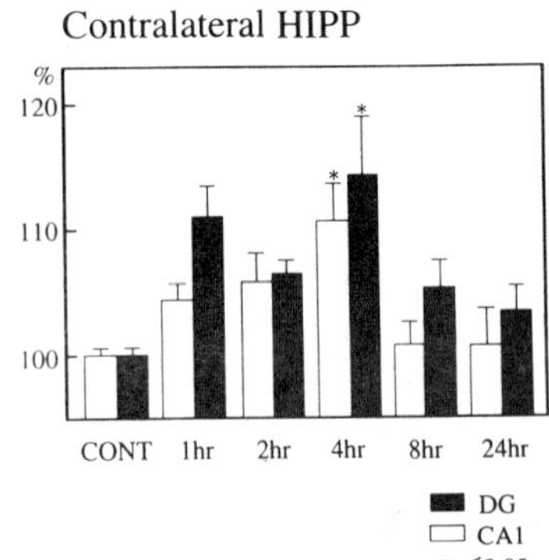

Figure 3. Time-dependent changes in mRNA of GABA transporter (GAT1) after amygdala kindled seizures in the dentate gyrus of the rat hippocampus.

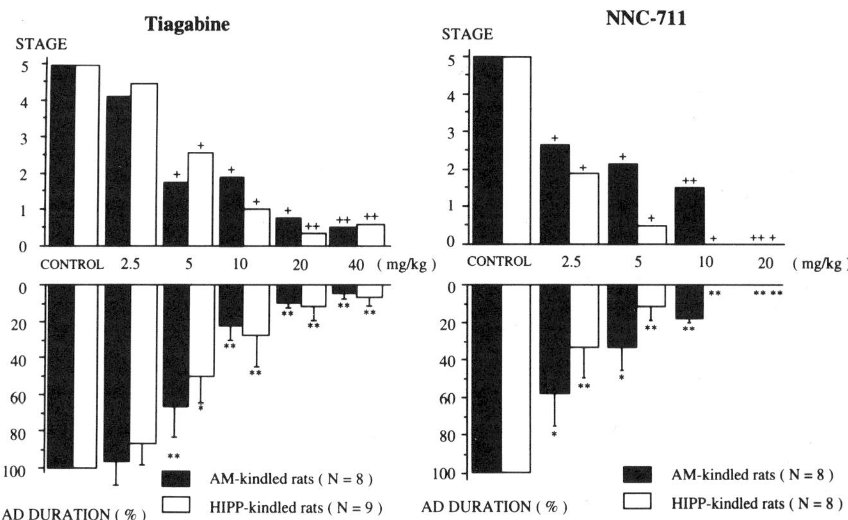

Figure 4. Dose-dependent anticonvulsant effects of selective GABA uptake inhibitors, tiagabine (left) and NNC-711 (right), on amygdala- and hippocampal-kindled seizures in rats.

Lamotrigine and its structurally related derivative BW1003C87 have been shown to primarily act at voltage-sensitive Na^+ channels and to stabilize presynaptic membranes, thereby preventing the pathological release of glutamate under certain conditions [17,18]. We have recently studied antiepileptic effects of lamotrigine [19] and BW1003C87 [25] in the rat kindling model. Intraperitoneally administered lamotrigine (3.35–13.4 mg/kg) or BW1003C87 (2.5–10 mg/kg) showed unusual long-acting (for 48 hours) and dose-dependent anticonvulsant effects against both amygdala- and hippocampal-kindled seizures (Fig. 5). Interestingly, the anticonvulsant profile of these agents showed that they act in an all-or-nothing fashion and that the effects were completely antagonized when stimulus intensity was increased up to twice or four times that of the threshold (Table 3). Furthermore,

Table 2. Comparison of behavioral adverse effects of tiagabine, valproate, and carbamazepine (CBZ) in amygdala (AM) and hippocampal (HIPP) kindled seizures

	Total adverse effects scores		
	Tiagabine*	Valproate	Carbamazepine
50% reduction of AD duration			
AM-kindled	1.5 (0–2)	3.7 (2–6)+	4.4 (0–7)++
HIPP-kindled	1.3 (0–5)	2.4 (0–4)	2.5 (0–5)
Block of GCS			
AM-kindled	1.3 (0–2)	3.7 (2–6)++	5.9 (4–8)++
HIPP-kindled	1.3 (0–5)	2.4 (0–4)	2.5 (0–5)

Total adverse effects included sedation, ataxia and muscle hypotonus and each score was measured by rating scale (0: non, 1: mild, 2: moderate, and 3:severe).
Values: mean (range), AD: afterdischarge, GCS: generalized clonic seizures, +: p<0.05, ++: p<0.01; Mann-Whitney U test, compared with Tiagabine.

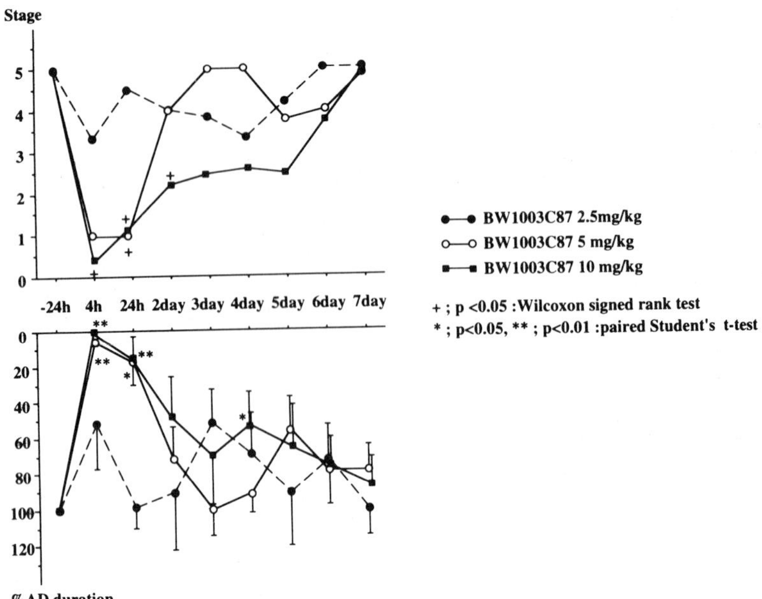

Figure 5. Time- and dose-dependent anticonvulsant effects of BW1003C87 on amygdala-kindled seizures in rats.

lamotrigine did not produce any adverse behavioral effects. From these results, it is suggested that lamotrigine and BW1003C87 have a unique antiepileptic mechanism, i.e., an elevation of the seizure-triggering threshold of the epileptogenic foci.

3.2.2. Glutamate Receptor Antagonists. In the rat kindling model, we have previously demonstrated that NMDA receptor antagonists, such as CPP and CGS19755 (receptor antagonists), MK-801 (ion channel antagonist), and 7-chlorokynurenic acid (glycine receptor antagonist), have potent antiepileptogenic effects, while their anticonvulsant effects were less prominent [20]. Consistent with our results, clinical trials of

Table 3. The effects of lamotrigine (13.4 mg/kg, i.p.) on generalized seizure-triggering thresholds (GSTs) in amygdala (AM) and hippocampal (HIPP) kindled seizures

	Seizure stage	AD duration	No. of GCS
AM-kindled			
Control GST	5.0 (5–5)	77.4 ± 7.6	6/6
Lamotrigine			
GST	0.0 (0–0)+	0.0 ± 0.0**	0/6
2 X GST	3.7 (2–5)	66.7 ± 24.4	4/6
3 X GST	5.0 (5–5)	78.9 ± 13.9	6/6
HIPP-kindled			
Control GST	5.0 (5–5)	74.4 ± 6.8	7/7
Lamotrigine GST	0.0 (0–0)+	6.5 ± 6.5**	0/7
2 X GST	1.3 (0–5)+	33.8 ± 19.3	1/7
4 X GST	2.9 (1–5)	95.2 ± 23.5	3/7

Values: mean (range) or mean ± SEM, AD: afterdischarge, GCS: generalized clonic seizures, +: p<0.05; Wilcoxon test, **:p<0.01; Student's t-test, compared with control.

NMDA receptor antagonists (MK-801 and CPP-ene) in epilepsy have so far been unsatisfactory because of the toxic side effects of these antagonists. MK-801 has been reported to induce psychiatric symptoms [21], whereas CPP-ene caused excessive sedation and motor impairment [22].

In contrast, a selective AMPA receptor antagonist (NBQX) had more potent anticonvulsant effects on kindled seizures at non-toxic doses [23]. Further investigations are required before clinical application of glutamate receptor antagonists in epilepsy can be attempted.

REFERENCES

1. Sato M, Racine RJ, McIntyre DC: Kindling: basic mechanisms and clinical validity. Electroenceph Clin Neurophysiol (1990) 76:459–472.
2. Engel J Jr: Seizures and Epilepsy. F.A.Davis Company, Philadelphia, 1989, pp5–6.
3. Wada JA, Sato M, Corcoran ME: persistent seizure susceptibility and recurrent spontaneous seizures in kindled cats. Epilepsia (1974) 15:465–478.
4. Cavazos JE, Sutula TP: Progressive neuronal loss induced by kindling: a possible mechanism for mossy fiber reorganization and hippocampal sclerosis. Brain Res (1990) 527:1–6.
5. Sutula T, Xiao-xian H, Cavazos J, et al: Synaptic reorganization in the hippocampus induced by abnormal functional activity. Science (1988) 239:1147–1150.
6. Cavazos JE, Golarai G, Sutula TP: Mossy fiber synaptic reorganization induced by kindling: time course of development, progression, and permanence. J Neurosci (1991) 11:2795–2803.
7. Cavazos JE, Das I, Sutula TP: Neuronal loss induced in limbic pathways by kindling: Evidence for induction of hippocampal sclerosis by repeated brief seizures. J Neurosci (1994) 14:3106–3121.
8. Racine RJ: Modification of seizure activity by electrical stimulation. II Motor seizure. Electroenceph Clin Neurophysiol (1972) 32:281–294.
9. Osawa M, Inosaka T, Nakagawa T, Sato M: Relationships of secondarily generalized seizures and morphometric change in dentate gyrus to the acquired seizure susceptibility in amygdala kindled rats. J Jpn Epi Soc (1995) 13:3–121 (in Japanese with English abstract).
10. Spiller AE, Racine RJ: The effect of kindling beyond the 'stage 5' criterion on paired-pulse depression and hilar cell counts in the dentate gyrus. Brain Res (1995) 635:139–147.
11. Morimoto K, Sanei T, Sato K: Comparative study of the anticonvulsant effect of γ-aminobutyric acid agonists in the feline kindling model of epilepsy. Epilepsia (1993) 34:1123–1129.
12. During MJ, Spencer DD: Extracellular hippocampal glutamate and spontaneous seizure, in the conscious human brain. Lancet (1993) 341:1607–1610. [13] During MJ, Ryder KM, Spencer DD: Hippocampal GABA transporter function in temporal-lobe epilepsy. Nature (1995) 376:174–177.
14. Suzdak PD, Jansen JA: A review of preclinical pharmacology of tiagabine: A potent and selective anticonvulsant GABA uptake inhibitor. Epilepsia (1995) 36:612–626.
15. Morimoto K, Sato H, Yamamoto Y, Watanabe T, Suwaki H: Antiepileptic effects of tiagabine, a selective GABA uptake inhibitor, in the rat kindling model of temporal lobe epilepsy. Epilepsia (1997) 38:966–974.
16. Ueda Y and Tsuru N: Simultaneous monitoring of seizure-related changes in extracellular glutamate and gamma-aminobutyric acid concentration in bilateral hippocampi following development of amygdala kindling. Epilepsy Res (1995) 20:213–219.
17. Leach MJ, Marden CK, Miller AA: Pharmacological studies on lamotrigine, a novel antiepileptic drug: II.Neurochemical studies on the mechanism of action. Epilepsia (1986) 27:490–497.
18. Lekieffre D, Meldrum BS: The pyrimidine-derivative, BW1003C87, protects CA1 and striatal neurons following transient severe forebrain ischemia in rats. A microdialysis and histochemical study. Neuroscience (1993) 56:93–99.
19. Otsuki K, Sato K, Yamada N, Kuroda S, Morimoto K: Anticonvulsant effects of lamotrigine, a novel potential antiepileptic drug, on amygdaloid and hippocampal kindled seizures in rats. Jpn J Neuropsychopharmacol (1995) 17:35–42 (in Japanese with English abstract).
20. Morimoto K, Sato M: NMDA receptor complex and kindling mechanisms. Epilepsy Res Suppl (1992) 9:297–305.
21. Troupin AS, Mendius JR, Cheng F, Risinger MW: MK-801 as an anticonvulsant—preliminary evaluation. In BS Meldrum, R Porter (Eds), Current Problem of Epilepsy IV: New Anticonvulsant Drugs, John Libbey, London, 1986, pp191–201.

22. Sveinbjornsdottir S, Sander JWAS, Upton D, et al: The excitatory amino acid antagonist D-CPP-ene (SDZ EAA-494) in patients with epilepsy. Epilepsy Res (1993) 16:165–174.
23. Namba T, Morimoto K, Sato K, Yamada N, Kuroda S: Antiepileptogenic and anticonvulsant effects of NBQX, a selective AMPA receptor antagonist, in the kindling model of epilepsy. Brain Res (1993) 638:36–44.
24. Hirao T, Morimoto K, Yamamoto Y, Watanabe T, Sato H, Sato K, Sato S, Yamada N, Tanaka K, Suwaki H: Time-dependent and regional expression of GABA transporter mRNAs following amygdala-kindled seizures in rats. Mol Brain Res (1997) in press.
25. Morimoto K, Sato H, Sato K, Sato S, Yamada N, BW100C87, phenytoin and carbamazepine elevate seizure threshold in the rat amygdala-kindling model of epilepsy. Eur J Pharmacol (1997) in press.

DISCUSSION OF KIYOSHI MORIMOTO'S PAPER

W. Loscher: Just to comment on your last slides, lamotrigine is not a selective glutamate release inhibitor. It acts by blocking sodium channels and can demonstrate exactly the same effect as phenytoin; so many of the effects of lamotrigine are similar to phenytoin. At higher concentrations it also inhibits GABA release also by the sodium channel blocking effect; so there are a lot of adverse effects of lamotrigine in the clinic, which to my belief can be explained by its nonselective effect on several neurotransmitters.

K. Morimoto: I quite agree with your suggestion. I think that previous studies showed that lamotrigine had relatively weaker inhibitory effects on GABA release or acetylcholine release but larger effects on glutamate or aspartate release. As I mentioned in my presentation, lamotrigine is not a selective glutamate release blocker, and I think the anticonvulsant profile of lamotrigine in kindling is similar to phenytoin or carbamazipine. In our unpublished studies, lamotrigine had very little effect on normal evoked responses in the rat hippocampus, indicating that lamogtrigine does not affect normal glutamate neurotransmission, but only affects it under pathological conditions such as ischemia or epileptic seizures.

C. Wasterlain: Lamotrigine of course has several characteristics which make it difficult to use clinically. Is NNC-711 going to be any better, or do you have any compounds coming down the line that will be more practical to use?

K. Morimoto: I think such selective GABA enhancers have some sort of advantage in controlling epilepsy, since GABA is the principal inhibitory neurotransmitter in epilepsy but noradrenaline and serotonin just modulate seizure induction. Among these GABA enhancers, GABA uptake inhibitors increase endogenous GABA, so little adverse effects would be expected. Clinical trials of tiagabine in epilepsy have just started.

M. Corcoran: If there are no further questions for Dr. Morimoto, I would like to invite two of our discussants, Dr. Fernandez-Guardiola and then Dr. Wasterlain, to present some of their recent findings to the group.

35

VAGUS NERVE STIMULATION

Effects on Circadian Sleep Organization and Kindling Development in the Cat

Augusto Fernández-Guardiola, Adrián Martínez-Cervantes, Alejandro Valdés-Cruz, Victor Magdaleno-Madrigal, and Rodrigo Fernández-Mas

Instituto Mexicano de Psiquiatría
Calz. Xochimilco 101, CP 14370 and
Facultad de Psicología
UNAM, México DF

1. INTRODUCTION

Vagal stimulation inhibits brainstem neuronal discharge and induces slow wave sleep (SWS) and rapid eye movements (REM) sleep in the cat[3,2,8]. It also inhibits motor activity[10]. Low-voltage vagal stimulation also significantly reduces EEG spiking activity of a cortical epileptic focus caused by topical application of strychnine[12] and prevents or aborts electrically and chemically induced seizures in rats[13] as well as PTZ induced seizures in dogs[14]. In a previous work[4] we described signs of paradoxical (REM) sleep that appear during the extinction of experimental seizures, suggesting a close relationship between the appearance of REM sleep and seizure arrest. The vagal stimulation as a novel approach for seizure control in patients who have intractable epilepsy has been recently documented[7,6]. In the present study we assessed the efficacy of vagal nerve stimulation on the development of electrographic and behavioral changes induced by kindling the amygdala (KA) as measured by the reduction in the frequency, duration and cortical propagation of amygdaloid afterdischarge.

2. METHODS

Seven freely moving cats weighing 3800–4100 g were studied. The left vagus nerve (LVN) was dissected, and a bipolar hook (5 mm separation) stainless-steel electrode was implanted. The animals were implanted for conventional sleep recordings, and bipolar stainless-steel electrodes were stereotaxically[11] placed into both Lateral Geniculate Bodies

Kindling 5, edited by Corcoran and Moshé.
Plenum Press, New York, 1998.

(LGB) and both Amygdalae. Surgery was conducted under sodium pentobarbital IV (33 mg/kg) anesthesia.

All animals were recorded during 23 hours twice a week (Tuesday and Thursday) and during 8 hours on the remaining days, starting at 8:30 a.m., in a light-dark (12:12 hrs) cycle. The amygdaline electrical stimulation (KA) was carried out daily (1 s train, 1 ms pulses, 60 Hz). Also, the LVN was stimulated during one minute (1.2 mA, 0.5 ms pulses, 30 Hz), just before the KA and thereafter every 60 minutes, for four times (from 10:00 to 14:00 hours), after KA. The sleep stages were analyzed by means of a specifically designed computer program for off-line cat sleep scoring[5]. The EEG electrodes were connected to Grass 7P511 amplifiers in a monopolar configuration. The signals were continuously recorded and stored on a hard disk as series of 4 s epochs. Off-line power spectra were computed and displayed in a tridimensional (3D) plot using hidden-line surface removal algorithms. This method permits the follow-up of the EEG during the experiment, showing both the effects of the LVN stimulations and the sleep changes in terms of its power spectral architecture and distribution as a function of time.

3. RESULTS

Kindling was significantly delayed during LVN stimulations; the animals remained in stages 2 and 3 for long time periods, and the duration and frequency of amygdaline afterdischarge failed to progress as in the sham LVN implanted animals (without stimulation). Moreover in the animals that reached stage 6, a failure of continuity of the LVN electrode was found (Fig. 1).

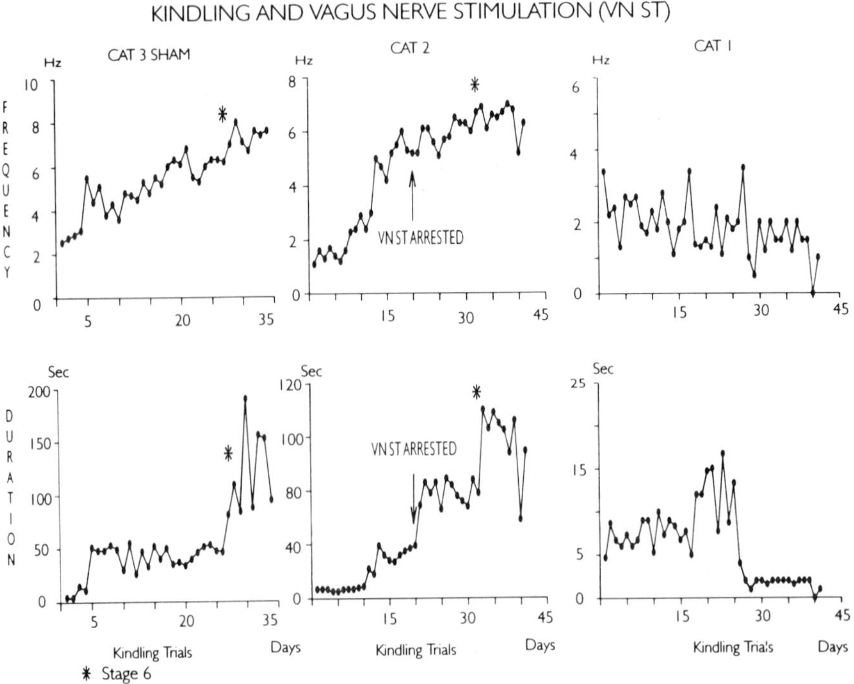

Figure 1. Effects of vagus nerve stimulation on the frequency and duration of afterdischarge during amygdaline kindling.

The LVN stimulation induced the following behavioral changes: Left miosis, blinking, licking, abdominal contractions, upwards gaze, swallowing, and eventually yawning, meowing and compulsive eating. Outstanding polygraphic changes were as follows: An increase of SPOL (Sommeil phasique à des ondes lentes) PGO waves and rapid eyes movements. The SWS and REM latencies were significantly diminished and REM sleep circadian shift to the light period was induced by LVN stimulation, despite of KA (Figs. 2 and 3). The density of PGO spikes was also significantly augmented. Interestingly, PGO appeared being the animal awake and quiet, with a pseudo hallucinatory behavior and moderate muscle tonus.

4. DISCUSSION

Description of the behavioral changes induced by LVN stimulation does not appear in the classical studies on vagal stimulation because most of the experiments were carried out in the *encephale isolé* or anesthetized animals[3,9]. The behavioral recording that we used is useful to ascertain mechanically induced damage of the vagus nerve especially when long lasting daily vagal stimulation is performed. The mechanisms for the induction of sleep and the antiepileptic effects of the electrical stimulation of vagal afferents are not fully understood. Early investigations in this area related these effects to the activation of the reticular activating system, which was regarded as the *locus* responsible for the sleep and waking cycle. Depending on the stimulation parameters, vagal afferent stimulation

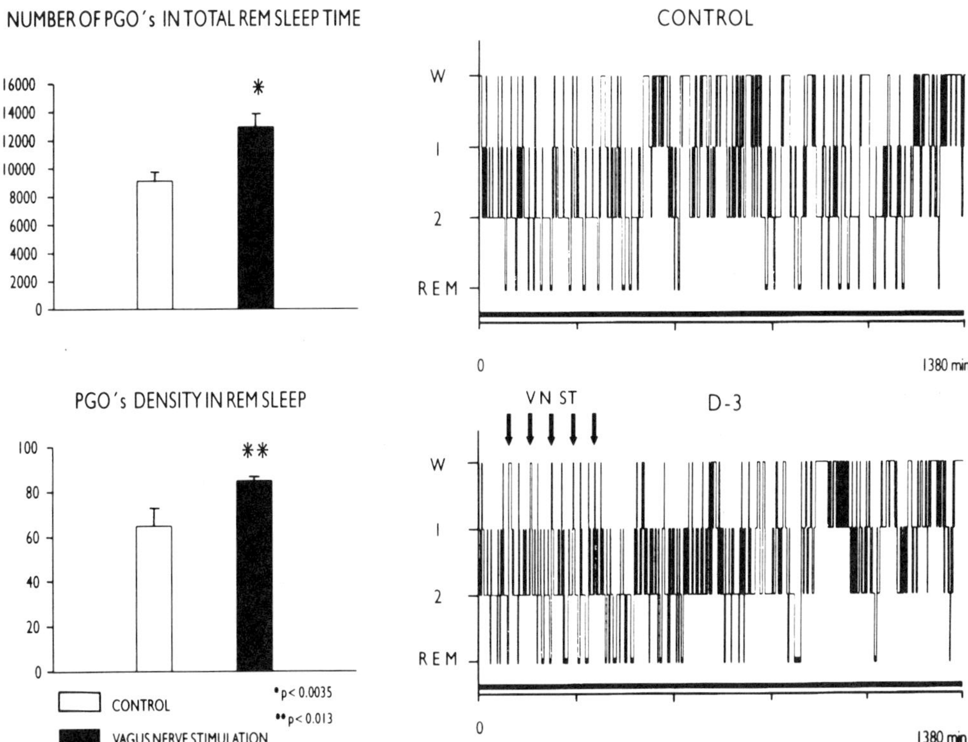

Figure 2. Effects of vagus nerve stimulation on measures of PGO waves during REM sleep in cats subjected to amygdaline kindling.

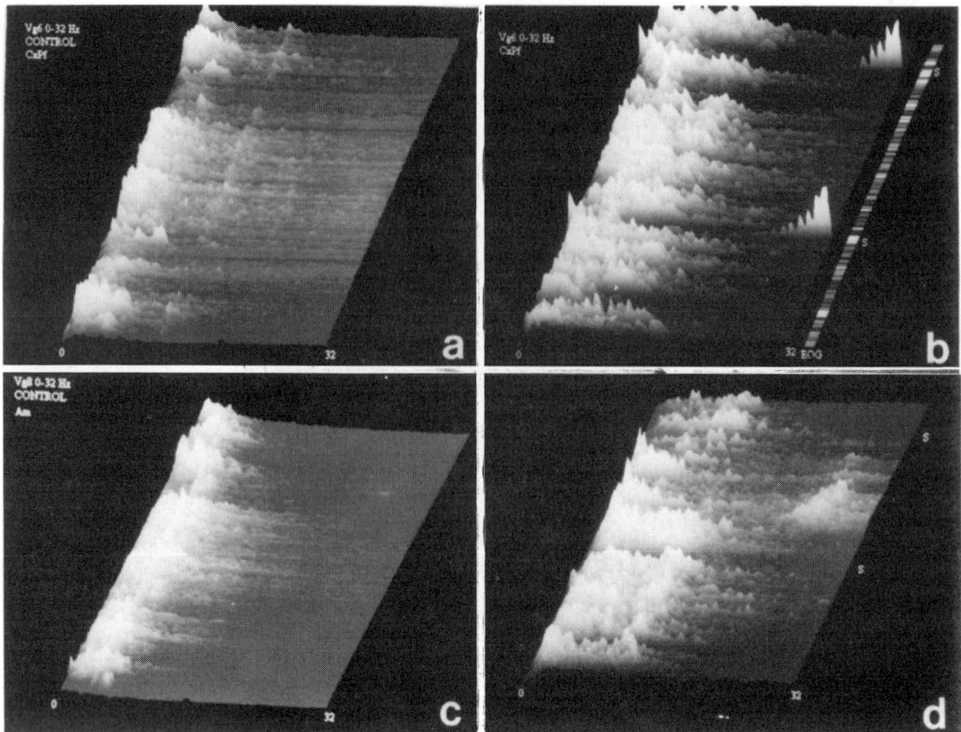

Figure 3. 3D EEG power spectra evolution (2 h, 0–32 Hz). a, Prefrontal Cortex (CxPf) control; b, CxPf during vagal stimulation (S). The band at the right, indicates the proportional EOG activity in the 3–7 Hz band.; c, Amygdala (Am) recording control; d, Am during vagal stimulation (S). Notice the power increase in the 8–16 Hz band induced by vagal stimulations.

produced EEG synchronization and affected sleep. Our results provide evidence that the pontine generators of PGOs might be directly activated by vagal stimulation. The electrical vagal stimulation might exert antiepileptic effects through the activation of PGOs pontine generators. The spontaneous PGOs apparition suppresses amygdaloid penicillin induced spikes[5]. Moreover, these actions are supported by the well documented anatomical data showing that the axons of the nodose ganglion enter the solitary tract and terminate in the nucleus of the solitary tract, which has a wide projection either directly with the amygdala, dorsal raphe, and hippocampus or, important for our hypothesis, via the parabrachial nucleus of which cholinergic direct activation induces phasic REM sleep phenomena[1].

ACKNOWLEDGMENTS

This work was partially supported by grant D111-903737 CONACyT and PUIS-UNAM.

REFERENCES

1. Calvo, J.M., Datta, S., Quattrochi, J. and Hobson, J. A., Cholinergic microstimulation of the Peribrachial nucleus in the cat. II. Delayed and prolonged increases in REM sleep, *Arch. Ital. Biol.*, 130 (1992) 285–301.

2. Chase, M.H., Nakamura, Y. and Clemente, C.D., Afferent vagal stimulation: neurographic correlates of induce EEG synchronization and desynchronization, *Brain Res.*, 5 (1967) 236–249.
3. Dell, P. and Olson P., Projections secondaires mesencephaliques, encephaliques et amygdaliennes des afferences viscerales vagales, *C. R. Soc. Biol. (Paris)*, 145 (1951) 1088–1091.
4. Fernández-Guardiola, A. and Ayala, F., Red nucleus fast activity and signs of paradoxical sleep appearing during the extinction of experimental seizures, *Electroenceph. clin. Neurophysiol.*, 30 (1971) 547–555.
5. Fernández-Guardiola, A., Martínez, A. and Fernández-Mas, R., Repeated penicillin-induced amygdala epileptic focus in freely moving cats. EEG, polysomnographic (23-h recording), and brain mapping study, *Epilepsy Res.*, 22 (1995) 127–136.
6. Hammond, E. J., Uthman, B. M., Reid, S.A., Wilder, B.J. and Ramsay, R.E., Vagus nerve stimulation in humans: Neurophysiological studies and electrophysiological monitoring, *Epilepsia* (Suppl. 2), 31 (1990) 51–59.
7. Penry, J.K. and Dean, J.C., Prevention of intractable partial seizures by intermittent vagal stimulation in humans: Preliminary results, *Epilepsia* (Suppl. 2), 31 (1990) 40–43.
8. Puizillout, J. J., Vago-aortic nerves stimulation and REM sleep: evidence for a REM-triggering and a REM maintenance factor, *Brain Res.*, 196 (1976) 81 184.
9. Puizillout, J. J., Ternaux, J. P., Foutz, A.S. and Dell, P., Phases de sommeil à ondes lentes avec déscharges phasiques. Leur déclenchement par la stimulation vago-aortique, *Rev. EEG Neurophysiol.*, 3 (1973) 21–37.
10. Schweitzer, A. and Wright, S., Effects on the knee jerk of stimulation of the central end of vagus nerve and of various changes in the circulation and respiration, *J. Physiol.* (Lond), 88 (1937) 459–475.
11. Snider, R.S. and Niemer, W.T., *A Stereotaxic Atlas of the Cat Brain*, University of Chicago Press, Chicago, Il., 1961.
12. Stoica, I. and Tudor, I., Effects of vagus afferents on strychninic focus of coronal gyrus, *Rev. Roum. Neurol.*, 4 (1967) 287–295.
13. Woodbury, D. M. and Woodbury, J. W., Effects of vagal stimulation on experimentally induced seizures in rats, *Epilepsia* (suppl. 2), 31 (1990) 7–19.
14. Zabara, J., Inhibition of experimental seizures in canines by repetitive vagal stimulation, *Epilepsia*, 33 (1992) 1005–1012.

36

FACILITATION OF KINDLING AND LONG TERM POTENTIATION BY HIPPOCAMPAL LESIONS

Claude G. Wasterlain, Andrey M. Mazarati, Yukiyoshi Shirasaka, Raman Sankar, and Kerry W. Thompson

Epilepsy Research Laboratory
VA Medical Center
Sepulveda, California 91343
Department of Neurology and Brain Research Institute
UCLA School of Medicine
Los Angeles, California 90095

1. INTRODUCTION

The relationship between kindling and chronic epilepsy with spontaneous seizures remains uncertain. Kindling is never observed as a natural phenomenon, but can easily be induced in any vertebrate species by stimulation of discrete brain sites. Focal brain lesions such as trauma or ischemia frequently lead to epilepsy after a delay of several weeks to months. Several models of status epilepticus (SE) which induce hippocampal and extrahippocampal lesions can also lead to chronic epilepsy after a delay of four weeks to four months (McIntyre et al., 1982; Leite et al., 1990; Vicedomini and Nadler, 1987; 1990; Lothman and Bertram, 1993; Shirasaka and Wasterlain, 1994; Milgram et al., 1995). This delay in the development of post traumatic and post lesional epilepsy has given rise to the speculation that lesions damage an antikindling filter, so that after some types of focal brain damage, kindling or over kindling (Milgram et al., 1995) takes place spontaneously, perhaps as a result of loss of inhibition around the lesion, and leads to chronic epilepsy. If this is true, epileptogenic lesions should lead to a facilitation of kindling and to an enhancement of long term potentiation (LTP) during the latent period between the occurrence of damage and that of spontaneous epileptic seizures. In the current study, we used the perforant path stimulation model of status epilepticus (Sloviter, 1991; Shirasaka and Wasterlain, 1994) and show facilitation of both kindling and perforant path LTP during the latent period following an epileptogenic hippocampal lesion induced by perforant path stimulation.

Kindling 5, edited by Corcoran and Moshé.
Plenum Press, New York, 1998.

2. MATERIAL AND METHODS

Techniques have been described in detail elsewhere (Shirasaka and Wasterlain, 1994; Mazarati and Wasterlain, in press). Male Wistar rats are subjected to 24 hours of intermittent stimulation of the perforant path (10 sec strains at 20 Hz, 20 volts, 0.1 msec, with continuous 2 Hz paired pulses, 40 msec apart, 20 volt, 0.1 msec) under urethane anesthesia (1000 μg/kg IV loading dose). Self-sustaining status epilepticus (SSSE) is induced by 30 minutes of similar stimulation in the awake state. Kindling trials use electrical stimulation from the angular bundle of the perforant path or from basolateral amygdala (60 Hz, biphasic square wave pulses, 1 msec each, 2 sec pulse duration, at afterdischarge threshold) three times a day, and seizures are rated according to Racine (1972). LTP is induced by tetanic stimulation (5 sec trains of single bipolar square wave stimuli at 400 Hz, 200 msec apart, with intensity sufficient to induce a half maximal population spike). The response to single square wave pulses is tested every five minutes, and the percentage increase of the population spike (PS) and its duration are recorded. Morphological studies are carried out in perfused-fixed brains, on serial sections stained with hematoxyline and eosin. Changes are evaluated by the repeated measure ANOVA followed by Student-Newman-Keuls test as post hoc.

3. RESULTS

Perforant path stimulation (pfps) by this protocol resulted in lesions of the polymorph layer of the ipsilateral dentate gyrus, and in milder lesions of the pyramidal cells (CA3>CA1) which were bilateral but considerably milder on the contralateral side. There were no extrahippocampal lesions. SSSE caused lesions in a similar hippocampal distribution, except for their bilaterality, and extrahippocampal lesions in pyriform and entorhinal cortex, the amygdala, and some neocortical sites. Using the paired pulse method, we found in the dentate gyrus, after both SSSE or 24 hours perforant path stimulation under anesthesia, a complete loss of GABAa- and GABAb-mediated inhibition, including long interstimulus interval(ISI)-dependent, short ISI-dependent, and frequency-dependent inhibition. The short ISI inhibition recovered substantially over a period of four weeks, frequency-dependent inhibition recovered partially and long ISI inhibition did not recover significantly during that time period.

3.1. Long Term Potentiation

LTP was tested in the SSSE group, one week after stimulation, and showed marked potentiation compared to pre-lesion status (Figure 1). In fact, a stimulus which induced long term depression in healthy rats sometimes induced LTP in the same animals after perforant path stimulation. In control animals, tetanic stimulation induced a 40 to 60% increase of the population spike amplitude lasting 30 minutes, and this increase was no longer significant 40 minutes or more after the end of stimulation. After SSSE, the population spike amplitude was increased up to 350% by the same tetanic stimuli, and a highly significant increase was still present one hour after tetanus in all animals. This enhancement of LTP was present 1, 4, 7 and 15 days after the end of SSSE, and a similar change was found after pfps under anesthesia (Fig. 1).

3.2. Perforant Path Kindling

When animals subjected to PFPS were kindled through the perforant path one week after PFPS, they failed to progress to stage five seizures even after 21 kindling trials,

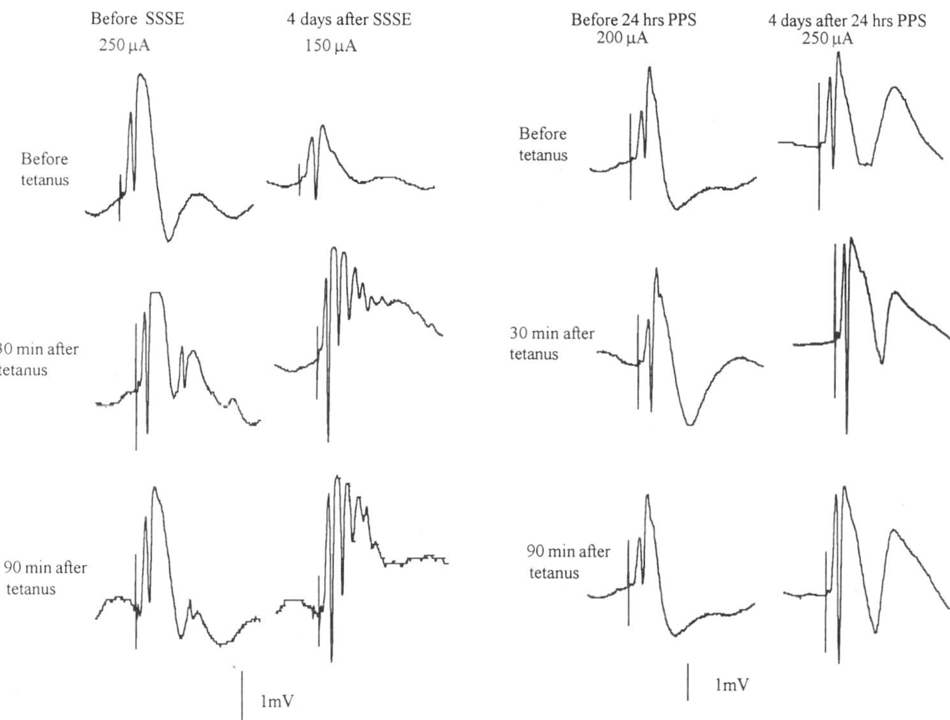

Figure 1. Representative tracings recorded from the granule cell layer electrode after tetanic stimulation through the angular bundle electrode. The same animals were tested before and after SSSE or 24 hr pfps.

while sham stimulated control rats required 12 to 16 stimulations of the perforant path to reach stage five (Table 1). After 21 stimulations, no change was observed in afterdischarge threshold or afterdischarge duration in PFPS animals, while the control animals which had reached full kindling showed a marked decrease in afterdischarge threshold and increase in afterdischarge duration.

Since it was possible that the failure of kindling in those animals was simply a post-ictal phenomenon, which would be expected to be transient, we repeated that experiment one month after PFPS, when post-ictal effects would be expected to have waned. The results were dramatically different. At that time, perforant path kindling produced a first stage five seizure in 3.3 trials ± 1.0 (range: 1–10) while a paired control group reached the first stage

Table 1. Changes in long-term potentiation in the dentate gyrus after SSSE induced by 30 min PPS in the awake rats, and after 24 hrs PPS under urethane anesthesia

Time after tetanus (min)	Before SSSE	4 days after SSSE	Before 24 hrs PPS	4 days after PPS
30	155 ± 12*	310 ± 12*	143 ± 12*	276 ± 14*
60	100 ± 0	261 ± 13*	102 ± 15	235 ± 11*
90	98 ± 10	226 ± 10*	100 ± 0	210 ± 22*

Data represent Mean ± SEM of posttetanic population spike amplitude expressed as a percentage of the population spike amplitude before tetanus. Each group contains 4 rats. The current intensity applied induced a half maximal population spike before tetanic stimulation. * $p<0.05$ vs population spike amplitude before tetanus, expressed as 100% (repeated measure ANOVA + NK)

five seizure in 11.0 trials ± 2.5 (range: 4–15), a highly significantly difference. The third stage five seizure (full kindling) was reached in 6.3 ± 1.1 trials in the PFPS rats (range: 3–16) against 18.0 ± 1.1 trials in a paired control group (range: 14–21), also a highly significant difference. In this same group, the first afterdischarge threshold decreased from 458 ± 71 μA in controls to 283 ± 35 ($\pi < 0.05$) while the first afterdischarge duration increased from 52 ± 14 seconds (range: 24–112) to 88 ± 13 seconds (range: 13–150). Thus it seemed that after the post-ictal depression had waned, there was an enormous acceleration of perforant path kindling of those animals. Indeed, around the same time many of those rats started showed spontaneous seizures and seizures on 2 Hz stimulation, never seen in controls (Shirasaka and Wasterlain, 1994). When we attempted to correlate loss of paired pulse inhibition, which at that time is in a recovery phase in many animals, with kindling susceptibility, there was a poor correlation between GABAa-mediated short ISI and frequency-dependent paired pulse inhibition and kindling rate. There was an excellent but not necessarily meaningful correlation between kindling rate and loss of GABAb-mediated long ISI-dependent paired pulse inhibition (Shirasaka and Wasterlain, 1994).

3.3. Amygdala Kindling

A single group of PFPS rats was kindled from basolateral amygdala one week after PFPS. While these animals showed no change in afterdischarge threshold or duration from the dentate gyrus at that point in time, they showed a dramatic decrease in afterdischarge threshold and a significant increase in afterdischarge duration from the amygdala at the same time. All animals showed a stage five seizure on the first stimulation of basolateral amygdala, and completed three stage five seizures in three trials (Table 2). While no efforts were made to record spontaneous seizures in those rats, three of the six rats were observed to display spontaneous seizures during handling incidental to kindling.

3.4. Change in Granule Cell Excitability

When we studied granule cell excitability using input-output curves, we found no change as an immediate result of PFPS. Thirty minutes after the end of stimulation, the ratio of the population spike amplitude induced by a 250 μA stimulation to the maximal population spike went from 0.4 ± 0.3 to 5.7 ± 3.9, and this small, nonsignificant change suggested that PFPS had not kindled the animals, since kindling would be expected to lead to a large increase in that ratio. Indeed, when control animals were kindled through the perforant path, their PS ratio increased from 10 ± 3.3 before kindling to 58 ± 14.9 after kindling ($p < 0.05$). In the two weeks following PFPS, this ratio increased to 74.4 ± 9.6 ($p < 0.05$, tested in the

Table 2. Effect of 24 hr PPS (under anesthesia) on kindling parameters

	First ADT	First ADD	First st. 5	Third st. 5
Group 1: PP kindling, 7 days post PPS (4)	1300 ± 470	13 ± 5	> 21*	>21
Group 2: PP kindling, 7 days, controls (4)	1270 ± 500	18 ± 5	12 ± 2	19 ± 3
Group 3: PP kindling, 4 weeks post PPS (12)	283 ± 35*	88.3 ± 13	3.3 ± 1*	6.3 ± 1.1*
Group 4: PP kindling, 4 weeks, controls (7)	458 ± 71	52 ± 14	11 ± 3	18 ± 1
Group 5: amygdala kindling, 7 days post PPS (6)	366 ± 88*	12 ± 5*	1 ± 0*	3 ± 0*
Group 6: amygdala kindling, 7 days, control (3)	633 ± 120	35 ± 4	9 ± 2	16 ± 2

ADT: afterdischarge threshold (μA), ADD: afterdischarge duration (s). First st 5: number of kindling trials needed to reach the first stage 5 seizure. Third st 5: number of kindling trials needed to reach full kindling (3 stage 5 seizures).
$p < 0.05$ vs. control.

awake state). Four weeks after PFPS, the PS ratio was 55 ± 12 (tested in the awake state) or 17.2 ± 7.9 (tested under anesthesia, $p < 0.05$). When these animals were kindled, no further increase in PS ratio occurred (post kindling in the awake state: 67.4 ± 11.8, no difference with four weeks, but $p < 0.05$ compared to controls). These results are compatible with the interpretation that spontaneous kindling occurred during the first two weeks after PFPS, a time when very little inhibition was present in the dentate gyrus, but a number of alternative possibilities might be equally plausible.

4. DISCUSSION

These data show a dramatic enhancement of LTP and kindling in animals with hippocampal lesions induced by seizure-like stimulation of the perforant path. We have no way of knowing whether these phenomena were the result of the hippocampal lesions, the result of plastic changes associated with these lesions, or the result of coincidental adaptive changes. However, it is likely that the enhancement of LTP was not the result of structural extrahippocampal lesions, since PFPS, which produced no extra-hippocampal lesions, was as effective in enhancing LTP as SSSE, which did produce more widespread extra-hippocampal damage.

4.1. Relationship between Kindling Rates and Hippocampal Lesions

Many reports have shown that mechanical or chemical lesions to the hippocampus frequently retard the development of kindling (Nakachi et al., 1988; Kryzhanovskii et al., 1985; Dasheiff et al., 1982) while a few have reported no effect (Mitchell and Barnes, 1993) and others yet found an acceleration of kindling (Grecksch et al., 1995). Of course, most of these lesions did not have the selectivity of seizure-induced damage, which affects neuronal subpopulations, such as the somatotastin- and neuropeptide Y-immunoreactive GABAergic hilar interneurons, while sparing the hilar basket cells and other interneurons in the same anatomical area (Sloviter, 1991).

4.2. Relationship between Hippocampal Lesions and Facilitation of Kindling

We previously postulated the existence of a "filter" which prevents the occurrence of kindling in response to routine daily brain activity (Wasterlain et al., 1986); this could be a frequency or intensity filter, and would be compatible with the fact that many brain cells (eg CA3 pyramidal cells) frequently fire in bursts at frequencies ideal to induce kindling but fail to cause that phenomenon. Kindling is easily induced in nearly every vertebrate species ever tested when natural defenses are bypassed by introducing an electrode into the brain, yet spontaneous kindling has never been described . According to that hypothesis, the delay before the appearance of post traumatic or post lesional seizures would represent the time necessary for spontaneous kindling after that "filter" is damaged by some lesion. The current results are compatible with the view that the hilar interneurons of the dentate gryus might represent part of such a "filter", and that their lesion might make the dentate gyrus susceptible to spontaneous kindling. Indeed, delayed changes in granule cell excitability compatible with that view were observed, but these changes were non specific and could be incidental. Nevertheless, the high vulnerability of hilar interneurons to many types of lesions (Lowenstein et al., 1994) and the notoriously slow kindling rates of primates (Wada et al., 1980) could explain the long delay that often precedes human posttraumatic epilepsy.

4.3. Relationship between LTP and Kindling

LTP is very likely part of kindling, although kindling appears to involve more than the sum of multiple LTPs. The decrease in inhibition observed by the paired pulse method is a potential explanation of the enhancement of LTP, which could itself explain at least part of the dramatic increase in susceptibility to kindling observed in PFPS animals. Dissociation between perforant path and amygdala kindling at one week might simply reflect the stronger post-ictal inhibition of the site of direct stimulation. However, our result would not rule out a key role for sprouting of excitatory fibers, or a modified "basket cell" hypothesis. A simple disconnection of the basket cells is not compatible with the delayed occurrence of increased granule cell excitability, increased kindling susceptibility, and spontaneous seizures reported here, but our results are quite easily reconciled with a modified basket cell hypothesis in which the basket cells would be actively suppressed because of the loss of inhibition of inhibition, or because of other plastic changes induced by PFPS.

In summary, hippocampal lesions associated with seizure-like stimulation of the perforant path are associated with a dramatic enhancement of LTP through the main excitatory synaptic circuit of the hippocampus, and with an equally dramatic enhancement of kindled seizures once the post-ictal changes have waned. These results are compatible with a hebbian mechanism of epileptogenesis, and with a role of kindling in epileptogenesis following hippocampal lesions due to trauma, status epilepticus, ischemia, or other causes. This speculative hypothesis is testable, and offers an alternative to those based on excitatory sprouting or to static changes in hippocampal circuitry.

Supported by VHA Research Service and by Research Grant NS13515 from NINDS.

REFERENCES

Dasheiff, R.M., McNamara, J.O., Intradentate colchicine retards the development of amygdala kindling, Ann. Neurol., 11(1982)347–352.

Grecksch, G., Ruethrich, H., Bernstein, H.G. and Becker, A., PTZ-kindling after colchicine lesion in the dentate gyrus of the rat hippocampus, Physiol. Behav., 58 (1995) 695–698.

Kryzhanovskii, G.N., Shandra, A.A., Makul'kin, R.F., Godlevskii, L.S. and Moiseev, I.N., [Effect of destruction of the hippocampus and caudate nucleus on the development of epileptic activity during corazole kindling], Biull. Eksp. Biol. Med., 100 (1985) 407–410.

Leite, J. P., Bortolotto, Z. A., & Cavalheiro, E. A., Spontaneous recurrent seizures in rats: an experimental model of partial epilepsy, Neurosci. Biobehav. Rev., 14 (1990) 511–7.

Lothman, E. W., & Bertram, E. H. D., Epileptogenic effects of status epilepticus, Epilepsia, 34 (1993) Suppl 1, S59–70.

Lowenstein, D.H., Thomas, M.J., Smith, D.H., & McIntosh, T.K., Selective vulnerability of dentate hilar neurons following traumatic brain injury: a potential mechanistic link between head trauma and disorders of the hippocampus, J. Neurosci., 12 (1994) 4846–4853.

Mazarati, A.M. and Wasterlain, C.G., Selective facilitation of kindled seizures from the basolateral amygdala after hippocampal lesions induced by perforant path stimulation. (submitted)

McIntyre, D. C., Nathanson, D., & Edson, N., A new model of partial status epilepticus based on kindling, Brain Research, 250(1982)53–63.

Milgram, N.W., Michael, M., Cammisuli, S., Head S., et al., Development of spontaneous seizures over extended electrical kindling.II. Persistence of dentate inhibitory suppression, Brain Research, 670(1995)112–120.

Mitchell, C.L. and Barnes, M.I., Effect of destruction of dentate granule cells on kindling induced by stimulation of the perforant path, Physiol. Behav., 53 (1993) 45–49.

Nakachi, R., Okamoto, M., Moriwake, T., Nakamura, Y., Sato, M., Effects of unilateral ventral hippocampal lesion on amygdaloid kindling in cat, Jpn. J. Psychiatry Neurol., 42(1988)625–626.

Racine, R.J., Modification of seizures activity by electrical stimulation. II. Motor seizures, Electroencephalogr. Clin. Neurophysiol., 32 (1972) 281–294.

Shirasaka, Y and Wasterlain, C.G., Chronic epileptogenicity following focal status epilepticus, Brain Research, 655(1994) 33–44.

Sloviter, R.S., Permanently altered hippocampal structure, excitability and inhibition after experimental status epilepticus in the rat: the 'dormant basket cell' hypothesis and its possible relevance to temporal lobe epilepsy, Hippocampus, 1(1991) 41–46.

Vicedomini, J. P., & Nadler, J. V., A model of status epilepticus based on electrical stimulation of hippocampal afferent pathways, Exp. Neurol., 96(1987)681–91.

Vicedomini, J. P., & Nadler, J. V., Stimulation-induced status epilepticus: role of the hippocampal mossy fibers in the seizures and associated neuropathology, Brain Research, 512(1990)70–4.

Wada, J.A., Mizoguchi, T., & Osawa, T., Secondarily generalized convulsive seizures induced by daily amygdaloid stimulation in rhesus monkeys, Neurology, 28(1978)1026–1036.

Wasterlain, C.G., Farber, D.B., Fairchild, D., Synaptic mechanisms in the kindled epileptic focus: a speculative synthesis. In: Basic mechanisms of the epilepsies. (Eds) Delgado-Escueta, A.V., Ward A.A.Jr, Woodbury D.M., and Porter R.J., Raven Press, New York, pp 411–433, 1986.

SUMMARY DISCUSSION

A. Fernandez-Guardiola: I would like to begin this discussion by congratulating all the participants for their excellent fine work in epileptogenesis and also on the pharmacology of the kindling process.

Unidentified questioner: For Dr. Wasterlain, as a control did you try to induce lesions in other fields of the hippocampus, to see if *any* lesion of the hippocampus would be able to increase the rate of kindling?

C. Wasterlain: No, we haven't done that, but it would obviously be something that would be worth doing. We are looking more at LTP, which is enormously facilitated. My prejudice would be that the hilus would not be the only site where this kind of phenomenon could be developed, that there could be other regions. Of course, as shown by Buzsaki and others, the biggest brake in the excitatory hippocampal circuit is the hilar interneuron, but it is not the only one.

S. Leung: Very exciting results, or I should say very epileptogenic results. How long do those spontaneous seizures last? I ask this because in the kainate model or maybe in the tetanus toxin model, spontaneous seizures don't last forever.

C. Wasterlain: The accelerated kindling that I showed is still present two months after the stimulation. As far as spontaneous seizures are concerned, we have not looked at how long they last.

D. McIntyre: Claude, has anybody looked anywhere else besides perforant path in this model? In other words, if one were to drive the amygdala instead of the perforant path, would you get the hilar loss and would you get the spontaneous seizures? I can easily envision the spontaneous seizures without the hilar loss.

C. Wasterlain: I don't have the answer, but I can easily imagine the involvement of one more site, including the site that you described.

F. Lopes Da Silva: Very interesting data. I just wonder whether you have followed the paired-pulse paradigm during the whole period of the delay, what type of evolution that you see, and whether there is any way of predicting whether you get spontaneous seizures at any particular moment.

C. Wasterlain: Well, we have measured paired-pulse inhibition throughout the evolution of the process. It is quite interesting, because the total loss of inhibition that you see at the beginning does not last. This progressive return of inhibition as measured by the paired-pulse technique seems to be corroborated by intracellular recordings carried out by Andy Obenhaus and Igor Spigelman, which are still preliminary. The paired-pulse results and the paired-pulse results clearly show a progressive return of inhibition over the next few weeks. We have gone out to 2 months, when the vast majority of animals have a lot of inhibition, but the recovery of inhibition may not be complete. In many animals there is one aspect of inhibition, for example GABA mediated inhibition, which is still abnormal, but overall there is a striking return of inhibition, which probably reflects sprouting and reinnervation of denervated areas.

Unidentified questioner: Can you relate this return of inhibition to spontaneous seizures?

C. Wasterlain: Well, I am well aware of Pete Engel's thoughts that perhaps inhibition can synchronize discharges and be a part of epileptogenesis. I have a feeling that the return of inhibition follows rather than precedes the development of epileptogenesis, but it is not substantiated by any solid numbers.

A. Fernandez-Guardiola: Which parameters of stimulation did you use?

C. Wasterlain: This is a straight Sloviter model stimulation, in which we give a 10 second train at 20 Hz once per minute, with the animal under deep anaesthesia. We use square wave pulses, and that continues for 24 hrs. I think that Bob Sloviter has shown that you need to stimulate for quite a few hours (more than 8 hours) to get lesions. We haven't broken down the duration of stimulation at all. For this particular purpose we use the model as described.

M. Corcoran: It is time to wrap things up. I would like to thank Lisa Armitage, Darren Hannesson, and Paul Mohapel for stepping in and assisting with the transcriptions of the discussions and with running the projectors. We all should also say thank you to Mary O'Rourke and Sarah D'Eath of Conferences Services, University of Victoria, for taking care of the molecular details of organizing this conference. Finally, thanks to Juhn Wada for continuing to inspire us.

I hope you all had as good a time as I did. Perhaps we can get together again in 5 years, at the beginning of the new millennium! For those of you who will remain in Victoria until tomorrow, I wish you a happy Canada Day.

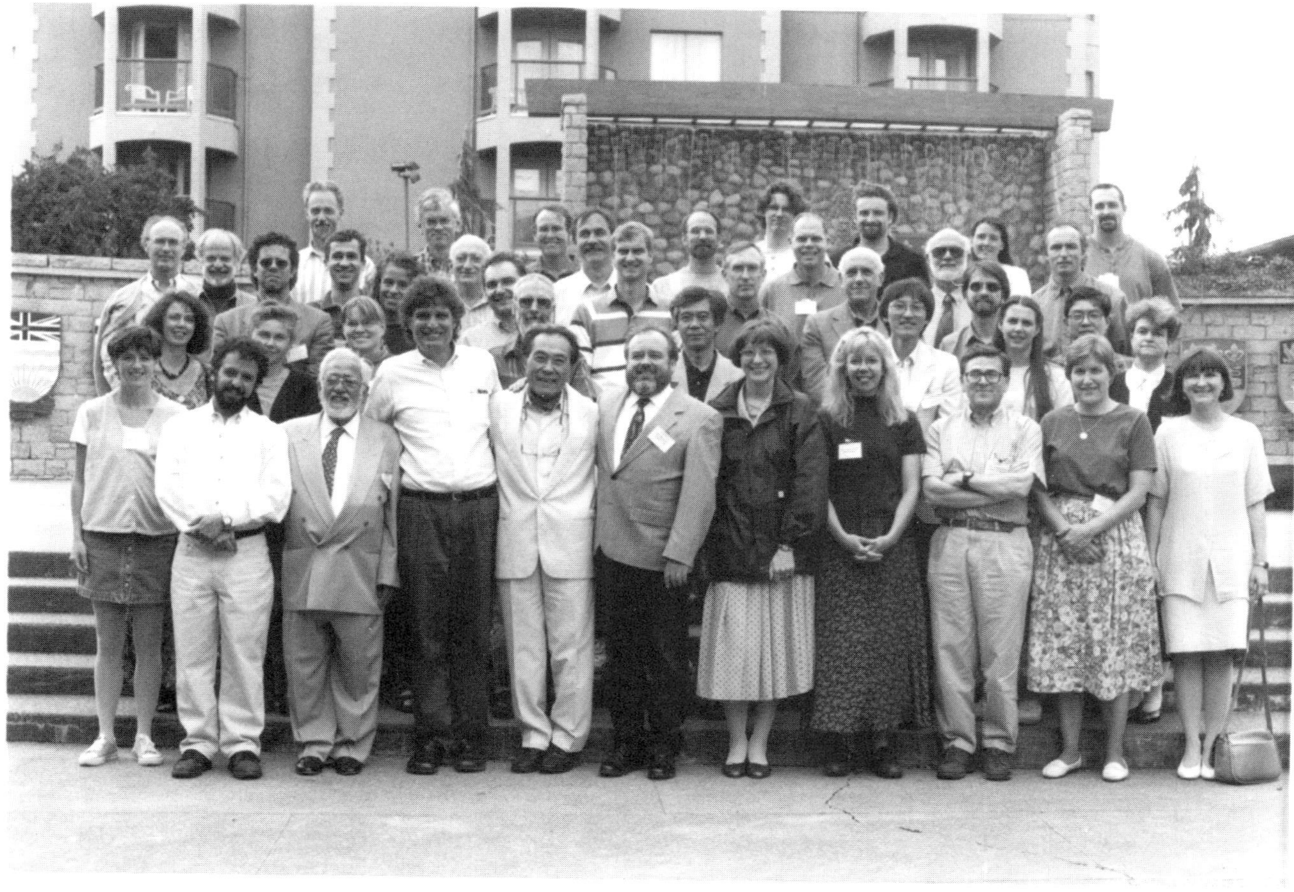

Participants at the Fifth International Conference on Kindling, Victoria, B.C.

INDEX